T0193059

Reimar Banis, M.D.

New Life
Through Energy Healing

The Atlas of
Psychosomatic Energetics

Translated from the German by
David M. Fogg

Reimar Banis, M.D.

New Life
Through Energy Healing

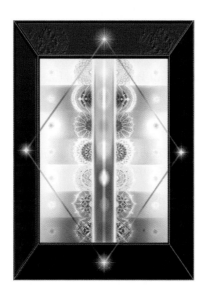

The Atlas of
Psychosomatic Energetics

Artemis Books
Nevada City, California

Picture credits:

Picture credits:

If not otherwise indicated: © Bildarchiv Preußischer Kulturbesitz Berlin, 2001.

Title page Klaus Holitzka; p. 18 "St. George and the Dragon" painting-by Uccello ca. 1460, London National Gallery; p. 24 author's photograph; p. 36 Dr. Stylianos Atteshli "Daskalos" (Inge Geissinger, Starnberg); p. 37 "Judgment of the Dead – detail from the Egyptian Book of the Dead," papyrus ca. 1000 BCE, Metropolitan Museum New York; p. 39 "Old Age and Death," painting by Hans Baldung Grien, Mardid, Museo del Prado; pp. 41-42 author's photographs; p. 43 "Two Ibexes and a Right-angled Symbol," Lascaux caves, France, photograph: Wolfgang Ruppert; p. 45 author's photograph; p. 53 Kurt Starz /Reutlingen; pp. 54, 57, 58, 68, 91, 102, 107 author's photographs; p. 108 Kurt Starz/Reutlingen; p. 115 Klaus Holitzka; p. 131 Prof.v.Holst /Bayreuth; p. 133 "The Nasty Boy is Thrashed by the Devil," woodcut based on a drawing by Moritz von Schwind, ca. 1860; p.137 "The Temptation of St. Anthony," painting by Joos van Caesbeek o.J., Karlsruhe Staatliche Kunsthalle; p. 145 Internet photos by eyewitnesses to the terror attacks of 11 September 2001 (Pentagon webpage, Washington); p. 146 "The Temptation of St. Anthony," painting by Hieronymus Bosch o.J., Museo del Prado Madrid; p. 155 "Ruggiero and Angelica" Arnold Böcklin 1873, Staatliche Museen zu Berlin, Nationalgalerie; p. 161 "The Young Witch," painting by Antoine Wiertz ca. 1850; pp. 170, 172 Leonardo da Vinci: grotesque heads, Windsor Castle/UK; p. 174 "Salome – The Dancer's Reward," drawing by Aubrey Beardsley 1872-1898; p. 185 photograph by pharmacist Manfred Kern/Bühl; p. 192 "Salome" painting by Franz von Stuck 1906; p. 193 "Napoleon I" woodcut based on a painting by Paul Delaroche 1797-1856; p. 195 "The Coquette," lithograph based on a painting by Gustave Dorè ca. 1860; p. 197 "Maja," painting by Anders Zorn 1900, Nationalgalerie Berlin; p. 200 "The Murdered Marat," painting by Jacques Louis David 1793, Brüssel Musées Royaux des Beaux-Arts; p. 203 "The Duisburger Merchant Dirck Tybis," painting by Hans Holbein the Younger 1533, Kunsthistorisches Museum Vienna; p. 227 New York from Empire State Building, author's photograph; p. 232 "View from the South of the Sphinx and the Great Pyramid," copperplate engraving by Schroeder based on a drawing by Conté 1812; p. 239 "Adam and Eve in Paradise (The Fall of Man)" painting by Luca Cranach the Elder; p. 240 Hell – (no author), p. 245 "Walpurgisnacht" woodcut 1861, Illustration to J.N.Vogl: "Twardowski, the Polish Faust"; p. 252 Hindu temple in southern India, author's photograph; p. 256 photograph by Kurz Starz/Reutlingen; p. 260 "Mona Lisa (La Gioconda)," Leonardo da Vinci 1503, Musée du Louvre; p. 264 Lucifer with the kind permission of © Venefizius, CH); p. 269 terror attack on 11 September 2001 in New York, photographs from the Pentagon, website, Washington, D.C.; p. 321 Swayambunath/Katmandu in Nepal, author's photograph; p. 329 author's photograph Graphic design of illustrations and tables: Fiore Tartaglia, Spectraweb Göppingen; Ideas conceptualized by the author.

Graphic design of illustrations and tables: Fiore Tartaglia, Spectraweb Göppingen, Ideas: © by the author.

Artemis Books layout and design by iTRANSmedia.

New Life Through Energy Healing: The Atlas of Psychosomatic Energetics - U.S. Edition © 2008 by Artemis Books **English text and illustrations** © 2008 by Dr. Reimar Banis

ISBN: 978-0645181-7

First published in Germany under the title: *Durch Energieheilung zu neuem Leben: Atlas der Psychosomatischen Energetik* by Verlag Via Nova, Petersberg, Germany, 2004

Published by: Artemis Books
P. O. Box 482
Penn Valley, CA 95946
USA

Printed by: Aegean Offset Printers, India

Dedication

This book is dedicated to the many patients who, through their openness in talking about their mental-emotional and energetic histories, have helped to form the basis of the book. I also dedicate this book to my three children and my one stepson, from whom I have learned a lot about myself and about my character. This book is also dedicated to all those children who, due to psychoenergetic imbalances, suffer conditions and diseases which up to now have not been diagnosed or treated – but which (it is my firm conviction) can be healed using the methods presented in this book, thereby giving those children a completely new and hopeful outlook for the future.

Disclaimer

Logo of Psychosomatic Energetics:

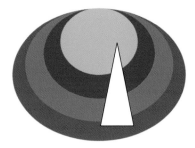

The logo designed by the author is intended to symbolize the four levels of the subtle-body force field: green for vital energy, red for emotional energy, blue for mental energy and violet for causal energy. The vertical white triangle symbolizes the healing power of homeopathic emotional remedies, that can influence and harmonize all four energy levels. Of course, any good holistic treatment stimulates all energy levels.

Table of Contents

Foreword

When kids fall down, they go running to mommy to be comforted. Mother fans the air above the injury and blows on it to cool it off. A clairvoyant healer observing this scene will recognize ancient healing wisdom in the mother's actions, now known as "energy medicine, laying on of hands and faith healing." With her hand motions, the mother removes bad energy from the injured child's Aura and speaks soothing words to the child's churning soul. Soon, the child is prancing about as if nothing had happened.

The holistic healing method that I'd like to introduce in this book is based on the same healing principles. In "Psychosomatic Energetics," we heal emotional wounds not just with words but above all by dissolving emotional blocks in the patient's energy field, so that the formerly blocked energy can again flow at full strength. Many diseases and emotional disturbances improve in this manner and, in many cases, disappear for good. The actual diseases and disturbances are not actually so important. Restoring blocked life energy represents a powerful universal healing principle that mankind has successfully used from time immemorial.

Now, every person has energy blocks to some degree, corresponding to unprocessed emotional experiences in the subconscious. This applies not just to the sick, but the healthy as well: nearly every person has these subconscious energy blocks. For healthy, emotionally balanced persons, healing energy blocks very often triggers astounding personal growth processes. Therefore, anyone wanting to develop spiritually, be it via meditation, working with the body or through conversations, can derive great benefit from the resolution of subconscious energy blocks.

We know that every spiritual path is indissolubly linked to improved self-knowledge, and the dissolution of one's own energy blocks makes it much easier to attain to a more profound and improved self-perception. One thereby much more easily gets close to one's emotional center and once again feels oneself to be more like the person one actually is. The system of Psychosomatic Energetics is thus suited for everyone, whether sick or healthy, to achieve spiritual depth and lasting progress and to approach one's emotional center.

At this point, many people have asked me why it is that such a universally valid and highly effective process is not more widely recognized. It is important to realize that modern medicine and psychology are, to this day, completely unaware that one can at all eliminate emotional blocks in the energy field. When I was a young med student, I was taught that the mind can be healed only with words. One exception to this generally valid rule is chemical medication: although patients who are upset or tired can indeed be influenced for a while with psychotropic agents, this is just a temporary solution. The therapeutic conversation must be introduced, according to the current perception, which, along with supportive medication, represent the load-bearing pillars of modern spiritual therapy. Current conventional wisdom has it that treatment with words is the undisputed royal road, the only sensible form of treatment. To wish to heal an emotionally ailing person without communication or psychotropics is a sheer impossibility for the modern western physician.

The fact that there are other promising treatment possibilities dawns only gradually on most specialists. Longstanding methods such as homeopathy and acupuncture have only recently been looked into more closely, and their astounding effectiveness recognized, after the curative results could no longer be denied. When such naturopathic procedures are used, there is often a general improvement and rebalancing of the entire person, which includes physical as well as emotional aspects. One speaks in this context of "holistic medicine" in order to underscore its broad comprehensive effect over the entire emotional-physical spectrum. At times, people find themselves transformed by these treatments in unexpected ways whose strength clearly goes beyond the usual healing effect. In all probability, the reason for this is the healing effect of energetic processes, through which the whole person is changed for the better in all dimensions of his or her being.

In my own work as a physician, it has been my experience that the healing effect is experienced by patients as being stronger and more holistic, the more the underlying energy blocks are taken into account and (of course) healed. Over time, I became aware that the oldest known healing methods – those of shamans and ancient priestly healers – had taken into account the subtle-body energy, but that this valuable knowledge is more and more being lost and forgotten. If you want to understand why we have come to such an unfortunate pass, and why most of the currently available healing methods are not very effective in this regard, it is worth taking a closer look at the history of medicine. Therefore, this book also includes a description of the historical processes that have led to the current inauspicious developments.

Many readers will no doubt recoil in shock at this announcement, and worry about getting drawn into a specialist's dispute. However, I am confident that I have been able to present the context in a manner that is accessible to a lay readership, so that all can grasp the underlying processes. Since we are dealing here with processes that are sure to be of interest to anyone interested in a more profound self-knowledge, it is worth the effort of looking in more detail into the history. It quickly becomes clear what is really meant by one's energy body, the meridians and Chakras, and what practical significance these systems have in our daily life.

It has taken me thirty years as a physician and naturopath to get to the bottom of this, and I have slogged through entire libraries in the process. I can now spare the reader all this effort – by giving it in this book, virtually a quintessence of the naturopathic healing arts and all of the background information with respect to the interaction of body and soul. In my opinion, it is extremely valuable for everyone (not just specialists) to understand the historical processes and their background – first of all because it very clearly explains the limits of the various therapeutic procedures, whether acupuncture or psychotherapy.

People have always sensed hidden connections between physical processes and emotional states – for example, in the ancient theory of temperaments. In earlier times, there was much that could not be explained, and so one had to make do with pure empirical descriptions of acquired experience. For example, the ancients knew that cholerics often had a dark-skinned constitution and gallbladder problems, but they didn't know why (which I will endeavor to explain in this book satisfactorily and understandably).

Unfortunately, much valuable ancient empirical knowledge has been lost over time, or has been altered beyond recognition by the passage of time. Therefore, I have attempted to revive this buried yet valuable knowledge, and to describe it in its wider meaning context. This is very important, because we can perceive many things more easily and clearly via our unseen body energies once we have been made aware of their actual existence. As on a foggy day, we need a clear plan by which to orient ourselves in order to be able to make sensible use of subtle-body processes. I'd like to make it clear, at the outset, that I am not here concerned with any otherworldly theories, but rather exclusively with practical everyday matters that can be very useful in leading a livelier and more sensible life.

It is easy to understand that spirituality and depth psychology are of utmost significance in arriving at a human picture that is as complete as possible, while remaining practical and taking into account all aspects of mankind. For if our human picture is incomplete, then important disease causes will be overlooked, wrongly interpreted and – worst of all – literally mis-treated. Regrettably, every age has ignored important areas of the overall human picture. For example, except for a few courageous pioneers such as C.G. JUNG, psychoanalysis has failed to integrate subtle-body and spiritual aspects into its human picture.

Yet only a truly all-encompassing human picture permits a sensible answer to such pressing questions as: Why are we in this world in the first place? What is our human mission? And: What possible sense does disease make? These difficult (even impossible) questions become, surprisingly, very clearly and sensibly answerable as soon as one chooses a wide enough contextual frame, to which the spiritual and the subtle-body aspects definitely belong. I will attempt to answer all these questions in this book in such a manner that readers obtain satisfactory answers, so that they (I hope) can draw useful conclusions for their own lives.

The most important key to healing and becoming whole seems to me to lie in the subtle-body system. "Tell me how you vibrate and I'll tell you how you feel and think" is the upshot of my decades of experience as an energy-medicine physician. When my patients are energetically completely exhausted and depressed, they are unlikely to be capable of much (if any) joyful sensations. Added to which, they get sick much more easily and – most important – heal with greater difficulty, as long as the energy isn't flowing! This sounds so simple and self-evident (although it has far-reaching implications for everyday life), but when it is examined more closely, it goes far beyond the significance of the disease itself, and should interest every person.

Ultimately, the mood of our subtle-body system determines our entire quality of life! It therefore makes sense, for entirely selfish practical reasons, to concern oneself in greater detail with the underlying processes. This book imparts basic knowledge about the various Aura levels, the seven Chakras and their interaction with our body and mind. Armed with this knowledge, it becomes easier for us to harmonize with our energy center and attain the worthwhile state of well-being and being charged up with energy that is only possible with a healthy energy system.

I have called the new method I developed "Psychosomatic Energetics," intending that the name convey that health is based on three factors – body, mind, and energy – and their harmonic interplay. I will describe this new method in more detail at the end of the book on the basis of practical examples. As we know, modern medicine still pays far too little attention to subtle-body energy. How patients feel and how much life energy they have seems to be a matter of little concern to most physicians, since (it would seem) "you can't measure that" and because most of my medical colleagues think that there's nothing they can do about such things anyway.

One of the main problems in working with subtle-body energy is that we have up to now been unable to adequately measure the so-called *Aura*. Working with a biophysicist, I developed a device that measures a patient's life energy and can determine, in just a few minutes, how a patient feels.

Now that may not sound like much at first, since one could of course simply ask patients how they feel and how much life energy they have. The trouble is, almost all patients have (amazingly) forgotten how to trust their own perceptions and to feel what is going on inside themselves. Another advantage to measuring subtle-body energy is that one quickly and precisely finds out how the patient is losing energy and what needs to be done to restore it. Later on, I will summarize some generally valid insights gained from thousands of such measurements. Readers can derive practical rules from these for keeping their energy levels as high and harmonized as possible.

Nevertheless, this book's main focus is not exclusively on subtle-body energy – about which there are already enough books – but rather on character and its subtle-body roots. It's well known that nothing is harder than insight into one's own character, with all its subconscious darker sides – and it's even harder to get rid of one's negative character traits. I think the reason for this has to do with subconscious energy blocks that give rise to subconscious conflicts. Since the energy blocks are not eliminated, most attempts at personal change – such as New Year's resolutions, or even expert assistance in the form of psychotherapy – understandably yield unsatisfying results: only treating the energy blocks can bring about significant and lasting improvements!

Traditionally, one tries to get a handle on and treat subconscious problems in psychoanalysis using words and internal images. Yet this approach is enormously difficult in practice. For the great majority of patients, long-term and costly psychoanalytic treatment is out of the question. Moreover, many patients refuse to realize that their disease might have anything to do with emotional problems – and even if patients are willing and open-minded, it is very difficult to ferret out conflicts and then heal them as well. Knowing the conflict does not make it disappear and heal up automatically, as one might casually think. Many patients know their own conflicts very well indeed, but are still not rid of them.

The main problem with the inadequate effectiveness of the majority of therapies is that they don't take into account the subtle-body energy blocks of the subconscious conflict. It gradually became clear to me in my work as a physician that the energy blocks correspond to undealt-with emotional processes stored in the subtle-energy body. As long as the energy block is not eliminated, it doesn't matter how well aware one is of it! However, as soon as the conflict is energetically extinguished, it triggers surprisingly powerful and lasting healing processes. In subsequent chapters, I will present numerous typical case histories from daily practice as graphic confirmation of my thesis. A fellow physician who had come to me for treatment once aptly remarked in this context: "Mr. Banis, it's absolutely incredible that you can spirit away my depressions with a couple of homeopathic drops! I am very grateful to you for this. As a physician, I

do not understand it and can only shake my head in puzzlement – but as a suffering patient, I don't give a hoot how you did it: the main thing is, it works!"

Yet another problem with emotional conflicts is the unfortunate tendency for them to remain completely mute and unconscious. In almost all cases, one loses the sense of one's emotional wounds, presumably so they will no longer cause pain. The mind withdraws into itself, in the form of an emotional conflict, like a snail into its shell. And then one no longer knows what is hidden away inside the snail shell and what kinds of emotions are lurking in there. As soon as the emotional wound is uncovered and brought into the light of day, it loses its at times demonic-seeming power over us: we recover our lost emotional component and once more become more our own self.

In fairy tales, emotional conflicts lead to the affected persons becoming literally bewitched creatures, as in Sleeping Beauty, or princes that have been enchanted and transformed into stags. Yet while the good princes and princesses remain morally upstanding beings despite their bewitchment, things are different in real life. In cruel daily life, emotional wounds often fester and lead to nasty behavioral patterns that have manifold unfavorable consequences, such as becoming the cause of destructive and evil actions. Or the person turns the destructive compulsion inward, making himself sick and driving himself to ruin. Thus, in the great majority of diseases, character weaknesses and practically all interpersonal disputes, one will find emotional conflicts that can be regarded as the actual cause of the disturbance, since they generate mental disharmony and unhappiness, block energy flows and upset metabolism.

In order to attain true emotional and physical health, we must ferret out the conflict, the real villain. To break out of the vicious cycle of unknown emotional wound and sick- and evil-making effects – comparable to enchantment in the fairy tales – we must break the spell and drag the conflict out into the daylight. Psychosomatic Energetics offers a uniquely effective opportunity to recognize an emotional conflict even when it is lodged deeply and silently in the subconscious – in children, for example, who cannot yet speak, or those conflicts that act as gigantic carriers of our character and whose portentous magnitude can be viewed as the true reason why we are no longer aware of the content of these conflicts.

However, these normally hard to uncover conflicts can be detected by measuring their energetic "fingerprint." I'll explain exactly how that works at the end of this book, but I'll jump the gun a little by revealing that the actual trick consists of uncovering the conflict's underlying energy block. In a sense, one nabs the energetic "packet" and knows at once, from its form, what kind of emotional content is hidden within, instead of having to laboriously poke around in the subconscious and, moreover, trying to puzzle out some questionable connections. Based on the kind of energy block, one can not only know which conflict it is and what contents underlie it, but also – fascinatingly – how great the energy of the associated conflicts is. This is very important in estimating how much the conflict is harming the victim and subconsciously influencing behavior.

When we have subconscious conflicts, the next question is when and how such blocks can have arisen. One tends to assume that most emotional conflicts have to do with early childhood traumas. My investigations have led to the surprising conclusion that even newborn babies come into the world with conflicts, even if the mother has credibly had a completely smooth pregnancy. One can't help asking from where the baby could possibly have acquired its conflicts, since no normal cause can be found for them. My researches indicate that these must be conflicts from past lives, as strange and shocking as that might seem. I have developed a system from this view of the matter that significantly expands on the current state of knowledge of depth psychology.

Our past lives' unresolved problems seem to have repercussions in our present lives. I have attempted to present, as logically and lucidly as possible, how to explain the secret processes, taking place behind the scenes, of Karma and Destiny. This inevitably leads to an overall picture of the emotional maturation processes that is in complete agreement with ancient spiritual ideas such as Aldous HUXLEY's *Perennial Philosophy*. The result is a fascinating grand panorama of human evolution that corresponds to the deepest insights of religion and the great spiritual traditions. By casting human history as a mirror of inner spiritual processes, we derive from the external world a reflection of our secret spiritual processes that corresponds to an often quite painful (but ultimately and inevitably integrative) spiritual growth process. We grow emotionally with respect to our external problems as well as our inner emotional conflicts, thereby uncovering more and more our true Self, so that our actual desires and drives emerge ever more clearly.

To aid the reader in attaining greater self-knowledge and in drawing the correct conclusions from it in order to develop into a happy and emotionally honorable person, full of energy and life, is one of the primary aims of this book. Lofty goals, to be sure, yet my daily experience with many patients has shown me that they are feasible. Ultimately, all people want the same thing: to lead a happy and meaningful life in harmony with their body and soul. The elimination of energy blocks can be a valuable step toward these ends, and in this process, becoming healthy means rediscovering the inner wholeness that we all once possessed and have only temporarily lost.

"Who am I?" — The Ultimate Question

'Experience' is the name we give to the sum total of our mistakes.

(Thomas Alva Edison)

I'd like to describe how this book came to be, first, from a private perspective – because this book's existence is directly related to my personal destiny. Yet I want to make it clear that I am not normally a fan of vain self-portrayal. I always find it embarrassing when people in encounter groups and the like publicly air their inmost privacies. There is a very natural sense of shame that should also extend to one's private life. Nevertheless, I need to bite the bullet and reveal private details about myself, for the simple reason that the content of this book also represents the end result of my own self-exploration.

As an established physician in middle age, I at one point came to the end of my rope. I had wound up in a miserable situation in which my private life was a complete shambles. A divorce had cost me my wife, my house with its beautiful garden, and above all the constant companionship of my beloved children. Shortly after the divorce, I remember sitting on a park bench, baby on my arm, watching my older child play with his toy steam shovel on the playground. My mood exactly matched the gloomy weather of this autumnal "father's weekend." It was an added challenge not to let the children get wind of my mood of infinite despondency.

Once the weekend was over and I had returned my sons to their mother, the endless hours of grief and loneliness in my bachelor apartment would begin. I played my electric guitar at top volume (to this day, I feel sorry for my unfortunate neighbors), anesthetized myself with all kinds of drugs and tried as hard as I could to distract myself with candies and sumptuous presents that I made for myself. But I just slid inexorably right down into a deepening and paralyzing despair that threatened to rob me of my sanity. At night, I was haunted by a thousand questions – How could it have come to this dreadful situation? What had I done wrong? And so forth – until, next morning, I would show up at my practice totally wrung out (where I had mere seconds to metamorphose from pitiable victim into mighty achiever, supposedly able to help others professionally, even though I was the one most in need of help). Months went by like this, my condition improving ever so slowly.

The miserable months after my divorce had set in motion a process of emotional change that led to further self-examination. Because, after all, what is it that causes interpersonal strife? How does the subconscious give birth to these problems in the first place? How does the whole process work? How had I slipped into the calamity that led to the divorce? I found the beginning of an answer to these questions at a medical convention that I'd like to report on here. A female psychoanalyst was discussing, with some physicians, *difficult patients* with which one has an above-average number of problems and disputes. The basic idea behind these medical get-togethers can be traced back to BALINT: in the '60s, the physician and psychoanalyst Michael BALINT discovered that the "problem patient" was usually an indication of hidden subconscious problems (including the physician's), and that bringing them into conscious awareness can help improve the doctor-patient relationship.

For me, the most amazing thing about these medical get-togethers was the unbelievable accuracy with which the female analyst was able to predict the behavior of certain patients, even when she had only heard a few descriptions of typical behavior patterns. Since this analyst certainly wasn't clairvoyant, but quite matter-of-factly coming up with her predictions, then the patient's behavior had to have a logical basis. This fascinated me enormously, because this meant that patient behavior could be predicted based on specific knowledge. For example, the psychoanalyst knew to predict that a female patient would be getting a divorce. From her description, one could at once see that the person in question was driven by her emotional dynamics to constant quarrel and strife which would culminate in a "big bang." This observation understandably hit me like a lightning bolt! I instantly recognized my own situation.

My curiosity piqued, I knew that I had to look into the entire process more closely. After all, knowing about these subconscious drives was bound to help not only me, but anyone else, a great deal. Much unnecessary suffering and misunderstandings could be avoided if each person were cognizant of his or her subconscious dynamics. Knowing the subconscious dynamic undercurrents, one could recognize the obscure rules that are the basis of our thoughts and actions. This way, we would no longer be mere "gofers" for our secret managers, but rather once again fully-conscious, autonomous, responsible human beings. The immeasurably valuable consequence of this is the fact that we can then recognize and avert, before it's too late, disadvantageous self-destructive behavior patterns in ourselves and in others.

Now, what generates these regularities in our behavior? Like a cannonball whose course can be calculated, control of our behavior is based on the already laid out "tracks" of our character. Character determines how we behave and what we feel to be right. As children, we are introduced to certain (of course extremely stereotyped) character types in fairy tales and puppet shows. The Hero is courageous and never at a loss for clever words, while his grandmother plays the part of the thoughtful, motherly protective and somewhat boring adult. The Devil, a cagey scoundrel, is always trying to get the upper hand by relentlessly taking on The Hero.

Even if we were to act out these roles for children in disguised form (say behind a curtain), the children would still easily be able to identify the individual characters, because, in the children's imagination, the Devil always behaves like a proper devil, a Hero like a hero and so forth. We adults can determine character in exactly the same manner. The difference between real life and the cartoony characters of the puppet show is that real-world character types are at first harder to penetrate. We need to become familiar with the various different types and their distinctive traits – but then it becomes remarkably effortless, and it requires no special abilities or specific training, just knowledge of the character types described in this book.

I was initially driven by curiosity, wanting to know my own character type. However, this made me increasingly uncomfortable! It got harder and harder to conceal from myself my unpleasant character traits. I realized more and more that, hidden behind the agreeable Goofy I had been playing all my life, there was a cagey devil (or rather, to be honest, more like a small yet very lively imp). I was by no means just the nice, innocuous young man; suddenly, I was peering down into depths of aggression and subtle peek-a-boo games that the evil in me impelled me to play in order to avoid being discovered. Of course, one at first refuses to believe that one is harboring an inner bastard. As the poet Christian MORGENSTERN put it: "Those who walk toward the Truth walk alone." The games people play in encounter groups, as they reveal supposed intimacies, begin to get uncomfortable as soon as they really do "get down to the nitty-gritty." North American Indians have a pertinent aphorism: *He who speaks the truth needs a fast horse!*

I had another problem in that, as a physician, you very much tend to believe in the idealized image that patients want to see in you. For this reason, the path to self-insight was particularly painful to someone like myself. To my mind, there's a reason why Jesus promised ordinary sinners a relatively easy time of it on Ascension Day, while coming down much harder on mendacious Pharisees. If Ascension Day has to do with repentance, even if one has previously sinned, then this is obviously much easier for regular sinners than for those sporting homemade haloes, who consider themselves to be better than the rest. I evidently belonged to the latter group, since confessing my character sins was extremely difficult for me.

I also made a surprising discovery, namely that confessing my sins and becoming aware of emotional abysses usually changed very little or (regrettably) even nothing at all! I experienced this in myself, as I – time and again – felt like boxing my own ears for doing the same stupid thing over and over. I saw the same thing in thousands of patients who all vowed that they were finally going to lose some weight and pay more attention to their diet – but who didn't lose an ounce. Or cut back on the booze, exercise more – and never turned good intentions into deeds. Basically, besides the sad fact that you have not reached your proclaimed goal, there comes on top of it the shameful feeling of having failed, making it all worse. Am I and all these people nothing more than spineless weaklings, inconsistent and unstable creatures?

It is precisely at this point that a very exciting new story begins, having to do with the discovery of conflicts. I found out that the subtle-body energy system contains subconscious emotional blocks (conflicts). Conflicts represent intolerable emotional content that we repress by pushing it down into the subconscious. Like a scratched record, stuck on the same melodic fragment, repeats it over and over, something comparable happens with conflicts. A conflict single-mindedly repeats its tune forever and thus forces us into harmful modes of action. A conflict generates negative moods and sucks energy out of us, so that, drained of energy and dissatisfied, we eat more, get drunk, or mistreat our fellow man.

But if conflicts have such catastrophic consequences in our lives, how do we get rid of them? Specialists long believed that simply becoming aware of conflicts would be enough to resolve and eliminate them – which, in almost all cases, has turned out to be wishful thinking, because *even if I become aware of my flaws, they don't just disappear.* This is a problem that has famously preoccupied religion and psychoanalysis right from the start. Even if I know what my problems look like, they usually stay right where they are. Why is that? At this point, the experts usually tell us that it's our own fault! We're too pig-headed, bigoted and weak to rid ourselves of our problems.

However, I have come to a completely different conclusion, thanks to certain investigations I made in my naturopathic clinical practice. When we are unable to lose weight and gorge ourselves instead, conflicts involving being hungry and profound frustration are the actual cause. This is by now quite well known and is indeed general knowledge. Yet experience has shown us that being aware of these conflicts helps just as little as if one knew nothing at all about one's emotional makeup. "Doctor, I know that I eat to fill an emotional void, but I still can't do anything about it," is what almost every (honest) overweight patient tells me. Nevertheless, this knowledge does nothing for the health problem, because as long as the emotional hunger in the patient's energy field is present to cause dysregulation, the knowledge will remain inconsequential!

So, if we want to free ourselves, quickly and permanently, from emotional misprogramming, the simplest way is via the subtle-body energy system. Instead of rummaging about in the patient's mind for years and delving into historical issues with no present relevance, the simple elimination of the conflict in the energy field leads to success in the least time. It's like deleting "buggy" software on a computer: when the defective program "being hungry" in the patient's energy field is deleted, then the emotional frustration (that makes the patient overeat and thus become overweight) also disappears.

We now know that certain character types have a strong tendency to obesity. Physicians speak of *pyknics*, who put on pounds very easily and thus tend to be overweight. As one might guess, pyknics, more frequently than the average person, have feelings of frustration that lead to them getting fat. At this point, one could let the matter be and move on to the order of the day. But if we really want to delve into the causes of diseases and turn them off, we cannot stop at this point – for the question arises: why do pyknics so often drag around with them so much miserable and frustrated inner emotional content? Is cruel fate simply punishing these people, so that they often have feelings of frustration? Or did they simply not get enough oral affection as babies, which is why they are so insatiable now?

My examination of thousands of patients has come up with another reason. The fact is, one can detect feelings of frustration in a newborn baby's energy field even before it has suckled at its mother's breast or had any frustrating experiences. Because of the inborn conflict "Frustration" in its energy field, this kind of baby will become a pyknic (and overweight) if the misprogramming is not deleted and the "Frustration" conflict removed. Evidently, the baby comes into the world with the frustration – but that means that the oral theory of traditional psychoanalysis cannot possibly be right! "Well, then it must have experienced frustration in the womb!" many readers will now object.

But now a new question comes up, having to do with the profoundest interactions of material body and mind. According to modern science, obesity is to a considerable degree a genetic problem. But how does the genetic programming in the womb manage to modify itself by means of feelings of frustration? Anyone familiar with the strict rules of genetics will find it highly unlikely that genes could be so radically altered by emotions. Fat people have inherited rigid, genetically determined natural tendencies that were fixed at the moment of conception. And here's another oddity: many mothers of overweight pyknics have assured me that their pregnancy was extraordinarily harmonious and free of frustration. Obviously, the theory of intrauterine frustration is untenable. There are actually only two ways that a genetically corpulent person could have inborn feelings of frustration: either they come from the genes themselves (in that certain genetic endowments impress very specific emotions on a person) or else the feelings of frustration are even older and long predate the time in the uterus.

At this perplexing point, I'd like to return to my own personal history. My research into my own history and that of my many patients has convinced me that our deepest emotions (i.e. our oldest conflicts) must have their origins in past lives. These deep emotions generate our character type and evidently lead to our prenatal choice of a body type that, for example, corresponds to a pyknic constitution in the case of feelings of frustration. **One of the most difficult puzzles of psychosomatics – the interplay of mind and body at the genetic level – is resolved by the assumption of a prenatally existent character type!**

Many questions and problems that have thus far engendered conflicting responses from medicine, psychology and religion can be answered simply and conclusively from this kind of higher viewpoint:

Character type and conflict are the two important poles that, like strong magnets, direct our lives in a usually undetectable manner. The individual character type is thus determined by the type of conflict (I will return to deal with this in greater detail later on in the book). Character type and conflict are thus intimately interlinked, which means that eliminating the conflicts automatically and favorably influences our negative character traits. The energetic dissolution of conflicts thus seems to me to be the primary key (and the indispensable precondition) for holistic healing.

What else we can do, besides resolving conflicts, in order to lead an upright life in accordance with our true desires, is one of the main concerns of this book. It has to do, above all, with truthfulness and love – the two foundations of a rewarding life. This book is thus a resource that can be used like a mirror to get to know one's concealed aspects and dark sides, primarily to assist one to better self-knowledge. To be sure, this kind of self-exploration can better be mastered with expert guidance, so that psychotherapists and other emotional assistants can be supportive attendants in this psychoenergetic birth process. Still, in most cases, one can do without specialists, especially if one's emotional problems are not too serious.

But in this book, I am pursuing yet another concern, having to do with a change in our customary, basically inadequate and way too short-sighted worldview. I hope to be able to show that our *Weltanschauung* is predominantly a psychoenergetic product of our general state of mind: **"I believe what I feel and how I vibrate energetically" is my basic thesis.** What we think is thus much less important than how we feel and energetically vibrate. As we know, psychology has long been aware that our perceptions are hugely influenced by subconscious and emotional factors – and it's not just emotions, but rather the totality of subtle-body vibrations and feelings.

Anyone who has observed – astounded – formerly embittered, emotionally emaciated people find their way back, in just a few months, to a positive life attitude once their conflicts have been eliminated, once again trusting in life (which is for me, ultimately, the essence of belief), realizes what all this is, at bottom, about. All new love affairs likewise affirm what amazing physical/mental changes are possible when people are energetically animated. Our subtle-body energy system plays a crucial role, as it guides and determines our thoughts and sensations, without our being aware of the full extent of it.

At this point, readers might be asking themselves skeptically whether they can trust my assertions. I'd like to make it clear that I have developed the main ideas in this book from the viewpoint of an active practicing physician who views his calling as consisting of helping his fellow man and alleviating distress. I am not, therefore, an unworldly theoretician, but rather primarily a practically-oriented healer whose motivation consists above all of explaining to my patients how I classify the background factors of their psychoenergetic problems, and what needs to be done for them to regain their health. This book is thus written first and foremost as a patient guide that provides all necessary explanations and models so that patients can, in private study, read it and then think through how their problems may have arisen.

I'd also like to tell critical readers that I pay allegiance to no sect or any other kind of organized religious view. To my mind, the highest principle of our thoughts and actions should not be determined by ideology but by compassion. Above all else, we should be persons who deal with each other humanely and with mutual respect! Many people slip up at this point, equating the social and humane with religion: God thus becomes for them a mere metaphor for a philanthropic attitude. In my understanding, however, mere humanity is far too paltry to serve as a surrogate religion, because the reality of God towers far above our human world.[1]

I'd here like briefly to describe some core ideas that I think are of fundamental significance, and which I will explain in greater detail later on as I get to them. On the way to ourselves and to God (ultimately the same thing), the very first thing we have to learn is to love ourselves. Now, this forthright self-love that comes from the heart must not be confused with egotism or narcissism! Self-love also has a selfless aspect directed at one's fellow man. We are separated from this broadly encompassing self-love, that includes our fellow man, by our subconscious conflicts. One consequence of this is that we succumb to our prejudices and project our subconscious problems onto others. Typically, we refuse to acknowledge (or eliminate) our own part in our misfortunes, which has to do with the dark side of conflicts – the so-called "evil." We cast about for a comforting excuse; we need a scapegoat as a most convenient pseudo-solution.

Respecting and loving oneself is a very difficult exercise, one which we all have to learn at some point! This has absolutely nothing to do with egotism, wrongly equated with a coarse overall attitude that does harm to others. Quite the opposite: self-love leads to more socialized and humane behavior, once we have fought our way past the dark aspects of the evil within. You can only forgive others after you have plumbed your own depths. Only when you value yourself can you value others. Only when you experience joy and pleasure in yourself can you share your *joie de vivre* with others. Through self-love, you automatically are more careful and loving in dealing, not only with yourself, but others as well. That's what I'd like to contribute with this book.

---

[1] It was the philosopher HEGEL who first made the mistake of shrinking the concept of God down to human scale: he believed that the world-spirit discovers itself in the course of [prehistoric] anthropogenesis and subsequent recorded history. MARX continued this fateful error in his dialectical Marxian view of man, which ultimately had to end in totalitarianism, since it lacked, from its very beginning, the humbling corrective of the spiritual God concept. MARX simply took HEGEL's ideas to their logical conclusion, even though his [Marx's] ideas were atheistic, for MARX (just like HEGEL) saw man as a godlike Titan, lifting up the universe – a narcissistic illusion that seems rather to have been a psychological problem of these two philosophers than to have originated in real-world facts.

A New Path to Self-Exploration

Although most people are fascinated by the unknown and eerie aspects of their subconscious, almost nobody is interested in the theory associated with it. Unfortunately, this attitude is totally wrong-headed and extraordinarily harmful, as I have shown in the preceding chapter. At some point, we must all grapple with the rules that subconsciously govern our thinking and behavior. Life forces us to! I, for example, had to pay an extremely high price for not knowing that my former partner and I were by nature diametrically opposed character types. Knowing the subconscious rules that govern behavior and are manifested in character type could have spared me a great deal of mental anguish.

This includes psychologists, psychoanalysts, and psychiatrists. It is tempting to turn over the tedious work on one's subconscious to these experts. Psychological help is sometimes unavoidable and certainly very helpful for the mentally ill, but it's simply not relevant for most people. Basically, I consider calling in a specialist, who's supposed to vicariously interpret and therapize one's subconscious, not to be a good solution for most of us "regular mortals."

For a long time – especially in the USA – the word was that each of us needed our own psychoanalyst, just as car owners are supposed to take their vehicles in for regular scheduled maintenance and cleaning. Gradually, though, we are beginning to realize that this is the wrong approach for most mentally normal people. Regrettably, analysis is not only very expensive, it has other drawbacks as well. As a physician, I have often noticed that it can generate detrimental dependencies and, many times, mental suffering flares up precisely when the analyst starts to rummage around in the subconscious, generating long-term confusion. I am aware, of course, that psychotherapy is very helpful for certain mental disorders, it's just that my experience has shown that this does not apply to most people.

But even for patients who seem to benefit directly from psychotherapy, the matter is not so simple. After psychotherapy, most patients can talk knowledgeably about their problems, yet in virtually all cases they still have them. There's a popular saying that refers to this well-known phenomenon, where a patient reveals the therapy's failure with the telltale sentence: "I still have my problems, it's true – but now they don't bother me any more." This is of course a result, just not a very satisfactory one, and not one that any reasonable person would seriously want. Ultimately, one consoles oneself with the thought that, as an uncured patient, one has at least been forced to learn to deal with one's own mental difficulties a bit better, even though the problems, for whatever reason, have not been resolved.

Contrary to what most people think, criticism of traditional psychotherapy is also widespread among specialists. In many confidential conversations with experienced medical colleagues, I am constantly told the same thing: "Sure, your criticism of traditional analysis is right on the money, but no one admits it openly, for fear of eternal disgrace!" No one is willing to admit publicly to a uncomfortable opinion because, for many people, psychotherapy is still somewhat holy. Apart from a few positive cases, the entirely word-based method of traditional psychotherapy is often unsatisfactory in terms of effectiveness. Very often, enormous amounts of doctor and patient energy are wasted vainly chasing after a cure, then afterwards putting a positive spin on the frustrating exertions.

A typical example from my practice:

Klaus W., a 20-year-old, extremely nervous slender young man, complains of anxiety states and the feeling that he's going crazy. He has been on the sick-list for quite a while already. I register very low values for his overall life energy (vitality). The cause seems to be a gigantic mental conflict acting as an "energy thief," robbing him of the greater part of his vital energy. Unfortunately, his situation deteriorates so much that we can no longer eliminate the conflict.

The patient stays for several months at a well-known special clinic; his condition on discharge is (in the words of the discharge report) "considerably improved." In the clinic, he has many regular individual psychotherapy sessions and takes part in group sessions several times a week. Based on my examination, the patient is just as bad off as before; his poor energy readings, as well as his conflict, are completely unchanged. He confirms that he indeed feels just as bad as my measurements indicate, except that that he is no longer so hectic and restless, thanks to the clinic's strong tranquilizers.

A great many patients report quite similar experiences with traditional psychoanalysis. They invest a lot of time, money and effort without experiencing the hoped-for improvement. Even more unfortunate, in my opinion, is when a patient, out of sheer sympathy for the analyst, feigns a gushing enthusiasm that has no basis in reality. I often get the impression that analysis has had a drug-like and rather unreal influence that, in extreme cases, can lead

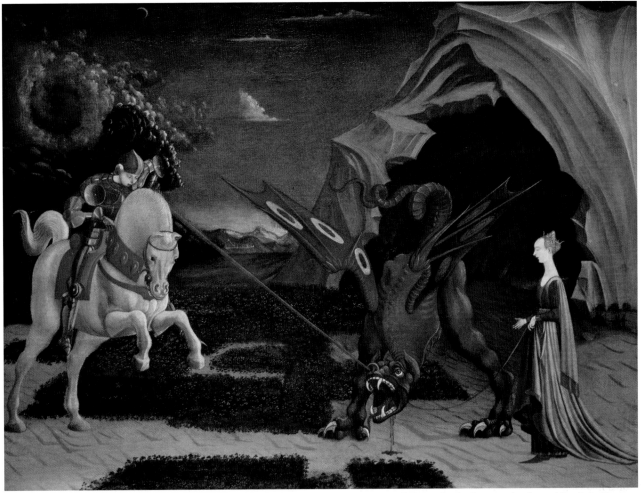

St. George fighting the Dragon depicts the archetype of "The Beauty and the Beast" (modern musical) or "King Kong" (Hollywood movie). Behind the voracious murderous Beast lurks Evil … indeed (and surprisingly) first and foremost the Evil in the Beauty's subconscious! This inner spiritual principle of the feminine psyche is known in Indian mythology as the destructive Black Kali. A later part of the book will make clear that Evil is actually inner spiritual conflict, here embodied in the Dragon. Actually, the valiant St. George liberates the fair damsel from her own destructive spiritual shadow-side. The painting symbolizes this by having the damsel lead the Dragon around on a leash like a house pet. If the Dragon were really dangerous, she wouldn't be standing there so casually with the Beast in her immediate vicinity, but rather would be showing some signs of fear or horror. On the second level, there is another depth-psychological interpretation, since the Dragon of course also symbolizes the Dragon-slayer's subconscious Evil, killing his own unruly and potentially evil lustfulness so that he may become a suitable lover and affectionate partner for his beloved.

to emotional dependency. Misjudging reality and many other problems sometimes crop up as well, such as are observed in actual addictive behavior. If my tone sounds a bit harsh, I'd just like to say that I am here simply presenting my own very personal opinion, and that I am aware that there are isolated individuals for whom analysis has been valuable and enriching. Still, in the majority of cases, the grandiose promise will not be fulfilled, that entire legions of intellectuals and brilliant therapists have invested in this kind of therapy, not to mention the multitudes of uncured and frustrated patients.

Psychoanalysis is, intellectually, an extraordinarily fascinating theory – it's just not suitable for the sensible treatment of the problems of most people. In this book, I'd like to propose a new approach, far simpler to apply, in my experience, and yielding much quicker and better results. I think that the reason why psychoanalysis (and many other procedures) accomplish so little has to do with the energetic nature of conflicts. Conflicts have to be ferreted out and erased in the energetic sphere, like erasing a schoolroom blackboard. The energetic dissolution of conflicts effects a strong and lasting mental self-healing that is not possible with other methods. I'll try to explain and substantiate this by describing remarkable patient destinies throughout this book.

Before getting more intensively into the treatment of emotional problems, I'd like first to dispose of two widespread preconceptions. The first one assumes that only specialists (i.e., psychoanalysts) should be permitted to probe into and treat the mind. This is utter nonsense, I believe, if only because every one of us does exactly this every day, even if we're not aware of it. We are constantly dealing with our own and other people's minds. One might just as well demand that every breath we draw be monitored by pulmonologists. Our subconscious is our very own private concern, whose analysis and treatment we should take into our own hands.

The second preconception concerns the common expectation that all forms of self-exploration are boring, hobbies for jaded neurotics who can't come up with anything better to do with their time. Actually, there's nothing more exciting than self-exploration. For instance, every crime novel conceals a gripping story, gradually revealed, that to my mind has aspects of self-reflection – because, through our excitement, we identify emotionally with the characters. We share with the murderer and his pursuers a part of life that reflects inner emotional tensions. Since we all – killers and victims, gangsters and upstanding citizens – have within us both bad and good aspects, we also reflect our own emotional makeup. This applies in particular to primordial emotional themes, such as *The Beauty and the Beast* or *Hero and Dragon*.

All theatergoers and crime novel readers derive excitement and enjoyment from a phenomenon that actually takes place in themselves. I claim that the same excitement will set in to the same degree when we concern ourselves with ourselves. In short, we follow the dramas and crime novels within ourselves. To do this, we just need an amplifier that makes visible the drama of our own inner emotional processes. A good way to get to know ourselves better is to notice our own enjoyment and excitement. The more something generates pleasurable excitement in us, the closer we are to our subconscious.

Desire and tension are well-known artful dodges that nature extravagantly uses everywhere. It does this with the subtle ulterior motive of inducing us to couple with other members of our species or to conquer new territories for living space. Nature makes use of special tricks, e.g. making desire much more intense when a partner has a particularly distinctive genetic makeup. This has been demonstrated in an experiment with the perspiration odor of male volunteers, using t-shirts they have worn as experimental objects.

The odor is more attractive to the female participants the more distinct certain immunity features are to them. Since specific genes increase the survival odds of one's offspring, the female therefore unconsciously seeks out partners that genetically fit her particularly well. As she is sniffing, that scent which most increases the female's desire represents, from nature's viewpoint, the one that yields the best individual procreative odds.

Man copies this tactic in a particularly subtle manner. For example, it always surprises me anew each time I notice how the number of blondes increases from year to year in predominantly brunette Italy. Anything unusual that catches our eye increases reproductive odds, so it automatically generates desire and tension. From the standpoint of discovering one's own subconscious, every disco, every park with amorous couples, and every group of flirtatious teenagers becomes a self-discovery site. As adolescents, we get to know ourselves as we associate with the opposite sex. In puberty, we begin to feel for the first time the vastness of just being alive. We fall in love and at some point start a family. The marvelous high points of our lives – first love, marriage, birth of children, career successes, moments of special happiness – are also times in which we get to know our subconscious in a very special way. Paradoxically, this also applies precisely to the unfortunate, miserable low points of our lives! Through these, we learn to look into our own abysmal depths.

In our mind, desire and tension increase most when the topics touch on strong internal emotional antipodes – those of life and death, "To be or not to be," subjugation and power, and so on. Incompatible concepts – inclination and disinclination, love and hate, sexuality and bloodthirstiness, ecstasy and ennui – clash particularly strongly. This collision of antitheses releases very large amounts of vital energy, which is why these opposites attract us so much. Every gawker at an accident site is thirsting for the horrific image of blood-covered victims to give him the secretly hoped-for "kick." All human curiosity, up to and including sensationalism, feeds off this phenomenon.

When opposites go to extremes, we worry about losing our mind. The deeper we penetrate into our subconscious, the more we are forced to confront emotional antipodes. We enter the dangerous territory of our emotional landmines, known in psychology as conflicts or complexes. Here we confront our mental abysses and emotional incompatibilities, which are coupled with great fear. For millennia, these inner mental areas were barred to the public by prohibitions and collective taboos that ensured that no one came into close contact with them.

These taboos and laws concern not only ecstatic and transcendental experiences, but also socially-proscribed behavior considered to be obscene, generally objectionable, and irritating. Looking back at the history of mankind, deep penetration into the subconscious has been an exclusive insider privilege for those who – as shamans, Egyptian priests, or meditation students – had special permission, with religious exercises and ceremonies, to press forward into these regions. Lately, though, the situation has changed drastically, and the taboos have largely fallen by the wayside. No one is prevented from meditating or attending self-discovery seminars.

Fear of the depths of one's own subconscious nevertheless persists in almost everyone, even if the warning signs – the social taboos – have been taken down. The very real danger of supposedly safe therapies such as meditation or Autogenic Training is that labile individuals can suddenly undergo profound borderline experiences that completely unsettle them and throw them way off course. Thank God this seldom comes to pass; I can count on the fingers of one hand the number of patients who have told me, in my practice, of such experiences. Still, these incidents show us that self-discovery is by no means an innocuous walk in the park.

Now, it is not my intention to stoke anyone's fears; I just want to point out that you proceed at your own risk and responsibility. Anyone who ventures into the subconscious without the trained assistance of a meditation master or psychologist should have a fairly stable personality and, at the first warning signs – feeling that things are spinning out of control, feeling too much fear and uneasiness, and suchlike – break off the "emotional SCUBA dive" and, if necessary, engage professional assistance. To clarify: my warnings are not directed at the average reader, but rather at those the medical profession designates as emotionally labile or borderline psychotic. Such people almost always know that, even in everyday life, they're "skating on thin ice." They need trained specialists in order to make any progress.

The path of self-exploration that I advocate in this book is, above all, enormously exciting but by no means anxiety-inducing. The self-discovery I have discovered and apply is called "Psychosomatic Energetics."

It represents a new natural healing method, in which the interplay of
- Material body (Soma),
- Mind (Psyche)
- And subtle-body life energy (Energetics)
is examined and harmonized.

The Greek word for mind is *Psyche*; for body, *Soma*; for the energy that flows through both, Energetics (*Prana, Ch'i, Orgone*). True health can only arise when the subtle-body life energy of our material body and our mind work together in harmony. The old Latin saying *Mens sana in corpore sano* (A sound mind in a sound body) is thus only partly right – since subtle-body life energy is absolutely part of it, too! We are only truly healthy when we have free and unblocked life energy that fills our body with vital energy and our mind with *joie de vivre*.

With Psychosomatic Energetics, we can ascertain that the great majority of people's vital energy is enfeebled. The overwhelming majority of all people are therefore only seemingly healthy and show light to severe signs of energy weakness. The main cause for this is almost always emotional conflicts. At the same time, it is my experience that phobias, in connection with the subconscious, are above all conditioned by our emotional conflicts! Actually, then, we are afraid not of our own subconscious but our emotional conflicts – the "demons and dragons" within us! When we track down the emotional conflicts and heal them with Psychosomatic Energetics, we lose the fear of our own subconscious. Paralleling the shrinking of our conflicts, our vital energy begins once again to flow unimpeded. We experience a previously unsuspected energy growth, and we feel good again, full of energy and sensuality.

Self-discovery only really gets going when we recognize our emotional conflicts, in order to dissolve them in the second phase. In the third phase, we begin to integrate the pre-existent emotional dark sides of our being. At first, this sounds quite logical and simple. Astonishingly, there are few "hang-ups" if we accompany the entire process with Psychosomatic Energetics – because we can ferret out deeply-hidden subconscious conflicts with simple energy medicine methods, identify them, and gradually heal them with certain homeopathic agents. I'll detail exactly how that works in subsequent chapters.

Getting Well and Feeling Well

Giving one's character some style – a great and rare art!
Yet one thing is necessary: that one achieve satisfaction with oneself.

(Nietzsche)

This book is about a form of medication. In the preceding chapter, I pointed out that almost all of us need this medication, since most people – at least 95%, by my estimate – are blocked in their subtle-body energy system and therefore hover in an intermediate state between health and illness. Because familiarity famously breeds contempt and blindness, we get used to our weakened energetic state. Many patients often notice only afterwards – i.e. after their recovery – how bad they had been feeling.

All good medications promote self-healing by providing profound stimuli for self-knowledge and for becoming truly healthy. Yet health never comes from outside, but rather is already implicit in us, needing only to be reawakened. We can therefore rightly say: "Nature heals." Getting well and feeling well is a comprehensive growth process that encompasses our entire humanity, together with our personality, our body and our inmost desires and yearnings.

In this deeper sense, getting well and starying well is one of the most important tasks in each person's life. Therefore, this book is aimed not just at therapists, but rather at any and all people interested in more profound self-discovery.

At some point, the day will come when we must face the truth about ourselves and our lives. We should therefore be proactive and deal early on with our self-discovery; otherwise, life itself will push us into this situation one way or another. Sooner or later, most of us experience a rude awakening: a disease, death of a family member or some other stroke of fate or shock that derails us and forces us to wake up. Or we grow old and one day realize that we have been unable to fulfill many of our wishes, because time has run out.

Actually, we cannot run away from ourselves, so the reasonable thing to do is stop and take stock: who are we really? The essential questions are: "Who am I? What do I really want? Who is really hiding behind the mask with the many roles that I am constantly playing? What are my real needs? What is preventing me from realizing my true feelings and wishes?" My experience as a physician is that people eventually become chronically ill if they cannot resolve these existential questions. This is why most diseases are bound up with these unresolved existential issues, even if it might not seem so at first (e.g.,

accidents or infections). To heal a disease from the ground up, the sick person must necessarily find sensible answers to his existential questions.

If we're honest, we have to admit that prefabricated answers aren't much help: they're pseudo-solutions that claim to be able to spare us the laborious task of coming up with real answers to our life-questions. By pseudo-solutions I mean seductive healing systems, religious sects, and fantastic sounding ideologies that would have us believe that our work is already done. The truth is, actually, that all of us have to answer the big questions of our lives for ourselves. To do this, we have to be quiet and learn to hear the still, small voice inside. Anything else is just running away, which accomplishes nothing in the long run.

In the process of self-discovery, the insuperable obstacle is often that we can no longer hear our inner voice. We have simply forgotten how to notice our deep motivations and genuine convictions. The main reason for this lies within us; we are wearing, as it were, dusty eyeglasses badly in need of cleaning, through which we can no longer see our true inner reality. The primary cause of our "dusty glasses" is our ingrained habits; we stick with the familiar daily grind and thus become dull and insensitive. In the background, it's ultimately the subconscious struggles that have to do with our emotional conflicts.

As soon as we have become internally clearer and more orderly, we can take the next step, which consists of **learning to hear the inner voice**. Only then are we capable of again perceiving it undistorted. We also understand the large and hard-to-solve problem allegorized in the image of the "dusty glasses." It is enormously hard for us to perceive the beam in our own eye, although we have no trouble at all noticing the mote in our neighbor's. We are known for being relatively blind to our own problems. Therefore, it is only with great effort that we can pull ourselves out of our own swamp. Despite that, the undertaking is not impossible, but is rather, with some help (which I will provide later), relatively easy and safe to manage.

However, self-discovery is not for healing and preventing disease. I have already mentioned that it is absolutely a worthwhile occupation for everyone, well or ill, to continue to mature mentally and truly to get well and feel well internally. So, if we examine people using subtle-body methods, we will find in practically every person certain subconscious emotional problems or conflicts that make him unwell, sick in some sense, and disturbed. Even if we feel well and healthy, these conflicts are buried deep in our subconscious. This is why I say that there is practically nobody who has no subconscious problems. The 5% seemingly healthy contingent – that does indeed exist opposite the 95% ailing or energy-deficient group – when observed over longer periods of time, are simply those who are enjoying the "calm before the storm." They aren't really healthy, just in a resting stage.

One can ask, of course, why bother about subconscious problems and conflicts, if one feels healthy. There are three reasons, in my experience, which I'll substantiate in more detail later on in the book. The first reason is based on subliminal pathological conflicts that throttle vital energy, burdening even seemingly healthy people. If we want to be truly healthy from the ground up, and full of vital energy, then there's no getting around eliminating our conflicts. I have yet to meet anyone who has not felt much better and healthier after the elimination of subconscious conflicts – and also much less susceptible to disease and much more resilient.

The second reason is based on perceptual distortion. The prevailing view of reality is limited by very large and distorting conflicts. Filtered by our subconscious conflicts, we see reality not as it is, but rather "through a glass darkly." Understandably, this is far from an ideal situation, both for ourselves and those around us, and it leads to constant misunderstandings and misinterpretations. In a certain sense, we misapprehend reality, while remaining firmly convinced that we are 100% in the right.

There is a third reason why comprehensive healing is necessary – for me the most important. It's no accident that "healing" [getting well] and "well-being" have, in the literal sense, such closely related meanings. In order to get truly well and whole, we must rid our mind of the garbage that many of us, out of fear and sheer inertia, drag around with us. But this can only work for so long, since the more we progress in our personal development, the sicker and more emotionally disturbed we'll be in our mental core if we have not cleared away the "mental rubbish" of our subconscious conflicts. And even if we'd like to slink silently and furtively away, life will force us – in the form of some unpleasant lessons – to recognize our emotional imbalance and to work on it. We should therefore begin the cleanup process as soon as possible.

Emotional healing of such conflicts is no walk in the park; it forces us to face deeply-rooted fears. Nevertheless, we need not "fear fear itself," because these fears are actually not nearly as bad as they feel at first. In fact, our emotional wounds are quite often no more than tender feelings of injury and pain, behind which we protect our extremely vulnerable spirit, like a princess, behind the high fortress walls of our emotional defenses.

This inner fortress corresponds to what psychologists call defense. Because a fortress must be constantly guarded and protected, life inside the inner fortress gets more and more unpleasant. This gives rise to all the characteristic deficiencies and excesses of personality distortions that can escalate to extremes of paranoia and evil. If we conceive of the fortress surrounding us as "sin" in the religious sense, we realize that the fortress walls seal us off from all of creation and even from God. If we view the inner fortress as a purely personal concern – as modern psychology does – then we cut ourselves off from our true Self. Ultimately, the entire view comes down to this: we erect mental walls to protect something that in reality cannot be protected – and (crazily and downright grotesquely) the protective measures then become the core problem.

For centuries, all of mankind's efforts at inner liberation were directed toward tearing down the fortress around the true Self – completely overlooking the fact that the inner fortress also has its good side, in that it leads to the development of a permanent personality, i.e. a firm character type. Therefore, one must not prematurely storm the fortress of the true Self. As the egg needs a shell to protect the growing embryo, we also need (for a while) the rigidity and steadfastness of this inner fortress in order to be able to develop a stable Self. Later on, I will explain more about the usefulness of our inner fortress.

However, at some point we must break through the eggshell and out of our prison in order to be able to continue and mature in life. Most people remain stuck in their shell like fledglings, which leads to a low-intensity atrophied life. For those stuck inside, those who have not ventured outside their fortress, it is much more unpleasant than for those around them. These people spoil their lives by cutting themselves off from all that is lively and from their true spiritual motivations. Flawed life in the inner fortress generates tensions and frustrations that are "burned off" externally as aggressive acts, destructive (and self-destructive) impulses, bitterness and rancor. Or else the shut-in will do the very opposite and become very quiet, withdrawn and inhibited, leading in extreme cases to complete apathy, insensitivity and even feigned handicaps. A third possibility is that physical diseases will appear to vent the inner tensions.

Now, most people seem normal and apparently healthy, yet a closer look reveals – except for a couple of saintly and enlightened ones – that they are stuck in their inner fortress, and they'll have to come out someday if they are not to get sick. Self-discovery is so important because it represents the most significant means with which to break out of our inner prison. Exploring our Self intensively, we get to know the rejected parts of our personality, with which we can again become "whole and hale." The conflict's occult power is thereby broken, and we become – as Sigmund FREUD so well put it – "master of our own house" again. Our true Self can emerge, and we once again live from our emotional center. This doesn't mean that all problems are solved and everything is now simple – quite the contrary: only from our emotional center can we really and truly begin to solve our problems and bring order into our lives.

The Spiritual Journey

The journey leads us back to ourselves.

(Albert Camus)

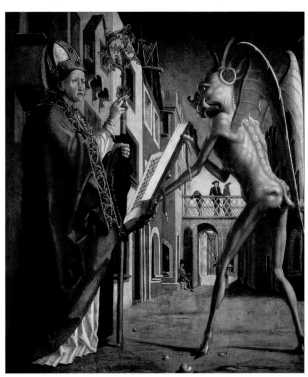

The Devil tempting Saint Wolfgang – allegorical representation of the subconscious demonic drives in us that dictate our world-view (represented by the Devil holding out a counterfeit Bible to the saint)

Right at the beginning of the descent into our emotional depths, we come face to face with great terrors. These are called the spiritual gatekeepers, and they live in the relative shallows of the subconscious. When we encounter such fearful figures in our dreams, nightmares (none too gently) interrupt our sleep. Like a car alarm that starts up with a bloodcurdling howl, the subconscious gives us a dreadful fright as we first approach it. For this reason, many people have a panicky fear of their own inner world. Later on in the book, it will become clear that the fearful figures are our own subconscious conflicts.

A surprising number of everyday phenomena serve to soothe our inner fears: life insurance, armies, police forces,

or other protective and defensive mechanisms – in all these cases, both the real utility and the unreal fears lurking deep within us are served by the defensive measures. And yet, upon closer observation, the inner recesses of our mind are really not scary: they are, all in all, a peaceful interior world whose spiritual abundance can enrich us with its living plenitude and latent purpose. But then there is also the topic of tension, that ultimately makes us good and lively, which is why the journey into our mental depths is one of the most exciting that this world has to offer.

The deeper we peer into our mind, the more our inner child surfaces, that – as in ancient Rome – wants *panem et circenses* (bread and circuses), fun and games, pleasure, and, above all, lots of excitement and suspense. We encounter this inner child at a particular stage in our self-discovery that is dominated by drives, passions and animal sensations. At some point it will become terribly clear to us that it amazingly resembles the audience of a gladiatorial spectacle in ancient Rome. At the first level of self-discovery, the fascinating yet shocking discovery consists of meeting this monstrously ravenous, utterly desire-oriented part of us. In Christian portrayals, the inner child is, from the outset, transformed into a devil that tries to lead us into temptation.

However, as we continue with our self-discovery, there is a question even more exciting than which gladiator will win and who the poor guy will be that the lions eat. What actually goes on in our mind to make us spectators find gladiator battles so fascinating when, down there in the arena, people are trying to kill each other? After all, we're talking about our fellow man, beings that we're supposed to treat with friendliness and empathy. Yet something seems to turn us into monsters that enjoy the suffering of others. We ask ourselves what turns people into torturers and tormentors. From a spiritual point of view, how do all these horrible things in the world come about?

We know that we project our wishes and yearnings, feelings and cravings onto the external world. Therefore, we find the actual reason for events out there within ourselves. With this, our spiritual journey begins, during which we can discover our true Self. It is not until much later, at the end of the journey and in very deep layers of the mind, that one finds gentle angels and divine vibrations. Then we feel at home again, and everything is idyllically peaceful and pervaded with heavenly serenity. But before we, after a prolonged odyssey, reach these Elysian Fields of peace, we first have to make our way through long stretches of our subconscious where the going is downright rough and unpleasant.

The following description of the "spiritual journey" contains a complete scenario made up of individual observations that I have knit together into a comprehensive whole. The observations depict experiences partly from my own self-discovery and partly from those of other people who have reported quite similar experiences with hallucinogenic substances. I have taken other parts of the spiritual journey from literature (DANTE's Divine Comedy), religion (particularly the Apocalypse), spiritual and cultural-historical works (mythologist Joseph CAMPBELL, and so on).

On our spiritual journey into the subconscious, we will encounter wild fellows and dramatic actions. We'll roam through infernos of animal drives and consuming passions. Down in the subconscious, many will confront (at first) grotesque, devilish aspects of themselves that have mutated into threatening monsters. At this upper level of the subconscious, it's all about "Sex, Drugs and Rock&Roll." On our inner stage unfolds a pandemoniacal struggle for power, love and desire. Erotic bodies writhe and intertwine in wild ecstasy, titans engage in titanic combat, and grotesque satanic masks, snakes and monsters threaten us most horribly.

The heroic Greek gods such as Hercules (or Shiva in India) can likewise be understood as projections of our subconscious, as can the erotic sculptures in ancient Indian and Nepalese temples, where everywhere sensual fantasies run riot. Demons and grotesque masks are thus the insignia of the subconscious. It's no accident that they are often used as temple guardians, to refuse foreign spirits' admittance to the Holy of Holies. From the viewpoint of the projecting subconscious, **the demons and grotesque masks guard the inner temple of the subconscious**. At the same time, they symbolize our displaced aggressions and the undesirable shadow sides of our character. They are thus nothing other than subconscious emotional conflicts that, because of their threatening and fearsome strangeness, are perceived as demons, snakes or insects. Our subconscious fools us into thinking that they look like that because they are, after all, formless shapes.

The fear-related contents of our subconscious will take on these eerie forms especially when we still have little experience with the subconscious and are confronted with it unexpectedly. This can be seen very clearly in children's frequent nightmares. When my brother was three or four, he would often scream horribly as he fell asleep, seeing some type of crocodile or tiger under his bed. As the fearless older brother, I would then have to look under his bed and scare the beasts away. I remember well how hard it was to convince him that there was really nothing under his bed. The frightful animals were clearly very real to him, and it took a great deal of effort to calm him down.

If there really are so many horrible things hidden within us, we can better understand all the horrors around us. "As the outer, so the inner." At this level of self-discovery, we understand that war, murder and hate are fed from this subconscious spring, as are erotic desires, creativity and love. If we really want to understand what really drives, inspires and motivates us and our fellow man, we need to take a look behind the scenes. This goes for the gladiatorial combats in ancient Rome as well as concentration camps and torture chambers. However, it also applies, in the positive sense, to everything having to do with beauty, peace and love.

We discover that all of the world's "theatrical" productions have a cryptic emotional background. At some point comes the significant turning point in our lives, when we realize that we are, each of us, spectator, actor and director in our own life movie: "Why does reality all of a sudden seem so oddly strange and dreamlike?" we ask ourselves as we rub our eyes in puzzlement. This can occur at a moment of particularly great emotional pain – or (quite the opposite) at an ordinary time of boredom and normalcy, when it suddenly becomes clear to us what a farcical façade this world really is. To call this "enlightenment" would be going too far – we should speak, instead, in terms of tearing away the veil of illusion (*Maya*[2]), of the habitual, that separates us from the world as it is.

The façade of the normal world conceals another greater and more momentous reality – and this other reality, tangible in fairy tales, dreams and many surreal perceptions, is closely related to our inner core. At this point, many people figure out that all this is actually part of their personal spiritual journey. Although the obstacles and problems along the way appear to us as sickness or cruel fate, we can in fact also recognize them as aberrations and deviations from the spiritual "straight and narrow."

So when certain problems arise in the material world, we should – using the insight "as within, so without" – look inside ourselves and check out what inner personal basis the problem has. This is why we most effectively change the world when we change ourselves. **We can designate our inner world as an "alternate reality."** The analogy of the nested dolls illustrates this very nicely. The reality we perceive with our five senses conceals another level of reality that is normally invisible and imperceptible to us.

---

[2] In Hinduism and among the Sikhs, *Maya* signifies the world of illusion, i.e. the way the material world manifests itself to us. According to this view, the world that we perceive with our five senses has no real significance. In a sense, the world only pretends to be real. In Mahayana Buddhism, this idea forms the core concept of enlightenment philosophy, in which attachment to the world of the senses (*Maya*) traps one in an endless cycle of rebirth. This view seems much less absurd in the light of modern nuclear physics, in which the atom has been revealed to be made up primarily of empty space and a little energy. Quantum mechanics goes even further, asserting the subjectivity of all seemingly objective points of view.

At this point, it is worth taking a closer look at the modern position on alternate reality. My basic conception is that our view of reality has crucially to do with our subconscious – an idea confirmed by modern perceptual psychology. When we compare our collective view of the external world to that of the inner world, the inner world seems at first relatively insignificant. From the point of view of the modern enlightened person, there's no profit potential in the inner world, nor any direct pleasure. To rationalists, the subconscious is mainly a "chest full of fairy tales" for occultists, unworldly types, and psychologists. In our modern secular world, shaped by egotism and materialism, this other reality (of the subconscious) has become more distant and invisible than at any other period in human history.

The esteem in which alternate reality has been held is quite different in the ancient world and the orient. It is part of general knowledge in all the world's great metaphysical systems that alternate reality is actually the true source of life. Many religions view alternate reality as the true secret entrance to the divine and the beyond. They know that it is basically a matter of our spirit and therefore affects an inestimably important part of ourselves. The great throng of seekers after wisdom who, in our modern society, occupy themselves with the esoteric and spirituality, actually represents the quest for this alternate reality. In this respect, such people are connecting up with ancient ideas – although still widely unpopular nowadays (at least in scientific circles) – whose significance will increase enormously in the future.

For us enlightened and clear-headed modern folk, our first access to alternate reality is, first of all, a completely private concern, a matter of health. No longer is the priest and shaman, but rather the psychologist in charge of this. I made it clear in a previous chapter that, as author, I do not agree with this hasty transfer of personal responsibility, this delegation of the exploration of one's inner life to some professional group. Yet I strongly suspect that, for many people, psychology has become a variety of surrogate religion, in that one bares one's soul to the analyst instead of the priest. This shifts too much personal responsibility onto other people.

However, delegating internal spiritual processes to a priest, as in the past, is something else entirely, because priests conjoin people collectively (as a congregation) with the divine. Today, by contrast, the official socially sanctioned access to alternate reality has turned into an intimate individual affair: the psychologist sits in isolation with the client in a closed room. The spirit is no longer regarded as something that unites us with nature, the Great Manitou, the divine; rather, it is a kind of mechanical gearbox in the brain, where hormones and neurotransmitters are busily at work. For the modern scientist, human consciousness is an emergent epiphenomenon from this piece of matter, whose complex workings

are seen as a kind of holographic structure. To modern science, the spiritual arises exclusively from the material.

Basically, this currently popular scientific idea that human consciousness is rooted in a kind of holographic structure, follows the simple logic that the whole has to be more than the sum of its parts. Because the psyche is quite complicated, one imagines it as a simulated three-dimensional image, a kind of virtual production of the brain. Therefore, modern science's conception of an independent intellectual reality is and remains an illusion. After his first spaceflight, the astronaut Yuri GAGARIN quite logically said that he wasn't able to find God anywhere "out there." To be sure, no one in his right mind would think that there was a bearded old wise man hovering about in outer space. GAGARIN simply meant to confirm what the materialistic scientists already knew: that God did not represent a materially graspable entity.

But the idea of a correct worldview first raises the fundamental question: who has the power to dare define the world? Not just astronauts, but (above all) physicists and other physical scientists as well, are granted the status of high priests, authorized to explain the world to the common folk. But where do they get the confidence to claim that neither God nor a meaning to life (in the transpersonal religious sense) exist at all? Psychology, the science of alternate reality, incorporates a pathetic remnant of spiritual knowledge, as much as remains in our modern world. Yet the great breadth and spiritual depth of alternate reality, which people of earlier times still knew and experienced, has been misplaced in our modern world. The physical scientist and the matter-of-fact person are particularly prone to the delusion of being the only entity in a godless world that presumes to know the important features of how the world works.

Scientists don't think in such limited terms out of any malice, but rather usually with the best of intentions, since they consider themselves duty-bound to honor Truth and the Scientific Method.[3] Neither the soul nor subtle-body energy can be measured or objectively veri-

---

[3] In the emotional background motivation of many scientists, one finds a not unreasonable fear of the overwhelming number of superstitions, inanities, and silly hocus-pocus that admittedly can also be found everywhere these days. For centuries, such superstition befuddled the mind of man and caused much misery. The world continues to be full of such follies. One need only open up a newspaper to the horoscope page, or study the ads for psychics and fortune-tellers. I don't for a moment deny that there are reputable people out there among the quacks. Yet despite everything, the fact remains that superstition – in this negative, short-sighted, and destructive sense – must be fought. I know from numerous conversations with scientists that they regard this as a great and serious task. You can't be too hard on them if they occasionally "throw out the baby with the bathwater" when they confuse dumb superstition with intelligent and loving belief in a higher power, and consider both to be the same.

fied. One comes up against the limits of science and finds oneself forced into the realm of belief. I'd like to mention the growing number of far-seeing scientists such as Albert EINSTEIN, Max PLANCK, David BOHM and Rupert SHELDRAKE, who view the whole matter quite differently and in a far larger context. For them, modern physics is by no means irreconcilable with the model of a spiritual world order. Quite the contrary: such scientists find a great deal of objective evidence of the existence of a spiritual and subtle-body world.

I was the recipient, in the last few decades, of a great and unexpected surprise. Most people believe, amazingly, in another kind of dimension to our reality! As a family doctor, I have spoken over the years with thousands of people who seem to know instinctively that we consist of more than just atoms and molecules. As a scientifically trained physician, I have learned a lot from my patients in this regard. Most people know that **we are actually spiritual beings animated with the breath of life**.

The mental and spiritual dimension of reality is very real to most people. To the great astonishment of scientists, in large-scale polls, over 60% of respondents stated that they had had extrasensory experiences (telepathy, precognition, out-of-body experiences [OOBE], and so on) at some point in their lives. Meanwhile, large meta-studies have shown clear indications that parapsychological phenomena generate meaningful results at a rate higher than random chance. Man's intuitive knowledge also includes that of a subtle-body vital energy. Surveys on this topic show this very clearly time and again – and are taken to be proof of how simple-minded and superstitious the ignorant masses are. It doesn't occur to any of the scientists that there might actually be something in all this.

Most people also know that many problems are due to emotional hardening and tension. They also know that healing and spiritual development are closely interrelated. When I told my patients about the (to me) new insights, almost all of them nodded: they had known this for a long time, and they were pleased that a physician such as I saw it as well. I came to a crucial turning point at a time when my delicacy of feeling was ever increasing. For example, I could correctly pick, on the first try, precisely the spot on a patient's back that was causing the most pain. How could I know this in advance? Or I would ask the patient something that came into my mind spontaneously, and it would hit the mark! Through these personal experiences, I came to understand my patients' intuitive knowledge better and better. We know that there is a huge difference between just knowing something abstractly and intellectually, and emotionally living it with all one's senses. Those who feel their own energy center and those of other people, who open themselves to the realities of these energetic-spiritual worlds, understand at once "at gut level"

what people have intuited and possess as prior knowledge.[4]

We physicians will soon have the chance of cautiously approaching vital energy and spiritual and energetic qualities without losing ourselves in wild fantasies, sectarianism, or other shallow waters. We can compare our experiences in clinical practice and our knowledge with that which we sensitively intuit, feeling our way forward slowly and cautiously, as in a darkened room. Bit by bit, we can use our critical faculties to separate the wheat from the chaff. To my mind, medicine (like religion) will have to open up, soon, to those areas that are currently descried as esoteric and "loopy." Energetic procedures such as homeopathy, acupuncture, and spiritual-esoteric knowledge are now so widespread that their significance can no longer be ignored. This will make many people more and more sensitive, exacting, energetic, and spiritually more open.

The new era of energy medicine thus challenges physicians and therapists to venture forward into unknown territory and open up their own sensibilities. After the discovery of the subconscious by FREUD at the beginning of the 20th century, I am convinced that the 21st century will see the discovery of the significance of subtle-body energy. We will only fully understand the complex interplay of psychosomatics once we take subtle-body energy into account. Our improved therapeutic understanding will result in better and more effective treatment, because we will be able to approach problems at a more profound level. Moreover, knowing about subtle-body energy has even more far-reaching consequences. For example, we acquire a new understanding of the liveliness of our planet (*Gaia* and nature). Through our perception of subtle-body energy, we develop a new relationship to spirituality.

It is part of mankind's ancient knowledge that life is a journey. It brings us into contact with a multitude of dangers and fears, and the resulting experiences help us mature spiritually. In this process, knowledge of subtle-body energy plays a very important role, as will become ever clearer in subsequent chapters. At all times and in all cultures, experience with and mastery of vital energy has represented a cru-

---

[4] Science is not made useless by spiritual and parapsychological perceptions, but rather is expanded. The laws of the higher world are just as present as those of the material world of the physical sciences. We can recognize this inasmuch as perceptions of auras and Chakras have, in a certain manner, an objective character: people from different cultures and continents perceive these phenomena very similarly. For example, a number of Swabian rural women, after meditative visualization exercises in our practice, drew pictures in which the seven Chakras and the aura were clearly recognizable. My astonished former partner, Dr. Ulrike Banis – who had led the exercises – asked whether any of these women had ever heard of Chakras or auras, or had ever seen pictures of such; the answer was a resounding and convincing no. Rudolf STEINER – coming from Theosophy – similarly took the objectifiable nature of the spiritual world as the occasion for viewing his Anthroposophy as an arts and humanities continuation of the physical sciences.

cial opportunity to access deeper spiritual levels. If we think of the importance of meditation and contemplation, then vital energy occupies a key position in accessing the subconscious and higher spiritual planes.

Vital energy was also important in our forefathers' medical science, for instance in acupuncture or Four-Element Theory. The healers of those times still knew that physical healing and being spiritually healthy depend directly on a person's vital energy. If patients have too little vital energy, then they cannot become healthy – physically or spiritually. In my own journey as naturopathic physician, this has become clearer to me over the years. Out of the fog has emerged, gradually, the outlines of a new model of energy medicine.

The *psyche* (spirit) and *soma* (body), normally kept separate in modern medicine, can be re-integrated via subtle-body energy into a comprehensive overall picture. In the process, I have come across many highly fascinating insights that combine ancient religious knowledge and modern scientific findings into a seamless integrated whole. But for me, the most impressive thing was finding out that applying this acquired knowledge confirmed spiritual occult wisdom and deep meditative experiences. Thus, for me, karmic ideas became more and more understandable and could be related to the new overall view with modern genetics.

Tests with subtle-body diagnostic methods in my practice showed, to my great surprise, that all persons have a certain energetic vibrational level. The vibrational level corresponds to the current level of spiritual development. Each of these developmental levels can be assigned to a specific subtle-body energy center (Chakra). I thus found a confirmation of the ancient idea of a spiritual journey, which also represents a journey through our energy centers. We do indeed seem, during the course of our life, to swing from one Chakra to another (ever higher) one. Condensations, in the form of turbulence and energy disharmony in a particular Chakra, are frequently associated with specific diseases. The psychoenergetic reason for the resulting energy disturbance – which has in turn led to a physical ailment – is based on an upward movement of the spirit, as it strives to attain a higher vibrational level. According to this interpretation, we often become ill in order to be able to reach a higher spiritual/energetic vibrational stage and thus a higher developmental level for our spirit.

The image of the larger dimension of our psychoenergetic development, as well as the underlying circumstances of diseases, inevitably leads to a search for meaning and purpose. Very trite the question: "What's the use of it? What's the point to it?" Modern science has long rejected "To what end?" thinking (**teleological thinking**) as unscientific. Lately, though, the importance of teleological thinking for the general perceptual process is on the upswing. An example is modern Bionics – the search for the reason why dolphins' bodies are shaped the way they are, which happens to be the most efficient form for swimming/streaming through water, leads only to the crucial insight after the "What for?" question has been posed. That which applies to biology and biophysics is also applicable to energy medicine. Because only when the question as to why human higher vibration exists is answered, or what the spiritual/energetic significance of illnesses might be, will we be able to find the crucial answers.

When we begin to understand the image of an upward movement of psychoenergy and the significance of diseases and conflicts, we encounter very deeply moving, highly spiritual messages – for, on our spiritual journey, we move incessantly in the direction of our true Self, hidden in alternate reality, which we must discover if we are to become truly alive. Ultimately, we are dealing with the yearning for our lost spiritual home, our true Self. **From this standpoint, disease and conflict are resources bestowed on us by a higher wisdom to lead us to our true Self and our true mission in life.**

Once we have understood and accepted that, we ask ourselves whether the laboriousness and endless anguish of the whole growth process might not be able to be made milder and gentler. Is it really true that only suffering can lead to true growth? Couldn't I acquire the insights and maturation processes of, say, a bout with cancer in some other less painful and self-destructive way? Personally, I am firmly convinced that an easier and better way is possible. We can structure our growth processes to be much gentler, less painful, and with more love and understanding, if that is what we want and are willing to work toward.

The main obstacle, however, is not so much our good intentions as the demons of which we have already spoken: their distortions of perception make sure that we don't perceive these harmful demons at all (like eyeglasses perched on one's nose). Moreover, their hypnotic suggestive power can make us, like a remote-controlled robot, repeat the same nonsense over and over again. These demons are the least well known and least understood actual disease causes. I will be discussing them in detail in the second part of this book, along with proposed solutions.

My Personal Pathway to Energy Medicine

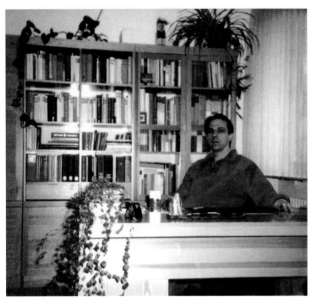

In my first medical practice in Achern in southwestern Germany, 1985

Much becomes clearer when one knows an author's personal background and history. Therefore, in what follows, I will be talking about myself and my life's trajectory. As a young physician with not much professional experience, I was at first not very familiar with many aspects of this profession. One important human aspect has to do with the physician's role as close confidant. Over time, one becomes for many patients a regular member of the family. Single retirees often make medical appointments purely as a way to escape their loneliness. Above all, they want to be spoken to and treated like human beings. Prescribing a series of innocuous injections or massage sessions gives these lonely people the longed-for excuse to pad out their empty weeks with scheduled "dates" and maybe to chat with some other patients in the waiting room.

Knowing this, a physician will, with increasing experience, no longer overwhelm people with all sorts of diagnostic and therapeutic procedures that could very well do more harm than good. Instead, one structures their weekly calendar with harmless diagnoses and therapies, and gives them the comforting feeling of moving toward a goal – even if it's

something as commonplace as a massage. After all (a patient tells me) this bothersome neck tension should ultimately go away again – after all, the massage sessions a year ago did so much good back then. And, especially in the imagination of older sick people, their doctor protects them in some unknown way from dying or from a wretched lingering illness. They will ascribe downright superhuman abilities to their doctor, abilities that have nothing whatsoever to do with the physician thus deified. Fantasies of this sort originate in the patient's deeply felt yet usually subconscious need for all-encompassing protection and constant care. From a depth-psychological standpoint, the physician is the powerful warder off of death and almighty rescuer in time of need.

In the early stages of one's career, you don't usually know, yet, about the subconscious backdrop of a patient's mentality. As a young physician, you view the world very differently. You follow up on each and every harmless symptom, and take yourself and every disease very seriously, the patient less so. Full of self-importance, you hang your stethoscope around your neck and put all your idealistic energy into the exercise of your profession. You discuss the X-ray results with colleagues, not noticing the patient in the thin hospital gown shivering out in the hallway. The finding is what counts, and it is viewed as a prize to be pursued, whose capture – if it is rare and hard to pin down – will mean a huge increase in collegial prestige. In the worst case, the patient degenerates to a mere delivery service of the trophy that the young doctor is stalking. Naturally, none of the ambitious young doctors admits this. However, the reality in today's clinics is that this situation has changed little over the years. The young doctor's desire to help is often misunderstood as wanting to fight diseases – rather than making sick people healthy. The ailing person sees things very differently, wanting to get well as a human being, not be reduced to a thing (lab result or X-ray or "the case in room 7").

Having a great deal of specialist knowledge can easily sidetrack a physician into self-important pomposity – and I had accumulated an enormous amount of technical knowledge. First, I worked my way through an intensive 2-year naturopathic training course. Then, I studied medicine and became a general practitioner. Even that wasn't the end of it. I also expended an enormous amount of energy acquiring, through additional private studies, comprehensive knowledge in all the important naturopathic disciplines. Added to this was detailed knowledge of orthodox medicine, culminating in passing an American State Medical Exam (the most difficult and scientifically prestigious exam). But all of this became secondary when it came to practical exercising of my profession! I was forced to realize that my humanity and the patience to listen calmly counted for more among patients than all my magnificent medical knowledge.

It dawned on me how impostors with no professional medical training could deceive their victims for years. Amazingly, this also applies to us physicians, because our university knowledge becomes relatively insignificant when it comes to daily practice. Considering the high doctor density in our latitudes, people don't become general practitioners, because they have to have solidly grounded, extensive medical knowledge – this is an automatic assumption. Anyway, patients go straight to a specialist the moment things get complicated. Besides professional competence, people expect family doctors, above all, to have compassionate character traits. Being able to listen, to empathize, to sense intuitively what has been left unsaid – all these become more and more important as one increases in professional experience. Often, nothing more was expected of me than to make myself (my time) available and to listen ("Thank you, doctor, for listening to me!")

Eventually there came a turning point in my life, when I was forced to get personally acquainted with the painful and severe hell of loneliness. It was only then that I knew in my heart what kind of emotional misery lay hidden in loneliness. Up until then, I had lived all my life surrounded by friends and a large family. But then I moved to a completely foreign place where I had no personal contacts. I made my profession my life and failed to notice the looming loneliness. All at once, I was struggling through weekends of endless emptiness, senselessness and despair. I often caught myself being thankful to the checkout girl at the supermarket for a few kind words, because she was the only person who spoke to me. It suddenly struck me what loneliness really means, and why solitary confinement is such a severe punishment – that many old people are undeservedly sentenced to by cruel fate! After this painful period of personally-experienced agonizing loneliness, I was more tolerant of patients who found themselves in the same situation.

As a human being and a physician, I learned some crucial things from these experiences that I wouldn't have learned in any other way. Physicians are taught to maintain a certain personal distance and a subtle yet perceptible) "emotional brutality." The desensitization process begins early on in medical training, namely in anatomy class and its cadavers. Later on, one finds it necessary to maintain emotional distance out of sheer self-protection, so as not to "lose it" when confronted with cases of horrible suffering. At first, it took me weeks to get images of torn-off arms and legs or desperately screaming children with severe burns out of my head.

Doctors need to build up a kind of emotional "callus" to protect themselves from the tormenting nightmares that, of necessity, are an integral part of their profession.

It is understandable, then, that many physicians, especially younger ones, exhibit a reserved attitude (that often comes across as arrogance) toward patients. It is (unconsciously) considered to be a sign of great professionalism – the way kids "casually" smoke cigarettes in order to look grown-up. Just so do young physicians, unsure of themselves, try to seem particularly professional and knowledgeable through their emotional coolness. Unfortunately, many of them cling to these behavioral poses well into their careers. It takes personally agitating emotional experiences to get them down off their "Demigods in White" pedestal. Many physicians who have gone through a severe disease have only then recovered a compassionate attitude toward their patients.

But my relationship with my patients changed for yet another reason, when I had acquired more professional experience. I am speaking of the emotional backgrounds to disease – of whose existence everyone is aware, but which are often very hard to detect in everyday life. This is mainly because emotional problems are usually buried deep in the subconscious. In virtually all cases, even the patient knows nothing at all about these causes, or puts a different meaning on them. I often found out the actual background only after extensive questioning, sometimes through intuition and many times thanks to sheer luck – when, say, I just happened to overhear some gossip.

A typical case history:

A patient contracted lumbago suddenly, shortly after getting a new, younger and arrogant boss at work. I only happened to find out about this from another patient's casual comment. The patient himself was totally unaware of this emotional disease cause, which is probably why he never mentioned it. Although the radiologist found a slipped disk that explained the disease, I couldn't shake the feeling that his new boss was the "slipped disk" pressing (so to speak) on his emotional sacral spinal region. And so it was, for after an extensive clinical stay, the disease disappeared at first, only to recur immediately once he returned to work, where the arrogant younger boss had been lying in wait for the recently discharged patient to reproach him for his absence. The patient at once returned to my practice, complaining of horrible lower back pains. I asked him if his boss had irritated him again, which caught him completely off guard: he had been totally unaware of any connection between being humiliated by his boss and his lumbago. Once he realized it, he quit his job and found a new one where he not only got the recognition he deserved, but his lumbago went away for good.

I learned from this that empathy and putting oneself in the other person's place is an extraordinarily important part of the healing arts – more so, usually, than "book learning." But I don't want to ignore what is by far the biggest problem in medical work, because it is indispensable to understanding the method that I developed out of this necessity.

It isn't all that often that we are handed such obvious and easily understandable causes as the one described above, with the arrogant boss who was such a "pain in the a**." More often, we are baffled by our patient's problems. We usually don't know which subconscious conflicts and suppressed feelings are behind the disease.

But there is an ever bigger obstacle to immediate insight into another person's emotional problems. Because of the human tendency to project inner problems outward, the actual cause is often to be found in the patient's emotional situation. I often get the feeling that the arrogant boss or the mean mother-in-law is not the real problem plaguing the patient. Actually, such projected figures are just catalysts of underlying conflicts of the patient's, far older than the current acute problems. For example, an arrogant boss just brings to the surface (and thereby revives) long-standing feelings of inferiority and unfairness. That projection is such a common practice is confirmed by the popularity among humans of gossiping and rumor-mongering, by means of which people frequently pass on their prejudices and hidden feelings. A society's marginal groups and (in)famous people are well-known and particularly popular projection targets.

Uncovering the emotional background in clinical practice is thus exceedingly difficult. This was one of the main reasons for developing a new healing method, which I have named Psychosomatic Energetics. This method can identify hidden emotional conflicts very quickly and accurately. Experience shows that only those conflicts are detected that are "ripe" and thus need to be treated. Another novel feature is that the gradual disappearance of the conflict can be measured during the course of treatment, thus making monitoring very reliable for the therapist. I'll return to this method in greater detail later on in the book. I'd first like to delve deeper into my personal development, which led me farther and farther away from being a mere "health jockey" in the direction of genuine physicianhood.

I'd like to describe another (at first irritating) experience, an astonishing one to our everyday understanding. It goes far beyond the conventional wisdom of psychosomatics knowledge. It also bursts the familiar confines of our usual sense of reality. It all started when an invisible bond formed between myself and patients, as we got to know each other better, that seemed to link us telepathically. I would think about a certain patient and that patient's case history; the next day, that patient – whom I had not seen in ages – would be sitting in front of me during office hours. This happened so often and in such a strange way as to exclude coincidence. It seemed kind of amusing at first, but I got more thoughtful as the instances piled up: they couldn't all be flukes!

From my studies, I understood enough of statistics and probability theory to be able to estimate the likelihood that something was due to random chance. My calculations put this in the neighborhood of the odds of winning the Grand Prize in a state lottery. The best proof in uncertain circumstances such as this is to turn the tables and put it to the test. Skeptically, I playfully tried out the telepathic connection a number of times and found, to my surprise, that I could indeed mentally summon patients to my practice.

At first this very weird phenomenon – that I could sense my patient 's symptoms and perceive their secret thoughts – annoyed me. It didn't always work, i.e., it wasn't reliably "on call," but rather only when I was in a state of intention-free tranquility. I had to enter into a peaceful "alpha state" (during which 10Hz alpha waves predominate in an EEG). I also had to be energetically disengaged and open, concentrated yet relaxed. At first, it surprised even me when, in a patient's presence, I would feel a previously unnoticed twinge on the left side of my forehead and would ask: "Are you feeling a twinge on the left side of your forehead?" Of course, my reputation went stratospheric as my astounded patient answered in the affirmative. "That's weird, doctor, I didn't say a thing about that to you!" From then on, that patient would regard me as some sort of mythical creature with magical powers at his disposal.

At the time, I was unaware that these phenomena are hard to repeat at will and call up spontaneously. So, I was made a laughingstock when new patients wanted to test my abilities; they had heard that I could perform diagnostic "miracles." At first, I was enormously flattered by these testimonials – which then led me, by way of penance, right into the trap, for I was ignorant enough to play along, whereupon I would fail miserably. After such disgrace, I decided to forego these little games in future, and I henceforth made use of these phenomena discreetly and in the background (where they work best anyway).

When we open ourselves up to things such as telepathy, we notice that there is always a link between people standing near each other, over which subliminal thoughts and feelings can be conveyed. This connection is always present as an invisible force, and sustains us in our work. Many therapeutic methods such as remote healing, Radionics, Reiki, faith healing and so on. specifically use this connection to channel healing energy and information to the patient. Amazingly, these methods work best when all persons involved strongly believe in them. The strength of the participants' belief in the efficacy of the treatment, and the amount of transferred healing energy, is crucial! The actual technique or technology (the "what") of the procedure seems to be secondary.[5]

---

[5] I suspect that a large part of psychotherapy's effectiveness is based on the existence of an invisible conduit of healing energy between therapist and patient. According to studies into the effectiveness of psychotherapy, it is not the "what" but the "how" that is decisive. Regardless of which psychotherapeutic procedure is applied, its effectiveness seems to be based predominantly on the human contact between therapist and patient – and, in my opinion, its curative efficacy is quite decisively influenced by invisible telepathic processes!

There were other experiences that helped me arrive at a new point of view for disease – a quite different one from that of orthodox medicine. For example, I would note an immediate and miraculous disappearance of numerous disease symptoms in patients undergoing an enlivening emotional-energetic experience. This might be falling in love and eroticism, or visits from faith healers who channel strong healing energies. As long as the surge of force from this healing energy held out, the entire symptomatology was markedly reduced – only to rise again afterwards, in most patients. For millennia, eastern medicine (acupuncture, Ayurveda) has known what a powerful healing force vital energy can exert. It's just that the healing process was, regrettably, limited and seldom lasted very long. Where did the energy go? I have since learned that emotional conflicts, acting as energy thieves, are to blame. I had not yet worked that out back then. At any rate, the mysterious healing process had greatly piqued my curiosity.

The other experience had to do with a years-long self-administered therapy with high-potency homeopathics and Bach Flowers. Add to this meditation and years of work with somatic psychotherapies (G. BOYESEN's Biodynamic Psychology and Bioenergetics). All of this sensitized me more and more. I learned the most from my patients, as I examined them using electroacupuncture and other energy methods. In so doing, a therapist learns automatically to be increasingly sensitive and energetically open. Amazingly, I also learned a lot from my own children's sensitivity and high-grade energetic openness while they were still quite young. Now, in researching subtle-body phenomena, it is understandably very important that one be as sensitive and energetically open as possible, since the investigator personally becomes the measuring instrument with which the investigation is carried out. The Japanese psychologist Hiroshi MOTOYAMA has described very well his increasing openness due to meditative practices (he is a priest in a religious order). His trail-blazing research of Auras and Chakras would have not been possible at all, had it not been for his own sensitivity, for which he thanks his energy exercises as a meditative priest.

My personal transformation ultimately culminated in a very revealing "enlightenment" experience. At the time, I was undergoing one of the most agonizing private crises of my life and I was in extreme existential distress.[6] I have already mentioned the dreadful loneliness that was just one of the many agonies plaguing me at the time. I just had to get out of this vicious cycle somehow! While doing deep meditation, I listened to recordings of Tibetan Lamas chanting their deep-drone ritual hymns. I used this, along with hyperventilation and meditative exercises, to "tune out and drop out." I was also using certain naturopathic agents (high-potency homeopathics, precious-stone vibrations, and the like) that I had tested out carefully, to improve my condition. All this raised my vibrational level in an unexpected

manner: after taking them, I felt as if I were "porous" and floating in midair.

On one lonely May weekend in 1986, I succeeded in raising my perceptive sensitivity to new heights. I had visions, I saw the fine Aural shimmer around freshly blooming trees, and I became so delicately permeable that leading a normal life got harder and harder; just the honk of a car's horn hit me almost like a physical blow. Even simple things like shopping or making a phone call were nearly impossible, because almost everything irritated and befuddled me. And yet, I was fully "with it" and felt fantastically better than I ever had in my life. I felt as if I had finally "come home" and was living in a glorious, downright supernaturally beautiful paradise. Every fresh flower sent me into rapturous ecstasy. A child's laughter filled me with the greatest joy. The entire situation affected me like the Pentecostal experience of Jesus' apostles. When I related the details to experts in these matters, they rated it as an extremely rare and precious enlightenment experience.[7]

Unfortunately, this magnificent state only lasted a few days, but it effected a lasting change in me. I was definitely a better person than before, but I had come in contact with a great power and wisdom that was bigger than I, which humbled me. Only then did I fully realize in what minuscule, limited orbits our lives and workaday consciousness normally move. When they had their Pentecostal experience, Jesus' disciples suddenly, mysteriously, began to "speak in tongues" – i.e., unknown foreign languages.[8] Quite similarly, many connections became increasingly clear to me, after this experience, that I had hitherto only understood

---

[6] In fact many people undergo great existential crises at the beginning of their spiritual development. A good example is Gopi KRISHNA, who thereby had his first life-transforming Kundalini experience. More recent examples include the American Byron KATIE (*The Work*) and the German-born Britisher Eckhart TOLLE (*The Power of Now*), both of whom discovered their causal body and its wisdom as a result of profound emotional crises – an experience commonly known as enlightenment.

[7] Contrary to popular opinion, such experiences seem to be not all that rare. I heard an amazing story from a friend of mine who taught meditation. A while back, a simple workman – rustic accent, blunt manner – showed up at the meditation class to pick up his girlfriend who was taking the course. Since he had come rather early, the leader invited him to sit in and meditate with the rest of the group at no cost or obligation. Since he had never done anything like this before, he consented gratefully. To everyone's surprise, he suddenly tipped over from his cross-legged posture, and all thought that he must have fainted. When he came to a few minutes later, he reported that he had been hovering up near the ceiling, watching everybody from above. The meditation teacher and students, some of whom had been meditating for decades, were astonished that an inexperienced newcomer was able to have that kind of OOBE (out-of-body experience) right off the bat, while they had not. On another occasion, a highly sensitive female patient told me that she had once had this same kind of experience while meditating, and was suddenly looking down from the ceiling at everyone. This startled her so much that she returned to her body with a bang, and the upshot was that she was plagued with headaches for days after.

abstractly – especially medical, philosophical, and spiritual questions. All at once, many formerly puzzling issues were effortlessly self-evident. I also developed a totally new sensitivity toward my daily medical work. I learned a great deal from this experience that I would never have gotten from mere "book learning."

Because this highly-sensitized state became increasingly incompatible with everyday life, I eventually took the advice of a well-meaning colleague and reached for "grounding" substances – namely cigarettes and knuckle of pork with sauerkraut and beer. This "grounding" restored my reality fitness in short order. I was then still too young and inexperienced to hold out for very long against the intensity of

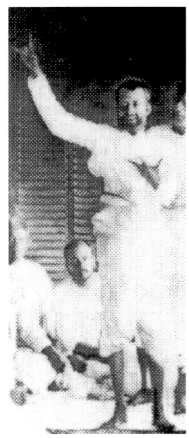

Ramakrishna in Samadhi on 21 September 1879, listening to Kirtan (meditative religious music).

---

[8] I want to firmly reject the notion that my transcendental experience had anything to do with Channeling or similar trance states. I believe, as a matter of principle, that all of these procedures are, potentially, extraordinarily dangerous, since one never knows what unknown forces one is exposing oneself to as a medium. Having examined many trance mediums with energetic methods, I feel I should sound the warning, because remarkably many of these people have become very sick emotionally and subtle-body blocked. One should reject methods that involve trances or drugs.

these circumstances; this is not a humanly viable situation over the longer term. For example, the Indian holy man Ramakrishna had to be artificially fed. Now, of course there are varying levels of such states, and Ramakrishna had certainly sunk down into an uncommonly deep one (*Samadhi*).

Surprisingly enough, shallower levels of such states are relatively easy to attain. If environmental conditions are favorable and one has a stable personality, one can remain in such a state of consciousness for a very long time. After studying numerous writings dealing with how to refine one's energetic perception, it dawned on me, in retrospect, that I had instinctively fulfilled the most important preconditions for attaining these "transcendental" states. I'd like to list them here, to encourage readers to reach these ecstatic states themselves:

Favorable conditions for bringing about transcendental states (of greater happiness and contentment)

1. *A basic mental stance of complete openness and acceptance is the most important prerequisite. Children have this attitude by their very nature ("If ye not become as little children …"). Also, an existential crisis can have a very favorable effect in breaking mental bonds and breaking out of the prison of circumstance. "Now I just don't give a damn what happens!" is what you tend to say in such a mood – a mood that initiation rites create artificially, using severe pain, frightening experiences that challenge one's most extreme courage, and so forth.*

2. *You have to be in top physical form: get plenty of sleep, do some moderate but regular sporting activity, eat well. The Buddha did not attain enlightenment until he gave up asceticism and began to eat and sleep well and be active, which, as the "proper measure" of a lifestyle, only then created the preconditions for an enlightenment experience.*

3. *You have to "turn off" the everyday world and work against the sensory overload of the daily grind – say, by enjoying the peace and quiet of nature. Important here is an attitude of unconditional openness and peaceful calm.*

4. *Awareness is important: a gentle openness that allows perceptions to flow unimpeded, a loving and tender relationship with yourself and the world.*

5. *Actions that activate the first Chakra are favorable, e.g., the droning, flowing singing of Tibetan monks as they chant Buddhist recitations (CD). Also effective is a deep, relaxing sexual experience, which activates the first Chakra.*

6. *Emotional conflicts should have previously been melted away and eliminated, in order to open up the energetic channels.*

Looking at all of these conditions at once can give the impression that they would be rather hard to implement. I disagree; my experience has been that it is pretty quick and simple to attain. If you can let go and let it happen, it's basically one of the simplest things there is, as easy as taking a walk. Many people are acquainted with these states, but are, amazingly, totally unaware of being in an elevated transcendental state. For instance, they might be stirring their coffee as, outside, the sun breaks though the clouds and, for a moment, they feel extraordinarily blissful and enraptured.

The trick, of course, is staying in this glorious state for a longer period of time. Usually, it's our own self-doubt and resistance that terminate it prematurely. Timid souls' objection that transcendental states might lead to insanity and lasting damage is highly exaggerated and is very rarely the case (applying mainly to mentally ill, highly labile persons). Actually, rapture states are among the most normal conditions that our consciousness knows in its deepest depths. The real problem is that our everyday human world, with its stress and grime, works against it. Another problem is the unfamiliarity of the state and the enormous force associated with the experience.

Anyone with normal intellectual and emotional disposition can experience transcendental states. Surveys show that a surprising number of people report having had parapsychological experiences and transcendent moods in their everyday life. A vanishingly small number suffered any lasting damage as a result. In fact, such states seem to be very healthful and inspiring and to promote spiritual growth. The social psychologist CSIKSZENTMILHALYI was able to show that people with augmented blissful states are better able to handle daily life, have more stamina, can orient themselves better and are better able to cope with strokes of fate. These flow experiences occur more frequently during artistic activity or while driving a car, as a kind of spontaneous, joyful contemplative state takes over. It seems to be crucial that the activity be challenging yet doable. It shouldn't be boring or intimidating, but rather should create an interesting tension that can be mastered fairly easily. With time, we get straight into the activity that lifts us out of everyday consciousness and allows us to be happy.

I myself was stuck in my search for deeper underlying disease causes. All around me, I heard colleagues raving about new methods that supposedly were better able to detect the true roots of disease. Borrowing the motto "Forewarned is forearmed," they also offered the requisite (profound and long-lasting, of course!) healing treatment. Since, as a naturopath and naturopathic physician of several decades' standing, I had mastered an especially broad spectrum of naturopathic healing methods, and tried out a great many others, I gradually became downright skeptical of these new healing promises. Many of them failed to deliver, and others worked only as long as the initial enthusiasm held out. As soon as the failures began to pile up, interest would abate, and the methods would no longer work.

For many patients, my general practice was the end of the line, the last graspable straw. Thus, it was not long before my waiting room was crowded with frustrated patients. Added to this, people came by the hundreds who had not been helped by years of psychotherapy, expensive acupuncture, single-remedy homeopaths, or what have you. In time, my former partner and I had one of the best-equipped and largest practices in southern Germany. Besides our health-plan practice, we had a large private practice full of chronically-ill patients whose exotic diagnoses would have flattered any university hospital's outpatient section.[9]

Despite great success, I couldn't shake the disturbing feeling that I had not really found the diseases' actual causes and, accordingly, was incapable of true healing. I began to delve deeper into my study of subtle-body energy. For decades, I worked with Chakras and energy levels. It wasn't until I read the Cypriot healer Dr. Stylianos ATTESHLI (also known as *Daskalos* , master – one of the great Christian mystics of our time) that I got the crucial impetus: it dawned on me that the main causes of psychosomatic disease are *elemental* ones (as *Daskalos* calls them). The term *elemental* is intended to illustrate the tenacity and durability of these emotional-instinctive internal structures, which are reminiscent of the physical elements. In everyday speech, we refer to hidden emotional conflicts, or complexes. As long as these conflicts remain unhealed, we cannot become truly and lastingly healthy.

---

[9] We performed the following in our clinical practice: various kinds of acupuncture, often in conjunction with the expensive Akabane Test (in which one tests, like the Japanese doctor Akabane, how long it takes a glowing incense stick being passed over a certain acupuncture point to trigger heat pain, which is supposed to correspond to an objectifiable pulse diagnosis), also ear acupuncture, single-remedy homeopathy with intensive remedy determination (Kent's Repertorization), related but likewise current compound homeopathy, Iridodiagnosis and Facial Diagnosis, Thermoregulation (measuring temperature at specific skin points before and after a stressful stimulus), Vegatest (skin-resistance measurement at acupuncture points), Segment Electrography (applying weak current pulses to various body regions) and Pulse Dermography (a variation of Segment Electrography), Kinesiology (measuring muscle strength for energetic testing), one-handed rod (dowsing rod held in one hand), Radionics (faith and remote healing with electronic devices), Mora (healing through vibration inversion), color therapy, colon hydrotherapy (colonic irrigation), Bach Flowers (healing system using flowers developed by Dr. Edward Bach), Neural Therapy (injection of local anesthetics) and Chirotherapy (bone resetting) including Dorn Massage (a special form of spinal-column therapy developed by Mr. Dorn), Phytotherapy (healing with medicinal plants), Orthomolecular Medicine (administering minerals and vitamins), Darkfield blood examination with color camera and TV monitor and using the Enderlein remedies (indicates blood slagging and hyperacidity), Ardenne's Multi-step Oxygen Therapy (oxygen supplied under stress), ozone (highly active molecular form of oxygen), HOT (blood irradiation with UV light), Niehans' Fresh Cell Therapy (injections of freeze-dried lamb tissue), Cytoplasmic Therapy (protein injections), Horvi Therapy (snake venom), Spenglersan Test (Dr. Spengler's detoxification therapy) and so on. As orthodox physicians, we collaborated with universities, surgical teams, and highly-qualified specialists. We retained some of these specialists for particular naturopathic problems: family therapists, Reiki instructors and, in special cases, even faith healers, exorcists, and Channeling mediums.

My initial question, as to what lay hidden behind most of the diseases of my patients as the true disease cause, eventually led to an even more profound question, namely: "What does the patient really want, in his heart of hearts?" Conflicts are known to harbor unfulfilled, suppressed desires that, for whatever reason, the patient doesn't want to experience or acknowledge. Thus, conflicts are created in order to deal with this compromise. This basic concept of modern psychoanalysis continues to occupy me intensely to this day, and accompanies me in my work. How much emotional potential is bottled up in all the inferiority complexes, diseases and symptoms? What capabilities, yearnings and possibilities lie buried, unable to be realized? What deeper meaning do these ailments and symptoms have, if one views them as compromises that the patient has entered into for some reason or other?

I learned to pay attention to subtle changes in tone of voice, gestures and posture, to moods and feelings as they arose in myself and the person I was interviewing. Above all, I learned that the patient's own spirit knows best what it really wants. The therapist can only be a cross between guide and midwife, helping the spirit express itself more easily. In this sense, healing is almost "close enough to touch" and its realization just needs to be made easier. This can often be accomplished through small, innocuous and seemingly unimportant things such as a few energetically harmonizing drops. After clearing away the obstacles to healing, one can see in the patient's changed behavior what kind of spiritual possibilities had been blocked – for I noticed that the true cause of blocked healing lay in the conflicts, and that these conflicts could be stimulated and cured with the right homeopathic complexes (about which more later on).

The truth is, in virtually all cases we make ourselves sick. However, we almost never notice this, because we have grown accustomed to our poor energetic condition and all its attendant consequences. Our true feelings, genuine thoughts and real needs are deformed, distorted and even turned into their opposite by deep-seated subconscious conflicts. Because we are unwilling to admit our inner deceitfulness either to ourselves or others, we suppress our subconscious conflicts even more vigorously. This triggers a vicious cycle that is extremely arduous to escape from on our own. Later on in this book, it will become clear that diseases, strokes of fate, career and partner choice, and many other things in our lives actually represent attempts at self-healing.

However, many self-healing approaches turn out to be very poor makeshifts or dead ends. Outside help is thus usually useful and often even imperative – when, for example, people can no longer extricate themselves from their plight on their own. Ultimately, healing is aid from outside, to stimulate self-healing powers and thus make self-healing possible. Surprisingly, often all that is needed is the simplest

of assistance, by means of which the subtle-body energy blockages are dissolved. It was to this end that I developed *Psychosomatic Energetics*. Many colleagues, when they learn about it, have trouble believing that cures can be so simply achieved ("That can't be right! It sounds way too easy!"). But my experience with thousands of patients confirms that it really is that easy.

Earlier, tracking down deep-seated disease causes was mostly an instinctive process, often quite subjective and therefore inexact. There are two reasons for this that, despite their simplicity, complicate things for the therapist right at the outset. For one thing, conflicts are situated in the non-verbal subconscious, which makes it extraordinarily difficult for patients to talk about them: how can you talk about something that you know nothing about? Understandably, most people reject psychotherapy, since they mostly feel healthy. There is, of course, that other group of people who sense their inner imbalance and disturbances. But even if they discuss these things for years with their therapists, experience shows that it usually remains pretty superficial. And there is yet another hitherto unsolved problem that I can get around by energetic testing of conflicts: inner resistance. Subconscious problems don't want to be brought into the light of day. This makes uncovering and healing subconscious conflicts very difficult and, indeed, usually impossible if energetic testing is not used as an aid.

Later on, I'll show, again with case histories from my daily practice, what fantastic healing effects are possible with energy medicine. I'd like to illustrate this by closing this chapter with a simple example:

The 61-year-old retiree (early retirement) first began to experience severe muscle and joint pain all over her body 13 years ago. Every muscle hurt, and she felt as if she'd been "beaten up" all the time. A rheumatologist diagnosed soft-tissue rheumatism. Ultimately, her suffering became so intolerable that she was forced to give up her career as a masseuse. Measurement of energy readings shows her vital energy down 50% (100% would have been normal), and her emotional-body reading (which reflects mood and emotional equilibrium) has sunk to a mere 10%!

As for conflicts, I test out a monstrous Rage in the patient's abdomen (the conflict is located in the 3rd Chakra). The Rage conflict, with 90% vitality and 90% emotionality, has far better readings than the patient herself. This is a huge energy thief, siphoning off a great deal of the patient's vital energy and equanimity.

I prescribe homeopathic remedies (emotional and Chakra remedies) to break up the rage. Some time later, she calls me up and reports enthusiastically that, after just three days of taking the drops, her rheumatic pain had completely disappeared! ("… like a miracle!") and to date had not returned! She had, she says, tried everything, but nothing had helped. She had given up all hope of being cured, and she now wants to know if, in most people live in a dream world that airbrushes out unpleasant facts – but also edits out a great deal of spirituality and emotional depth that could help them in unsuspected ways to confront their true Self.

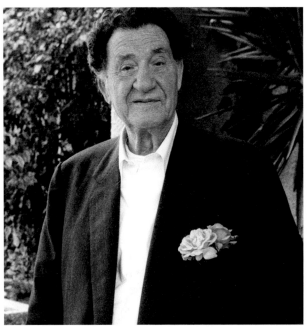

Dr. Stylianos Atteshli (Daskalos, i.e., master) – Greek author, philosopher, and Christian mystic teacher

my experience, the results would last: she's worried that the pains might return.

I reassured her that, in our experience, the results are usually long and lasting. And so they were: she has remained healthy for quite a long time now. As a postscript, she later suffered a relapse when a fear-filled conflict theme in the heart region became active. She was impressed that, after taking the "rage drops," she had vivid dreams involving strife and conflict, such as she would have never allowed in her normal life. Now she can say "No" in everyday life, and express her needs, where before she had just swallowed hard and put up with whatever happened. Thank God that's over and done with, she said, and she can now say what she really means.

The next chapter delves into the deepest dimension of medical life, a topic with which every doctor has to deal every day, but which also touches him or her personally eventually: the inevitability of death and dying. As we know, in our modern world, nothing is suppressed and denied as vigorously as death and mortality. No one wants to die, and everyone clings to the illusion that dying happens just to other people. The psychological term is "narcissistic self-overestimation." Even children exhibit this mental attitude when they feel invincibly strong and that the world revolves around them and their concerns. For children, this has an important emotional protective function, but it leads in adults to illusionary misjudgment of reality. To this extent,

Spiritual Experience in Medical Practice

It is not death we should fear, but rather that we might never begin to live.

(Marcus Aurelius)

ne of my most extraordinary experiences as a medical student was to be present at a person's death. I was all alone on the ward, doing the night watch to earn some extra money. It was unusually quiet in the long hospital hallways, their gray linoleum flooring weakly lit by the overhead neon tubes. The only sound was an occasional groaning that would stop for a moment, only to resume after an anxious interval. These were the noises of a dying man, whose bed had been shoved into the broom closet where the ward's cleaning supplies were kept. The dying man had been put there so as not to disturb the other patients' sleep with his dying moans.

At some point, the moans ceased. As I entered the room and saw the dead man in his bed sheet, it once again struck me how shriveled the dead seem compared to just moments before, while they were still alive. This impression of sudden weight loss never fails to astound me: one gets the unmistakable impression that people get lighter at the moment of death. Of course, this is not really so. As far back as the Middle Ages, people had weighed the dying in an attempt to "weigh" the soul that was leaving the body. But no weight change was ever noted. The dead only seem lighter because the vital energy triggers something weighty in the observer.[10] When the body loses its vital energy, it thus seems lighter to us.

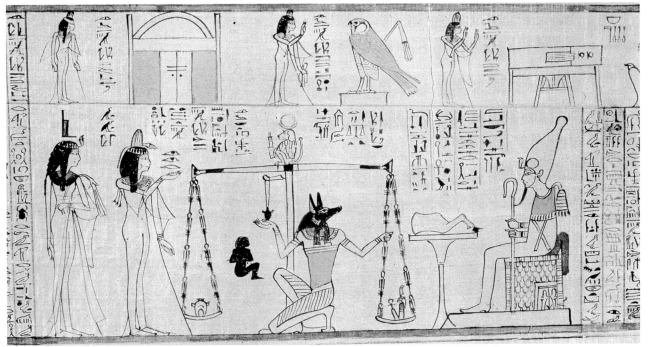

Egyptian Book of the Dead – Anubis, the jackal-headed God of the Dead, weighs the heart ("… the Soul or the Self," in the terminology of this book about the causal body) of the deceased. If he has led an honorable life, then it will balance with the feather of the Goddess Maat, and he is allowed into Osiris' kingdom, to accompany the Sun God on his celestial journey, and live among the polar stars (in Christian terms: "Enter into the Kingdom of Heaven"; in the language of this book: live on as individual soul in the causal body). Evil persons and liars, however, are sacrificed to the "devouring monster" (… in other words, they fall victim to their inner demons, the conflicts). The monster, a cross between crocodile, lion, and hippopotamus, is not shown here, but it lurks in the vicinity of the scales. One just needs to imagine it there.

---

[10] We often perceive someone as having a physically lighter body if they exhibit a weak or very transparent, lightly-flowing aura. You then often hear: "Boy, you look thin! Have you lost some weight?" Actually, the altered aura generates an impression of lightness that had not existed before.

When you first walk up to a dead person, the most shocking thing is the speechlessness. Of course, there's nothing more to be said. Since I was familiar with the *Tibetan Book of the Dead* and had spent many years studying Buddhism and reincarnation, I sometimes felt like doing something useful in this situation (if I had time and the inclination, instead of whiling away the long night reading magazines). I therefore spoke to the dead man in a soft whisper, words of advice and encouragement. I was like the prompter at the theater, to remove the dying man's fear when he moved toward the "great white light" – because, according to the *Tibetan Book of the Dead* (and, since 1975, the *American Book of the Dead*), shrinking back from the white light means the beginning of a descent to lower forms of existence, until finally one is reincarnated.

Even though I am still not sure whether my supportive words were of any use to the dead man, I am firmly convinced that one should speak to the dying and, above all, the recently dead. Whether you speak out loud or merely think the words is probably not so important, since the dialogue takes place in the spirit world. It seems to me crucial that one convey one's friendship and sympathy, instead of (as family members are prone to do) weeping and wailing and basically staying wrapped up in one's own grief. For the dead one is, in reality, not dead at all! Plus, in all likelihood – according to the reports of many a medium – the dead are very confused by the onset of death, not knowing what's going on or where they are. They need to be reassured and have the situation explained to them.

But just as the dead can profit from the living, if we turn to them and give them emotional support, the living receive something extraordinarily valuable from the dead. I have always experienced something remarkable in the presence of the dying. It is always with a curious mixture of jubilation and melancholy that I leave the hospital after these dying escorts. You rejoice in the gentle dawn mood – which is particularly striking when death occurs at night – and you're happy still to be alive. At the same time, you're overcome by melancholy because you have had to confront mortality – including, of course, your own. The Middle Age's *memento mori* (Remember you must die) is stamped with this mental attitude. People back then were explicitly prepared for death by the clergy. Back then, death was a constant companion, thanks to famines, plagues, and dreadful wars. Yet another reason was that medieval man did not deny death with our present-day persistence. Instead, they all lived in the certain knowledge that they would have to die someday.

Another experience with the dying has to do with the odd observation that the dying are frequently alone at the moment of death. I thought about this a lot, until I realized that the dying person's soul needs solitude to be able to exit the body. It must be alone in order to venture into the unknown condition of death. When death comes without their presence, this is experientially hard for the relatives to take. At some point, relatives have to go to the bathroom, or go home to catch up on lost sleep. When they return, he is dead whom they had sat next to for hours. "Why did he go without me?" Emotionally, it feels like a kind of betrayal, even though the dying one had no choice in the matter.

Relatives then tend to reproach themselves, especially when children die, who (as the parents believe) now have to embark on the journey into the Hereafter all alone. The grieving parents' protective urge seems to lead them astray here, since numerous near-death experiences consistently report that the dead one's soul is greeted by relatives who had died earlier, and taken into their midst. The dead are not forced to wander about in a lonely Hereafter, but rather return to the bosom of their family. To grieving patients of mine who are skeptical of this, I recommend the books of the death-and-dying expert Elisabeth KÜBLER-ROSS, and I try to impress on these patients the idea of a "good end."[11]

However, our modern society's denial of death takes its toll in yet another nasty way which has nothing to do with lack of faith or the Hereafter. In fact, it has to do with something crucial in the here and now. I strongly suspect that a great deal of our culture's emotional aloofness and alienation is rooted in our denial of death. In a very elemental way, knowledge of death is related to how we basically feel about life! **Amazingly enough, it is only knowledge of death that can really bring us to life.** Why that should be so is something one can long ponder; I'd like to just leave it as an assertion for now, since I have experienced this striking psychological fact time and time again.

Knowledge of death makes us humane and humble deep in our heart of hearts. I have experienced this many a time with grieving relatives. They perceive in their sorrow an overwhelming truth that transforms their own life. **The point is that death above all confronts us with the truth of our own life.** For instance, many cancer patients radically alter their life when they learn about their illness. Many mourners find a new meaning in their life, because they sense what an infinitely valuable gift their own life represents. The general atmosphere of leave-taking after wars or catastrophes underlies the same purifying transformational process.

---

[11] My grandmother told me that her son paid her a visit the night he died. He came to her in a dream and said "Mother I must bid you farewell." The next morning, my grandmother was very upset, and she made a note of the time and the day of the dream in her diary. Six weeks later, a friend of her son's returned from Stalingrad on front leave. He brought with him the sad news of her son's death and his watch, which had stopped at the moment of death. The date and time agreed perfectly with my grandmother's diary entry. Later on, I heard many similar reports from patients of mine. The archives of parapsychological research are likewise full of such reports, whose consistency makes it hard for skeptics to deny, and which, in my opinion, provide clear confirmation of life after death.

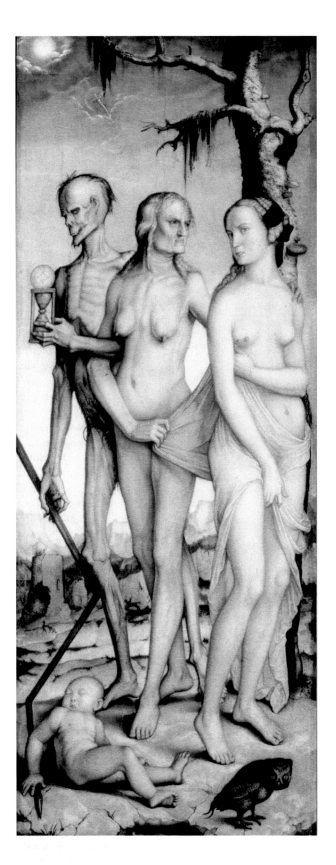

Medieval representation of the Ages of Man and of Death, holding an hourglass and whose staff already touches the infant (who must likewise die someday despite being so young). The owl in the lower right corner, a symbol of wisdom, exhorts us to be wise and remember to reckon Death as part of our own life.

To get back to my spiritual experiences as a physician, I'd like to say something in this context about consolation. One of the greatest duties a doctor has – and for which one's studies usually do not at all prepare one – is the pastoral function. As a rule, the doctor is the first to be confronted with the pain of grief, and he must comfort the relatives and instruct them about death. This might at first sound a bit overblown, but it is based on very real, tough problems. It has to do with emotionally extremely agitating experiences. How, for example, do I console a mentally handicapped woman whose husband had been a blend of surrogate father, beloved and best friend, and who is now completely on her own? How do I help a mother get over the death of her child? These problems are much rarer for those who are devout believers or are spiritually oriented. In these existential crises, the only help that I can offer as a doctor is, ultimately, religious belief.

Rationalist patients then ask me, curiously but also a touch provocatively: "Do you really believe in this rubbish?" In the meaning of life? In a higher power that wishes us well? In life after death? My "Yes" is often not at first convincing, so I have to provide proof. I point to the numerous persuasive reincarnation experiences, especially in children (since they can more easily recall their former lives). Also, the books of the death and dying expert KÜBLER-ROSS provide numerous stories relating life after death.[12]

Another transcendental-seeming experience in clinical practice is the accumulation of certain kinds of improbable occurrences.[13] The most ordinary type of these coinci-

---

[12] An Indian child dying in New York City told KÜBLER-ROSS that her sister was going to pick her up. Normally, relatives who have already died fetch dying children (I like to tell this story to desperate parents). "That's odd, her sister is still alive," thought Ms. KÜBLER-ROSS – but then, after the child's death, she heard that the sister had died a few days before in a fatal traffic accident on the reservation. Now, the news of this accident had not reached New York City, so that the dying child could not have known of it (Ms. KÜBLER-ROSS subsequently confirmed all this in a thorough inquiry.).

[13] Another fascinating topic that magnifies the dimensions of medical routine into the spiritual, is telepathic contact with patients. Over the years, a close human connection is established between doctor and patient – and this strong bond, according to parapsychology, seems to be a good precondition for telepathy. With this invisible long-range form of communication, I have acquired experiences that continue to surprise me – for one thing, because they are so astonishing, but also because they work so well. After having introduced a new healing technique – it was, I believe, colonic

dences are accumulations of illnesses relating to certain meteorological phenomena, times of day, and so on – such as leg thromboses when large low-pressure areas gather, or biliary colic at 3 in the morning. All these unlikely collections of phenomena are, nevertheless, scientifically explicable and have a completely understandable basis. Thus, the flow in leg veins is reduced by physical weather influences. Biliary colic is more likely at night due to the high level of parasympathetic activity (i.e., part of the autonomic nervous system) which inhibits gallbladder activity and thus attenuates bile flow.

About twenty years ago, an even deeper spiritual dimension opened up for me when I turned to energetic testing of the deeper spiritual levels. I was particularly interested in the level of truthfulness, humanity, and honesty, that becomes visible during very profound experiences. This is the level of the causal body, where we encounter the deep spiritual or collective unconscious. This level will be treated in detail later on in the book. The causal body level has a strong healing effect and cleanses us of "sins," emotional complexes, and diseases. Spontaneous remission in cancer cases and "miracle cures" have to do with this level. On the causal body level, we experience great honesty, in which there are no excuses and no masquerading. Miracle cures are always characterized by the people involved being completely honest and clearly cognizant of what they truly want in their heart of hearts. This spiritual opening-up releases unsuspected healing powers that enable a dramatic turn for the better.

In the encounter with death, we come into closest contact with our own causal body, which is why death affects us so powerfully. It is here that we encounter the greatest enhancement and intensification of reality experience that we humans are capable of perceiving. We must learn once again to accept death, regarding it as an important step into another phase of our existence, namely life after death.

In the next chapter, I take up the topics of shamanism and magic. These are the oldest therapeutic methods known to mankind. In Africa and in numerous primitive tribes, these systems are still alive. Magic and shamanism arose at a time in mankind's development in which, according to developmental psychology, people still had a magical or animistic worldview. To these people, everything was animated by occult forces that could be channeled by shamans or magicians to suit their purposes.

Modern man today characterizes such beliefs as "superstition" and smiles condescendingly at the use of horseshoes and other lucky charms. For skeptics, the widespread use, even today, of such magic amulets and rituals is just added confirmation of the ineradicable foolishness of many of their contemporaries. I'd like to make a different judgment and say that the use of magic simply cannot be equated with foolishness and superstition, for the power of spiritual forces is, in my opinion, indisputable – and magic is simply the practical application of these spiritual forces. Why magic should nevertheless be rejected is one of the topics of the next chapter.

---

hydrotherapy – in my practice, I thought about several patients, some of whom I had not seen for a long time, who could definitely benefit from this procedure. At first, I thought of sending out a circular, but then thought that might be too pushy. Weeks passed, and I caught myself, over and again, saying to certain patients: "It's good that you came by: I was on the verge of writing you when you showed up on your own." At some point, most of the patients I would have written came by "quite by chance." Doing it this way saved me a lot of effort and postage. I recently tried out telepathic communication again – almost for the fun of it – as I was landing at Frankfurt airport. I thought of a patient who had not been to my practice for many years, and "purely by chance" he called two days later to make an appointment.

Western Psychotherapy, Shamanism, and Magic

In our modern high-tech society, nearly all our forefathers' healing art in the curing of psychosomatic diseases has been lost. People don't go anymore to shamans, believe in the "evil eye," have themselves exorcised or a spell broken. We consider all this to be useless superstition. On the other hand, ethnologically active physicians face insuperable diffi-

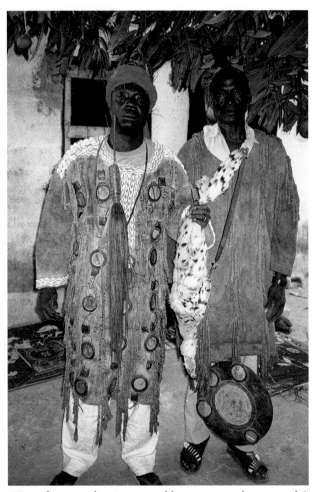

West African medicine man and his assistants; the mirrors he's wearing are supposed to ward off evil spirits. He wears the fur coat of a beast of prey as a sign of his spiritual powers. We saw him pierce his cheek with a large needle with no visible sign of pain; when he removed it, there was no trace of a puncture wound.

culties introducing our modern psychosomatic worldview to native cultures and talking them out of their superstitions. Clearly, there is a wide chasm separating these two medical worldviews.

Since I am a Western-trained physician, the occidental point of view and attitude seems initially quite normal to me. Shamanistic practices have always interested me peripherally, though, as a curiosity, the way one reads adventure novels. To set the mood, I'd like to relate a personal experience: the time I first met a genuine shaman in his native habitat. During a visit in western Africa, my former wife and I had our native Jeep driver take us to a real medicine man. His practice was in a hot corrugated-iron hut behind a filthy entrance curtain, and he was squatting on the dirt floor. Despite the dismal surroundings, he was said to be very famous and possess great powers. The man we met was reserved and looked tired, but he radiated a sense of superiority and serenity.

Our lack of language skills made conversation nearly impossible. Still, he gave us some herbs to take back for our patients – which turned out later not to be very effective, possibly due to our having misunderstood how to use them, or to the loss of volatile ingredients. The climax of our meeting was when the shaman poked something like a shishkebab skewer, without first disinfecting it, through both cheeks with no pain reaction whatsoever. When he pulled it out, there was no bleeding, nor could we see a puncture wound.[14]

Now, traditional shamanistic practices result in numerous paranormal phenomena and astounding cures that always flabbergast unbiased ethnologists. If one believes in the shaman, his magic seems to work. Evidently, belief plays an important role in magic. Amazingly, many shamans are aware that this belief is not omnipotent and that their powers have a limited effect. When they come up against their

---

[14] This cheek-piercing procedure, used by many healers, was reproduced by many skeptical rationalists (such as the leading American skeptic James RANDI, who has made it his job to unmask charlatans), with the ostensible result that a puncture wound is not seen because the cheek muscles at that point have a high intrinsic tension that pulls the wound shut and prevents bleeding. This seems to me not very credible, since my former partner, Dr. Ulrike Banis (with her years of intensive surgical experience) was, like myself, unable to find the slightest trace of a wound on the inside or outside surface of the cheek, even though the skewer had a diameter of 2-3mm and, in addition, had had a relatively heavy object hanging from it for about a minute.

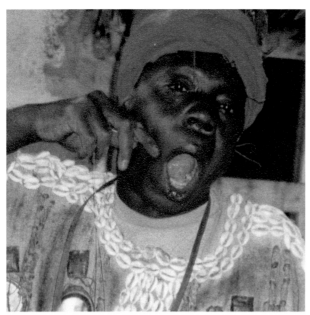

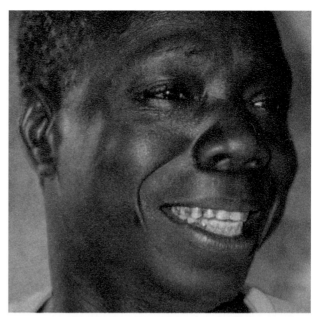

An African medicine man pierces his cheeks with a thick nee-dle. Right after the needle is removed, my former wife and I – both experienced physicians – inspect the facial skin and the

buccal mucosa. There is not the slightest sign of a wound to be seen anywhere. The right-hand photo was taken immediately after removal of the needle.

own limits, they advise patients to have an operation in a Western hospital, or to use antibiotics,.

As in every healing discipline, shamanism also has something like a "dosage/effect" relationship. The experienced shaman knows when he and his powers have come up against insuperable obstacles. To my mind, this is a persuasive indication that magic really does work – for effective powers have different intensities, whether it is our bodies' muscle power subject to our conscious will, or the healing power of a shaman. As with every power, some people are endowed by fate with more of it than others, so that there seem to be especially good, less good and even relatively ineffective medicine men.

But there is other evidence that can convince us of the effectiveness of shamans' healing powers. We note, among medicine men of the most diverse cultures, something like a common speech and basic approach that turns up in widely-separated regions of the world in amazingly similar form. Shamans everywhere seem to act on the same principles. Also, shamans by no means heal entirely with magic, but also use very down-to-earth medications. They collect plants that contain active substances. This shows that shamans do not rely purely on their magical rituals and the power of their healing charms, but rather are acquainted with a broad palette of healing methods. Still, the core of their therapeutic methods is magic itself. **Magic** is understood as an action or conjuration that in some allegorical way anticipates a particular goal in order to attain it in connection with unseeable power sources and forces. For example, a bullet that has caused an injury is ground into a rem-

edy. Ingesting the "bad" rifle bullet as a remedy is supposed to make the wound heal faster.

Other kinds of magic make use of animal sacrifices. In his book *Hidden Africa*, the Italian researcher Attlio GATTI tells of a Zulu shaman who very quickly cured a half-blind man with severely inflamed eyes. First, chanting incantations, he places a hypnotized rooster on the sick man's head. He then beheads the rooster, places a herbal bandage over the eyes, removes it after a few minutes – and the old man has been completely healed! Confronted with such cures as this, we say "witchcraft" because we don't understand what's going on behind the scenes. The best medicine men achieve outstanding and immediate results with their magical practices that border on the miraculous. The American Max Freedom LONG describes seeing a Hawaiian magic priest-ess (Kahuna) heal a serious bone fracture, before his very eyes, in mere minutes. The leg bone had been broken in a car accident and protruded from an ugly flesh wound. After a few minutes, no trace of the accident was to be seen and the young man was completely restored![15]

Magical healing rituals continue to be practiced throughout the world, to undeniable success. Accordingly, the World Health Organization (WHO) a while back asked third-world countries such as India to provide more support for

[15] In his fundamental work Quantum Man (see Bibliography), Michael HARNER has brought together from various sources an abundance of well-documented miracle cures that make the phenomenon of miracles seem quite credible. Also, at Lourdes and many other religious sites, there are notes of scientifically-trained observers documenting a great many miracle cures.

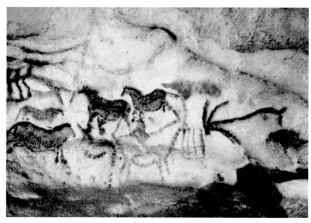

The hunting magic of prehistoric man follows the basic magic rule of anticipating what is hoped for, thus ensuring its manifestation.

traditional therapeutic methods, because traditional therapies are more accessible and affordable for the poor of the world than expensive Western medicine. But the main reason for the WHO's recommendation is studies that substantiate the excellent effects of traditional therapeutic methods. Shamans have proven particularly successful when it comes to psychosomatic diseases. Why this should be so, I will deal with shortly.

How do the shaman's healing practices differ from those of our modern psychotherapists? The most striking difference has to do with sharply divergent worldviews, in that shamans and their patients view everything as being imbued with spirit. To them, there is no mind-body split. Our modern Western conception of a division between body and mind (soul) seems quite arbitrary to shamans and their tradition-oriented patients. Because the shaman distinguishes no dividing line between a sick person and his clan – or the natural world around him – a medicine man actually treats not just the patient, but his entire milieu as well.

To a shaman, family and workplace are just as much part of a disease as the surrounding nature. Family ghosts and local spirits at sites where houses are built can be upset and furious, and need to be calmed down. To accomplish this, the shaman makes a sacrificial offering as a clear sign of contrition for the wrong committed; this is meant to put the spirit in a peaceable mood. Of course, the very best thing is not to let things get so far in the first place by means of preventive rituals, altar sacrifices, and prayers.

To us modern Westerners, this might at first seem outlandish, but if we open up and become more sensitive, we will feel a certain "spirituality" at certain locations. The ancient Romans expressed this as the "spirit of a place" (*Genius loci*). Moods and vibrations are different at certain locations. Amazingly, places with a violent past seem cold to us and make us feel anxious. Then again, there are places

that feel especially peaceful and calm – known as *areas of power*) – where one feels refreshed and can "recharge one's batteries." Chinese *Feng shui* and Geomancy in Europe have investigated and described these kinds of places in detail. I will go into this in greater detail in a subsequent chapter on geopathic stress zones.

The most striking difference in viewpoint between modern psychology and traditional shamanism has to do with the differing significance ascribed to external influences. Shamans see diseases as coming almost exclusively from outside. From this viewpoint, the sick person is above all a victim of unfavorable circumstances. The disease has befallen the victim because social and emotional differences exist within the tribe or with nature. A neighbor might be envious, for instance, of some witch or wizard who has the "evil eye."

Western critics like to emphasize the childlike nature of this animistic worldview, thereby disposing of the entire subject. Animism means viewing the world as being imbued with spirit. Typically, this kind of worldview characterizes the spiritual feelings of children. Revealingly, when children clumsily run into a table, they'll kick it and swear at it as if it were a sentient being ("Bad table! Just for that, I'm gonna hit you!"). Scientists think that primitive tribes view the world much in the same manner.

This viewpoint holds that everything bad comes from outside – as a spell or curse, say. It is easy and convenient to pass off the responsibility to someone or something else. Even today, we find that patients prefer to blame anything bad on external causes instead of looking within themselves for the source of the problem. To shamans, external disease causes are almost always responsible. Even if we assume that a shaman is not doing so deliberately, he is still cleverly taking advantage of his fellow man's naïveté and laziness. Because patients and shamans alike view the environment and their disease as imbued with spirit, that evidently leads to an inability to perceive their own contributions to the overall problem. For this reason, I consider shamanistic procedures and methods to be totally unsuited for us modern Westerners! We know that projection – i.e., blaming external circumstances – is not going to get us anywhere.

Still, I don't wish to reject shamanism's healing methods out of hand, because its healing repertoire contains an extremely valuable "pearl" that will, I suspect, prove to be of inestimable value for us in the future. It has to do with viewing the conflict as a demon in the subtle body, which offers the shaman substantially better healing possibilities – because if something harmful indeed exists in the real world, you can get hold of it and neutralize it. On the other hand, if we believe, as does modern psychology, that the conflict exists only as a diffuse, intangible, purely mental construct in the patient's subconscious, then we have nothing by which to grab hold of it! At this point, I'd like to make clear up front that disturbances in the subtle-body field (the Aura) are real and tangible, and can be healed by means of specific healing methods (homeopathy, for example). How that works in practice I'll get into later on.

Let's take a closer look at the shamanistic worldview. The ethnologist (now deceased) Carlos CASTAÑEDA describes the shamanistic trance in his books. He notes that, in their visions, shamans see patients' diseases as snakes, spiders and such. Sometimes, they also see them in their visions in the form of diabolical demons, poisons, or harmful objects that attach themselves to patients or are located in their bodies. We must be clear that we are dealing here with allegories, i.e. symbolic transformations of spiritual subtle-body phenomena. Thus, an Eskimo shaman will see dangerous polar bears, whereas a jungle shaman will perceive a tiger. Visions thus depend on preformed images in the imagination of the person in question, and have no objective form as such.

The shaman sees, in a very real manner, that these evil spirits live off the patient's energy, draining away his strength. This way of looking at it will have far-reaching significance for our later analysis, which is why I am once again bringing up this important point. To the shaman, disease demons torture and occupy their victims and cause them to fall into perdition. Also at this important point, we should not hastily assume that these are pure fantasy or simplistic projections – because shamans perceive the entire drama of spiritual conflicts quite clearly and correctly, just translated into a symbolic language. The visualized demons are in all likelihood a visualization of the spiritual contents with respect to the "conflicts," about which more later on in the book.

Psychoanalysts go about it very differently: in conversation sessions sometimes lasting for years, they view the conflict from the outside, tracking it down in the patient's subconscious, so that the patient, once made aware of it, can resolve the conflict. The shaman, on the other hand, claims to be able to eliminate and heal conflicts by driving the demons from the patient's body or energy field via magical rituals. The patient need do nothing more than keep still. The shaman invokes the conflict demon, grabs hold of it, and pulls it out of the patient.

The big question now is, who is right: the shaman with his magic or the analyst with his rational procedure? Critical modern man and psychoanalysts (our modern "shamans") don't think much of the traditional healers' procedures.[16] At any rate, that's what I keep hearing, over and over, in numerous conversations with a variety of people. If it works

at all, it must do so only among the primitive folk who believe in the shaman's magic. Basically, these cases are nothing more than "placebo effect" cures. I then hear the exact opposite from shamans and energy healers: the analyst really doesn't heal at all, patients just fool themselves into thinking that they're making progress and being cured. Because the analyst busies himself so with the conflict (the demon), hovering around the associated problems, he thereby gives the demon added strength, often making the problem even worse.

And so there is a very deep chasm between these two worldviews. Nevertheless, this can be overcome, and great progress made in the direction of holistic medicine, by extracting the best from both views. What that means specifically will be explained in later chapters and substantiated with convincing patient case histories. At this point, I'd like get into the phenomenon of **magic** in greater detail. Magic is a very important (yet often misunderstood) key to comprehensive healing. First, I'd like to describe some of my own experiences and mention some inspiring books that clearly describe the essence of magic and its attendant dangers.

I got my first dramatic lesson in the effectiveness of magic when, as a medical student, I read the fascinating autobiography of the English physician Aubrey T. WESTLAKE . All his life, this surgeon and GP had occupied himself with topics like this that also interested me. He carried out experiments with Wilhelm REICH's Orgone Box. He dealt extensively with PARACELSUS' confusing multiform Cosmos. WESTLAKE was particularly interested in the shamanism of the native Hawaiians and its Huna doctrine. These are all topics that have especially inspired me as well. Near the end of his life, WESTLAKE gathered a group of like-minded people around him to search out completely new therapeutic methods. In typical British manner, the group met in a house trailer complete with potbellied stove and tea trolley, so that they could pursue their research in peace. The focal point of the magical circle was a *channeling medium*. Her messages were supposed to yield crucial information indicating a new therapeutic method.

According to the medium's messages, the new system consisted of geometric figures. This included, the ancient symbol of the *Celtic Cross*. As the "Cross of Life," it symbolized the union of the spiritual world (vertical axis of the cross) with the material (horizontal axis), bound together into a unified whole by a circle. Certain remedies (homeopathics, Bach Flowers,

---

[16] C.G. JUNG was one of the few psychoanalysts of note to believe in spirits and other ghostly phenomena and, moreover, to admit it openly and freely. It is less well known that FREUD, near the end of his life, was able to overcome his rigid rejection of the parapsychological, because proof to the contrary kept on accumulating. (In fact, he was heard to say that, given the chance to start his life over, he would concentrate on parapsychology instead of psychoanalysis.). JUNG's doctoral dissertation even dealt with possession by a spirit he sensed in his

cousin, who was secretly in love with him. This only came to light recently in some biographical material; Jung was either unaware of this crush, or else suppressed it (he didn't find his cousin particularly attractive). Critics might object that this particular demonic possession was nothing more than a case of repressed sexual desire. I think otherwise, having carefully studied the available material. Parapsychological phenomena demonstrably took place that have no purely rational explanation. That at least speaks in favor of Jung's thesis.

precious stones) were positioned at the corners of the graphic so as to attain a virtually perfect energetic harmony with the patient's specimen. The patient specimen could consist of blood, hairs, a photograph, or any other personal object, and was placed in the center of the graphic.

One of course asks oneself how that can work. In principle, it is a magical arrangement that works via sympathetic magic. According to this view, objects or persons that are similar or mutually sympathetic (i.e. they "like each other") relate directly with each other independently of time and space. Now, there are two scientifically proven facts that make the possibility of such a relationship credible. The first relates to parapsychological research, which has shown that telepathy functions quite reliably and reproducibly in numerous cases. There is now a great deal of solid information about this. By mentally concentrating on a person, one can very well imagine that not only is mental contact taking place, but possibly a subtle-body energy exchange as well. The second fact comes from modern quantum physics, which says that *entangled* particle pairs (that had once been in contact) react in synchrony no matter what their subsequent separation.

Sympathetic magic is as old as mankind and is found in all cultures. The Navajo Indian medicine man, for example, heals the patient body and soul by means of sand drawings (geometrical healing symbols). In this case, it is white magic that does good and enables healing to take place. In the Voodoo cult, on the other hand, we encounter the black magic (destructive and evil) aspect of sympathetic magic, in which a doll is pricked with needles. The doll represents the victim upon whom mortal pain is to be inflicted.

WESTLAKE himself practiced white magic, using a pendulum in his healing arrangement. Radionics originated in England around the beginning of the 20th century – a method that traces back to the American physician ABRAMS. Along with his pendulum, WESTLAKE made use of radionic tables to examine and heal patients. The simplest kind of radionic table is a sort of speedometer (as in an automobile). A table of this kind can be drawn up, for example, with a few strokes on a piece of paper (see illustration). One concentrates on the question to be answered (e.g. "How healthy is the patient, percentage-wise?") and notes the direction of the pendulum's excursion.

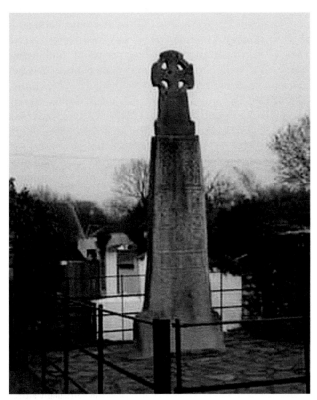

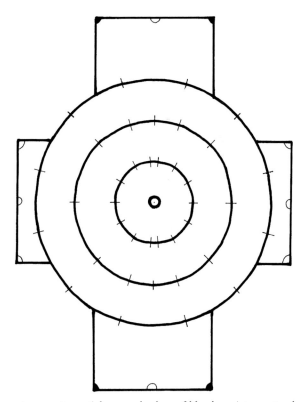

Celtic Cross – On the left a monolith from the early Middle Ages in Carew (Wales); on the right the precise arrangement for a healing cross, as per Aubrey T. WESTLAKE, including the small semicircles where the healing ampoules are placed. The

patient specimen (photograph, drop of blood, etc.) is put in the middle. This is the original picture from my experiment with Johann (described in the text).

Back then, I wanted to try out WESTLAKE's simple arrangement right away on one of the students in the commune. Johann seemed to me a suitable test subject, since he was often sickly and suffered occasional migraine attacks. I didn't tell him a thing about what I had in mind. But the silly thing was, I didn't have WESTLAKE's drawings. WESTLAKE said, falsely, that he had destroyed them right after the strength of the effects forced him to recognize the danger of abuse. A few weeks later, I was browsing an art book dealing with magic practices that a theology student friend of mine had "somehow accidentally" brought with him to the university. And look there! Miraculously, here were reproduced all the most important of WESTLAKE's supposedly destroyed drawings!

At this point, I'd like to point out the significant circumstance that magic practices frequently lead to self-reinforcing coincidences that are, in reality, not coincidences at all. The thing is, these ominous accidents are examples of *synchronicity* (increased probability somewhat in the sense of the "celebrated coincidence"), which aims at reinforcing our intentions and luring us into continuing our magical activities. How that happens and why it does will become clearer later on.

I first copied the drawings out of the book: the original book illustrations would have been too small to put ampoules on (These glass ampoules are about little-finger size and are used in energy medicine to test out which remedies a patient needs.). After that, it was easy to implement the rest of my plan. For an entire night, I let a carefully selected ensemble of Bach Flowers and homeopathic LM potentiations work their effect on a photo of my fellow student. The test ampoules were lined up like little tin soldiers on the DIN A4 sheet of paper with the "Diamond" drawn on it.

The next morning, I was enormously curious to see the healing results. Unfortunately, my test subject Johann was (against all expectation) white as a sheet and felt sick as a dog. He said he had lain wide awake all night, feeling horribly miserable. I have to admit that, at the time, I was too cowardly and confused to confess my magical séance to him. I was possibly also trying to avoid a dreadful Donnybrook and continuing unpleasantness, which would have made my emotional situation – quite aside from the therapeutic debacle – even more insecure. To be sure, I didn't feel outright culpable because my intentions had been honorable. But I had evidently done something wrong, or else the effect was simply too strong. To be on the safe side, I destroyed the photograph and terminated the healing ritual I had secretly set up in my room.

To this day, I have not repeated those practices. The shock of the unexpected effectiveness shook me to the bone in a beneficial way. Since that time, I have known magical practices from personal experience. From my own experiment and numerous other experiences and reports, I am

convinced of the effectiveness of magical practices. I am, notwithstanding, an avowed opponent of magic. My reasons have directly to do with the bad outcome of my experiment. Of course, I have thought long and hard about what the actual reason for Johann's awful night could have been,

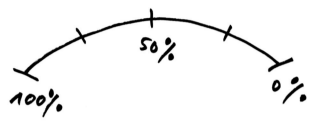

Simple pendulum template with 100% scale gradation.

as I was secretly "irradiating" him. At some point, I realized that, way down deep, I really didn't like Johann; he had all the character traits that I considered abhorrent.

My subconscious had taken advantage of the situation to "let off steam," which is why the healing séance had such a tragically poor outcome. The transmitted healing energy had got mixed up with my negative feelings for my housemate, and the negatives won. **When it comes to magic, there is thus always a danger of so-called "lower astral energy" mixing into the healing ceremony and being conveyed as well!** Now, magic fans will no doubt accuse me of overdramatizing and elevating an isolated instance into a general rule. As a matter of fact, it is many further experiences that have persuaded me generally and totally to reject magic – at least in our Western high-tech civilization, where magic is no longer culturally integrated and its unusual situation tends therefore to generate abstruse and dangerous results.

Contrary to universal opinion, magical practices are widespread in modern naturopathic medicine. Therapists and patients alike often underestimate the danger posed by unintentionally conveyed negative energies – just as, on the Internet, "hackers" get into the act as demons and black-magic powers. Of course, a therapist has only the best of intentions, but that often seems not to make much difference. The at-risk methods include all forms of remote healing, Radionics, Mora, Bioresonance, and the computer-aided transmission of healing vibrations. These are all methods that, at first glance, don't seem to involve magic at all. Also to be avoided are also such obvious things as conjurations, healing séances, and any other recognizably magic-based rituals.

The following story, told me by a patient, illustrates how strongly black-magic practices can be unintentionally amplified:

Mr. M had a rough childhood. His depressive father committed suicide when the boy was still in his teens. His mother was also emotionally disturbed and imposed a great emotional burden on the youngster, since he always had to take care of his parents from childhood on. On top of which, as the oldest, he had to look after his siblings, making his studies (in between familial duties) very difficult. Life for him had always been a constant struggle that he had been forced to fight alone. He is now happily married, has healthy children and a successful career – but the shadows of his past caught up with him.

For more than a decade, he has become increasingly certain that he has inherited his parents' depression. Medications prescribed by his psychiatrist make life tolerable, but they don't take away the emotional pain. Years of psychotherapy have no effect. Family Constellations yields good insights from a systemic standpoint – but change nothing regarding his condition. A few years back, a somatic psychotherapist made some progress with muscular relaxation techniques and emotional resolution, but wound up doing more harm than good, because he bound the patient strongly to himself emotionally: he insisted that every important step in the patient's life be coordinated with him first. In the end, he became totally dependent on the therapist, phoning him many times daily.

The therapist was very spiritual, and at one point spoke of a curse he had detected which had cast a black-magic spell on Mr. M's entire family. The curse needed to be worked off and counteracted slowly and gradually. The patient was terrified and, in this condition, caused a serious multi-car collision that put the entire family in the hospital (they were going on vacation). After this, the catastrophes just kept piling up, making the curse thesis more plausible. In his desperation, the patient went to another therapist, who recommended that he disassociate himself from the earlier one. He was told to write this therapist (who had come up with the curse thesis) a farewell letter and then burn it. Shortly thereafter, the chain of catastrophic events came to an end and the patient felt markedly better.

We can clearly see in this story how black-magic practices befell first the therapist and then the patient. First, the therapist got on a "lousy ego trip" – which is unfortunately not all that uncommon when therapists make clients mentally or physically dependent and then abuse their position of power. Next, the therapist projects his own emotional problems onto the client's family as he talks about malevolent energies and curses. After this, the mishaps pile up as the self-fulfilling prophecy works itself out, until the curse theory seems totally believable to all concerned. As for exorcisms and witch-burnings, it is easy to see here how evil branches off independently and spreads out as soon as it is acknowledged as a present danger and its importance thus confirmed. This initiates a process of projection and identification that is very hard to bring to a halt.

I had another instructive experience with an acquaintance who was a talented medium. She is highly sensitive and can,

for instance, perceive essences in a person's Aura. Once, while giving her a tour of a house we used to live in, wonderfully situated, she stopped at the veranda. She was picking up, she said, "very, very negative vibrations" radiating directly from the neighboring house through the dormer window to our house. The vibration she felt was a mixture of jealousy and envy. Now, she knew absolutely nothing about the extremely negative relationship we had with our neighbors back then, the cause of which we had never been able to figure out. Possibly we were, as a married couple of doctors with a large practice, simply too successful not to generate some surreptitious envy – for the neighbors had big financial problems, although we didn't know that at the time.

Another crucial experience illustrates a further important energy phenomenon long known to shamans, namely the **transmission of emotional qualities**.[17] As with a vaccination, one is "infected" with emotions that are not one's own. The prerequisite for this seems to be relaxed openness and a certain susceptibility to the emotion in question. My former wife and I had gone out to eat with a couple who were friends of ours. The women, seemingly in the best of moods, kept up a marvelous conversation throughout the evening. And yet, the next day my wife felt oddly weak, discontented, and irritable. Eventually, I tested my wife energetically and, while looking for the disturbance, found a compound homeopathic (emotional remedy) that responded to a specific subconscious conflict. The conflict's content had absolutely nothing to do with my wife's life at that time. Nevertheless, it was an emotional topic that was not totally unfamiliar to her. To that extent, there was a resonance based on some affinity, so it was easier for the conflict to gain a foothold in her. But we were still puzzling over how this strange conflict had come about. As I thought about it some more, I remembered that I had tested out exactly this conflict some weeks earlier in the woman my wife had been talking to. We then went out to dinner again with them a few months later.

This time, it was my turn to sit next to her. It would have been easy for me, as a robust male, to ward off such **emotional transmissions**. But I found the whole thing a bit much, and I wasn't 100% convinced that there was anything to it. Possibly we had let our imagination get the better of us. All the same, I shielded myself, as a precautionary measure, by visualizing a white light, and by wishing the woman peace in my thoughts. So I was downright annoyed

---

[17] Brazilian trance therapy (Captaçao) includes similar observations as an essential therapeutic element. Around 1970, the physician Dr. Mendes noticed that patients improved when nurses "adopted" certain of the patients' symptoms. With the aid of sensitives, Mendes developed a trance therapy that combines Afro-American elements of possession and spirits with modern hypnosis techniques. The sensitive lets the hidden spirits speak, after which the therapist (placatingly/pleadingly or energetically/urgently) attempts to influence the spirits to leave the patient.

when, a few days later, the same lassitude and listlessness overcame me as had befallen my wife earlier. Now it had nabbed me, eh? This was particularly awkward to me since it forced me to confront, first, my weakness and, second, my unbelief. Even more annoying, it absolutely did not fit in with the difficult stage of life that I was trying to cope with at the time. Not to mention that the same emotional topic was in play as the first time. It was also clear that I was dealing with a familiar yet unresolved spiritual theme.

We influence not only ourselves with these subconscious conflicts, but also those around us. Thank God this emotional transmission (my name for this phenomenon) is, in my experience, relatively rare among adults. To that extent, the incident with our friends was a rarity, only possible because all those involved were unusually open energetically and who, in addition, were carrying around the same "emotional baggage." Energetically open people in particular (children, healers, highly sensitive persons) can be subliminally influenced by emotional transmissions, as can people who, for whatever reason, share a close personal relationship. Children frequently have the same conflicts as their parents, and I do suspect that the parents have (without anyone noticing) transferred their conflicts to their children.

In the worst case, influencing other people can cause serious illness. First, these negative influences trigger psychoenergetic blocks, frequently without any detectable disease. In this phase – which can last quite a long time – the victim just feels a bit out of sorts and queasy. Interestingly, the "emotional donor" (who is now partly free of his conflicts) often feels noticeably better! I have often observed that these emotional donors cling like limpets to their victims – masquerading externally as caring concern. Once the psychoenergetic block is broken up, the process can almost always be resolved fairly quickly (more on this later). Victim and perpetrator are separated energetically, since the conflict – the "docking station" – has been healed and eliminated. Of course, this means that the emotional donor no longer has the option of saddling someone else with his excess baggage; he has to haul it around himself.

In the next chapter, I'd like to describe vital energy in greater detail – something about which we know very little, even though it is the most important basis for our existence. **The quality of our vital energy is, first of all, crucial to our quality of life.** Nothing else influences our existence as much as our vital energy!

The Significance of Life Energy

Since ancient times, man has sensed an invisible vital force. According to seers, shamans, and sorcerers, life is bound up with a particular force. To be alive means to be pervaded with this life force. The more life force streams through one, the better off one is. Therefore, this life force has long been viewed as the source of health, well-being, sexual desire, and feeling alive (and lively). Yet the significance of the life force extends far beyond this – as mankind has known since time immemorial. In many animistic and magical cults, life energy is even elevated to the Godhead; this is true of practically all aboriginal cultures. All fertility cults (literally) idolize the life force. In the cult of the Egyptian sun god Aton, the life force is prayed to in the representative form of the sun.

A serious elementary error underlies the attempts of modern theoreticians to *equate* life force with light quanta (photons) or physical phenomena such as tachyons, zero-point energy, magnetism, and so on. This error is based on an impermissible simplification and, in my opinion, on some totally false basic assumptions. Life force is more than light quanta or other physical phenomena. Plus, there's another problem that's much harder to penetrate, because its roots are completely subconscious: the great and enormously fascinating dynamics of these hypotheses rests on their magical aspects. However, the magic thinking is largely subconscious and tends toward fanaticism – for who would willingly renounce a kind of thinking that is so directly associated with desire (i.e., the gratification thereof) and magic (i.e., power)?

Before mankind developed the concept of monotheism, the practice of magical idolatry was, from a spiritual standpoint, not a problem. Idolatry fits the magical worldview of the aborigine and thus does not cause the damage that we see later, when people have progressed to higher psychoenergetic developmental stages in which the enlarged individual ego leads quite easily to the abuse of magical ritual. I alluded to this in the preceding chapter, when I warned against using magic for healing purposes.

Even if we mean no harm to anyone and our intentions are good, there still exists a considerable risk potential due to our large (compared to aborigines) individual egos. These dangers are depicted in the Bible as the worship of Mammon (dancing around the golden calf). At that time, the Israelites' religion was already monotheistic, but famine and desperation caused them to lapse back into their old rites. The dangers lie not so much in idol worship itself as in the long-term damages that can be conjured up thereby. I'll come back to this in a later chapter about Karma. Ultimately, the person responsible winds up hurting himself as the egotism of magic turns on him.

From here on out, I prefer to speak mainly in terms of **energetics** when referring to subtle-body (invisible) life force. Older terms for life force are *Prana* in India, *Ch'I* in China, *Pneuma* in ancient occidental medicine (GALEN), *Archæus* (PARACELSUS), or *Fluidum* (MESMER). Often, the reference is to *Spiritus* or *vitality* or *Æther*. When we survey the history of the West, life force doesn't seem to have the central significance it had in the ancient East. Amazingly, though, there have been modern thinkers who were aware of the great importance of the life force. One of these is the German philosopher SCHOPENHAUER, who made the concept of the life force, in its full scope, the cornerstone of his worldview.

SCHOPENHAUER fulminates against the omnipresent distortions of the philosophers, who *"make of perception a fundamental entity"* and *"would have the will issue from perception."* What does he mean by this? For SCHOPENHAUER, *Will* means the life force itself. The life force incorporates an enormously strong survival instinct. In order for life to arise and exist, life force must be present. Therefore, life force (the Will) is the primary and first primeval cause from which the world issues – *not* some theory thought up by man *(perception)*. SCHOPENHAUER also recognizes the subconscious and concludes: "That which the heart resists the head will not admit." He also recognized the subjectivity of human worldviews and our tendency to deny and suppress that which is emotionally abhorrent to us. These days – about 150 years after SCHOPENHAUER – we understand ever better that we are decisively controlled by, and dependent on, subconscious emotions and subtle-body energy states.

The developer of homeopathy, Samuel HAHNEMANN, also considered an immaterial alteration of the life force to be the beginning of disease – and at the same time the crucial key to its cure. **According to HAHNEMANN, diseases arise when the life force gets upset.** HAHNEMANN was hardly the first to say this, since this was also the official medical opinion back then. Life-force doctrines culminated in the theory of the Scottish physician John BROWN *(Brownianism)*, with the simple basic assumption that understimulation cripples the life force, whereas overstimulation exhausts it. Either extreme causes disease, while health is a balance between the two. Based on this, the doctor's task is to harmonize. According to Christoph Wilhelm HUFELAND, GOETHE's personal physician, disturbance of the life force is the elementary basic precondition for every disease. His multi-volume basic work *The Art of Lengthening Human Lifespan* already contains all the elements of the modern naturopathic movement.

I mentioned previously that, about 200 years ago, life-force theory was respectable science; it was a recognized part of medicine. Yet some critics were already raising objections back then. They were bothered by the fact that "life force," ultimately, couldn't be defined. The indefinability and "sponginess" of life force was contrasted with the "scientification" of modern medicine. At the universities, there were regular skirmishes between life force fans and materialists. Still and all, it was obvious what the outcome of these confrontations would be.

The rise of the physical sciences meant that (in medicine as well) all that counted was what could be weighed and measured; everything else was deemed subjective and, ultimately, denounced as irrational. It was banned from the "orthodox medicine" taught at the universities. But we know that not everything significant in medicine is measurable. Since the tenet of ignoring the incommensurable continues to be upheld, these issues eke out a marginalized existence at the universities. Thus, by the end of the 19th century, there was no longer any room for life-force theory. So-called "Vitalism" was last championed by the biologist and philosopher Hans DRIESCH, who died in Leipzig in 1941, leaving behind no influential disciples.

For many enlightened and rational persons, life-force theory has in the meantime taken on an air of mysticism and esotericism. They reflect, sadly, the truncated worldview of the physical sciences, true to the motto: "If respectable scientists do not concern themselves with these topics, then there is nothing to them." Few are aware that, until EINSTEIN's time, physics made use of the concept of the *ether*, which agreed in many essential aspects with those of subtle-body life energy. At some point, this old-fashioned hard-to-define concept passed into oblivion. With all his might, EINSTEIN initially resisted the elimination of the ether concept, but was eventually brought around by distinguished colleagues such as Max PLANCK.

There have been more and more signs, lately, that scientists – the primary pace-setters of our current worldview – are gradually beginning to rethink their position; but then critics darkly infer a relapse into magical mumbo-jumbo and downright mysticism. To my mind, these critics are guilty of propagating nothing less than stick-in-the-mud propaganda, because it's specifically the brightest scientists who are beginning to realize that the world is made up of far more than the merely measurable. Chaos theory and the discovery of cybernetic holographic models give one a good

idea of these developments. Within the physical sciences, we are making progress away from a rigid, mechanistic viewpoint toward more functional thinking that embraces concepts such as unseeable formative powers. Researchers such as Rupert SHELDRAKE and his *morphogenetic field* represent a modern science that can once again deal with the concept of life force.

If observer and world are as closely coupled as modern physics' quantum theory (likewise SHELDRAKE's morphogenetic field) tells us they are, then the observer of course becomes hugely significant. If everything is resonating and interacting, then it would seem, at first, that the observing person defines the world – but this is so (I believe) only to a very limited extent. This view fails to take the overall state into account and, above all, the energetic aspect or, loosely put: "… what kind of a mood the scientist is in." A depressed and frustrated scientist will obviously view the world differently than a happy, optimistic one. I have already mentioned SCHOPEN-HAUER, whose position was much the same. When a scientist has a broad intellectual horizon, it has less to do with his genius or intelligence and more with his energetic openness; energetic openness in turn reflects the state of his spiritual maturity.

Later on in this book, **I'll try to prove that our worldview can be conceived of as a predominantly energy-driven process!** Taking the saying "You are what you eat," it would be more accurate to say: **"As a human personality, you perceive, think and act (according to) what you energetically are in your totality."** The German philosopher FICHTE put it succinctly: *"The philosophy one selects depends on what kind of person one is."* As long as a person is stuck, say, at the level of the 5th Chakra in his thinking (the usual Chakra of the great majority of intellectuals and scientists), that person will tend to react narrow-mindedly and, regrettably, blindly to many phenomena. As modern people at a 5th Chakra developmental level, we pigeonhole the world into mutually independent compartments. People at the 5th Chakra level (the typical Chakra of the modern) perceive the world from an intellectual perspective that divides and differentiates. Reality is unduly diminished in this manner. When a scientist's spiritual development increases, his viewpoint and worldview will change automatically. Thanks to greater spiritual advancement, he will comprehend larger contexts and acquire a more objective worldview.

Comparable phenomena exist in energy medicine, where the healer whose energy system is most harmonized and balanced will make the best diagnoses – i.e., healers whose own energy situation is good can arrive at the most objective diagnoses. The point is whether the healer can be objective while remaining energetically balanced and staying free of presuppositions or expectations. If so, then objective results that stand up to scrutiny are possible. I will go into this in more detail in the next chapter.

When we realize that modern man's psychoenergetic vibration puts him at the level of the 5th Chakra, where the tendency is to think in terms of stereotypes and rough over-simplifications, it comes as no surprise that something as immediate and intimately binding as life force has been so long forgotten. Amazingly, this is not at all true of naturopathy and empirical medicine. Here, the naturopathic physicians, homeopaths and naturopaths invoke the ideas of vitalists such as HAHNEMANN or HUFELAND or the worldview of oriental medicine. Because of the great importance of life force in these medical systems, an extremely valuable resource of medical knowledge has accumulated over the millennia, as found for example in acupuncture, Ayurvedic medicine, homeopathy, and energy medicine. The existence of the life force and its healing has always been a direct part of such therapeutic methods.

We can perceive the existence of subtle-body energy as a subjective phenomenon. We feel "something" – and that is the feeling the life force triggers in us. The opener we are, the better our perception. We constantly perceive subtle-body energy, usually without being consciously aware of it. We can best train our perceptivity by becoming spiritually open, inwardly calm, and watchful. The more concentrated yet intention-free our watchfulness, the better we'll be able to perceive the subtle-body energy in ourselves and others. The EEG will then show Alpha waves, then Theta and Delta waves, all of which are observed during relaxation processes.

Mental relaxation is an important precondition for perceiving subtle-body energy. However, the most important thing is re-developing a perception of one's own life force. That sounds harder than it is – for, with some hours of concentration to acquire the necessary delicacy of feeling, virtually anyone can perceive another person's *Aura* as a tingling in the palms or some similar sensation. One can similarly perceive one's own energy flow. In the next chapter, I will give some practical tips on how most simply to achieve this.

The perception of subtle-body energy is, amazingly enough, a very normal everyday process, so much so that we regard it as completely self-evident. It's just that we normally use different terms when speaking of the perception of subtle-body energy. For instance, **well-being** or **sympathy** are energetic phenomena that we perceive in ourselves or in our contacts with others. When we feel good, our energy is flowing well. When we like someone, then our energy flows even more. We feel better and therefore feel a liking for the other person. Clairvoyants describe the process as an energy exchange between congenial people that enlivens and strengthens both parties. "It makes me feel good to be with him!" we then say.

Since our culture has forgotten how to perceive energetically, we lack the related energy concepts as well. When we tell someone "Wow, do you look bright and lively!" that

simply means that this person has especially much stored-up life force and is also radiating it. Energetically charged-up people not only seem livelier to us, but also more sexually attractive and dynamic. Moreover, congenial people are those with whom our own life force connects particularly playfully and pleasantly. The more energetically open and genuinely friendly a person is, the more people are going to like him.

Wilhelm REICH, the discoverer of Orgone energy, went so far as to say that *only* energetically free and relatively unarmored people are capable of perceiving energy. Orgone is REICH's designation for life force. As in acupuncture, REICH is aware of the negative consequences of pent-up life force, which he calls DOR. His assessment of DOR as the primary cause of sexual function disorders – the basis for authoritarian (life-hostile) personalities – on up to his discovery of the cause of cancer as a consequence of DOR, are above all a symptom of the black-and-white intellectual climate of that fascistic and totalitarian era (1930–1950). Added to this were REICH's subconscious savior fantasies. In my experience, DOR as such does not exist, or at least not as described by REICH. It is a product of the imagination, which wrongly interprets correctly perceived facts – which, by the way, applies in large part to REICH's entire body of work. Nevertheless, REICH is one of the foremost pioneers in humanistic psychology, and the forefather of Bioenergetics, Biodynamic Psychology, and many other psychotherapeutic procedures.

My clinical practice experience totally contradicts REICH's extreme statement that only unarmored people are capable of perceiving the life force. In fact, neurotic and vegetatively severely disturbed patients often develop enormous energetic sensitivity. Therefore, sensitivity to energetic phenomena only permits to a very limited degree drawing any conclusions with respect to a person's spiritual health and energetic openness. Also, many people try to deceive by basing their supposedly higher spirituality on their energetic sensitivity – but the two don't have all that much to do with each other. Although every spiritually advanced person is also highly sensitive to the life force, not everyone who perceives the life force (or manipulates it in some way or other) is spiritually advanced.

There are other deceptive practices, in an energy context, that one should be aware of. For example, you can simulate sympathy and friendliness by reducing your energetic force field. This can be achieved by means of perfume, for example, which makes the force field smaller and thus makes us seem more congenial. Critical and highly sensitive people (as well as energetically open children) see right through this trick, and find over-perfumed people quite repulsive. They instinctively sense the large, rowdy Aura of strongly perfumed persons and their veiled intent to deceive. The same goes for certain kinds of especially "sexy" clothing, by the way. Erotic attraction can also hamper the energetic evaluation of another person, since sexual desire boosts our energy flow enormously. This might have to do with one of the main reasons why amorousness so often ends abruptly, if we see the other person's true energy situation. We then have the painful realization that we have allowed our sexual feelings to lead us astray.

The more civilized and cultivated a person becomes, the greater the filter between the subtle-body energy and its perception. In the language of social psychology, the term is alienation: estrangement from one's own body, its sensory perceptions and its being part of the natural world. Parallel to this, subtle-body energy is less and less perceived. For many, sexuality is the only part left where they allow themselves to be themselves fully, and be sexual in a non-alienated manner. If we regard desire as something that has to do with strongly flowing life force, then sexuality becomes a special exception in which one, as a civilized person, can still come into contact with one's own life force unfiltered and direct. Other than that, one lives an inhibited life on "simmer" – as far as spontaneity, *joie de vivre*, and desire are concerned. To those tempted to preach the sexual revolution as a solution: this cannot lead very far, for the reasons given, because sexuality remains an island even if its extent is magnified, say by granting it greater meaning in one's own life; the "ocean of alienation" will still surround the sexual island. This is why many of the attitudes of the sexual revolutionaries were so odd and unconvincing.

If we now turn to mankind's beginnings, we get much new and valuable information regarding perception of the life force. The human race had different problems in its early stages than it has now. Back then, the most important issue was sheer survival. We observe in primitive cultures a much greater openness to energetic phenomena than today among us. In fact, for primitive hunters, having an expanded sensorium was a survival necessity. Good hunters feel a psychoenergetic bond with their prey, calling it their hunting instinct. This is likely a real phenomenon, not superstition. The famous cave paintings of the wild game of stone-age hunters seem to us like naïve, credulous magic – but they derive from the knowledge that the animals painted are thereby "half caught energetically" and thus easier to hunt down.[18]

Animals, by the way, are energetically extremely open – in the wild, anyway. Among domestic animals, openness seems to decline as neuroses set in and internal emotional conflicts block the energy flow. Because of their unblocked energy flow, the cancer rate among wild animals is much lower. Their energetic openness allows them to perceive the Aura of other creatures. This is easy to confirm by reaching out to touch an animal's Aura and observing the animal's reaction. Practically all animals sense the Aura and exhibit appropriate reactions when

the surroundings allow a free energy flow, i.e. when a calm, friendly and relaxed atmosphere prevails.

In earlier times, life was generally calmer and more relaxed. For that reason alone, subtle-body energy was sensed by significantly more persons than in our stimulus-saturated modern world. Calmness wasn't the only reason, of course; there were also special techniques taught in secret cults. The esoteric teachings of ancient Egypt, with its targeted use of energetic forces such as pyramid energy, demonstrate that, in the ancient high cultures, knowledge of energetic phenomena was central to their understanding of the world. The same applies to acupuncture in ancient China, or traditional medicine in India *(Siddha, Unani-Tibb, Ayurveda)*, in which subtle-body energy provides the key to true understanding.

Subtle-body energy plays a great role in the West as well. In the Middle Ages, cathedrals were built on top of former heathen places of worship because the strong energy fields emanating from them favored inner collectedness. Of course, the Christian builders were also saying, with their choice of location, that Jesus was superior to the earlier idols. Yet the medieval people did also know about the extremely strong *geomantic zones* over which the heathen places of worship had once been built – because the baptismal font and the pulpit locations were chosen with extraordinary accuracy, as investigations using dowsers have shown time and again. At these concentrated energy zones, it is much easier to enter into a meditative state and perform religious rituals with the requisite ardor. These are what are known as *areas of power*. This applies as well, by the way, to pyramids, whose true significance is revealed only after one has allowed them to exercise their energetic effect. The strong energetic radiation of the Cheops pyramid or the Chartres cathedral is the reason why these structures exert such a tremendous fascination on us.

I learned more about the **energetic effect of ancient heathen places of worship** from a patient, a geobiologist, who had explored the Oracle of Delphi in Greece. Underneath the present-day sacrificial altar, partially reconstructed and open to the public, his dowsing rod found an enormously strong geobiological zone. In his

---

[18] I suspect that, like primeval man, the aborigines probably live more in the so-called *emotional body* than modern "rational man" does ("head cases," as the idiom has it – or stylized head/foot creatures, as many children so correctly draw us!) By the by, this explains the *dreamtime* of which the aborigines tell, in which they claim mostly to live – or to have lived, that is, before they succumbed to the white man's drugged and alcoholized nightmare-time and were delivered into the present-day aborigine underdog existence. The emotional body is also said to permit *Out Of Body Experiences* (OOBE), e.g. telepathy, time travel and such. The discussion of the emotional body will come later; I just mention it here because it's thematically part of the aborigine subject. By the way, *hunting magic* really does work, according to numerous eyewitness accounts, and was almost certainly known to the cavemen painters.

words, this area of power was "the strongest one in his life!" Evidently the area of power's strong energy had been crucial to the Oracle's effect. That he had instinctively found this externally so unsightly and inconspicuous zone simply astonished the local guide ("Who told you the secret?") – because, prior to a frightful earthquake a long time ago, the original Oracle had stood on this inconspicuous site, said the guide. Of course, tourists are not told about this deception.

With the ascendancy of modern science, knowledge of the life force has faded into obscurity, as I have shown in detail. However, the so-called "simple folk" never forgot subtle-body energy. Much traditional knowledge at first looks like absurd superstition. Think about the familiar story of the stork bringing babies. Few people today realize that there's more to this stork tale than we might think. We know that storks build their nests on houses that are free, in a wide radius, of geopathic stress zones; this is exactly what the stork tale is trying to tell us, because geopathic stress zones are a common cause of infertility. Therefore, the number of storks is related to the number of children in an area. The townsfolk noticed, quite correctly, that particularly many babies are born in houses with stork nests.

A typical example from my daily practice that makes clear the fateful (and often unrecognized) influence of geopathic stress zones in cases of infertility follows:

Ms. W., a 25-year-old salesclerk, is a lovely, slim and sporty woman who has been vainly trying for quite a while to get pregnant. Her problem is a hormone-producing tumor of the pituitary gland (hypophysis), which had been surgically removed 5 years ago. Ever since, she has had to swallow a varied mix of hormone tablets to make up for the hormonal deficit. At the university clinic, they explain to her that experience has shown that women with this disease seldom if ever get pregnant, so she should simply give up wanting children.

But the feisty Ms. W. is not content with that. She asks me if I can come up with any other options. I suggest energy testing, and I find a geopathic stress zone burden in the pelvic region (a homeopathic test ampoule for this reacts in the pelvic region). I suggest that she hire a good dowser, who indeed finds a severe burden in the pelvis.

He recommends that she change the location of her bed.

Since I never make any arrangements of any kind, nor pass on any information, before an investigation, with the dowsers I work with – and since the dowser does not ask about the patient's symptoms – the results are always more surprising. But I can confirm, from years of experience, that my suppositions and the dowser's results agree to about 95%. After an examination of the bed site, a good dowser can almost always recite the patient's ailments off the top of his head!

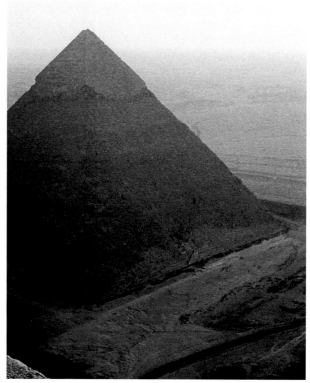

Cheops pyramid, built ca. 2500 BCE

I prescribe for Ms. W. a homeopathic-herbal compound preparation (with Agnus castus, *or Chaste tree) to harmonize the female hormonal cycle. A year and a half later, I received a photo of a beaming mother. She had, against all expectation, become pregnant!*

Modern man's problem is that we have largely forgotten how to perceive energetic phenomena. This applies especially to so-called **geopathic stress zones**, which have to do with a change in the earth's subtle-body force field. An enormous number of people don't sleep well and feel exhausted, without knowing the reason for their problems. Following the conventional wisdom, they assume their sleeplessness and morning lethargy is caused by stress – or else pin the blame on conflicts with people close to them, or private worries. When it comes to restless children with concentration problems, parents tend to think of excessive TV watching or food preservatives, wasting not a single thought on geopathic stress zones. Yet they often overlook the main reason why their child is grouchy in the morning and can't concentrate in school! The next chapter deals with the significance of subtle-body energy in everyday life. I'll return, in more detail, to the topic of geopathic stress zones and tell how to recognize bad locations – with some advice on how to find a good location.

Amazingly, most people are sensitive to subtle-body vibrations. With proper training of their sixth sense, they can perceive the slightest changes of their energy field, even if they had previously not noticed anything for years. **This means that perceiving energetic phenomena is trainable. With a little training,** more than 95% of all people are able to carry out simple psychoenergetic tests (Kinesiology, dowsing rods, pendulums, Aura sensing). Perception of energy as such, and in contact with others, can also be trained and enormously enhanced.

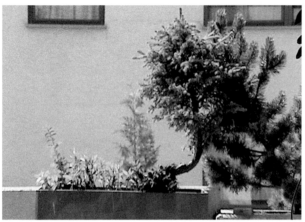

The small pine on our balcony, by growing sideways, is trying to evade a disturbance zone. Weeds grow on the disturbed site, and ants are seen there over and over (both typical signs of disturbance zones).

I note in myself, and others in situations like mine, a remarkable ambivalence that runs parallel to the finer perception of energetic phenomena and leads to strange, opposing sensations and observations. On the one hand, the coarseness of the environment often drives those who are more receptive to subtle-body energies to sheer desperation. This is particularly so for the dull insensitivity of many people, leading such people to adopt a "Prince(ss) and the Pea" attitude. Eventually, sensitives begin to get upset by a fly on the wall. Luckily, there are also opposing tendencies – for greater vitality means that one can accomplish much more and endure much more. Therefore, on the one hand, one becomes more sensitive and even hypersensitive, but on the other hand more vital and capable.

There are of course special cases where people who are just naturally larger than life and extremely vital scarcely notice an energy increase, but instead fidget all the more with their nerve-sapping sensitivity, which they downright curse. At the opposite extreme are former shrinking violets whose increase in sensitivity is barely noticeable. Instead, they have problems with the driving force of their new-found vitality. However, the most important cause for the problems of sensitive and energetically open people is not so much whether they're based not so much on whether they're hypersensitive or, on the contrary, incapable of being "too dynamic." The core problem almost always has to do with unresolved emotional conflicts. As soon as they are eliminated and broken up, they feel "really good" again.

Also in interpersonal contact one finds similarly opposing and confusing experiences. If, prior to one's "becoming energetically aware," other people seemed congenial, this presumed congeniality is not really sincere in many cases, and doesn't reflect the actual situation. Possibly the congeniality consists merely of a subconscious projection, an attempt to gain social prestige or suchlike. Once one becomes more sensitive and energetically more open, one can no longer stand such people. One feels them to be intolerable "energy vacuum cleaners" or insensitive contemporaries that get horribly on one's nerves. This is contrasted with other experiences where previously overlooked persons take on a new significance and esteem. One suddenly notices how much energetic vitality and sensitivity quite ordinary people have, that previously one would not have thought them capable of. Before, one was simply too blind to see how friendly and open the bus driver, the cleaning lady, the salesclerk are at the core of their being.

Increasing energetic openness initiates various highly unusual phenomena that manifest a kind of consciousness and self-dynamism of energy. Practically all people who have experienced these opening-up processes tell of miraculous coincidences that accumulate in the most unlikely manner. C.G. JUNG calls it *Synchronicity* . As soon as we tap into the flow of psychoenergy, changes begin to take place in and around us that seem downright improbable to outsiders. More and more miracles happen! Evidently, the resonance for previously hidden qualities and occurrences in us and our environment is elevated. In a kind of magnetism or amplifier effect, subconscious processes are so amplified and concentrated that coincidences pile up.

When you know that these unlikely-seeming coincidences are a kind of **resonance**, the situation becomes clearer. It has long been known that **energy follows mental attention**. There were examples of this in the previous chapter. This aspect of energy, which reaches up into the spiritual, could well be the main reason why the phenomena described in the previous chapter took place – say, in the sense of emotional transmittal. In the same manner, the Indian medicine man uses symbols to transmit healing energy. The symbols concentrate and amplify psychoenergy. As "courier" for the transport of healing energy to the patient, the shaman calls upon helpful spirits to assist him. The effectiveness of the ceremony is based on the fact that the energy goes where the healer's attention directs it.

When we modern naturopaths deal with energy, as a rule we no longer do so directly, but rather use energetic procedures. Among the best-known healing methods of energy medicine are acupuncture and homeopathy. Empirically, these methods are always only as good as the therapist applying them – since, independently of any technique and procedure, the physician uses subtle-body energy to heal even if he is totally unaware of it. The more energetically open and energetically trained a healer is, the greater his healing success will be. Actually, the therapist doesn't heal: nature does. The healer is merely a channel through which healing energy flows. Thus, the physician is only the assistant of a greater force and wisdom latent in nature itself.

Subtle-Body Energy –
Everyday Significance and Testing

It is very important for us to be well acquainted with our own subtle-body energy and to be able to manage it intelligently. I have already mentioned that no other factor is as important to quality of life. I am here of course assuming that basic needs, such as food, sleep, shelter are met, as well as freedom from enervating ailments or strong emotional burdens, thus permitting a state of normality. Starving people or those with tuberculosis of course first need food, antibiotics and a lot of rest. Those being harassed at work or suffering from other emotional stress factors of course need to eliminate first these burdens before trying to get on an even keel energetically. I don't consider subtle-body energy to be a panacea for all conceivable problems, but rather a "master key" once basic needs are satisfied and the goal is a decent quality of life – or even really good and permanent *joie de vivre*.

If we take a look around at today's industrialized nations, we are forced to note the frightful fact that a relatively high percentage of the population is energetically weak and thus potentially sick. A clairvoyant once told me that, on the subway, he noticed to his horror that most of the passengers had considerable energetic disturbances. My energy tests on healthy volunteers rarely yield normal, healthy results – and if they do, it's mostly happy, healthy children, or the truly few people who lead an energetically conscious life. In recent years, I have been noticing more such people, so I'm very optimistic that the number of spiritually highly developed and energetically open people will continue to grow in the near future.

The main reason for poor energy states is, as I see it, the manifold burdens we are subjected to. Geopathic stress zones and subconscious emotional burdens are the most significant of these. Helping one recognize one's own emotional burdens and offering solutions for their healing is the main goal of this book). There are also an abundance of other stress factors that inhibit and damage our subtle-body energy. Geopathic stress zones and electrosmog are important damage factors that one should be aware of – but there are also a number of other burdens whose importance often goes unrecognized.

It might sound bewildering at first that just about everything can have an influence on our subtle-body energy system. Because the life force is all *around us* as well as *within us*, we are swimming in an energy ocean in which all participants and objects are networked together. Like a fish in water, we are swimming around in an ocean of life force. Just as fish are forced at some point to swallow tiny current-borne traces of the garbage we have dumped in the far reaches of the oceans, so too does everything influence our body's energy. Still, there are huge differences between the consequences of, say, peeing in the ocean and dumping overboard highly toxic substances such as mercury compounds.

The fact that even the tiniest of burdens can throw a pre-sensitized person off-kilter is, of course, another matter entirely. The principal causes of such pre-sensitization are almost always subconscious emotional conflicts that destabilize their victims even in a resting state. It only takes the smallest stress for such people to slip into horrifying disease and ailment states. I am thinking here of the legions of people who are made ill by preservatives, electrosmog and pesticides. As a rule, they are already extremely psychoenergetically sick even in the absence of the suspect substances. They then completely lose their balance when the least burden is added, which is then taken to be the main cause. We have now arrived at the core of the basic problem that permeates all work with subtle-body energy. It is: "**What is important and what is not** (or only of secondary importance)? What must be changed to heal the sick (or to prevent the healthy from becoming ill)?"

Before listing the most important influences that affect us energetically in our daily lives, I'd first like to present some common testing methods, because subtle-body energy is undetectable to most people. We therefore need tests as amplifiers, to make subtle-body energy visible. In my experience, anyone can learn these procedures and make practical use of them. Depending on sensitivity and talent, some may pick it up faster than others, but eventually it almost always works. People with great emotional blocks, severe muscle cramps, and/or considerable emotional resistance need to eliminate these blocks first, before they can do any energy testing.

In the so-called muscle test (**Kinesiology**), for the basic position the arm is extended out to the side horizontally. The tester attempts to push the arm down, exerting a gentle yet constant force. If the arm has been weakened by some incident, this signifies a **test reaction**. The test reaction means that the test subject's energy system is indicating a stress, like a red alarm indicator light. The arm's becoming weak says: "What you are doing to me is stressing me out!"

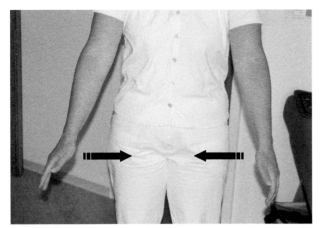

1. Bringing the outstretched hands together (in this photo, the therapist is demonstrating a self-test as she observes her own reaction).

2. Evaluation: On the left a neutral (negative) test reaction (arms the same length), on the right a positive test reaction (arms different lengths).

Other easily-learned methods include pendulum swinging and dowsing rods. Physicians and therapists make use of methods such as electroacupuncture and other measurement procedures at acupuncture points (Mora, Vegatest, and so on) or NOGIER's pulse diagnosis.

I personally recommend a variation of Kinesiology in which one extends the arms out diagonally at approximately a 45° angle to each other, then brings them back together while pulling lightly on the arms. It sometimes work best if one doesn't pull on the arms at all, but rather simply brings them together. Beginners tend otherwise to "pull away" the test reaction. The whole process looks to the uninitiated like a kid's kindergarten game – or like you're trying to teach the test subject how to clap hands by grasping the wrists and then bringing them together. While bringing the hands together, note the position of the thumbs, because when there is a test reaction, the thumbs will noticeably (1/2 to several cm) change their position relative to one another. A test reaction means that the test subject has become stressed (the energy system is reacting to something, either the test or something else you're wanting to check). In a certain sense, you get the feeling during a positive test reaction that the arms are different in length. The test is quite objective, not very interference-prone and not too tiring.

I am often asked where the different arm length comes from. In my opinion, the test reaction begins in both sides of the brain, each of which holds one of the body halves under constant muscular tension. Think of a coachman guiding a two-horse team with reins kept as equally taut as possible: the

two horses correspond to arm lengths. If the brain gets stressed, maintaining the same even muscular tension in both arms will be harder, like horseflies distracting the coachman. Therefore, the test reaction in an energy test is above all a phenomenon whose outcome takes place in the brain.

Critics are fond of objecting that energy testing with dowsing rods or Kinesiology involves eidomotor movements. One sees this in twitching or other negligible tics and tremors that, in the opinion of these critics, are being over-interpreted. I admit that meaningless movements in the sense of involuntary eidomotor motions can occur. These are usually found with beginners or people under mental strain, as when critics or skeptics watch a dowser at work.

The biggest obstacle to the acceptance of subtle-body testing procedures is their lack of objectifiability. Now, this does not mean that the converse is true, namely that such procedures are purely subjective! As long as we perform the procedures with a basic attitude of relaxed openness, and concentrate, they almost always yield good to excellent results. I mentioned that my results and those of my dowser agree 95% of the time; similarly high percentage values are also found in medical contexts. Things start to fall apart if we become mistrustful; that is when big testing errors accumulate.[19] **Mistrust is pure poison for energy testing!** Therefore, anyone who performs it with a skeptical attitude – which is of necessity a given in scientific experiments – is guaranteed to fail. One needs to know this in order not to succumb to error.

---

[19] I have noticed an above-average quota of compulsive types among the critics of energy testing. Compulsives are by nature mistrustful, insisting on a detailed "User's Manual" for everything in life – but this just isn't possible for spontaneous and intuitive phenomena such as energy testing. As soon as a compulsive begins to doubt the correctness of the examination, testing errors will multiply, in turn magnifying the doubt. In the end, the test becomes totally ineffective, thanks to subconscious sabotage triggered by a hypercritical attitude.

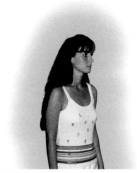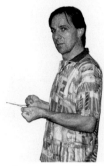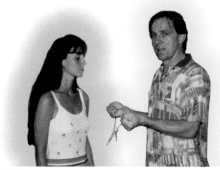

The dowsing rod (the author's in this photograph) dips as soon as the energy fields come in contact

Basically, I believe that everybody should master and use some testing technique or other, regardless of occupation. This applies especially to sensitive and energetically open persons, since, if they haven't mastered an energy test, they're like blind people in a labyrinth! Because energy tests are the simplest and best way to find out about, say, the energetic quality of a particular food or bed location or medication. It has been shown that energetic tests provide very reliable and valuable information, not otherwise available so quickly and easily.

When we test medications, the procedure is called a remedy test. Normally, the basic principle of Kinesiology is demonstrated with the counteracting food substances salt and sugar. A sugar cube in a bodybuilder's hand can be enough to cause him to lose all his strength in a few seconds, and the extended arm will be like pudding, and can be pushed down effortlessly. But if we give our bodybuilder the antipolar substance salt (a saltshaker, for instance), his arm will immediately be strong again. There are thus fortifying and debilitating factors – but they are not necessarily the same for each test subject.

How we react depends crucially on what our "polarity" is – like a battery, we can react antipolarly. As the saying has it: "One man's meat is another man's poison." In acupuncture, we call the polarities Yin and Yang. It can happen that another testee (other than our bodybuilder) will react quite differently to a substance (like sugar) and his arm will remain strong. What enervates one person can invigorate the antipolar type. This can be illustrated with the metals gold and silver: there are gold and silver types. The significance of this will become clearer later on, in the discussion of the autonomic nervous system (ANS). By the way, time of day also plays a role, so that test results can vary depending on constitution and time of day.

If we ban sugar consumption for every patient who reacts to it in an energy test, then we have fallen prey to the error in reasoning of the **pseudo test reaction**: we promote a minimal stress to the pathological. In my experience, many allegedly allergenic substances (wheat, sugar, milk, gluten) give an indication only because they are responding to this digestive stress. In reality, many patients have no intolerances or allergies whatever. Often, the underlying cause is an energetic disturbance due to subconscious emotional conflicts. Besides that, there are many people with poor intestinal flora full of fermentative and putrefactive bacteria, causing the intestinal tract to react hypersensitively. A simple **acclimation test** can determine whether a substance is truly harmful. You wait a few minutes with the patient holding the substance in one hand. When you test after the familiarization period, almost all substances will now test neutral and no longer show any test reaction. On the other hand, if there is a genuine allergy or intolerance, the body does not get used to the substance.

Basically, I'd like to advise every energy tester not to overrate test reactions. It takes a lot of practice and experience to separate the wheat from the chaff. Many testers resort to imagining something along the lines of a quality scale or formulated questions such as "good / bad," which are then checked out. This is so-called virtual testing, in which one mentally pictures a scale, for example, and then asks oneself: "How severe is this disease in percent?" Or: "How debilitating is this toxin in percent?" This very often leads to considerable error, because most people lack the concentration and inner collectedness needed for good results. I therefore recommend estimating the harmfulness of a factor (such as a geopathically disturbed location) or a substance (such as a medication) based on the change in how a person feels who is exposed to it. One develops, amazingly quickly, a feeling for which factors are detrimental (or beneficial) and in which manner, and can draw conclusions from this.

Let us now address the factors that burden our subtle-body energy system the most, and with which one should thus be familiar. The commonest and most harmful environmental influence is the pathological location factor *geopathic stress zone* or *geopathy*. **Geopathic stress zones are among the most important triggers of carcinosis!** Geopathic stress zones do not of themselves cause cancer, but they do make it much easier for it to occur. It is thus not a risk factor in the traditional sense (such as smoking cigarettes), but is instead a stress that impairs or inhibits cellular repair of genetic damage. If I have no genetic burdens or damage, geopathic stress zones will not increase my cancer risk. This is why there will always be cases where people remain healthy despite being exposed to geopathies. But the stronger my genetic cancer predisposition, the more I smoke and so on, the more genetic damage will occur – which, in the presence of geopathic stress zones, will be repaired ever more poorly until a cancer develops.

Many people puzzle over the processes that play a role in geopathic stress zones. I don't claim to know in detail what is going on; still, my study of the available technical literature, discussions with competent researchers, and my own experiments have led me to some very reasonable hypotheses. Geopathic vibrations are modulated upon the earth's magnetic field and cosmic rays. They are sources of a laser-like radiation whose strong structure disrupts membrane-potential-based intercellular communication that makes use of environmental background noise (chaotic noise) to transmit its signals correctly. But if a physicist tries to measure geo-radiation, he'll turn up nothing outside of a few minimal deviations, because the signals to be measured are masked by the measuring instruments' intrinsic noise level (these include minuscule changes in atmospheric ionization and magnetic field). Since geopathic stress zones are not directly graspable materially, but rather represent information, they are of course much harder to verify and measure physically.

Cellular repair seems to be much more easily disrupted by highly-structured geo-radiation, which makes carcinosis significantly more likely. On the other hand, in geo-radiation-free locations, the aforementioned chaotic noise predominates that does not impede intercellular contact. These processes are best compared to a radio: if the radio is tuned to the static (noise) between stations, we can carry on a conversation – but not if it's tuned to a talk show. The cells evidently need and like a chaotic energy environment, and the more structured and ordered energy becomes, the worse it is for the cells ("Chaos good, order bad."). Applied **chaos theory** has been able to verify something like this for a number of diseases. For example, the spasmodic *synchronous* discharge of large numbers of brain cells triggers an epileptic seizure. There is a greater risk of a sudden fatal heart attack in the presence of *ordered*, non-chaotic cardiac dysrhythmia.

Besides cell repair, geopathic stress zones disturb the body's entire energetic system. The specific information of various different geo-radiations plays an important role in the genesis of many diseases. For example, there seem to be specific geo-radiations for specific diseases, such as lattice systems at earth fissures for multiple sclerosis, and many other geo-radiation patterns that are specific for cancer. Rural inhabitants who can look back over entire generations know about "cancer beds," in which all family members who sleep there for any length of timeget cancer.

In general, women are much more sensitive to geopathic stress zones than men. This is because the female Yin structure reacts more strongly to the geo-radiation's predominant Yin principle. Generally speaking, women in our culture are much more open to subtle-body energies. Most patients who are unaware of their geopathic stress zone burden are men. I believe this is a very important, totally overlooked reason for the shorter life expectancy of males vis-à-vis females – because if men don't realize how much their own bed location damages their energy system, then they'll hardly do better in dealing with other risk factors. Many heavy smokers, alcoholics, workaholics, and those who take psychoactive drugs (such as tranquilizers) never notice their geopathic stress zone burden. Of course, they likewise fail to notice the constant energy damage to and overexertion of their regulatory systems caused by their unhealthy lifestyle.

If one has a geopathic stress zone burden, only its elimination will restore health. The bed must be moved to a radiation-free location – shielding mats (all of them) are useless! Therefore, every energetic and naturopathic treatment should begin with the clarification of geopathy. This is most simply done with the aid of a geopathy test ampoule (Geovita© – a homeopathic compound remedy[20]) that I developed for global testing of geopathies. With this, you can diagnose very reliably. When patients have a geopathic stress zone burden, their arm will weaken when the test ampoule is put in their hand and arm strength is tested kinesiologically.

If you want to test a bed location, you can perform a very quick and reliable test on the spot. You first kinesiologically test the patient's arm strength before he lies down. After a ten-minute lie-down, the strongest muscleman's arm will test out quite weak if the bed is in a geopathic stress zone. So you can tell right off whether the energy system has been weakened and made long-term sick by a bad bed location. Another option is to simply move the bed 3–6 feet, or into another room, to see if, after a few weeks, the patient now sleeps better and feels fresher in the morning. It usually takes 3–4 weeks for the geo-radiation impregnation to fade away. If the Geovita test ampoule no longer evokes a response and the patient feels markedly better, then the geo-

---

[20] Available from Geovita – cf. Appendix

pathic stress zone problem has been solved. Now and then, strong terrestrial movements (caused by earthquakes or heavy street-building machinery) will temporary alter the bed-site situation. However, this seldom lasts long, because the original situation usually reasserts itself.

Basically, there are bad, neutral, and good locations. The latter are places that enable unbelievably deep regeneration and recuperation during sleep. Many people recall farmhouse beds in the mountains, where they slept like logs and woke up totally refreshed. In these good locations, our energy values rise markedly as we literally "fill 'er up" energetically. Good ascends to *extremely good* at locations of power and of healing, where the energy is frequently so strong that, over the long run, one can even get sick again due to energetic overcharging. The same goes, by the way, for many magnet pads and energizing disks that, if used for too long, supply more energy than is good for us. I therefore reject all artificial energy amplifiers, which includes copper bracelets and the like!

Electrosmog also plays a significant morbific role, although its contribution is greatly overrated by the critics of electromagnetic pollution – while those who would have us believe that electrosmog from cell phones, transmitter antennas, high-tension lines, and so on, plays no role whatsoever go to the opposite extreme. As so often, the truth lies somewhere in the middle. Based on dowsers' experiences, the electrical field's 50Hz (60Hz USA) frequency induces a subtle long-lasting contraction of (for example) the neck musculature when clock radios or other electrical devices are situated closer than one yard from the head end of the body: the musculature mistakes the electrical field for nerve impulses.

Many patients work in front of a computer screen all day and are surrounded by countless other electronic devices with high-voltage static fields (up to several thousand volts!). At night, these patients then lie down in iron-frame beds that act as antennas for numerous radio waves and static electrical charges, with clock radios and nightstand lamps at the head end. Even metal eyeglass frames often act as antennas, as do dental braces and other electrically conducting parts (such as fillings). Because of their electrical heating systems, waterbeds are extremely potent sources of electrosmog stress. To make matters worse, the latticework of iron reinforcing rods in the concrete ceilings of today's homes amplifies electromagnetic waves. One recommended measure is installing AC power disconnect switches in bedrooms; also recommended: maintain a large distance from high-tension lines, substations, and overhead electrical cabling for trolleys and trains.

In my experience, electricity is only marginally responsible for carcinosis. Children, with their sensitive and still growing organism seem to be an exception. Infantile cancer in particular seems to occur more frequently in the vicinity of high-tension lines, as has been shown in a number of studies. At any rate, electricity is indeed harmful to the autonomic nervous system, even if it no longer triggers cancer in adults. In my opinion, single-frequency vibrations are especially harmful. Many therapists work with signal generators and test out which frequency the patient needs. Some also make use of fixed vibrational patterns (e.g., Hulda CLARK) in order to ostensibly heal diseases such as cancer and eliminate parasites from the body. I am not convinced that such procedures deliver long-lasting and truly curative results. I therefore recommend relying less on experts and more on one's inner voice and how (good or bad) one feels, when applying these kinds of electrical therapies

Cell phones are particularly bad in that they upset the entire energy system. The disruptive effect persists even after they are switched off, so it is recommended to transport cell phones at a distance of at least 50cm from the body and use them only in emergencies. Those whose job requires their use should at least use a speakerphone setup and choose a low-emission model (lists of wattage ratings for various makes and models are available from consumer protection groups). Cell phones, pagers, and beepers all seem to have a disruptive effect. Noise or interference suppression measures do nothing to reduce electromagnetic pollution: the transmitted wattage is not reduced at all. On the other hand, many interference suppressor chips can have an energetically attenuating effect. Trusting in this (and, moreover, spending a lot of money in the process) seems to me justified only if one absolutely has to use a cell phone a lot. In quartz watches the built-in battery is a factor.

Buccal currents from amalgam fillings – or, less often, other metals (usually metal denture brackets) – are disruptive in two ways: first by increasing the release of heavy-metal ions that are then carried away to be swallowed and thereby ingested; and second through the proximity of vegetative control centers to the upper palate. These highly sensitive vegetative centers (hypothalamus) react at least as sensitively to electrical disturbances as computer chips. Many patients, who were much improved after the buccal-current batteries were removed, can attest to this.

Personally, the influence of nature, architecture and interior furnishings in Chinese **Feng Shui** has always seemed downright strange to me. Many of its tenets seem very artificial, too rigid and static – but this could just be my personal prejudice. Still, it should be welcomed that Feng Shui promotes sensitivity toward energetic aspects. Basically, energetically healthful architecture leads to a house that keeps us in a happy mood and lifts our spirits. At the same time, it should not create any energy blocks, such as a calamitous latticework of iron reinforcing rods in a concrete ceiling that acts as an amplifier for geo-radiation. When we feel good at home and even a prolonged stay doesn't disturb us or "bring us down," then the energetic situation is very likely OK. The best case is for our home to be a power location where we can recuperate and recharge our energy reserves.

Clothing has an effect on our energy state that is often underestimated. Dark clothing lets in exogenous vibrations and lowers our own. Black mourning clothes are viewed as a symbol of depression and of voluntarily remaining in a state of sadness, but also of openness to consolation and sympathy. In the extreme case, black absorbs all environmental vibrations, while at the same time not letting any endogenous vibrations out – an "energy vacuum-cleaner " effect. For the same reasons, dark clothing is warming. White and light-colored clothing, on the other hand, raises endogenous vibrations and blocks external ones. In addition, white clothing lets out healing vibrations, which is why medical personnel are usually clad in white.

In my experience, it also matters which colors are worn in which layer of clothing. Dark underclothing absorbs foreign energy much more strongly than outer layers do, which is why sexy lingerie is very often of a dark color. In a sexual situation, energy exchange is of course desirable – which is almost always not true of everyday life, where we would rather be shielded from disruptive foreign energies. In general, therefore, one is best advised to wear white underwear for its shielding properties. Dark outer clothing, on the other hand, is energetically less harmful (dark pullover, etc.). Silk and Gore-Tex® act like light-colored materials, in that they let out endogenous energy while shielding exogenous ones. Cotton is neutral, whereas nylon-type synthetics (older synthetic fibers that hold a static charge) often act (on me, at least) like dark materials do.

Scents, with their links to the deepest, evolutionarily oldest parts of the brain (reptilian brain), are closely tied to strong emotions, sexuality and instincts. Scents are also related to karmic memories, as they store particularly old memories. Scents have a much more profound effect than other sensory modalities. Psychoneuroimmunology has been able to show the great significance of scents when it comes to partner selection. Based on scent, women instinctively select the partner best suited to them. By means of the major histocompatibility genes (genetically preformed markers on the surface of the cell), by which self/other can be identified, the sense of smell evidently entices us into especially good couplings. Interestingly, partner selection fails if the woman is taking birth-control pills – which vividly illustrates what fine antennae we can unwittingly turn off.

Perfumes "attract" because the force field of the perfume-wearer shrinks, making the person seem easier to conquer, more vulnerable, erotic and friendly. Essential oils have a particularly strong relationship to the subtle-body energy system and the energy centers (Chakras). The more pleasant a scent is to us, the more harmonious it is for our energy system. In my experience, resinous scents in particular have a generally enlivening, harmonizing, and cleansing effect (e.g., tree resin, myrrh, and frankincense). I'll return to essential oils in greater detail in the discussion of energy centers (Chakras).

Jewelry has different effects (depending on polarity and kind), and many precious stones such as quartz can be energetically charged up. To charge quartz, place it first in bright sunlight for a while and then on ailing body regions. After 15 minutes, the absorbed disease energies can be discharged by rinsing the quartz in running water. Since crystals can preserve negative vibrations, I am generally quite skeptical and cautious with them. Of course, one's own sensitivity and energy reserves are crucial to being able to cope with disturbances of this sort. This applies especially to used jewelry: I would always advise cleaning this kind of jewelry thoroughly, then rinsing it for a long time in running water.

Crystals in particular are a two-edged sword. Besides their beneficial effects, crystals can also have harmful ones. This can be the case, for example, if they are absolutely unsuited to the patient or are charged up with harmful energies. In this context, I can relate a personal experience that clearly illustrates the possibly devastating influence of precious stones:

At a seminar, I once bought a piece of tiger's eye crystal and put it in my upper left coat pocket. I sat in a circle with some other attendees and listened to a lecture. After about half an hour, I felt dreadful and threatening stabbing cardiac pains and a constricted feeling. In a flash, all the buried hypochondriac fears of the experienced physician welled up in me. I thought it might be an imminent cardiac infarction (which had claimed both of my grandfathers), and I lived through some agonizing minutes. I thought feverishly about how to get to a hospital as inconspicuously as possible. While stroking the region – as one does involuntarily during heart attacks – I hit a big bump: the cherry-sized tiger's eye! I placed it to the side at a distance and the cardiac symptoms ended in five minutes. Despite my initial skepticism that the tiny piece of rock could conjure up such dramatic effects, it did just that!

By the way, I have experienced similar incidents with patients now and again. If a piece of jewelry tests out bad and the patient puts it away, many symptoms disappear as if by magic! Skeptics might think I am imagining things, but I am convinced that these are due to actual energetic effects. After all, in secret societies, crystals have always been known to store up and pass on energy. The latest example of there being a deeper truth in these claims is quartz and transistors in modern technology: here, too, one is dealing with crystals!

The general practitioner and geo-radiation researcher Ernst HARTMANN many times pointed out the **polar effect of Gold and Silver**. Some people are *gold* types and get charged up energetically by gold; others are *silver* types who will get weakened by gold. So you can't just recommend gold fillings for all patients , to replace harmful amalgam. The gold wedding band on the ring finger, by the way, helps stimulate the Circulation/Sexuality meridian. This seems to work independently of polarity. This stimulation of the Circulation/Sexuality meridian is said to ensure sexual potency and the fulfillment of "marital obligations."

Postures such as interlocking the arms behind the back shrink the force field much like the way perfume does. Adolf HITLER frequently made use of this minimizing posture to seem friendlier and more trusting, as if he were really just a shy, awkward, ingenuous person. By putting his aggressively active arms behind his back, he made his body language say "Why, I wouldn't hurt a fly." Yet it's precisely through postures and gestures that we betray what is really going on in us. The subtle-body energy system plays a great role in this, because it provides information about qualities such as sympathy or antipathy, strength or weakness, stimulation, or rejection.

In discussion groups and such, one will see that people sitting next to each other cross their legs in the same way. They then vibrate similarly and subconsciously express their sympathy to their neighbor. Of course, the opposite can also be observed, when opponents emphasize their hostility with a contrary posture. Therefore, anyone who carefully looks at the people around him can learn a great deal, from their body language, about their subtle-body constitution and psychoenergy. However, the HITLER example also illustrates the limits of this, because some people practice deliberate deception. Body language is fairly clumsy and direct, so that, with a little practice, one can misuse it to conceal and deceive.

Movements and postures, as well as **breathing techniques** have for ages been enormously profound ways to regulate energy. Chinese *Ch'i Gong* and shadowboxing are both based on the realization that gentle, flowing movement patterns increase energy. Indian *mudras*, specific (formerly occult) hand positions and signs, can channel and influence energy. Linking movements with positive/healing and spiritual thoughts charges up our overall energy. This applies especially to Indian Yoga and many forms of meditation. Entire healing systems and religions, as we know, build on this.

In particular, flowing and gentle movements ensure that life energy flows optimally. A completely unforced, comfortable and flowing feeling is crucial. Our movements must be accompanied by enjoyment and feeling good in order for the best possible effect to arise. We must never forget that, despite manipulative and prideful tendencies, subtle-body energy often flows better the less forced, more loose and free it is. This is why laughing and fun are so effective, making us feel freer and better than before. Many believe that reward can only come from sacrifice. Yet overly rigid and impatient effort throws away a lot of possibilities, since fun, enjoyment, and happiness are the best energy providers.

Stress, coercion, and pain, on the other hand, prevent energy from flowing!

Meditation systems are almost never checked out with respect to quality. Automobiles of various makes or commercial services are tested by product testing firms. This is fully in the consumer interest of the consumer, who wants the best product for his hard-earned money. In my opinion, this will also be possible in future for meditation systems, with the proper energetic measurement methods. One would then know right off which systems guarantee the most progress. My former partner and I have performed energy measurements on about a dozen people before and after Yoga sessions. Surprisingly, a third improved energetically (by about 10–20%), a third remained the same and the final third actually showed deterioration! After years in clinical practice, I can confirm that meditation doesn't benefit every practitioner every time. It's highly likely, moreover, that the type of meditation chosen plays a large role, and whether it matches the person's character type (more on this later in the chapter on types of therapy).

One is always meeting people who react hypersensitively to everything imaginable. I have had highly sensitive patients who, given the smallest possible homeopathic high potentiations, react as if an earthquake had hit them. In my experience, the true cause of this extreme hypersensitivity is often found in a substantial dysautonomia, behind which lie (very often) subconscious emotional problems. Instead of *neurasthenia* (weak nerves) or *vegetative dystonia* (autonomic nervous system disorder), the newer medical terminology refers to *somatoform disturbance* (incorporated or bodily disturbance). This means that a churned-up, disharmonically reacting nervous system can evoke all manner of bodily symptoms. A patient might thus complain of heart or lower-back pains, but in reality a disrupted nervous system is behind it all.

Most people (approx. 60–70%) with **hypersensitivity** are not spiritually highly developed, but rather simply neurotic. They will doggedly attempt to get you to buy the fairy tale of their spiritually advanced status – but experience has shown that their source of misery is themselves, since they have a disturbed ANS and many emotional conflicts. This makes them miserable, highly overwrought, and extremely sensitive. Because as soon as you calm down their high-strung ANS and melt away their conflicts, they become as normal as anyone else. In retrospect, their hypersensitivity turns out to be a figment of their imagination. Of course, they love to exploit their hypersensitivity as a means of exerting pressure to get special treatment. In medicine, we speak of a "disease benefit" that some patients extract from their status as sick person. For children, the disease benefit comes in the form of toys and extra TLC; it is a privilege for adults to be "put on the sick list" and be allowed to take it easy. The disease benefit also includes pensions and the attention and care of family members and one's doctor.

Hypersensitives also include many people suffering excessively from chemical toxins. Tragically, they often exhibit a rigid fixation on the purely environmental aspects that has downright dogmatic overtones. The inner emotional disturbance and problem is projected outward to evil chemistry, lurking everywhere and causing skin rashes, provoking headaches or shackling one – exhausted – to one's bed for days on end. In an American naturopathic magazine, I read about "Chemical Sensitivity Disorder – CSD" patients who live a life of isolation in remote desert regions of the USA. These victims of our modern high-tech civilization develop terrible day-long pain syndromes if, for instance, a farmer thirty miles away sprays his fields with chemicals while the wind is blowing toward the sufferer. This is no April Fool's gag. In their perplexity, doctors recommend this hermit lifestyle because they don't know what else to do to help the victims. In my experience, these people virtually always suffer from considerable emotional disturbances. These minuscule amounts of toxin are the straw that breaks the camel's back.

As to cause and effect, my experience has shown that when you have a disturbed nervous system, you have to seek out the primary disturbance cause (the patient often feels quite the opposite!). If you calm down the nervous system and cure the underlying emotional conflicts, many hypersensitives are quickly able to tolerate much more than before. This applies as well to a great many pain patients, and those who feel very badly for no discernible objective reason. Many paranormally talented patients also belong in this category: their ANS has become hypersensitized by chronic cramps. This facilitates the emergence in them of paranormal phenomena, such that their clairvoyance is an expression of their hyperstimulated nervous system.

Of course, not every highly sensitive person is automatically emotional disturbed and in a state of chronic ANS tension. There are also natural **sensitives** (as they are called) who are emotionally in fine shape. People with spiritually highly developed energy centers and open causal bodies are by nature highly sensitive, even if they had earlier (before their spiritual development) been robust average persons. There are thus two kinds of *sensitives*: those who are born that way and those who become so as part of their personality development. Both kinds generally know to which group they belong. Sensitives are recognizable in that they feel completely normal, at ease with themselves and content. Sensitives may have to endure the world (above all coarse and brutish people) but not themselves. This is not the case with those who are vegetatively disturbed, because their basic mood is predominantly negative and depressed.

In recent years, I have noted a sharp rise in the number of sensitives, particularly in children (so-called indigo children, supposedly with a violet Aura). These people have causal body readings, as measured by the REBA® Test Device, of 70% or greater. These sensitives' biggest problem is being misunderstood by their fellow man, since they represent a small minority: they are thought to be "cranks" and "weirdos." Children are branded as twitchy hyperkinetics or some such. Sadly, these (often highly talented) children don't fit in any of the conventional pigeonhole categories. Because most teachers are spiritually much less developed, they simply cannot understand such advanced children. When sensitives meet others like themselves, who have had the same experiences, the result is great emotional relief all around. It always surprises me how people on the same level of development get along and understand each other right off the bat; in no time at all, their minds are in tune with each other.

The quality of **food, air and water** is very important to energetic health. In my experience, there is a lot of misunderstanding when it comes to nutrition. Crucial – but often forgotten – is, it seems to me, the enjoyment that is a part of any meal. Food must taste good if it is to be well digested. As a rule, the more sunlight our food receives, the better it is for us. This is because the sun emits very high vibrations. Sunbathing is a very simple way to energize oneself. The higher one's energy level, the higher in quality one's nutrition needs to be. In particular nuts, high-grade spring water, and wild fruits are very good. I personally do not think too much of water purification devices: natural spring water is much better, even if it costs considerably more.

As for air quality, I recommend to all who would become energetically healthier to move to a place with cleaner **air**. Smog and cigarette smoke depress the overall vibrational level. Long walks in the woods or lakeshore and mountain hikes supply important subtle-body energy. As the altitude above sea level rises, so does the vibrational level, which is why monasteries and hermitages are often located at higher elevations. Therefore, mountain vacations are twice as healthy as seaside stays, since the energy is higher in the mountains.

The fact that the energetic radiation of foods has a clearly perceptible influence on our energy system is in all probability the origin of the saying "*You are what you eat.*" The energetic vibrational level of a food is an expression of its material quality – so high-grade food vibrates higher. Thus, as we progress spiritually, we get more sensitive when low-vibration foods "bring us down." On the other hand, there's the inverse phenomenon, in which our progress in spiritual development makes us more independent of external influences, whether it be nutrition or other influences.

In daily clinical practice, I have noticed time and again that many strict vegetarians quite often are, energetically and with respect to intestinal flora, much less healthy than the average person. Now, it might be that sicker people turn instinctively to vegetarianism – but that seems to be only one of the reasons. The real reason is likely that the diet of some vegetarians is too high in raw fruits and vegetables, which causes the intestinal contents to ferment and generate fusel oils that irritate the intestinal walls. Therefore, pre-cooked tasty fare – also well seasoned and good-tasting (such as Indian curry/curcuma) – is surely the most healthful. I'd also like to mention that whole grains (particularly wheat germ) contain natural antibiotics (phytins) that are extraordinarily hard to digest, and they have caused severe intestinal damage in animal experiments. One should therefore basically be very cautious about too much wheat germ and similar whole-grain products.

One of the most important sources of health is restful, recuperative **sleep**. In the discussion of geopathic stress zones, I've pointed out the importance of sound sleep. In my opinion, there are two main reasons for poor-quality sleep that make all other reasons negligibly secondary: the aforementioned geopathic stress zones, along with other structural biological problems (noise, filth, electrosmog...) and subconscious emotional conflicts. From a subtle-body standpoint, a good sleep is analogous to recharging a battery, by which means we regenerate our life-force reserves.

When it comes to **sexuality**, subconscious emotional conflicts have an immense significance that puts all other disrupting influences in the shade. I here characterize sexuality in its broadest sense as the ability to create enjoyment and psychophysical wellbeing relatively autonomously and self-determinedly. So, a quadriplegic or a monk could have a healthy sexuality as long as he manages, in this sense, to feel good and create contentedness and pleasure. Sexuality is a basic function, independent of the sexual organs, which can be defined as the capability for pleasurable, energetic self-regulation. Everything that, from an emotional standpoint, *truly* feels good and increases our wellbeing also increases our energy flow. In this sense, children also have sexuality – although, in children, sexuality is experienced almost completely separate from the sexual organs. Nevertheless, children do have sexuality, in that they enjoy themselves and constantly strive for wellbeing.

Our personal **life rhythm** plays a big role in our wellbeing. Many people feel their life is either too hectic or too monotonous, drifting either into crippling boredom or chronic hyperstress. But I believe that our achievement-obsessed society greatly undervalues inactivity. By *inactivity* I mean simply aliveness without having to do anything in particular. Many people lead a defiant life of constant struggle with their superego (the moral code instilled in us by our parents and society). The superego is what tells you that you must behave like this or do that in order to amount to anything. In this process, you can miss hearing the still, small voice inside that knows best what is good for you. Finding your own life rhythm means learning to listen to your inner voice. This is usually a tedious process that has no final answers and constantly necessitates new solutions.

The closing issue at the end of this chapter is, for me, how to stay as energetically healthy as possible. How can this succeed in view of a prevalently unhealthy lifestyle?

How can we maintain harmony when all around us emotional tensions prevail, with ever higher divorce rates, psychosomatic disorders, and diseases on the rise? I know many who are convinced that everything will inevitably continue to get worse. I, on the other hand, am one of those optimists that believes in a better future. Of course, much progress is incessantly wearisome, with many setbacks and struggles. Yet I believe – unlike many pessimists – that most people in the affluent industrialized regions have never had a better chance to lead an energetically healthy life as today. Never before in the history of mankind have there been so many opportunities for personal development. There is the option of satisfying sexuality without having to worry about off-spring. There are delicious foods and pure water. One can spread one's spiritual wings to a degree that has never been possible at any earlier time in human history.

The main reason that everyday life is nevertheless so unsatisfying and disappointing for most people so much of the time is, I believe, subconscious emotional conflicts. **Our inner frustrations get in our way and prevent us from leading a happy and meaningful life!** The more we listen to our inner voice, the more demanding will we be regarding our true needs – the less demanding with respect to pseudo-needs that only lie to and deceive us. We thus need to do something to gather up and dispose of our emotional garbage. Only then can we discern what it is we really want and who we really are. Undeniably, this is a lofty ambition. Surely we have not been put on this earth by divine wisdom to err cnstantly, forever floundering about and leading a dreary life. The quickest, best and most lasting way to personal enlightenment, the ability to know what is right and the vigor to do it, consists of clearing out our emotional garbage!

Before explaining in later chapters what is meant by "emotional garbage," I'd like to elucidate in this next chapter how energetic healing works. I'd also like to provide some supportive advice for energetic healing.

Magic and Energy Work

In all things of nature there is something of the marvelous.

(Aristotle)

It's natural for anyone whose business is healing to wonder how it is that nature can heal. How does nature do it, when a disease heals up and the battered body regenerates itself? In my opinion, that is above all due to the fact that life force intrinsically includes the notion of health. When the life force goes into action, the right things needed for healing automatically happen.[21] We can imagine life energy as a stimulating and vitalizing power permeated with intelligent concepts of health.

For example, we know from out-of-body excursions [OOBEs] during near-death experiences that blind persons can see and the deaf hear. As the soul hovers above the operating table, a patient blind from birth can see a tattoo on the surgeon's forearm; or a previously deaf person can suddenly recite in detail the surgeon's conversation with the scrub nurse. What may we conclude from this? Simply that, in reality, the health of their eyes and ears had never been lost, but simply stored away in the matrix of their personal life force – but the "healthy idea" contained within their subtle-body energy was not enough to repair the defective organs during their existence in the physical body. However, as soon as subtle-body energy leaves the physical body (… the soul hovers …), the deaf or blind person can once again respond in a healthy manner; there is no longer a defective organ hindering healthy, normal operation.

In the case of phantom pain, this is precisely the core of the problem! Here, the life force is desperately trying to resuscitate the amputated limb, resulting in pain similar to what we feel when thawing out frozen hands. Phantom pain is thus a self-healing attempt that cannot succeed, since the limb is gone. So the healing attempt goes around in circles and causes pain. In my estimation, in phantom pain cases you have to work with the Aura of the severed limb and get the energy flowing there again, while at the same time soothing the brain's pain regions (with subtle-body medications that heal Chakras and conflicts – this is covered in later chapters).

---

[21] We consider it a "miracle" when healing takes place with unexpected rapidity (after extremely large quantities of life force have been provided). The life force can sometimes overcome the inherent inertia of material processes, accelerating them enormously, so that suddenly all is well once again. Still, I am firmly convinced that miracles do happen, and that they are crucially dependent on belief. If I believe in miracles, then my life force can go about its work without hindrance. If I don't, the healing flow is blocked and cannot flow as needed.

Basically, two things are needed for healing:

1. **An ailing organ must be capable of regeneration if it is to regain its original state.**

2. **The quantity of supplied life energy must be enough for healing to begin.**

If a patient is too weak, energy must be supplied so that healing can take place. By "supplied energy" I mean food and fluids, if the patient has a deficiency of such, or other substances such as hormones, vitamins, and minerals (which can also be viewed as a kind of energy supply). But by "too weak" I also mean that it will often be necessary to help the patient from the outside in some other manner. This can include excision of inflammation foci, cancer nodules and such, or the use of chemical agents (allopathics) to combat pathogens. The patient's weakness is here the inability to regain health without external assistance. A doctor is usually called on these cases: sometimes a disease can't be beaten without bringing in the heavy artillery.

The following has to do with non-medical people also being able to help their fellow man by supplying healing energy. This is known as **energy work**, because providing the ailing person with enough life force is an extraordinarily important and helpful opportunity for the sufferer to be able to regain health. For incurable patients, energy work can see to it that they do not get any sicker by at least stabilizing the situation for as long as possible. Later on, I'll touch on a second healing option having to do with emotional conflicts that diminish and block life energy. But let me set that aside for now and first explain the main features of psychoenergetic healing.

Many people confuse **energy work** with **magic**, but these are completely different concepts, although they use essentially the same processes. Unlike magic, in energy work one has a different awareness of what should take place, and in what context it should act. Which of the two therapeutic methods one prefers depends primarily on one's level of Chakra development. Magic is a healing method of the lower Chakras, and so its effect is more destructive the more spiritually developed a person is. Frequently, a person at a higher Chakra level will register less and less what actually is happening, and more and more wants to impose what should be happening. An image occurs to me here, that of a wild bull trying to be ridden by someone who's never done it before. Magic should be left to aborigines, who know how to use it much better.

I have already warned of the **dangers of magic**. By means of particular rituals, magic causes something to happen that would not otherwise take place. Of course, an astonishing part of our everyday behavior is to some degree magical, if you look at it closely. When we attach a horseshoe to our car's radiator to ward off accidents, or wear amulets, those are examples of magic. It gets dangerous if we try to manipulate others to our own advantage. This kind of magic can very easily become polluted by our own emotional negativity. If we are honest about what goes on inside us, we have to admit that we are "of many minds," so to speak. It is thus pretty easy to contaminate our healing energy with negative emotions if we operate primarily on the magical level.

We often have repressed, negative feelings toward our fellow man that we are, at first, totally unaware of. Tragically, these negative feelings sneak totally unnoticed into our subconscious, where they can cause great harm to others (and to ourselves in covert, long-term, and karmic ways). For instance, you might not be able to stand a certain person, but you want his money. Your subconscious hostile thoughts will be conveyed even against your will. Even if you are neutral with respect to someone, avarice is still an emotional pollutant that can impair the healing process. For this reason, many healers refuse to charge a fee, leaving it to the patient to make a donation. In this manner, they avoid the risk of damaging – even losing – their healing energy with impure motivations.

Energy work, on the other hand, involves the higher Chakras, in which one becomes a servant of higher spiritual powers ("Thy will be done."). This is why we moderns should make use of this higher form of energy work exclusively. The prototypical form of energy work is **prayer**! True to Jesus' saying "*Ask and ye shall receive*," we ask the divine power to make of us a channel for healing. This doesn't mean that we need do nothing more. Our task is to feel our way into sufferers' Auras and try to supply them with psychoenergetic strength (by laying on of hands, say) and to dissolve harmful blockages. Generally speaking, this kind of procedure is also known as "spiritual healing" because an indiscernible spiritual force is at work.

Surprisingly, energy work operates independently of distance. Of course, it is better to be near the patients, but it also works at a distance. Healing energy is transmitted between sender and receiver by resonance. EEG measurements taken at therapy sessions have revealed that the brain waves of therapists and patients adapt to each other during the course of the healing procedure. This resonance phenomenon can be likened to a telephone conversation. As with telephoning, the addressee and his unchanging attribute (i.e. telephone number) must be known. Just by thinking of someone, I am at that moment linked to him. Every mother knows the instinctive feeling of being intangibly bound to her child. We are linked with people who affect us emotionally by a very special invisible bond; our patients should be like that to us, because this strengthens the contact.

The next step seems to me the most difficult, because the more ardently we consciously desire something, the less likely it is to be fulfilled. The American internist and "prayer researcher" Larry DOSSEY has carried out controlled experiments using prayer whose statistical results improve when the prayer content is formulated less specifically. "Please see that John gets better" is more effective than "Please see that John recovers fully from his heart attack." A precisely formulated prayer request seems to block the subconscious more strongly. If you want something too much, the prayer cannot be answered so well – but if you don't want anything at all, that's not good either: total passivity leads to the opposite extreme. You need to "knock, and it shall be opened" – just not too loudly and insistently. You must of course want what you are asking for, then make the request somewhat open-ended and leave its fulfillment to the higher wisdom of the universe.

If we try to force healing by commanding "Now get healthy, and I mean now!," then it's guaranteed not to work. It's like many subconscious processes that function less well the more we force them. We're all familiar with the futile attempt to will ourselves to sleep. Communication via energy work is a similar situation. If we try too hard to transmit thought-modulated energy, the attempt is bound to fail. The secret is to go at the healing process with a kind of nonchalance.

I did some experiments of my own to clarify this matter. They involved measuring brainwaves and energy levels, and they yielded enlightening results that shed some light into the obscurity of these healing processes. The thing is, the more brain waves (of the kind that correspond to everyday conscious reasoning) I generated with a small electronic device, the more the energy field shrank. Evidently, abstract thinking and the life force are highly (yet inversely) interrelated. It's a simple phenomenon, familiar to every gradeschooler who has felt half dead after six classroom hours. Strenuous (abstract) thinking and life force are antipolar!

A number of conclusions can be drawn from this simple experiment. First, one should be aware that too much strenuous rational mental activity saps life force. We need to counteract this, for instance by taking long walks in natural surroundings, in order to "recharge our batteries." Thinking is healthier and more advantageous the less we strain at it and the more enjoyment we derive from it. It is then that alpha waves appear, which don't block the life force as much. There is more to learn about life force itself from the experiment with the brainwave device and energy levels. Basically, the less we consciously (try to) influence it, the more subtle-body energy flows, because it's not being blocked by our mental apparatus. The more open-ended healing prayer sentence ("Please see that John gets better.") works better than the more explicit formulation ("Please see that John recovers fully from his heart attack.") because a term such as "heart attack" is a bit abstract and thus tends to block the healing energy somewhat. This is why the two sentences – the open-ended and the precisely specified request – lead to different healing outcomes.

We can say in summary that healing effects always have a co-component derived from energetic-mental healing power. It is based mostly on the implicit faith that therapists and their healing methods engender in their patients – as well as, of course, the faith that therapists have in themselves and their methods. The faith of the two parties generates a common field in which life energy impregnated with healing information flows. In a broader sense, therefore, all medical procedures are permeated with such processes, and they generate effects that exceed normal expectations. This can be seen most clearly in the well-known *placebo effect*.[22]

Then there's the wonderful story from Africa's colonial period. A Christian mission was once sent an X-ray apparatus, a really impressive piece of equipment. No one there had ever seen anything so magnificent and modern. The mission doctor checked out the device's mechanical functioning, without turning it on, on one of his black servants. Next day, there was a long line of natives waiting outside, all wanting to be X-rayed. Evidently, the word had spread like wildfire that a miraculous device had arrived, since the servant who had first been "X-rayed" had been improved by it. That the device had not even been switched on was viewed as a lame excuse by those seeking relief. They only calmed down and went home after each of them had been allowed to stand in the X-ray device. Subsequent queries confirmed that the miracle device and its healing powers had led to some unexpected cures.

---

[22] Critics will object that I am making inadmissible use of the placebo concept. After all, scientists should have long since noticed that placebos have to be a kind of prayer or remote action. The rejoinder to this is: how are scientists supposed to notice something that, from the outset, they consider to be nonsense and that they do not include in their calculations? The placebo effect in animals and small children is explained by saying that zookeepers and mothers are particularly caring and kind after administering placebos. They smile very lovingly or do something else especially nice. Subliminal signals are thus the ostensible reason why a certain percentage of healing takes place in these suggestive little beings. I think this is quite plausible as an add-on argument, but it is way too thin to serve as the main explanation for the placebo effect. Because if we turn the tables and look at the entire process from the premise that the subconscious healing signals (as in prayer) are what really heal, what acts in the placebo, then the usual explanations come across as lame excuses.

Psychosomatics, Energetic Polarity, and the Four Elements

For healthy functioning, the human organism needs not only food, water and oxygen, but also (and above all) life force. Life force is an invisible yet absolutely necessary working substance. When we are dead, we have no more life force, even though our body just before and after the moment of death is made up of the same material particles. Like the soul, life force has no weight in any conventionally measurable sense. Despite this, we can evaluate the character (the personality-shaped "soul") and the vigor of somebody by describing the effect that person has on us.

Later on, I will use case histories to illustrate that it is actually possible to measure life force and character relatively objectively. I say "relatively" because the measurement is somewhat interference prone (which is intrinsically true of all energetic measurement methods). I have already pointed this out in the previous chapter, identifying mistrust as an important source of error. Additional factors include the tester's psychoenergetic health and talent (the latter being trainable, of course). Experienced testers arrive at virtually identical results – barring negligible (hence tolerable) discrepancies – which is why I say "relatively" objective results.

For this measurement, I use a subtle-body measurement method called *Psychosomatic Energetics*. Using a lectern-shaped measurement device (REBA® Test Device), I administer increasing amounts of a frequency mix via a spiral cable attached to the test subject's wrist. These frequencies resonate with the subject's brainwaves and Aura, thereby subjecting him to increasing stress. A stress reaction is produced when the energy system can take it no longer. This reading corresponds to the percentile Aural charge, and with this one can say how much life force (in percent) someone has. I will describe the procedure in detail at the end of the book.

Psychosomatic Energetics makes it possible, for the first time, to

- measure life force;
- detect subconscious conflicts and character;
- define health and sickness energetically.

When it comes to maintaining health, the life force is of paramount significance. Nothing is as important for warding off disease! In this context, character and the underlying subconscious conflicts play a major role, since their faulty vibrations disrupt and partially block life force. When our

life force flows freely and in large quantities, then we will be (and generally remain) healthy.

However, in daily orthodox medical practice, neither emotions nor life force play much of a role. This applies, with qualifications, even to psychiatry and psychoanalysis, which – although they don't take the life force into account – at least accord character some degree of importance. We know that character plays a certain role in pathogenesis. For example, slender persons with a schizoid character structure more frequently suffer from schizophrenia or tuberculosis, while corpulent persons tend to depression and gallstones, and athletic types to neuroses. It is unclear, however, why this should be so. Modern psychoneuroimmunology is finding some preliminary answers, but is as yet in the initial phases of its investigations, which consist mostly of collecting detailed material that lacks a perceptible wider context. Deriving disease tendencies from blood groups, popular among medical amateurs, plays no role in day-to-day medicine. Primarily, it is a matter (here as well) of a classification

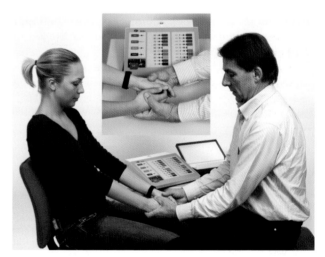

Typical Psychosomatic Energetics test situation: the patient's stretched arms are pulled gently at the wrist and guided by the tester (here the author). With each test step, the REBA® Test Device is switched 10% higher, beginning with 0, until the patient shows stress by significantly changing arm length (noticeable by thumbnails gaining distance of about 1-2 cm – see detail).

system based on mere commonalities devoid of any discernible overarching context.

The beginnings of psychosomatics reach back over two thousand years. The pioneers in the occident were the Greek HIPPOCRATES and the Roman GALEN, who noted that melancholic and choleric types more frequently got cancer. In their opinion, the cause was poor bile flow. This represented the first attempt to link bodily traits and metabolic characteristics with emotional factors. We call the interplay of mind and body psychosomatics (where *psyche* = mind and *soma* = body). Modern psychosomatics arose in a wave of initial enthusiasm with the discovery of psychoanalysis.

The German physician Victor von WEIZSÄCKER, one of the leading pioneers, described in his magnum opus *Gestaltkreis* [Form Cycle] the collaboration among subconscious motives, personal destiny, and the emergence of specific diseases. Sick people shape their destinies and their diseases based on subconscious motivations. WEIZSÄCKER had the insight that people often choose physical disease as a relief from emotional suffering – because physical suffering is easier to take than mental. Physical disease is also used as a safety valve, to prevent getting even sicker in an overall mind-body context – as when a woman in an unhappy marriage has asthma attacks (physical disease) instead of cracking up and becoming psychotic (mental disease).

Modern medicine takes a different view of disease – and therefore goes at it differently as well. In conventional medicine, the strict separation of body and mind leads to the regrettable circumstance that both of these human aspects (psyche and soma) are viewed as component parts and not as wholes. The psychosomatic physician WEIZSÄCKER set out in the 1930s to overcome the calamitous mind-body division and once again view the patient as a whole. In reality, however, psychosomatics has mostly proven a failure – with a few laudable exceptions. This person-based medicine proved unable to gain widespread acceptance against the *zeitgeist* of the scientific paradigm. Whereas a century ago, stomach ulcers were considered to be a purely psychosomatic disease, we now know, thanks to the discovery of the stomach bacterium *Helicobacter pylori*, that most ulcers represent an infectious disease. The same goes for diseases such as asthma, Neurodermitis, or migraine, that are now less considered mental and more somatic.

As a young doctor, I once got a living illustrative lesson in the insoluble dilemma that modern psychosomatics finds itself in. I was working in a well-known psychosomatic ward that was affiliated with the internal medicine division, while at the same time being looked after by "mind-oriented" professors. The discussions in the ward hallways between the "soma" and the "psyche" doctors were grotesque performances. Every contentious professor was convinced that the other professor was wrong and taking a completely false approach to the problem. At the same time, for tactical reasons, each professor kept his opinions to himself, so as not to get the other side up in arms. Normally, an uneasy truce was maintained in which each professor did what he thought right. However, integrating these two conceptual approaches was impossible, and this approach was praised only in (the frequent) ceremonial speeches. On this ward, as later on in my life, I found confirmation, time and again, that true psychosomatics is very seldom practiced: it's usually just an irreconcilable standoff between somatics and psychosomatics.

One of the main reasons why psychosomatics has such a hard time of it is its disappointing diagnostic and therapeutic situation. When I, after hours of interviews and tests, have finally put together a halfway reasonable picture of the patient, there still remains the possibility that I might be wrong. Psychosomatic diagnoses are quite subjective because they depend on the physician's psychotherapeutic school of thought and his way of looking at things. But simply arriving at a psychosomatic diagnosis is a long way from healing the patient – because now begins the long trek down the road of talks, relaxation exercises, body perception exercises, and much more. It's relatively rare that a patient is released completely cured from a psychosomatic clinic; relapses are an ever-present possibility. The entire effort is time and money intensive – and, unfortunately, in many cases fails to produce the desired results. Despite this, I'd like to make it clear that I consider psychosomatic therapy to be far better than a purely symptomatic haphazard approach that ignores the mental backdrop. What I'm getting at is that psychosomatics is in dire need of change; it needs to include the energetic component and thereby improve its healing results.

I'd next like to undertake to found a new psychosomatics that brings together metabolism, subtle-body energy and depth psychology into a single unit. This may seem, at first glance, harder than it really is; all the important components of such a new structure of subtle-body psychosomatics (which I call *Psychosomatic Energetics*) are already known – there is, after all, very little that is truly new under the sun. The individual factors just need to be weighted against each other and joined correctly – but we first need to understand how the life force "docks" in the body. In explaining this, I cannot avoid peppering the reader with details from the history of medicine, religion, and philosophy – because, as we know, we only know who we really are through our history. Added to which, modern energy medicine is based on ancient knowledge. One must be familiar with this knowledge in order to work with it.

Our first key question is: how does the life force manage to mesh with all the cogs and gears of the physical body? How, specifically, does it do that? Initially, the various viewpoints mix together into a virtually opaque muddle of the most varied theories regarding how the life force intervenes in the body and attaches to it. Every naturopathic physician and every school of naturopathic medicine – whether

Ayurveda, acupuncture, Tibetan medicine, or Western naturopathy – has its own very specific concepts. Superficially, all these viewpoints may seem to have little in common, but if we look below the surface and ask what the actual substance is, we find amazingly many commonalities.

It quickly becomes clear that all these systems can be traced back to certain very similar basic concepts, based on the ancient idea of polarly organized *humors* or elements. These ideas originated in ancient India around 1000 BCE, from whence the element theory spread via the Silk Road to China and Arabia, then on to Greece and Rome. In this diffusion process, information was lost; not all the knowledge about humors and energies was preserved. On the way to China, the Chakras (Aura levels) were forgotten, but even more was lost during the journey to Arabia and Europe. The theory of humors was correctly conveyed in all directions, which is why it forms the common scaffolding of all ancient medicine systems: Traditional Chinese Medicine (TCM), *Ayurveda*, and Arabic-Occidental humoral pathology.

This doctrine originated in India and Persia, where seers such as India's *rishis* perceive, in clairvoyant visions, how and why people get sick and how they can once again be healthy. The *rishis* discover previously hidden energy centers (Chakras) that are closely linked with important nerve plexa and hormonal glands. They discover the subtle body with its various gradations. They see that the Aura looks unclean, discolored, or porous before diseases develop. Chakras rotate in the wrong direction or become very small when disease is imminent. They also discern that metabolic disorders in the form of maldistributed humors provoke disease. If the underlying Aura and Chakra disorders are eliminated, disease disappears. From their visions, the *rishis* developed an internally logical spiritually-oriented healing system.

Unlike shamanism, which proceeds purely on the basis of intuition and vision, we have here, for the first time in human history, the origins of a medicinal system that can be formally taught and containing the beginnings of scientific structure. This is the doctrinal system that lives on in present-day *Ayurveda* and traditional *Yoga*. The great success of this system continues to this day, thus confirming impressively that a universal healing principle has been found. The insights of this healing system are the basis for the following exposition:

The common foundation of all ancient medical systems is the Four Humors Theory (Humoral Theory, Four- or Firve- Element Theory) found, in various varieties in diverse cultural groups:

- As the complex system of traditional Indian medicine (*Ayurveda*)
- As a highly developed metaphysical/philosophical theory in ancient China (in Traditional Chinese Medicine / TCM as Five-Element Theory – in which life force,

designated as Æther, is erroneously counted as the 5th element);

- As humoral theory under GALEN and HIPPOCRATES in ancient Greece (as **humoral pathology,** it dominates Occidental medicine on into the 18th century and includes the four constitutions: melancholy, choleric, sanguine, and phlegmatic).

The big plus of element theory is that mankind for the first time had developed a medical system that contained logical elements and produced predictable results. This meant that, from now on, healing was no longer dependent on the will and mercy of the gods – which is why the profession of physician was able to split off from that of priest-shaman. Logically, the priest only intervened when the physician could do no more, to administer the last rites to the dying patient. This is the context for VOLTAIRE's witticism that "the profession of physician is the only one in which the practitioner is allowed to bury his mistakes." The Olympian air of omniscience that once characterized priests clings to physicians to this day.

With element theory, healing no longer depended on the talent of individual healers or other unknown factors. Instead, medicine became a predictable and self-confident science. It's no wonder that modern medicine proudly invokes HIPPOCRATES, considered one of the fathers of Western medicine. The Greek physician HIPPOCRATES and, centuries later, the Roman GALEN developed a complex system known as *humoral pathology*. It is based on the four elements, and so is also known as *element theory*.

Hardly anyone today is aware that element theory is by no means a dusty obsolete medical system, but rather a reliably functioning therapeutic method. This could be seen quite well in the success of the Viennese gynecology professor Bernhard ASCHNER who, a Jew, had emigrated to New York during World War II. In many hundreds of cases, ASCHNER successfully applied the ancient prescriptions and methods of humoral medicine. In no time at all, ASCHNER gained a reputation as a miracle doctor. Sadly, ASCHNER did not live long enough to exert a lasting influence in the USA, nor to pass on ancient element theory to younger physicians.

In Indian *Ayurveda*, as well as in Tibetan and Chinese medicine (all operating according to the classical rules of element theory), we can see similar tremendous successes. It is thus very rewarding to work with element theory. Along with energy medicine, it ensures that we get a comprehensive medical worldview that leads to noticeably better healing results. This by no means devalues modern medicine, but rather enriches and expands it with these once-lost insights and techniques. Therefore, I am convinced that, in future, besides scientifically oriented medicine, three additional types of healing arts will experience a rebirth and become very important: element theory, energy medicine, and body-oriented (to some extent behaviorist) psychotherapy. They each cover different areas of hidden disease causes that can much better be healed with these procedures. Above all, they enable true disease prevention (prophylaxis) to be practiced. *Psychosomatic Energetics*, which I discovered and promote, and which will be presented in detail at the end of this book, constitutes a harmonious connecting link between element theory, energy medicine and psychotherapy. I do not claim that their associated procedures thus become superfluous.

Element disturbances are normally totaled up by experts into an overall picture on the basis of physical signs (body shape, skin color, eye color, and so on) pulse diagnosis (soft hard, etc.) and the body's excreta (urine color, skin odor, and so on). This is a kind of diagnostic art that is, however, quite teachable and learnable as a craft – although it takes a top-notch practitioner to attain true mastery. When I was studying naturopathy in the 1970s, I and another student (an electrician) developed a device to measure acupuncture meridians. Our results agreed excellently with those of other students who were skilled in Chinese pulse diagnosis! Later on, as a doctor, I continue to check my diagnoses against those of my colleagues, often finding very good agreement, even though a superficial inspection might consider them to be subjective evaluations. Thus, all in all, element theory is an amazingly objective science.

We can now take a deeper look at element theory. The first thing we need to understand is how subtle-body life force incorporates itself into the material and coarse-body realm. When we consider how the life force operates in the organism, we come up, first of all, against the law of polarity. As in a battery, tension (voltage) must build up between polar opposites for life and movement to be possible. Polarity not only enables data transmission (e.g., in reproduction), it also represents the primordial basic condition for life force to begin to flow. Without polar opposition, our organism would meander about aimlessly, a leaderless lackluster chunk of stuff. The true dynamism of our being alive only arises due to opposed tensions. Because opposites attract and animate each other, the whole machinery gets into gear. Life force *must* therefore become polar if anything is to happen. Polarities are found everywhere in the form of opposed pairs: light and dark, hot and cold, acid and alkaline, oxidation and reduction, positive and negative polarities of nerves and muscles. All of these polarities see to it that "something happens."

For data transmission in the world of opposites, nature makes use of a binary signal sequence much like that used in both computers and the genetic code. To be sure, a simple on/off language seems at first pretty unimaginative, like a simpleminded person who only answers "Yes" or "No" because that's all he's capable of. But nature is by no means stupid – in fact it is enormously clever! A yes/no answer is hard to manipulate or falsify. Moreover, binary codes allow an immense, virtually inconceivable amount of information diversity. We can see this very clearly in the huge variety of creatures that the genetic code's binary symbols have been able to bring into being. Polarity enables practically any

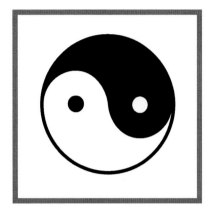

Yin-Yang-Monad

kind of information to be conveyed, because fine gradations and complexities can also be binary encoded .

In this context, **sexuality** forms the foundation of polarity. Virtually no other human activity generates so much tension as the sex act – nor, in the organism, so much cathartic release. The life force that then flows refreshes our psychoenergetic system. After satisfying sex, we are not only physically relaxed and contented, but we also have a sense of spiritual wellbeing and peace. According to the Indian Kama Sutra, romantic tension is said to be particularly high when the woman is a particularly gazelle-like Yin female and the man is a decidedly bull-like Yang male. Sexual compensation is all the more delightful the greater the contrast – i.e., the more masculine the man and feminine the woman.

Sexuality presents us with yet another life-force phenomenon, in which we can discern elementary patterns and regularities in the connection between sexual desire and life energy. **Desire arises when large quantities of life energy flow.** Sexual satisfaction allows a lot of life energy to flow, which charges us up psychoenergetically and nourishes us. This applies not only to adult sexuality, but also to the breast-feeding baby. Desire/pleasure is not just nature's clever trick to seduce us via our senses into eating or sexual coupling; it is, rather, an expression of a stronger flow of life force in us.

Every person has an innate tendency for a specific polarity. Basically, we can first distinguish men and women as antipolar beings. The Chinese speak of Yang (male) and Yin (female). Since these are superordinate principles, there are types within the sexes that are more Yin or Yang: there are manly and effeminate men, and there are feminine and mannish women. An effeminate male can still be a real man, just as a mannish female can be a proper woman. The cru-

Polarity concepts	Source/ Classification	+	−
General Polarity	Ancient China	Yang	Yin
Sexual Polarity	Everyday Concepts	Man	Woman
Human Polarity Types	CERVANTES	Don Quixote	Sancho Pansa
	HUTER	Sensory Temperament	Nourishment Temperament
	CURRY	K-Type (cold-front sensitive)	W-Type (warm-front sensitive)
	KRETSCHMER	Leptosome	Pyknic
	Hollywood Film	Stan (goofy)	Ollie (chubby)
Polarly Oriented Bodily Functions	Acid-Base Balance	Acid	Base
	Muscle Tone	Contraction	Atony
	ANS	Sympathetic Nervous System	Parasympathetic Nervous System
	Sleep/Wake	Waking	Sleeping

cial aspect in this arrangement is the fact that the Yin/Yang division represents a superordinate polarity which contains the sexual one. Naturally, a "Yinny" man will come across differently from a "Yangy" one. A male with more Yin tends to have a curvier female physique (A good example of this is the rock singer Elvis PRESLEY.). On the other side, a high-Yang female will be more muscular and angular (Many female athletes are this type.).

The psychiatrist KRETSCHMER uses the division of physique into slender and chubby to relate them to psychiatric disease tendencies. These are concepts that are still in use in psychiatry today. The chubby pyknic is often found among depressive types, while the slender leptosome tends to schizophrenia. The German discoverer of psychophysiognomy, Carl HUTER, makes a fundamental distinction between feeling types and feeding types. Today, this formulation seems badly chosen, since a feeding type can be very sentimental (and vice-versa). In his polarity, HUTER means those emphasizing eating and sensory perception. Feeling types are thus those who, when busy, forget to eat, which is much less likely to happen to a feeding type.

The American physician CURRY classifies people based on weather sensitivity (to warm or cold fronts), calling them

W and C types. Another classification scheme is based on the fundamental tone of the autonomic nervous system (ANS). In this system, there are sympathicotonic types, known for their bustling excitement, nervousness and inner tension. Sympathicotonics often have overlarge pupils. The opposite parasympathicotonic type (vagotonic) is calmer and more jovial, and tends to constipation and all manner of cramps, spasms, and seizures. Vagotonics can easily be identified by their undersized pupils.

People with relatively equal parts of Yin and Yang are designated as **harmony types**. Their effect on us is balanced and harmonious, whereas pronounced Yin or Yang types seem more interesting and dynamic. A strong Yang type exhibits a lot of masculine combative restlessness, while a strong Yin type radiates a powerful sense of groundedness. Actors are rarely harmony types, since that type generally comes across as somewhat boring and way too "normal." As in daily life, harmony types in movies are generally balancing characters around whose calm center the more lively types run riot.

A tripartite classification – into Yin, Yang and harmony types – makes sense because this results in a fundamental pre-characterization of the ANS and metabolism. Physicians then know how patients will react to diseases and what kind of therapy is called for. When sick, Yang types usually tend to move to a state of even more Yang and thus need Yin in order to re-center. This might involve sleeping more and relaxing, as well as high-Yin foods (e.g., alkaline and sweet substances) and Yin medicine (calming and relaxing remedies). The situation is exactly reversed for Yin types, who need stimulating and animating (tonicizing) foods and remedies such as bitter and acidic substances and stimulating medications (ginseng, *Echinacea*, camphor) that enliven depressed circulation and metabolism and counteract exhaustion. Acute crisis cases of infectious diseases almost always lead to extremely polar states in either the Yin or Yang direction. This is why the cold sufferer feels so miserable. The simple yet extremely useful tool of polarity compensation can do a lot of good against colds. If we maintain the patient in a harmonious state as much as possible, the healing process will begin more quickly.[23]

Colds disrupt the **autonomic (vegetative) nervous system,** which energetically then has an underlying disturbed polarity. This applies particularly to viral colds, which severely disturb the ANS. The vegetative nervous system regulates physical processes such as sleep/waking, respiration, and digestion, all of which run without conscious intervention (autonomously) and are crucial to well-being. The headquarters of this vital automatic process is the hypothalamus in the brain. Fortunately, the ANS relieves us of the need to consciously regulate life-critical physical functions. We don't need to worry whether our skin pores are dilating when we need to perspire, or whether our intestines should be active. The ANS thus makes daily life easier by doing a lot of regulatory work for us.

The simplest way to understand the anticyclical polarity of the ANS is to consider cows. In ancient times, cattle were under constant threat from predators. As is known, sometime during the course of bovine evolution, multiple stomachs (rumens) were created to aid digestion that had to be frequently postponed out of fear of predators. Cattle grazing in meadows had to be constantly on the alert and eat quickly (sympathicotonia or Yang state). Once they were safe – for instance in a hollow or other secure place – then the pleasant digestive state could take over (parasympathicotonia or Yin state).

Although we're not cattle, we humans are subject to very similar laws and regularities. In the daily stress of **sympathicotonia,** everything is set for immediate flight or fight:

blood pressure is elevated, heart rate accelerated, muscles tensed and mind running at full speed. People with sympathicotonia or excess Yang are thus, in a certain sense, always "on the run" or – if a more combative, offensive type – in a state of constant battle alert. Modern research into cardiovascular risk factors views the behavior of the Type A personality as particularly damaging with respect to ailments such as heart attacks and such. People belonging to this behavioral type are full-time warriors living in constant tension. Psychodynamically, they tend to badger and goad other people. They secretly feel they are superior because they see themselves as the "doers" in a developing situation.

However, the opposite, ***parasympathicotonia,*** by no means leads to a relaxed state, but rather overshoots the mark. Such people tend to atonic states such as cramps, exhaustion, and low blood pressure. To stay with the grazing cattle image, the opposite of fight/flight is the completely exhausted, almost-chased-to-death cow that hardly has any energy left for digestion. The entire metabolic system runs very slowly and under great strain. People with parasympathicotonia or in a Yin state tend to constipation, gallbladder cramps, and depressed metabolism, which predisposes to fatty degeneration and flaccidity. Psychodynamically,

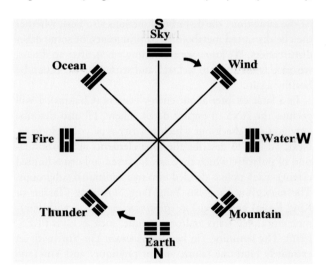

"Pre-world" order (from BACHMANN)

Yin types often exhibit flight tendencies and tend to view themselves as harassed victims.

Just as the grazing cow in our example doesn't feel well either when surrounded by predators (medically *sympathicotonia*) or when, completely exhausted from running away, it reaches shelter (*parasympathicotonia*), so also is it not good for us humans when we find ourselves at one of the extremes of our ANS. According to the stress researcher SELYE, we speak in these cases of distress. We feel best when things proceed at a moderate pace, without becoming boring. This is known in psychology as eustress, when we

[23] Appropriate remedies include Simvita© for Yang states (often at the beginning of a cold with high fever) and Paravita© for Yin states (often in a later phase of healing). One tests kinesiologically for what responds best and then administers as many drops on the tongue until the patient doesn't need any more drops. This can be repeated every 1–2 hours until healing begins. With this easy method, 90% of all plain infectious diseases can be treated simply and quite effectively.

feel stimulated without being overstressed or bored.

Compared to the cow in our example, the harmony type is a member of the species that feels best in *eustress* – i.e., when things are proceeding neither too aggressively nor too calmly. Yang types, on the other hand, are most contented and at their emotional center when their lives are constantly under some pressure. One can imagine a steer that, up to a point, enjoys predators creeping around him – just as long as it's not too many of them! The Yin type feels really comfortable when (think female cow) it is in safe company and can graze peacefully and "moo the fat."

If we mentally put ourselves in the place of these three types, we can understand how each type can get sick and feel unwell. Overemphasis on one's own type and falling out of one's center to tip over to the opposite extreme are the different ways one can feel bad and even become seriously ill. Thus, knowing one's type is the first step to real and profound prophylaxis! **Disease almost always begins with disturbed polarity.**

Basically, it doesn't matter all that much what the symptoms are, whether disturbed acid-base equilibrium, muscle cramps or whatever. It's not the label that matters, but rather recognizing the disturbed polarity. For if we can normalize upset polarity, we'll heal and prevent many a disease. At the same time, the disturbed functions also heal, whether they be disrupted metabolism, painful joints, or some other disturbances. We know we are healing when, after an illness, we once again begin to feel well and sense that we'll soon be healthy again.

In a later chapter about energy centers (Chakras), I will go into the ANS in greater detail. There, I'll also describe how you can check out which polarity type you belong to. Next, I'd like to describe the **four elements** as a continuation of polarity (which they are, however, only to a limited extent). Each pole is divided into two additional subgroups. The masculine Yang has Yang-Yang *Superman* (Tarzan or King Kong) and Yang-Yin *effeminate man* (one with feminine emotional traits and/or physique, such as Elvis PRESLEY). The feminine Yin has *Superwoman* Yin-Yin (with an extremely feminine nature and/or physique) and Yin-Yang *masculine woman* ("dominatrix" type with masculine physique and/or nature).

However, the four elements go beyond mere polarity variation and exhibit qualities of their own. In ancient China, the elements were represented by so-called trigrams (three lines). Interested readers can learn more in the book of oracular wisdom, the *I Ching*. Personally, I am reluctant to accept this division, because it is too easily downgraded to a rigid system in which the original dynamism gets lost in the shuffle.[24] Still, it provides us – with some reservations – with

fascinating and profound insights. In casting about for a suitable metaphor, we can best liken the four elements to the four seasons. To the polar seasons Summer and Winter are added the two additional seasons of Spring and Fall. The seasons are self-contained qualities, each possessing something uniquely its own.

The four elements are aggregate states of the energetic and material world, each describing a self-contained preliminary stage of an energetic and material basic state.

Thus

- **Wood** can, through
- **Fire**, become
- **Smoke** and gases (**Air**), in which the soot particles at some point
- Condense with **Water** molecules into rain and
- Make the **Earth** wet and fruitful.

Another possible image is that of a prism, as when a cloud of light-scattering raindrops creates the colors of the rainbow when the sun shines through. Colors are likewise closely related to the elements (though not identical).

Life energy is split up by the energy centers (Chakras) and our innate disposition (genes) into various humors or elements, giving rise to the **four constitutional types: phlegmatic, choleric, sanguine, and melancholic.** This constitutional matrix ensures that, with our metabolism as well as our temperament, we display a specific preset reaction and behavioral pattern. Four-Element Theory is a thousand-year-old doctrine concerning the interplay between body and mind, which, from birth, *places* people into certain constitutional typologies. Each of us thus has a constitution, whether we want it or not, while our modern concept of *psychosomatics* comprises a freely chosen element that, despite its limitations, nevertheless allows for drastic reversals and even complete healing. The psychosomatically ailing patient can therefore get well, whereas the constitutionally sick patient can only do things that fit within the borders of his constitution. Thus the constitutionally ill person can only become well within constitutional parameters, and never transcend its predefined borders.

Cancer provides us with a good example for the viewpoint and the chosen procedure of the ancient theory of humors, according to which cancer was viewed as predominantly a problem of specific flawed humors. Thus, so-called *black bile* was said to be responsible for melancholia. Of course, other constitutional types can also have *black bile* disturbances, it is just more common in melancholics, according to the doctrine of humoral pathology. Along with the general metabolic disturbance of *black bile*, the melancholic tends to gloomy thoughts (melancholia). Modern psychoneuroimmunology confirms the idea that a pessimistic basic mood and long-term sorrows predispose to cancer. Melancholics who already have cancer have a markedly worse prognosis than those with a more optimistic nature.

---

[24] China's Five-Element Theory counts metal as the fifth element. There's more on the Chinese system in the next chapter.

Basically, the ancient physicians viewed cancer as a kind of ineluctable fate. The attitude was fatalistic and discouraged any kind of treatment. According to HIPPOCRATES, therapy would only serve to hasten the inevitable end; this was the cautious standpoint of the ancient physicians – and they were indeed right in most cases. If they were unable to heal their cancer patients, their prognoses were at least correct. HIPPOCRATES was the first, by the way, to use the word *carcinoma*, because the congested chest veins of breast cancer were said to resemble a crab. The Roman physician GALEN, whose concept of humoral pathology (four humors doctrine) dominated medicine on into the modern age, was the first to initiate cautious therapy for cancer, proscribing anything that produced *black bile*: meat, cheese, vinegar, wine, and so on, and made his cancer patients fast. We can see from this that hyperacidity had already been recognized as a pathogenic element. Also, GALEN said that

turbed blood composition is the cause of a tendency to thromboses and vascular diseases, as well as mood swings.

We can most easily understand the nature of the elements if we view them as aggregate states possessing their own inherent dynamics. Each of the four elements has a tendency to compensate. Like a hot/cold temperature gradient that leads on our planet to compensation of climatic zones by means of high and low pressure regions, the four elements also give rise to various *transformational states* of energy. This concept of *transformational states* first shows up in ancient China. I have chosen this concept because it unsurpassably illustrates that life energy actually is "transformed" by means of the four elements. As with a drive belt, imperceptible life energy is conveyed to the physical organism via the dynamics of the transformation that inheres in the four elements.

Now, the first and most important fundamental rule of element theory says that **we remain healthy for as long as**

Theory of the Elements and Constitutional Types

Element	Air	Fire	Earth	Water
Constitutional Type	Sanguine	Choleric	Melancholic	Phlegmatic
Character	Walking on Air Ecstatic / Deathly Sad	Brooding Worried Enraged	Irritated-inappropriate behavior	Rigid-fixated Bored
Psychiatric Types	Manic Depressive	Endogenous Depression	Schizotyhmic Antisocial	Rigid Obsessive-Compulsive, Fear
Appearance	Pyknic		Leptosome	
Disturbed Bodily Processes	Plethora	Cholestasis		Hydogenoid (Mucous Membrane)
Disturbed Organ Systems	Cardiovascular	Digestion	Nervous System	Connective Tissue

emotional agitation was to be avoided, which is also amazingly modern advice.

According to ancient humoral doctrine, each constitution is based on a specific, fundamentally disturbed mixture of humors. In melancholics, it is the black bile humor that is disturbed, which predisposes to cancer and melancholia. In cholerics, the humoral mix of the *yellow bile* is the cause of a volatile temperament and sluggish metabolism (including lithogenesis and other metabolic deposits such as arthrosis). Phlegmatics have poorly flowing phlegm, making them susceptible to diseases of the mucosa, and representing the cause of their inertia (phlegm). Finally, the sanguinic's dis-

life energy flows normally within the elements. Ultimately, this means that, when life energy flows normally, the elements appear at normal strength. For example, in an ecosystem where one season is overemphasized and another is present in severely abbreviated form, there will inevitably be disturbances. If a winter is short and mild, then insect pests will multiply – the more so if spring lasts for a very long time. All the sprouting greenery will immediately be gobbled up by the insect pests. We can observe very similar phenomena in the human organism if the interrelationship of the elements gets shifted and disordered. Life energy no longer flows evenly and disease results.

Specific elements have come to be empirically associated with specific organs and metabolic systems. For example, in Chinese medicine, the element water corresponds to the kidneys and mineral/water equilibrium. By means of specific pulse qualities, skin/mucosal changes, tongue coating, patient body odor and unusual behavior, the Chinese physician can detect a disturbance in the *water* element, for instance. The qualities of disturbed life energy that then appear can be reduced, amplified, irritated, or dammed up, be stubborn or ephemeral, and so on. The Chinese physician will attempt to cure the disease through the use of medications that normalize the disturbed element *water*, by diverting life energy, e.g., with moxibustion (therapy that uses a kind of incense stick) and acupuncture. If the disease is not too advanced, the treatment will be successful.

Those who work in Traditional Chinese Medicine (TCM) do not treat the kidneys or disturbed water/mineral metabolism in isolation, but rather in the context of the associated water element disturbance. (By the way, our ancient Western healers also proceeded in like manner as the traditional Chinese physicians: they too treated the disturbed element underlying the disease.) However, if the kidney is incapable of recovering on its own, then it's time for Western medicine to step in. For example, a large kidney stone can be pulverized with sound waves (shock wave lithotripsy). If the kidney is completely nonfunctional, then we need dialysis or a kidney transplant. Modern scientific medicine is justified, then, when the body's self-healing powers have failed.

To appreciate the logic on which element theory healing is based, picture a conductor directing an orchestra composed of body cells and metabolism. The "element theory conductor" wields a much better and longer lever than one who starts at the body-cell and metabolic level, since the elements represent a superordinate system, one that we might compare to a computer program that controls the material plane.

An example from daily practice can help clarify the pluses and minuses of both medical systems. Consider a nervous, highly stressed man with constant headaches and frequent nausea. Let's assume that this man has the option of going to see two different doctors: an acupuncturist or a mainstream neurologist. Which one would be better for him? In my experience, the great majority of patients would prefer the neurologist for diagnosis and the acupuncturist for therapy – because from the neurologist, they would want the reassurance that their headache is not due to some possible underlying organic disease, such as a brain tumor, that could also cause one to feel stressed all the time and suffer from nausea and vomiting.

Yet most people know that neurologists don't really do etiological (causal) healing as much as acupuncturists do. Only elimination of the elemental disturbance can permanently cure the headaches; the added nausea often indicates

Element Theory and Scientific Cellular Medicine

Element Level

According to Four/Five Element Theory
  – Energy combines with metabolism
  – The humors are basic states that transition into each other
    like the four seasons (energy transformation)
Healing through humoral medicine (Galen, Hippocrates), Ayurveda, traditional Chinese medicine

Influences

Cellular Level (Level of the Cells)
Influenced by
  – Allopathy (forces cell reaction)
  – Genetics (alters cells)
  – Surgery (removes cells)
  – Fresh cells (stimulates cells)
  – Orthomolecular Medicine (influences enzymatic processes)

a problem with the *earth* element, associated with the liver/gallbladder functional system. Then, via the bile meridian – whose acupuncture route runs from the shoulder via the temple – it gives rise to headaches, while the nausea relates to digestive disorder (caused by weakly flowing bile). The nervousness is usually provoked by mineral disturbances, also due to underlying reduced bile flow that hinders adequate mineral uptake.

In my own practice, I have been detecting "humoral disorders" more and more frequently as my experience increases. Soon, I was prescribing liver/gallbladder remedies for over half my patients. These are innocuous bitter substances, often derided as "granny remedies" because older women take them as digestives and mild purgatives. Markedly weaker, but with a similar action, are the bitter schnapps liqueurs taken to aid digestion in countries such as France and Italy. This also includes bitter fruits such as avocado and artichoke. In my opinion, they're a little noticed yet nontrivial part of the "French paradox," according to which life expectancy in France and Italy is unusually high, even though risk factors such as high cholesterol, obesity, and cigarette smoking are prevalent in both countries. It seems to me that red wine explains just part of the "French paradox" effect (the bitter pigments also play an important role).

Much to my amazement, these bitter substances had surprisingly great energetic power. From migraine (a downright classic "bile disease" in the view of element theory) to the most varied skin diseases (hives, Neurodermitis, *Pruritus sine materia,* and so on), I often observed well-nigh miraculous healing results. In time, I began to understand what humoral theory meant by *melan**cholia*** and **chol**. These were evidently patients with bile (Greek *chol*) disorders that, in Four-Element Theory, occupy two element categories. About half of all patients belong to these two types.

The remaining two humoral types, the sanguinic (plethora) and hydrogenoid types (skin/mucosa with disturbed connective tissue) usually require other remedies. Sanguinics, for example, benefit from bloodletting and spleen/pancreas therapy. This organ system is closely associated with the formation of red blood corpuscles (hematopoiesis) and the sanguinic's energetic problems. Hydrogenoid types benefit most from therapy of the intestinal mucosa, detoxification of the upper respiratory tract and fortification of the stomach and pancreas. Step by step, my own experience as a naturopath was telling me that ancient humoral theory is still a very modern and up-to-date therapy. Anyone taking a closer look at the composition of successful naturopathic preparations will automatically encounter humoral theory. Iridodiagnosis, especially popular among naturopaths, owes its great success to the fact that it makes possible constitutional therapy of the various element types.

Humoral medicine offers the terrific possibility of attacking the roots of a disease at a very elemental level. Humoral medicine, also known as *milieu therapy*, views a disturbed milieu as the root of all disease. Naturopathic medicine attempts to improve the milieu with all manner of "detoxification" techniques such as fasting, dietary modification, sweating, and elimination of metabolic waste byproducts via the natural excretory organs (skin, lungs, kidneys, intestines). This is based on the conviction that healthy humors in a healthy metabolic environment are the best protectors of health.

In the next chapter, I describe the first psychosomatic system known to medical history: ancient Chinese element theory. The ancient Chinese were the first to make the connection between passions and extreme emotional states on the one hand, and the corresponding elements on the other. The Chinese conception of psychoenergetic interrelationships is so important, it seems to me, because it continues to be relevant to this day in the system of acupuncture – for Chinese medicine operates in largely unaltered form to this day, based on principles that are thousands of years old.

Passions as Disease Causes
in Ancient China

The more logical our actions, the freer we are – and the more enslaved,
the more we allow our passions to rule us.
(Leibniz)

In ancient China, as in many other early cultures, emotional disturbances and conflicts were often personified in the form of fearsome demon, dragons and monsters. These demons often took on godlike attributes simply because they seemed so powerful and terrifying. Yet the demons and dragons were not the products of pure imagination, since dinosaur bones had been found by Chinese farmers in their fields, thus seeming to confirm their existence. The enormous size of these creatures was quickl- associated with the tremendous untamable magnitude of human passions. Just as a big roaring lion generates enormous fear in us, so too do the enormous dragons and demons give rise to monstrous passions. From there, it is but a short step to equating demons and passions.

In ancient times, man's thinking was much more magical, which accordingly magnified the tendency to externalization and projection. There is no reality as such in magical-animistic thought. When virtually everything is viewed as being imbued with spirit, as it is in the worldview of so-called primitive cultures, it is known as *animism*. Animistic religions are practiced to this day throughout Asia; they are even found in modern-day Japan. Animism fuses man's inner and outer world into a single universe. Dreams thus herald real events, just as magic acts can partly – or almost entirely – anticipate actual realization. The priestly oracle derives enormous power from this. Likewise, imagination's magical figures take on very real shape with comparably enormous inherent power and importance.

In ancient China, as in ancient Greece, we encounter a prototypical form of rational thinking mixed in with animistic residues. In this process, the gods characteristically metamorphose into humanoid beings. In ancient Greece, the gods lived on Mount Olympus and behaved like humans. This means, of course, that they often "misbehave" – which makes them more sympathetic and human. The ancient Chinese took another (much more practical) route, conferring demigod status on spiritual leaders such as Lao-Tzu and Confucius. In Lao-Tzu's *Taoism*, the wisdom of nature becomes a goal worth striving toward, while *Confucianism* locates human happiness primarily in conforming to social norms. However, the Chinese gods never acquired individual character traits in the Western sense.

In my opinion, this reflects the general tendency of Asian cultures to elevate the communal over the individual. Of course, this makes understanding individual mental processes difficult right from the outset, in comparing such an attitude with that of modern Western psychology. For Asians, "going too far" in the sense of stronger passions is more unusual than the internal emotional processes which play out in the individual. By the way, Buddhism and Hinduism have very similar approaches. I'll return to the role of passions in the context of enlightenment.

The entire energy and medicine system of ancient China has always seemed outlandish to me. Despite years of intensive involvement, I have never been able to "warm up" to it nor feel comfortable with it. Part of the problem is surely the pictorial nature of written Chinese. To my mind, the Chinese have for this reason a different way of thinking, which some modern linguists have confirmed. What follows should therefore be taken in part as an expression of my problem in "getting into" Chinese thought. I admire physicians such as the American Leon HAMMER who, as psychoanalyst and psychiatrist, managed to fashion Chinese medicine into a functioning instrument which he uses to good effect.

Part of the problem with comprehending Chinese thought is its enormous intellectual intricacy. **Five-Element Theory** combines religion, philosophy and medicine into a highly complex whole. In intellectual sophistication, it is at least the equal of our Western philosophy. When the Chinese emperor Huang Ti (about 3000 years ago) asked his personal physician how long it took to become a good acupuncturist, Chi Pa's terse reply was "Seven hundred years." Of course, he meant: for a true understanding of Five-Element Theory, not for the ability to stick in acupuncture needles hither and yon according to certain rules.

The Chinese consider metal to be the 5th element; this is unknown in Western humoral theory, which only has four elements. Strictly speaking, metal is a manmade entity, not a naturally-occurring element, since it is found in the earth as an unrefined ore. I would assign the Chinese metal element to the Earth. The *metal* element is considered to be different from the others because it possesses transformative aspects lacking in the other elements. By the way, in the so-called pre-worldly order – a kind of primordial world that preceded the world of man – there are only four elements.

The aforementioned personal physician Chi Pa located the cause of psychosomatic disease in an unhealthy excess of passion: normal human emotions are exaggerated, leading to disease. He describes the process to the emperor as follows:

- **Anger** drives energy upward,
- **Joy** calms the energy flow, energy becomes peaceful.
- **Sadness** reduces energy by weakening lung energy.
- **Fear** drives energy downward by closing down the upper heater.
- **Worry** concentrates energy, so that it ceases to circulate.
- **Excessive physical exertion** expends too much energy,
- **Excessive mental energy** blocks energy circulation."

(Cited from Guido FISCH: *Akupunktur*)[25]

The named feelings are predominantly those emotional states that we would locate in the area of the superficial subconscious – for I am capable of telling if I'm sad or angry. After some reflection, I am always aware of sadness and anger. The personal physician Chi Pa was not referring to suppressed emotions. We would thus assign these extreme passions to current superficial conflicts. There is no question that these extreme passions can be suppressed and driven down into the subconscious, from which depths they will continue to act – yet it is precisely this that is largely unknown in traditional Chinese medicine. This omission leads inevitably to grave diagnostic and therapeutic errors, since if I allow something to drop out of my field of view, then it can no longer be seen or assessed – and thus is not treated.

Later on, I'll adduce even more viewpoints that can be taken as weak points and gaps in ancient Chinese medicine, when we compare their qualities to modern depth psychology. Next, I'd like to take a closer look at the individual passions, whose value for comprehensive psychoenergetic health is for me unquestionable. These are also known as the "seven demons," which aptly expresses their malign, out-of-control, and overly intense aspects. We can learn a great deal from a closer look at the pathological passions of ancient China.

It seems odd to us that **excessive physical exertion** is reckoned as one of the passions in ancient China. This is by no means due to laziness on their part! In our modern society, physical exertion includes, above all, high-performance sports. These lead to the release of endorphins that, so say addiction specialists, are very similar to addictive opiates. Many marathon runners become utterly addicted to the resulting euphoria. It should thus come as no surprise that so many professional athletes die uncommonly young. Thus, the Chinese disapproval of physical exertion refers to any kind of unhealthy exaggeration.

The second surprise is that **excessive mental exertion** is also counted as a passion. If we consider the extreme intellectualization (in the sense of excessive mental effort) that is endemic in our Western high civilization, this contradicts the Chinese ideal of moderation. I already mentioned that I undertook my own attempt to substantiate this thesis. In experiments with brainwave generators (so-called *mind machines*), test subjects' life energy sank when exposed to brain waves (11-30 Hz). We feel that subjectively when mental overexertion, over the longer term, tires us out and, like all heavy work, completely exhausts us – as any intellectual worker can confirm. One would have to be terrifically clever or an energetic powerhouse not to notice it much. One conclusion to be drawn from this is that school rest periods should be made longer than they currently are, and filled with more fun and physical activity.

Today, we would no longer count **joy** among the passions. One can only speculate why, keeping in mind that the Chinese understand joy to be any intense excitement ranging all the way up to shocking experiences. Since such emotions are known to be a burden on the heart – which goes along with our Western thinking – one can define joy more comprehensively as encompassing all intense excitement, both positive and negative (Nervousness falls within this purview.). **Sadness, fear, worry,** and **rage** are all passions whose morbific effects are beyond question.

What is much more surprising is the total lack of those concepts that are known by psychoanalysts to be sick-making emotions. This includes ideas such as jealousy, lust for power, inferiority complexes, greed and hate – to name just the most important ones. Incredibly, all these passions – without which no individual pathology is conceivable – are missing. My feeling is that the true roots of this perceptual gap are to be found in Asian cultures' fundamental anti-individualism. Anyone who has a chance to experience an Asian tourist group will be surprised, time and again, by the uncommonly strong group cohesion. On our many vacations to Hawaii or Switzerland (where Asians are fairly common), my partner and I have virtually never noticed any "loners" in these groups. The few we have seen are almost always extremely westernized group members who ostentatiously display their individualism.

The second point deals with the rigorous self-discipline that is an immutable basic requirement in Asia. It imprints itself on the Asian character to this day, and is also one of the most important religious demands. To this extent, the control of passions continues as a religious commandment.

---

[25] These seven passions (in boldface above) were later reduced to five, presumably to bring them in line with Five-Element Theory. Orderliness is certainly "half the battle" – even when it comes to classifying chaotic and anarchistic emotions. I think, however, that this Chinese tendency has the disadvantage of leading to rigid and formulaic thinking. It lacks final, dynamic, and linear aspects, as well as chaos and imperfection.

This is seen most clearly in Tibetan medicine, which combines Chinese medicine with Indian Buddhism. The Tibetan priest-doctor equates the passions with spiritual sacrilege (corresponding to our idea of *sin*). In this context, "Calling negative attention to oneself" or "losing face" are among the worst things that can befall an Asian. Those who indulge their feelings and lose their nerve are seen as weaklings and lose status and respect.

If we take a look at the relationship between the passions and the elements, we see correspondences whereby organs (as functional systems) can be symbolically associated with elements(see table below).

One can interpret the associated passions as something the germ of which is already contained in the respective element – except that a passion overdoes it to a pathological degree. If we understand the elements to be emotional states that we all experience at some time or another, then we can tell which emotional states will harm us during a particular phase. In the following description, I make use of additional concepts that are likewise associated with the elements (such as seasons, colors, and taste).

We must not think of the liver in the modern sense, but rather as a functional unit to which the material organ liver belongs. Belonging above all to the liver is the energy that is characterized as "woody" in the sense of "growing dynamically." If we grasp the rest of the liver assignments such as *wind*, *spring*, the color *green*, the taste *sour*, then we'll understand liver as a big metabolic factory, to be sure, but also as a symbol of everything that grows, that is fresh and newly sprouting. Understandably, tender shoots and interwoven growth processes do not respond well to rough handling. If we think of the awakening soul that each of us bears as a tender young shoot, then we'll understand how the emotional tornado of the passion *rage* blows everything away that is trying to grow. In a certain sense, rage represents an exaggeration of the dynamics inherent in the power of growth and regeneration.

In the summer of our emotional life, agitation and nervousness are harmful to the maturing process we are under-going. Anything trying to take on a final structure is harmed by chaos. In late summer, we find ourselves in the *Thanksgiving Celebration* phase. We are rewarded for all the efforts that life has laid on us. Our predominant feeling should be equanimity, while sorrow and worry are the very opposite thereof. In the autumn of our life, we need, once again, to learn something different, namely to bid farewell and dissociate ourselves from things. If we don't do this voluntarily and with good grace, then sadness results. In the winter of our emotional life, everything living comes to a standstill. If the standstill triggers fear, that is the worst possible reaction.

We now have an idea of how we should **not** react in certain situations. But why is it only the negative passions that are overemphasized? One may well ask, in the words of the humorist Erich KÄSTNER: "*Where does that leave the positive, Mr. Kästner?*" After all, positive and good feelings should also have some meaning. The health-promoting effect of positive feelings – being in a good mood, laughing, gentleness – are acknowledged even by science. Since the ancient Chinese didn't specifically mention these good feelings, I'd like here to make good the omission. I have related the positive health-promoting feelings to their corresponding elements. This idea first came to me when an acupuncture instructor mentioned that energy disturbances could be healed with taste qualities. I thought about the possibility that one might also be able to heal with good emotions instead of good-tasting food. But above all, these good emotions would be important health donors, by keeping our energy system harmonized.

There is, of course, the fundamental question: Why do negative things always generate the most interest, be they newspaper headlines or medicine? This has largely to do with stress focusing our attention: good and normal things are, after all, boring! In medicine, the "interesting" case is the very sick patient. A patient who makes an unexpectedly speedy recovery does not get as much attention. Healers and physicians have an inborn fascination for the morbid and broken-down. Therefore, the possibly natural and obvious

Passions, with their organs and energies (acupuncture)

Passion	Organ	Element
Wrath	Liver	Wood
Nervousness	Heart	Fire
Sadness	Lungs	Metal
Sorrow	Spleen	Earth
Anxiety	Kidney	Water

good, harmonic, and friendly healing principle does not immediately occur to us.

In what follows, I'd like to iron out these widespread errors of our profession by listing the emotions that are particularly good for us and best stimulate energy flow. You can never get enough of these emotions, since they make and keep us healthy. These positive emotions also harmonize us psychoenergetically. Drawing on the ideas of the medieval physician Hildegard von BINGEN, I'd like to call them *virtues*. To Hildegard, virtues play a significant role in the prevention of disease. Moreover, she knew about more virtues than I have listed here, of which the Love of God is foremost. I would place Love of God under the rubric *happy*, because (in my experience) people who believe in God and have a strong spiritual orientation are often very happy and joyful emotionally.

When we look at the five named virtues, the selection at first strikes us as unusually old-fashioned and un-modern. In today's society, virtues such as *being able to keep quiet or still, or being happy or contented (modest)* seem very quaint and boring. Our mind's eye pictures a person from long-ago times, living in peace and contentment with himself and nature, perhaps a somewhat reclusive farmer. Chinese society is known to have been an agricultural society whose survival and *virtue* consisted specifically of doing the right thing at the right time – so our farmer does make sense.

In fact, we moderns tend to look down on and put down "hillbillies" and other old-fashioned types that exemplify such utterly important virtues. Thus, keeping still can mean that someone is in reality a lazybones in disguise ("Don't just sit around so much: do something, for goodness' sake!"). Someone who is externally happy and contented can actually be a naïve dummy who doesn't know enough to worry – and so forth. In so judging, we are confusing form and content. We should relearn how to appreciate these good feelings, and try to produce these very valuable traits as often as possible. Our hectic modern life, with its cynicism and unremitting avarice, often stands in diametrical opposition thereto. Psychosomatic specialists agree that our

emotionally unhealthy lifestyle makes us sick. We mostly experience the negative passions, namely the vices such as *anger, nervousness, sorrow, and fear*. What we desperately need, however, are virtues such as *direct (vigorous), patient (relaxed), happy (good-natured, jolly) and quiet (peaceable)*.

All manner of people would have us believe that only they have the key to true happiness. **The truth is, our happiness is already within us!** It is the buried treasure of a happy life that we need to salvage. For this, we have to learn to have these feelings without external assistance, i.e., from within ourselves! Daily immersion in a meditative exercise, in which one pictures to oneself the named feeling-states and enters into them, can be very helpful. Practice makes perfect: in that the more we do the exercise, the better we can maintain the desirable feelings.

The search for happiness raises the crucial question that accompanies our life from its first day to its last: "How do I find lasting happiness and well-being?" Even a baby needs constant care and feeding to grow and prosper. Because of our dependence on the environment for basic needs such as food, drink, shelter, etc., we become (in the extreme case) susceptible to extortion and subjected to a social pressure to conform, which inhibits our personal development. Personal happiness can founder on the most elementary conditions, which have to do with our social powerlessness. It is naïve and hasty not to take note of such omnipresent problems. Another obstacle to personal happiness is our internal opposition. We have subconscious passions and emotional conflicts that impede our life. We can therefore approach our personal state of happiness only up to a point, limited by pre-existing inner blocks and obstacles. Recognizing and eliminating inner conflicts represents the very first and most important step in self-liberation! How to detect and heal inner conflicts will be explained in a later part of this book.

Regrettably, the Chinese tradition has little to say concerning individual emotional needs and depth-psychological dynamics. Although normalization of disturbed body energy has positive repercussions on overall somatic/mental

Good adequate emotions (virtues) along with their organs and energies (acupuncture theory)

Good Feeling	Organ	Element
Purposeful	Liver	Wood
Cautious	Heart	Fire
Happy	Lungs	Metal
Contented	Spleen	Earth
Calm	Kidney	Water

well-being, the underlying emotional conflicts nevertheless are generally not eliminated in this manner. This considerable drawback of Traditional Chinese Medicine is found in exactly the same form in all other kinds of humoral medicine. The next chapter takes a critical look at the limits of these techniques, which do not make depth-psychological uncovering and healing of subconscious conflicts unnecessary, but rather can (at most) complement them. However, the exaggerated pretensions of these techniques often cause this to be overlooked, giving rise to new problems.

Some Critical Comments on Humoral Medicine and Naturopathy

Diseases do not befall us out of a clear blue sky, but develop out of our daily sins against nature. When these have accumulated sufficiently, they break out unexpectedly.
(Hippocrates)

In the preceding chapters, we retrospectively traced the history of medicine. From shamans and priests there developed a professional caste, that of the physicians, which split off from theologians and priests, who dealt more with matters mental and spiritual. Every development has its good and bad sides, and the current separation of religion and the healing arts is an unfavorable one, secularization having led to the loss of much comprehensive and important knowledge. One of the important concerns of my book is to reanimate a sense for these buried and largely forgotten disease causes.

We can only truly make people healthy if we have an underlying vision of man that encompasses spiritual and subtle-body disease causes. Of course, one must also be aware of the limits of the healing methods used. We've already seen that, for too-far advanced processes, element medicine can no longer accomplish anything on the material plane. This applies to fractures or appendicitis, irreversible metabolic dysfunctions such as diabetes, and many kinds of hypertension. For many infectious diseases such as malaria, tuberculosis, and anthrax, the use of antibiotic treatment is often unavoidable when the disease process is too advanced.

Yet another ancient bone of contention is the dispute as to whether the milieu or the bacterium is more important. The renowned French physician and adherent of the milieu theory, Claude BERNARD, at the height of the mid-19th-century quarrel between cellular pathologists and milieu devotees, defiantly phrased it thus: "*The bacterium is nothing, the milieu everything!*" In this he is surely right, in many cases. Recently, a professor sought to prove this controversial thesis by means of a heroic experiment performed on himself before an audience, in which he drank a reagent glass full of infectious intestinal bacteria and, against all expectation, remained completely healthy. But one should not view the issue too absolutely. In my opinion, a patient can get sick despite being in a good state of health (i.e. good milieu and good energy situation) if the bacterium is aggressive enough.[26] Still, the possibility of disease is much less than for a person who is already latently ill.

Naturally, the idea of putting the internal milieu and the environment into diametrical opposition is tempting for a number of reasons. Many therapists and their patients unshakably believe in simple formulas of health and illness – first of all because (of course) many people more readily accept simple solutions (out of ignorance or laziness), or as artifice on the therapist's part, in order to more easily mobilize the patient's own healing powers. Because if healing depends on oneself (and one's therapist), then this makes all involved more confident.

Added to which, therapists have, since time immemorial, been susceptible to the occupational disease of self-overestimation. Thus, many physicians are attracted to radical theories because this lets them subtly to magnify their own power. Yet many times, the healing profession is possessed of the opposite of power madness, as many insecure therapists cover up their subconscious fears and feelings of inadequacy with radical theories and measures. My point here is not to beat up on my professional colleagues, but rather to shine a light on some typical professional weak points – for an astonishing number of physicians and therapists are themselves psychoenergetically ill to a considerable degree, as my own investigations have revealed. These people are prone to suppress their own emotional problems in the process, all too often transferring the evil to be combated to the hostile external world, while remaining "untainted" and "safe and sound." Thus, all the bad chemicals, parasites, and hostile toxins are lying in wait out there in the environment, while the healer rids himself and the patient of these with *detoxifications*. Evil is thus *externalized*, to use the specialized jargon of psychology.

Besides limitations having to do with the therapist's person and his inner emotional problems, there are other important restrictions one should be familiar with, inherent in the naturopathic healing methods themselves. The main

---

[26] In shamanistic thinking, being free of demons (emotional conflicts) is considered the best and most important condition for health. The only exception that shamans recognize are epidemics, when even demon-free shamans armed with protective health spirits can get sick – i.e., when bacteria are highly virulent and are present in great numbers.

reason is based in the history of medicine, **because at some point, the medical profession simply "forgot" that emotional conflicts exist at all.** This problem was delegated to priests, who became responsible for them from then on. In some rural regions of Italy, China, India, Korea, and Brazil, it is still customary to call the priest or shaman to deal with spirits, possession and exorcism.

Yet there is no doubt that subconscious emotional conflicts play a role in most diseases, yet at some point it became repugnant and difficult for physicians to occupy themselves with this. Therefore, conflicts were simply forgotten, or delegated to other professions. A similar phenomenon from medical history can also be seen in surgery, which was similarly felt to be repugnant. Thus, in China, the emperor banned it outright. In the West up through the late Middle Ages, surgery remained the province of army field surgeons and highly specialized barber-surgeons. A profession as highly regarded and elegant as that of physicians would have nothing to do with such lowly activities. Anyone who reads attentively in element medicine won't find much in there about emotional conflicts.

Holistic naturopathy, i.e., comprehensive psychosomatic medical science that includes the emotional, is encountered much less often than one might think out there in the harsh real world. The next interesting issue is, above all, what the natural healer who fails to recognize the conflicts does instead. What are the consequences of ignoring the actual cause of a psychoenergetic disturbance? This important question is a very topical one, since (in thousands of practices all over the world) acupuncture, homeopathy, fasting cures, etc. are being done — without the underlying emotional conflicts being adequately recognized and treated. The burning question is: What happens to the patient if we balance out the humoral and energy system without breaking up and healing the underlying conflict?

I here view the conflict in a twofold manner: as a problem that is suppressed in the subconscious and that, at the same time, has its own subtle-body existence. The conflict's dual nature makes healing downright difficult, since just talking about a conflict does not heal it energetically. Therefore, conventional psychological techniques are quite unsatisfying from an energetic standpoint. Often, conflicts are neither detected nor healed, regardless of which methods a patient had previously used:

- Patients who had seen a psychologist, might be aware of a part of their conflicts – which, however, changes nothing about their existence in the subtle-body energetic realm.
- With orthodox physicians, patients' conflicts and energy system have mostly been artificially sedated and throttled down by pharmaceutical agents (allopathics).
- For patients who had gone to naturopathic healers, the energy system is usually harmonized and the milieu detoxified, but the conflicts continue their existence down in the subconscious depths.

In order to exemplify this dilemma, let's take a look at disease genesis from the perspective of an acupuncturist (keeping in mind that this perspective applies equally well to all other naturopaths). In our example, disease is viewed by the acupuncturist as an energy disturbance, i.e., disturbed *Ch'i* or energy flow. Our acupuncturist can distinguish various kinds of energetic disturbances. A therapist taking a pulse can tell whether too little or too much energy is flowing, whether the energy is congested, wrongly constituted, or qualitatively disturbed. Empirically, chronic and serious illnesses are mainly evoked by too little energy; inflammatory and acute ailments, on the other hand, usually arise due to an excess of energy, which then gets congested and provokes inflammation and pain.

Our acupuncturist deals mostly with chronic diseases evoked by energy deficiency. Collectively, these are serious long-term disturbances that show little inclination to heal up on their own. So, a chronically ill patient is being examined by our acupuncturist. The first question that the patient will have for the acupuncturist has to do with the significance of the energy deficiency. As with all defects in daily life, we in medicine also ask ourselves what the actual underlying cause of the disturbance might be. Unlike the modern Western physician, who searches either for measurable material disturbances or emotional causes, the acupuncturist moves in an intermediate realm, seeking out deeper disease disturbances in the area of humors and energetics – and the resulting success in combating chronic disease seems to validate this course of action.

An acupuncturist will seek out the energy deficiency in a mixture of humoral disorder and energetic problems. One or more of the elements have gotten disordered. But, in my opinion, acupuncturists cannot detect with sufficient clarity that emotional conflicts are the true cause of the patient's diminished energy flow. Why can't they detect subconscious conflicts? Because most people's emotional conflicts are completely subconscious, so they are not perceived – and that which one cannot perceive one will of course not be reporting to the doctor. Nor can you blame acupuncturists either for failing to see something that lies beyond their perceptual horizon.

Still, if we were standing in judgment here, we would nonetheless assign the primary blame to the therapist. Acupuncturists are supposed to find out what's wrong with their patients – but they can only make out disturbances at the humoral and low-vibration life force levels. Regrettably, the ancient Chinese physicians were completely blind to disturbances at the higher vibrational emotional or even Causal Levels. In this respect, they were no different from their ancient Indian, Greek, or Arabic colleagues. Amazingly, the situation remains essentially unchanged to this day in the area of traditional element medicine!

Let us now turn to the therapeutic scenario: the patient looks pale and sickly, feels constantly unwell, and has numerous vegetative symptoms. Where do they come from? If we recall the image of the conductor from the previous chapter, directing the elemental orchestra, we'll understand the acupuncturist's motivation, who is thinking in terms of a humoral disorder or disturbance of subtle-body energy at a point where the lever's fulcrum can be applied and the patient "redirected." Using certain acupuncture needles and healing herbs, this in fact succeeds quite satisfactorily. The actual, deeply hidden disease cause – the subconscious conflict – has come through unscathed, however, and is once again skulking about in the depths of the system. Even though the patient feels good again and looks rosy-cheeked healthy, an unhealed conflict smolders, unnoticed, in the depths … and it will, at some point, break out again (see illustration below).

Visually, we can picture the patient's total energy as a vessel into which less power can flow because of the conflict.

Unfortunately, the patient is not a transparent object, as the depicted vessel might lead one to think. In this puzzling situation, the acupuncturist in our example actually only notices the end result, namely that the patient lacks energy and that the elements and humors are all mixed up. The acupuncturist supplies energy and balances out the elements/humors, restoring the system's equilibrium. The patient is better and healing processes begin. The patient seems healthy and is enormously grateful to the acupuncturist. The problem is that the still undetected emotional conflict crawls back into its shell, from which hiding place it secretly continues to affect things and can, at some future time, make the patient sick again (see illustration on next page).

One can take the attitude, of course, that "*He who heals is in the right.*" But we already suspect a pseudo-cure. Now, I have no doubt that genuine healing takes place now and then, when subconscious conflicts heal spontaneously and disappear thanks to a well-chosen energetic/humoral treatment. Still, my years of experience indicate that this is rather the exception. Therefore, in most cases, the holistic healing that therapist and patient were striving for with naturopathic methods simply does not take place. Another exception is when a therapist has the rare gift of being able to ferret out and energetically heal conflicts while discussing the conflict theme with the patient – but this kind of highly intuitive "healing artist" is as scarce as hen's teeth.

Actually, it's not always appropriate to dredge up the deepest disease causes: if someone suddenly has a severely inflamed appendix, it should be operated immediately, even if triggered by an emotional conflict. Further reasons can likewise be presented as arguments against uncovering conflicts. Bringing up conflict themes is to be avoided when dealing with people who basically consider the idea of emotional causes to be hokum. Also, some people are simply totally incapable of self-insight, e.g., children, the mentally handicapped, and the severely neurotic. Sometimes, in cases

Energy deficiency due to emotional conflicts

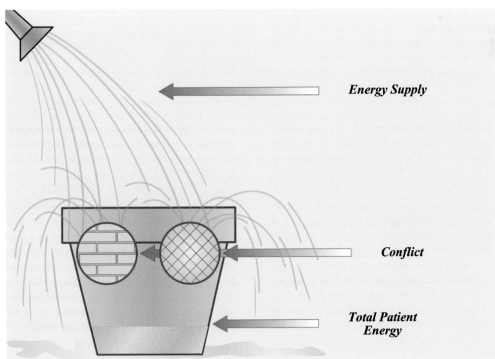

Energy Supply

Conflict

Total Patient Energy

involving suicide proneness, psychoses, and other kinds of emotional volatility, one has to worry that uncovering conflicts might constitute a real danger for the patient.

Despite which, it is definitely a good idea, in most cases, to uncover the underlying conflicts. Of course, this is not enough to heal the conflict: purely psychological therapy is no panacea either, since, besides becoming aware of the conflict's contents, it must also be dissolved energetically. I'd like to illustrate, with a typical case, how conflicts are uncovered, their content discussed, and then energetically dissolved:

The 53-year-old woman, bookkeeper, 6 years ago was struck, out of nowhere, by a horrible anxiety attack that kept on escalating. She cannot recall there being any reason for it. She is happily married and had an untroubled childhood. The ago-

flict tests out in the Brow Chakra: No. 24 (Uneasiness). The conflict has energetically huge values (with extremely high values of 70% Vital, 80% Emotional, 20% Mental and 70% Causal). Based on its size, the conflict is a so-called Central Conflict, which has the significance of a life theme. Discussing the conflict theme, she relates that, for as long as she can remember, she has always felt uncomfortable in her body. I explain to her that the energetic treatment of the conflict can lead to intense dreaming, and advise her, moreover, to learn to accept her feeling of discomfort, and to try to become aware of the beautiful and pleasant aspects of her body. Medically speaking, what she has is generalized anxiety syndrome (GAS). Evidently, the hormonal shift of early menopause was in part responsible for activating her Central Conflict and making it her dominating life theme and most important emotional problem, which then began to generate symptoms. Like many patients

Energy/humoral disturbance and a hidden emotional conflict as the true cause

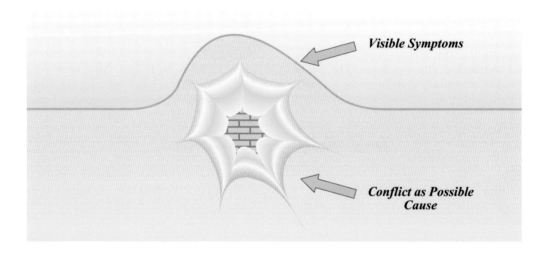

nizing anxiety has come to dominate her life. She has trouble sleeping, is incapable of relaxing and has lately been feeling more and more depressed. She is often unable to concentrate on her work because the anxiety is so bad. Her family doctor prescribed a tranquilizer that proves to be of little help. She doesn't want to go to specialists such as psychiatrists and psychologists because she considers herself completely normal mentally. A naturopath tested out some minerals and vitamins (so-called orthomolecular remedies) on her, which helped for a while but did not lead to any lasting improvement. An acupuncture series and foot reflexology massages helped temporarily. Measuring her energy levels shows a sharply (40%) reduced emotional Aura value. Emotional body values that low are found in cases of incipient depression; to that extent, the value matches her depressed mood. The rest of the readings are relatively normal (70% Vital, 100% Mental, 60% Causal). A subconscious con-

with this kind of anxiety syndrome, she reports that relaxation exercises just intensify the anxiety. Her thyroid and everything else had been thoroughly examined, but no physical cause was found for her anxiety. In the remedy test, placing the homeopathic complex for the Brow Chakra and the conflict Uneasiness in her energy field completely normalizes the energy picture at 100/100/100/70. Because of these good healing prospects, I recommend discontinuing the tranquilizer. Eight weeks later, a beaming patient is sitting in front of me: the anxiety is almost gone, she says, and life is once again beginning to be enjoyable. Her emotional readings have risen to a normal 100% and the conflict has been reduced by half. To be on the safe side, treatment for it is continued for a few more months, after which the patient is completely cured.

The above example makes it clear that eliminating emotional conflicts leads to lasting healing. Any other kind of treatment is mere patchwork with, at best, transitory improvement. As with any therapy, it is crucial to identify and eliminate the true cause of the disease. Only then, when the energy blocks caused by the emotional conflicts are eliminated, can the natural healing powers once again do their work to full effect. The patient is free of anxiety and again becomes a cheerful and energetic person.

The next chapter deals again with subtle-body energy and its stratification into different levels. Understanding the Aural Levels constitutes the basic precondition for being able to grasp the subconscious conflict over its entire spectrum – for a conflict is layered energetically very much as we are. In a certain sense, one can think of a conflict as a small independent being. The multilayered nature of conflicts can only be understood with reference to their psychoenergetic structure. Therefore, conflict origins will be discussed later, once the Aura and energy centers (Chakras) have been thoroughly covered.

The Aura

The envelope of subtle-body energy that surrounds each of us is called the *Aura*, (Greek "air" or "breeze"). Generally, the Aura is viewed as an invisible copy of the body, surrounding our coarse-body physical vehicle and towering above it.[27] The extension of the Aura's first layer (Vital Level) is usually about 20 inches – but it can fluctuate considerably. Many people's Aura barely reach an inch or two, whereas other's extend out three to six feet. It is not yet known very well what the significance is of the Aura's extension. Basically, a small Aura seems to be associated with exhaustion or hypersensitivity (Yin state), while a large Aura typifies robust, resolute persons, as well as (often) the early stages of cancer (Yang state).

The Aura's extension – which can fluctuate considerably within seconds – has fairly little to do with the Aura's charge. This is fortunate, since the Aura's extreme fluctuations are hard to measure and standardize. My recommendation therefore is not to ascribe all that much importance to the Aura's extension. Instead, it is much more useful to deal with the Aura's quality – figuratively, its *luminosity*, represented in paintings of Saints as a circular ring around the holy person. The Aura exhibits amazingly stable and reliable quality readings, with virtually no day-to-day variation, which therefore yield very practical and usable results.

From the standpoint of practical medical usefulness, the Aura seems at first to be quite insignificant. Only Yogis in the Himalayan hinterlands seem to be interested in such exotic phenomena. As a physician, however, the statements of a number of clairvoyants, some time ago, made me wonder if diseases might be observable in the Aura long before they manifested themselves physically. This would of course represent a terrific opportunity for the early detection of diseases! Moreover, the Aura seems to offer the possibility of influencing the coarse body by using it as an access route. Thus, many clairvoyant healers claim that healing blockages within the Aura has beneficial effects on the material body. All of these medical possibilities have fascinated me, and led me to occupy myself intensively with the Aura for about three decades now.

If you imagine the Aura as a kind of software that controls the material body's hardware, then this presents an outstanding and elegant possibility of influencing the processes of the coarse body. We are reminded of regulation by the elements (humors), which we learned about earlier. Because of its invisibility, this kind of healing process is often referred to as ***faith healing; energy work*** is another term that means the same thing. There are well-known healers who transmit their own healing energy through the laying on of hands, at the same time eliminating disturbances in the ailing person's Aura.

By now, a great many scientific studies of faith healing have been conducted that consistently confirm the effectiveness of this healing method. This tells us that people can exchange energy and information invisibly, in a mental/spiritual manner. The resulting exchange process can be consciously controlled, and often has a healthful effect. The clearly demonstrable successes have resulted (especially in Great Britain) in faith healers being allowed to operate in normal hospitals. Earlier, I pointed out the attendant risks of practicing magic; here, I would like to emphasize that modern faith healers are generally aware of the risks inherent in magical practices, and repudiate them. Practically all faith healers that I know have a serious spiritual background that guides them to operate in a responsible manner.

The Aura represents the linkage between such disparate procedures as faith healing and modern naturopathic techniques (homeopathic, light/color therapy, etc.). The actual influence of all these procedures rests on their effect on the Aura, which is harmonized thereby and rid of disturbances; this in turn harmonizes the elements and humors, which normalizes metabolism and heals the energy system as a whole.

The depiction of the three only possible healing levels clearly shows that the energetic healing level represents the highest one. We attain this level by means of any therapy that influences the subtle-body energy system. This includes, in the West, homeopathy first of all, with which "life energy's discords" (in the words of homeopathy's discoverer, Samuel HAHNEMANN) are to be healed. Also, certain kinds of classical acupuncture can be considered to be energy medicine, because they don't so much influence metabolism (humors) as emphasize harmonization of energy itself. This includes acupuncture of the miracle meridi-

---

[27] In modern medicine, *Aura* refers to those symptoms that, for example, precede an epilepsy or migraine attack. Aura in the subtle body sense, however, is completely foreign to modern medicine.

ans and certain special points that can influence emotional-energetic health states.

Since energy medicine's triumphal procession continues unabated, the Aura will in all likelihood be hugely significant for the medicine of the future. It thus makes sense to get into it intensively. The Aura represents the deepest and strongest access to the actual regulation of our organism as a whole, which includes the material body as well as the subtle-body/energetic and emotional/intellectual.

The following chapters discuss the four most important Aura layers and how they are interwoven with the material body, as well as their relationship to the soul. I here make use of a representation that follows the nomenclature of traditional Yoga, modifying the system and adding some colloquial terminology to make it more understandable. The system presented here also includes my practical experiences as a physician.

Healing Level Layers and Associated Healing Methods

Energetic Level

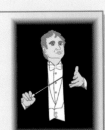

Energy (Ch'I, Prana, Orgone)
  – *Gives cellular level health concepts (positive ideas)*
  – *Influences cell metabolism (enzymes, hormones) as power donor*
  – *Gives "power" to make cells viable (primordial energy)*
Healing of disorders on this level through "energy work" and healing of conflicts. Energy supply from healthy lifestyle, fresh air, vital nutrition, regular sexuality, abiding in the natural world

Influences

Element Level

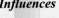

According to Four/Five Element Theory
  – *Energy combines with metabolism*
  – *The humors are basic states that transition into each other like the four seasons (energy transformation)*
Healing through humoral medicine (Galen, Hippocrates), Ayurveda, traditional Chinese medicine

Influences

Cellular Level (Level of the Cells)

Influenced by
  – *Allopathy (forces cell reaction)*
  – *Genetics (alters cells)*
  – *Surgery (removes cells)*
  – *Fresh cells (stimulates cells)*
  – *Orthomolecular Medicine (influences enzymatic processes)*

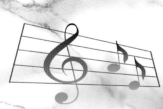

Now, when we turn to medical practice, the biggest problem is **perceiving the Aura** itself. As nice as it would be to be able to discern the Aura, most of us have to rely on clairvoyants. But this, over the longer term, is not a realistic solution in daily practice. I know a few medical colleagues – whose ability I envy – who can see the Aura. I usually don't see the Aura; when I do, it's only after weeks of meditation when I enter into an unusual state of extreme sensitivity. If we were able to perceive the Aura easily and relatively objectively, that would clearly be an immense advance, since we'd then be better able to detect diseases earlier. However, objective perception of the Aura seems to be very difficult. Normally, we assume that clairvoyants see the same thing and describe it in the same words. Unfortunately, that is almost never the case: clairvoyants see highly subjective phenomena that deviate sharply from each other.

In this context, I'd like to report on some experiments with clairvoyants. I was fortunate enough to actually find two unusually sensitive mediums, women of middle age, of which one is regularly consulted by the police in murder cases. I mention this to underscore the level of quality of this highly sensitive woman's abilities, whose paranormal abilities have often led to amazing success.

Right at the beginning of our first meeting, she told me her tale of woe: "*You know, doctor, it's horrible to be able to foresee so much. Let me give you an example: once, I was in a bakery and I saw a neighbor woman. At that time, I was still just a beginner as a clairvoyant, and so I wasn't yet very confident in my abilities. And yet, I knew at once that my neighbor only had a few days left to live – but I couldn't bring myself to tell her. As I said, I was still unsure of myself and didn't want to disgrace myself. Two days later, she died in a traffic accident!*" Since then, she understandably blames herself for not having said anything to her neighbor; she has conscience pangs every day when she sees the widower and his flock of children. In my experience, therefore, being a medium is often an extraordinarily stressful matter.

During numerous energetic experiments testing out homeopathics on patients, I asked the two clairvoyants to describe the resulting phenomena: "I see a reddish gleam in the 3rd Chakra that was not there before," one of them said. "The force field is brighter overall and lights up more, but I don't see a red gleam in the 3rd Chakra. Instead, the entire body is brighter." After a while, it became clear that the two women had perceived different phenomena. Later on, I tried a different experimental setup, in which a faith healer with known strong healing powers transmitted his energies to an ailing person – but they repeated their differing descriptions in this case as well. The most disturbing aspect was that the one clairvoyant sometimes saw major changes while the other one barely noticed anything. Subsequent experiments with other clairvoyants turned out much the same.

So it is that clairvoyance seems to me to be an extremely subjective phenomenon, very dependent on the individual person. To be sure, clairvoyants now and then see particular phenomena very similarly, and agree as to their meaning – but this seems to apply to inexperienced clairvoyants who adopt the other's interpretation. Evidently, the clairvoyants in question subjectively filter the Aura in their heads. For this reason, clairvoyance is, in my opinion, a so-called *synæsthetic phenomenon*. Medically, synæsthesia is the mixing-up of sensory impressions, as when for example one hears music while eating. We now know from numerous interviews that synæsthesia is a surprisingly common inborn trait. In this sense, clairvoyance would be the transformation of an Aura feeling (in the sense of a "breath of air") into an optical perception. The clairvoyant thus doesn't actually see the Aura, but rather transforms another kind of perception into a visually-sensed one. Because of the strong subjective component, Aural perception is to my mind therefore unsuitable as a measuring instrument.

There are of course other ways to perceive the Aura. With enough sensitivity and training, we can feel another person's Aura. We'll perceive it, for instance, as a gentle breeze that often seems to give off a type of vibrating motion and cool freshness. This same phenomenon can often be experienced in a crowded bus or subway car. Many people turn around when you look at them from behind, because you have mentally touched their Aura. Or someone approaches us from behind, and we suddenly get another feeling, in the immediate vicinity of the other person (starting at a certain distance and point in time). Our discomfort is often a sign that a fellow traveler has come near whom we are not congenial to. It is much harder to detect a fellow traveler with whom one is spontaneously sympathetic. From this we learn that, energetically, sympathy means the admixture of the two Auras, whereas Auras repel each other in the case of antipathy.

We can of course also picture the Aura using energetic test procedures. For example, if you approach another person, a dowsing rod will dip at the moment that the two Auras make contact. An earlier chapter, **Subtle-Body Energy – Its Everyday Significance and its Testing**, photographically captures just such a situation between myself and my assistant at the time. You can also experience the same phenomenon with a so-called *one-handed rod* or a pendulum. In the thereby ascertainable Aura extension, one speaks in terms of *reaction distance,* i.e., the magnitude of the so-called *Vital Level* that corresponds to the lowest-vibrating Aura level. The other Aura levels are difficult (if not indeed impossible) to detect in this manner.

In the supposed Aura detection by the high-frequency fields of *Kirlian photography*, electrical skin discharges are captured by photographic paper. However, the discharges in Kirlian photographs by no means represent the Aura, being simply biophysical phenomena. So-called "Aura cameras" artificially convert bioelectrical skin phenomena into colors whose composition and hue is attuned to that which a clairvoyant has previously seen – but the "Aura camera" doesn't show the actual Aura either! There are by now countless photon, magnetic-field, and other kinds of devices, all of which are (wrongly) supposed to detect/portray the Aura. If we keep in mind that subtle-body energy is of a kind that has yet to be verified physically, then it's logical that the Aura will not be detectable or measurable **directly** in any form as a physical phenomenon.

The biophysicist Dieter Jossner (of Medical Electronics in Rheinau in southern Germany) and I co-developed a microprocessor-driven measuring instrument that can measure the Aura **indirectly**: the REBA® Test Device. Measuring the Aura with dowsing rods or the sensitivity of our hands are also indirect methods, in that the examiner's own Aura is used to portray another person's. The downside of these methods is that they are subjective and extremely interference-prone. The predefined signals of the REBA® Test Device, on the other hand, make relatively objective Aural measurements possible, in that different examiners arrive at essentially the same results. In this context, that means deviations of no more than ±10%, which permits meaningful and usable Aural measurement results.

To measure the Aura, one still needs the person as display instrument, such that the new test device cannot function without the examiner's sensitivity and reactive capability. The REBA® Test Device emits certain frequencies that resonate with the Aura and, like a tuning fork, stimulate it into co-vibration. The REBA® test device emits transverse waves, scalar waves similar in their physical characteristics to sound waves in the audible range. In all likelihood, scalar waves play an important role in conveying biophysical signals. The frequency spectrum of the REBA®Test Device corresponds to that of brain waves.

The four EEG wave types of deep sleep (Delta), dreaming/REM sleep (Theta), awake/alert (Alpha) and stress (Beta) correspond, according to my research, to the Aura levels of vitality, emotionality, mentality, and causality:

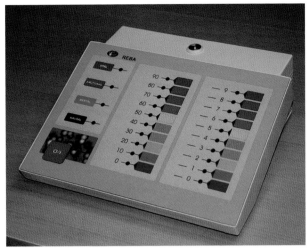

REBA® Test Device for measuring Aura levels

The REBA® Test Device measures the Aura indirectly by using the brain as a resonance system, whose spectrum exhibits a direct resonance with the Aura. The better the Aura reacts to and co-vibrates with an ever larger frequency mixture, the healthier the subject is on the corresponding Aura level. The measurement result is expressed in percent, which intrinsically leads to a "self-explanatory" understanding. Anyone can do something with this who has a vitality of 30%. At such low values, patients realize right away that they feel pretty puny and easily fatigued. At a vitality of 100%, on the other hand, most patients report feeling good and in top form.

The measured values match up very well with patients' subjective feelings. Often, the measurement results are confirmed after the fact, since surprisingly many people have not learned to be aware of how they feel, much less describe it in detail. For this reason, many examiners often have the correctness of their test results confirmed only in retrospect. Sometimes, other factors are involved, such as when time con-

Brainwave Frequency, Aura Level and Significance of Existing Relationships

Brainwave frequency	Aura Level	Function
Deep Sleep (Delta)	Vital Level	Vital levels regenerate
Dreaming (Theta)	Emotional Level	All levels regenerate
Awake (Alpha)	Mental Level	Throttles back Vital & Emotional Levels
Stress (Beta)	Causal Level	Programming of deep-rooted dogmas

straints prevent taking a detailed anamnesis and the measurement results are only discussed afterward. The measured values are amazingly objective when compared against the patient's sense of well-being. In many thousands of measurements, I have been able to establish (with very few exceptions) that patients recognize themselves in their measurement values, and they confirm the accuracy of the tests.

In this situation, critics might suspect that an experienced physician basically gets confirmation of that which his observation of the patient, and years of practical experience, has already intuited. To this I can only reply that I myself am very often surprised by the test results. If I then ask the patient whether my test results are on the mark, the answer is almost always in the affirmative. It also happens now and then that I don't get to question the patient before the examination. This is often the case when administering tests to colleagues as part of their training – but even then, the correctness of the test results is almost always confirmed (except for a very few exceptions, as will be encountered with any testing method). For me, the most conclusive test results are those that agree with those of other examiners, as is the case with very minor exceptions (in over 95% of cases).[28] I therefore conclude that examinations with the REBA® Test Device are very reliable and largely objective.

Up to now, I have been emphasizing Aura measurement because, of course, only a reliable perception of the Aura and its disturbances can create the indispensable basic conditions for subsequent medical activity. For we require of any good diagnostic instrument that it be, above all, reliable. I would like next to explicate the Aura's structure in greater detail, because we have to understand the structure and significance of the individual Aura levels if we are to arrive at a deeper understanding of the associated structures and the resulting disorders.

At the beginning of our involvement with the Aura, there is the (initially very vague, then ever more distinct) development of a consciousness of *Aura Reality*. As time goes by, it becomes clearer and clearer to us that we don't **have** an Aura; rather, we **are** our Aura. This is a process of ever finer self-perception, one which becomes easier the better we get to know that which our perception is directed at. Our Aura constitutes a part of our overall person, which – along with other parts such as the material body and the immaterial soul – unite to create a whole. The Aura is especially tightly bound up with the subconscious, an important part of the mind that is reflected in the Aura (in particular the emotional and causal bodies, which will be discussed

in greater detail shortly). In other words, getting involved with the Aura is a kind of self-exploration.

Following C.G. JUNG, we can liken the totality of our mind to a house whose stories correspond to different levels of our perceptual ability and consciousness. Everyday consciousness would then be the ground floor in broad daylight. All the other floors are located in the dark cellar of our subconscious. A key problem with our involvement with the subconscious has to do, initially, with the overwhelming dominance of normal everyday consciousness. This can be compared to a sunny summer day whose brightness at first makes the interior seem pitch dark because our eyes have not yet adjusted to the darkness. It's just like this with our subconscious, the perception of which needs to be practiced, because normal everyday consciousness so totally dominates our perception.

Ancient India (1000 BCE) already knew about the four layers of consciousness, with a direct relationship to the Aura. Most likely, the most important insights were gained by extremely clairvoyant, energetically open Yogis who had practiced meditation all their lives (so-called *Rishis*, i.e., Masters). I have already mentioned the pioneering knowledge of these wise men – that changed the medical (and religious) world – in the discussion of the theory of the elements. However, the *Rishis* didn't discover just the four elements, but also the energy centers (Chakras) and the Aura levels. During meditation, the Indian wise men entered into the various Aura levels and afterward noted what kinds of feelings and experiences were associated with each level.

According to these Indian sages, there are differently ordered layers of the Aura, each having a higher vibrational intensity and extension than the previous one (these are also known as *vibrational bodies*). In the ancient Indian writings, the material body (which vibrates energetically the lowest) is designated as the Aura's first body, followed by (in the view of the ancient Indians) four nonmaterial – and hence invisible – subtle bodies, as in the chart below.

The West, meanwhile, has incorporated the idea of four energy levels, and views the material body as something separate. Whether or not this approach is justified is open to debate, since it naturally involves the risk of our thinking taking a

The Four Aura Levels and the Five Bodies of Yogic Tradition

1. Annamaya-Kosha
   – the physical body
2. Pranamaya-Kosha
   – the vital body
3. Manomaya-Kosha
   – the emotional body
4. Vijnanamaya-Kosha
   – the mental body
5. Anandamaya-Kosha
   – the causal body

---

[28] In several hundred control measurements performed over the past few years at seminars for physicians and other health-care professionals, talented examiners who concentrate well come up with nearly identical test results for the same subjects more than 95% of the time, and this with no prior knowledge of the others' measurement results. By the way, this same reliability can be observed in testing disturbed Chakras and their associated emotional conflicts.

wrong turn due to an incorrectly represented structure. For instance, it is then easier to overlook that, from the standpoint of quantum physics, the material body can basically be conceived of as mostly empty space. Once we realize how much empty space there is between individual atoms, then our dense, solid-seeming material body turns out to consist almost entirely of imperceptible emptiness. We are thus fully justified in viewing the material body as a vibrational body as well.

Despite this, I can adduce two serious reasons for regarding the material body as a separate entity independent of the Aura. As we know, matter is relatively stable, motionless, and not very moldable.[29] Unlike the material body, the subtle body is in all likelihood not tied to a specific location. This applies at least to the astral or emotional body that, according to spiritual masters, can move about relatively independently of any particular object. These phenomena are known as *astral journeys*, whose symbol in fairy tales is the magic carpet. The nonlocality of the subtle body is, it seems to me, a valid reason to consider the four Aura layers separately from the material body. The second argument is based on the very first description of the Aura by the theosophist LEADBEATER, whose nomenclature has become widely accepted, and according to which the *coarse body* was always to be viewed as separate from the subtle-body Aura – presumably so as not to confuse readers who were grappling with these ideas for the first time.

Basically, there is not just one, but several Auras.[30]

The energy levels in man are four:
1. Vital (= ethereal)
2. Emotional (= astral)
3. Mental and
4. Causal

There are even higher levels, but I am omitting them here in the interests of simplicity and clarity. These higher levels have no significance in everyday life, since they are fairly inaccessible, rarely attained levels of enlightened consciousness.

---

[29] Occult phenomena – faith healing, teleportation and dematerialization, in which solid matter is suddenly and miraculously healed, moved large distances as if by magic, and at times even made to vanish – are rare exceptions that I'd rather not dwell on here because they are so insignificant. I leave it to the individual to decide if such phenomena are even possible, and I only mention them for the sake of thoroughness. There are numerous observations of independent witnesses describing such phenomena being performed, not only by the living Indian holy man Sai Baba, but also by numerous other persons on many occasions.

[30] The Cypriot sage DASKALOS makes use of a different classification scheme in which every level has an ethereal double. The Vital Level would then be the double of the material body. According to DASKALOS, the Emotional and Mental Levels also have ethereal doubles, since they too need ether (vital force) to live. The Causal Level is not mentioned by DASKALOS, but it probably corresponds to his idea of the Holy Ghost. From a pragmatic viewpoint, DASKALOS' classification is essentially congruent with mine. I mention his only because it seems to me somewhat more complete and, in the subtlety of its gradation, actually the correct one.

There is no need to describe the first level of everyday consciousness, since it is the one we all live in all the time. If you lower your consciousness and begin to descend into the subconscious, you first enter the dream region. In the Indian view, we are much closer to our True Being there, because we are much freer and unconstrained: in dreams, we can imagine and even wish into existence things that would be impossible in normal reality. The next level down is the dreamless state of deep sleep, also the predominant state of Yogis in deep meditation (as verified by EEG readings). Consciousness is even freer here than in the dream state. But there is yet a deepest level of enlightened consciousness, very difficult to attain. Anyone moving about on this enlightenment level can go to any other level at any time – but the opposite is not true. Enlightenment thus means being the most free of limits and limitations.

The sequence of the four Aura Levels derives from the vibrational pitch at which each respective Aura layer

Aura and Chakras in Modern Western Representation

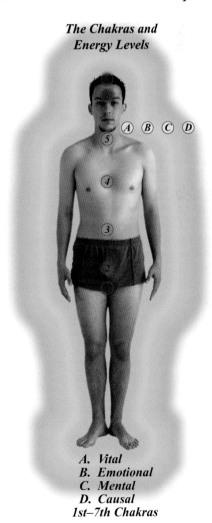

The Chakras and Energy Levels

A. **Vital**
B. **Emotional**
C. **Mental**
D. **Causal**
1st–7th Chakras

vibrates. The Vital Level vibrates the lowest and the Causal Level the highest. The higher the Aura vibrates, the finer and at the same time larger the energy field becomes that fills it out. There is also, inside the Aura Level, a variable degree of radiative force or intensity, akin to a light bulb that is made more or less bright with a dimmer control. Each Aura level can thus "shine" weakly, moderately or strongly. The stronger the Aura radiates, the more subtle-body energy its carrier has – and more energy automatically means more health, well-being, and liveliness, while low energy leads to tiredness, illness, and bad moods.

If we take a look at the four energy levels in order, then the subtle body begins with the

- **Vital body**

In the vital body, the vital force vibrates the lowest of all other levels. At the same time, our vital force expresses itself most straightforwardly and primordially. Everything material having to do with organ and metabolic functions is regulated by this level. Because of its central importance to life, I like to designate it the **Vital Level** (synonym: *vitality level)*. All life (Latin *vita*) needs vital force, and in fact life is inconceivable without vital force. Therefore, all living beings have a vital body. The Vital Level is most strongly associated with the phenomenon of respiration. Specific breathing techniques thus have a particularly great effect on the Vital Level. In death, not only does breathing depart from us, but also the *breath of life*, and we become more and more an inorganic clump of matter. Another close relationship is with water: all life – whether plant, animal, or human – needs air and water to live.

The next emotional (synonym: *astral*) level corresponds to the emotional body and the instincts. We share the

- **Emotional Level**

with animals, who also have this Aura level. We are now in the emotional sector of the subconscious, the part that gives our life its subjective tone and meaning. Without feelings, we would be soulless robots, not enjoying anything really, and bereft of any meaning in our life. The Emotional Level can be disturbed by emotional conflicts, which block contact with deeper emotional levels. A large portion of this book will concern itself with the problem of subconscious conflicts. Yet conflicts do not have negative characteristics only, just because they make us emotionally ill; they are also, in a sense, "the spice of (our) life."

This is because the conflicts become the actual points of departure for the shaping of our personality and the development of our Self. Without conflicts, we cannot mature emotionally.

The next higher vibrational region, the

- **Mental Level**

is only found in fully developed form in the human species, although domestic pets and trained animals can have a minuscule rudimentary mental body. From the Mental Level on, we are dealing with levels that only appear in man. The Mental Level is the expression of our consciousness of Self and of rational mental activity. Daydreaming states or short-term lapses of consciousness (*Absénces*) aside, we spend most of everyday life in the mental body. Our mental body gives us the sense of being an "I" and having free will.

The highest vibrational region is known as the

- **Causal Level**

and is also found in man only. It is the very deepest subconscious, the contents of which have instinctive, archetypal, and normative character. The conviction of spiritual gurus is that this level creates cause (Latin *causa*) in the karmic sense. It is at first very hard to grasp why the Mental Level doesn't increase upward into a kind of super-consciousness, but instead sinks down into an especially deep unconsciousness. I'll return later on to this initially confusing circumstance. The reason that the Mental Level transitions to the Causal Level is that we are situated in a sea of vital force in which the Causal Level and the Vital Level are very tightly interrelated (see illustration below).

We thus find ourselves, as individuals, in a sea of vital force consisting of causal and vital energy. The vital energy more corresponds to the "fuel" and pure vital energy, while the Causal Level is related to the intellect-like informational aspect of the "life ocean." As individuals, we have, within this life ocean, separate mental and emotional bodies that can be equated with our personal boundaries. In the mental body, the vital force flows predominantly as causal energy, which is why the emotional body merges into the vital body.

Energy Level Transitions

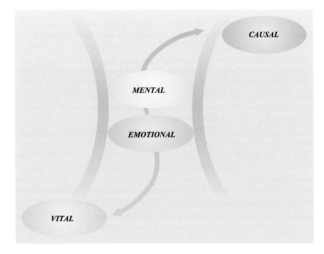

It seems to me that we can at this point make out, in the arrangement of the Aura layers, the rough outlines of an evolutionary principle, which I will go into in greater detail later on. The general consensus of opinion among esoteric teachers is that animals have no mental or causal bodies. Animals have no higher energy levels that would correspond to rational mental activity (mental body) or the deep subconscious (causal body). If we look at plants, we find that they have one body less than animals do: they lack the emotional body.

Each of the four energy levels of the subtle-body force field is linked to different developmental stages of the living being:

- The Vital Level operates in the lower forms up through plants
- The Emotional Level is added for animals and
- The Mental and Causal Levels belong exclusively to man

If we view each of the energy levels metaphorically as software, then the complexity and mental degree of freedom of the associated hardware would increase steadily from one level to the next. This becomes clear in the difference between thoughts and emotions. "Thoughts are free," as the song so aptly puts it, while each of us is familiar with the constricting influence of certain emotional states. As wonderful as many feelings (such as falling in love) might indeed be, feelings can also degrade us right down into slavery. Many poets and animal experts have described a particular form of being closed in that turns animals into despondent prisoners of the emotional body.

On the other hand, being imprisoned in this manner does not exist in the mental body. I have already mentioned that the Indian sages of antiquity understood the Aura Levels to be degrees of consciousness associated with increasing freedom. The highest degrees of freedom are thus also associated with the highest Aura levels. We can view the Aura Levels not only from the standpoint of freedom, but also from that of uniting consciousness. This would be a way of looking at the matter that could explain phenomena such as meditation, telepathy and the like.

If we think of the energy levels as forms of consciousness that link us with other fields of consciousness, then the four energy levels connect us, in a certain sense, with all of creation. Like a TV with innumerable channels, our perceptual capabilities thereby become virtually limitless. It is just the habitual use of certain narrowly-limited channels that limits us, be it due to sensory perceptions or rational convictions. From this viewpoint, we can understand the utility of meditation: it expands the consciously perceived bandwidth of the Aura levels as "reception channels." We

The Aura of Plants, Animals, and Humans

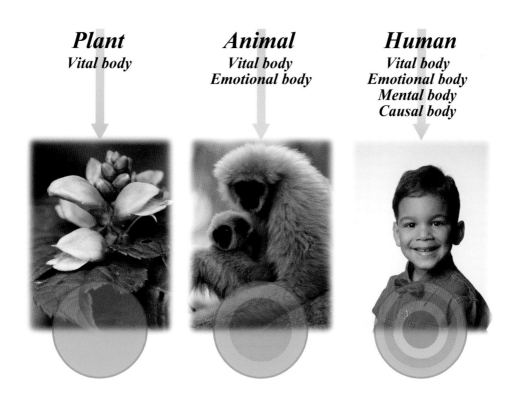

Plant
Vital body

Animal
Vital body
Emotional body

Human
Vital body
Emotional body
Mental body
Causal body

immerse ourselves in ever deeper consciousness and Aura levels, which expands our perceptual capabilities. People who practice deep meditation report, in consistent agreement, that they have acquired an expanded consciousness horizon.

The four Aura levels will be presented in order in the next chapter. I will begin with the lowest Vital Level, the *vital body*, which contains our vital force in its strongest form and which most directly shapes our overall life feeling. The following saying applies most of all to the vital body: "Tell me how you vibrate energetically and I will tell you how you feel." The more vitality we have, the more lively and authentic (more centered) we feel. Compared to the other energy bodies, the vital body most strongly determines our general life feeling. It is thus worth the effort to deal with it intensively.

The Vital Body

Our lowest energy level is the so-called vital body. In discussing the life force in earlier chapters, I have already touched on many of the vital body's characteristics. Because it is so important, I'd like to go over some of these points again. The vital body is the most primitive, direct and dynamic form of the life force (synonymous with C'hi, Prana, ether, od, Orgone). The vital body defines our basic feeling of well-being and liveliness. Clairvoyants describe a strong and vital Aura as particularly brightly illuminated, vividly colored, and lively. According to the ancient energy medical traditions, the most important and essential thing that the body needs for life is vital energy; life simply is not conceivable without it.

The organism receives its daily ration of vital energy through respiration and nutrition, but also from interpersonal exchange. A vibrant sexual life is an especially intense energy donor. As well, deep sleep, with its vitalizing dreams, refills our reserves of life energy – as do all sensuous dreamlike experiences, be they movies, being in love or pleasant imaginative activities. Anything that is pleasant, enjoyable and makes us feel good supplies us directly with life energy. Since the life force is an omnipresent cosmic energy which permeates us at all times, we basically can never be cut off from it.

The more life force we have, the more vital we feel. Vitality means a feeling of strength, but also lightness and dynamism, of desires and pleasant flows coupled with the ability to concentrate on our work (EEG Alpha state). We feel well and comfortable in our skin. Pure life force itself feels fresh, lively and new, tingly, flowing, and light. It generates pleasant tugging flows in the body, which we can perceive when we luxuriously stretch our arms and legs. Regrettably, as adults, many people no longer know these states that they experienced spontaneously as children – or, when such states do crop up, unexpectedly and abruptly, in our adult lives, then it is during those rare moments of falling in love, or sumptuous feelings of happiness. It is at times like this that we feel a hint of that heavenly *joie de vivre*, like a clear blue sky suddenly bursting forth on a gray and overcast day.

Because the vitality charge is so strongly tied up with dreams, sexuality and drug receptors (opiate, nicotine and cannabinol receptors, among others), there is an understandable need, particularly for people with low vitality charges, to induce these states artificially – because these joyous states can be simulated and faked through drugs and other artifices, as in the notorious trio of "Sex, Drugs, and Rock&Roll" (formerly "wine, women, & song"). The harder it is for people to achieve a high and lasting vitality charge on their own, the greater their frustration and dependence on surrogate techniques will be, thereby ratcheting addiction ever upward.

At this point, I need to mention some fundamental differences in the conception of life force between psychoanalytic and ancient ideas. Sigmund FREUD designated life force as Libido, but limits it to the sex drive, which can gratify our basic need for desire and being alive. Accordingly, for FREUD, it is only sexuality that is the primary driving force of our thoughts and actions. Amazingly, this narrow and old-fashioned view is still considered valid by most psychoanalysts. They view the secret motives and the "form-speech" in their patient's symptoms exclusively from the aspect of concealed sexual desires (e.g., they construe "fear of mice and spiders" as "fear of the penis" and so forth). To exaggerate a little, I would call this a "pornographic world-view" in that it, exaggeratedly and inaccurately, oversexualizes the situation.

In his first exchange of letters with FREUD, C.G. JUNG expressed his reservations with viewing sexuality in such an overt and exclusive manner. For JUNG, the libido is what differentiates the living from the dead, known variously as "*Odem*, breath of life, *Vis vitalis*," and so on. He viewed the libido as the actual essence of liveliness, which of course encompasses much more than just sexuality. JUNG's conception thus more resembles the ancient worldview, in which the life force is a universal phenomenon extending far beyond sexuality. My own conception, like that of most people I know, agrees with JUNG's.

Yet in another sense, I'd like to "rehabilitate" FREUD, because, in his assessment of sexuality, he has quite correctly intuited something which the ancient Indians had called Kundalini energy. Of course, FREUD, as an atheist and anti-mystic, never spoke this way about Kundalini. And yet, for me, his overvaluation of the libido expresses this knowledge intuitively. Kundalini energy has an enormous dynamism, and contains the explosive force of the condensed libido, visualized as a coiled snake in the pelvis, there holding at the ready an enormous reservoir of strength deriving from the cosmic ocean of energy. In the experience of enlightenment, this mass of condensed energy is released and shoots up into the head, enabling the highest spiritual insights and a mystical feeling of oneness with the divine (*Unio mystica*).

In Tibetan and Indian Tantra, orgasm and enlightenment are viewed as essentially similar experiences, based on similar processes. Orgasm, with its brief interruption of consciousness, is known in French as the *petit mort* (little death). The enlightenment experience is based on similar phenomena, having to do with loss of consciousness and strong energy flooding. In Tibetan Buddhism, the process of enlightenment is symbolized by the Buddha in the Yab-Yum position with his female partner. This of course also expresses the unification of the Yin/Yang polarities. From the Buddha's own enlightenment (that took place without a female partner and thus no sexual act) we realize that the unfolding of Kundalini is by no means bound to the sexual act. The life force is available to all living beings independently of sexuality and can thus flow full strength in any individual who, like the Buddha, meditates quietly and alone.

In deep relaxation states, we can get a part of the life force to flow that is normally tied up in the form of permanent muscular tension. We are normally unaware of these tensions that hold us captive in a subliminal cramped state. After a while, we can get a feeling for our rigidity in the jaw, tightly clenched anus or tense neck muscles. At some point, these cramps dissolve and the life force begins to flow more intensely as relaxation increases. We experience a pleasant flowing in our arms and legs. As the flowing life force continues to increase, we eventually discover the channel of desire, as I like to call this phenomenon. There exists a similarly pleasurable energy exchange of a circular worm-like structure between mother and nursing child, in which the breast is the exit gate of maternal energy, and tugging instreaming pelvic sensations arise. The channel of desire thus reverses direction in the mother. In the child, the direction resembles that of later genital activity, in which the mouth takes in and the pelvis gives off.

We experience a pleasurable flow from mouth to pelvis, i.e. from the central erogenous zones, that of the mouth (passive sucking, Yin, devotion) to the anal and genital region (active giving, Yang, tribute). in my opinion, the channel of desire is a preliminary form of Kundalini energy, to some degree a more "everyday" little brother (as it were) of the great enlightenment experience. Internally, we feel, from the region between anus and genitals, via the intestines, chest and neck to the mouth, a streaming, pleasurably relaxed tingling feeling resembling a snake or channel of desire.

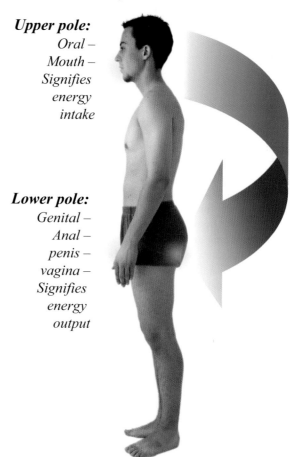

The "Channel of Desire" as a Kundalini Stream

Upper pole:
*Oral –
Mouth –
Signifies
energy
intake*

Lower pole:
*Genital –
Anal –
penis –
vagina –
Signifies
energy
output*

In the view of many spiritually experienced people, we are abundantly and literally surrounded by life force. The Creator has superabundantly blessed and gifted us with this force. Visually, we swim in an inexhaustible ocean of life force. Healers and saints are said to be able to tap optimally into this reservoir of strength and transform great quantities of vital energy with which to effect cures and other wonders, including materializations. The appearance of such phenomena usually involves emotional opening up of deeper layers of the subconscious. These are above all the subconscious layers belonging to the causal body, which is where the great channel is located through which life force streams into us.

Healers and spiritually advanced persons have been shown to have high vitality and causal values; this is made possible by the fact that such people have worked on themselves and their basic fears. Since their life force streams through them unimpeded, healers can pass some of it on to other people. When healers establish a good connection with the highest energy levels (i.e., have a causal body that is as open as possible), they do not get tired prematurely when healing others because they do not give too much of their own energy reserves; instead, the healer, being open to the highest energy levels, can tap into the inexhaustible energy reserves of the Cosmos – basically, becoming a channel for cosmic energy.

When we turn to the everyday importance of the life force, no other factor has as great a significance in our lives. Unfortunately, the overwhelming majority of people are totally unaware of this. As a rule, most people don't concern themselves with life force as they should. The more I as a physician deal with energy medicine, the clearer it becomes to me that it is life force above all that determines our fate and quality of life. No other factor has greater significance in our lives! – neither the quality of the food we eat, the air we breathe, nor social relationships are as important as most people think they are. Naturally these factors are important, but less so than the life force.

Since most people have a relatively low energy level, external influences assume a fairly great significance for them. However, because such influences are overvalued, this leads to a distorted perception of them. One erroneously takes the overlarge number of energetically ailing persons to be the standard. As long as we are supplied with enough vital energy (and are not harboring any serious genetic defects), there's not much that can harm us health-wise. An exception is the infamous brick that can land on our head, or the rare circumstance of highly-infectious pathogens in individual cases, against which there is often not much that can be done.

Moreover, people with high levels of life force lead a pleasurable, lively and meaningful life. This is because the life force includes all of these qualities. So, when statistics show that people who enjoy life and have structured their life meaningfully are less often sick, one can justifiably say that these people are full of vital force. The life force is in fact the primary life-promoting and health-maintaining factor. Joie de vivre and a meaning-filled worldview arise automatically when the previously low life force once again flows freely and fully.

Emotional conflicts are among the greatest thieves of our life force, and I will deal with them later in great detail. Their elimination should be our very greatest effort – for that alone can enormously increase the flow of life force. Since life force is usually available in sufficient quantity all around us, our problem is actually that we don't take in enough of it, nor allow it to circulate harmoniously within us. Plus, the larger a conflict is, the more it saps our life force. Conflicts are thus the most important reason that we are cut off from the vast ocean of life force.

The biggest conflict is the so-called Central Conflict. Entwined around it is our greatest fundamental fear, which is why it is so deeply buried in our subconscious. Because of the resulting fundamental fear, the Central Conflict is the starting point of our character formation – a process which I will describe in detail later on. All conflicts can be dissolved with certain homeopathic remedies, and this of course includes the Central Conflict. The entire process of conflict healing usually takes a few months. After all the methods that I have checked out to date, the best and most economical seems to be to act so as to increase life force permanently. Conflicts are dissolved with homeopathic energy medicine, thus allowing the life force to flow fully once again. Nothing boosts our life force as much as healing conflicts!

The Emotional Body

Who steals our dreams gives us death.
(Confucius)

The next higher vibrational level is known as the *Emotional Level* (also Astral Level). Energetically, it corresponds to feelings, emotions and drives. Our nightly dreaming activity takes place on this level. The Emotional Level correlates with our personal subconscious. It contains all suppressed and uncomfortable consciousness contents, which psychoanalysis subsumes under the rubric of the personality's shadow. Yet the Emotional Level also has many positive traits, such as creativity, imagination, intuition, and the ability to become enthusiastic. So, the subconscious by no means consists only of pathological material from which neuroses and other emotional diseases derive. In fact, the Emotional Level contains extraordinarily valuable material that has healing capabilities and that lends variety and vivacity to our lives. The Emotional Level is also the level on which most hypnotic phenomena take place. Deep contemplation takes us directly to our emotional body.

But above all, the Emotional Level holds our feelings (emotions). According to C.G. JUNG, emotions may be viewed as precursors of consciousness. This is also known as "emotional intelligence," of which there are various degrees. Many people are rationally dumb but emotionally brilliant; with others, it's just the opposite. Since pets often have an unusually highly-developed emotional intelligence – as do many mentally handicapped persons – their masters often consider them to be quite clever. But "clever" in this case refers to emotional intelligence, which has nothing to do with abstract reasoning intelligence.

In animals, pre-wired programs known as *instincts* run the show in the emotional body, forcing them to act in certain stereotyped ways. These instinctive programs represent something like a pre-consciousness (later on in the course of evolution, these programs develop in man into full mental consciousness). But feelings are of course also a kind of consciousness! Feelings are something like content-laden energy units that want to be perceived and become conscious. We can think of them as packages with labels on them that say e.g. "I find you sexually very attractive!" when we encounter a desirable sexual partner, or "I hate you! Get lost!" when we meet someone whom we simply can't stand. In the case of the attractive sexual partner, the instinctive message is "Go on, sleep with him/her!" and it wants to be implemented at once. Thus, dogs start right in copulating without much foreplay. With like vehemence, a dog will start to growl and bite when it has received the instinctive message that it

doesn't like us, because we've taken away its bone or invaded its territory.

Human beings are also subject to these instinctive sequences. However, most of them proceed subconsciously, for we are ashamed of many of our secret feelings, wishes and drives, and we hide from other people. Behaving like an animal, as a reproach, is an insult. In medicine, we speak of behavior-disturbed individuals' lack of inhibition or impulsiveness – people who will more than likely run afoul of the law sooner or later. Often, there are genetic or organic brain disorders behind this kind of behavior, e.g., brain damage in a serious traffic accident, brain tumors, congenital brain damage, or infections such as syphilis.

We react subconsciously and instinctively upon encountering an attractive sexual partner. Rather than initiating copulation right off the bat, as an animal would (or possibly a sexual offender with no inhibitions), we send out certain signals that announce our interest to the sexual partner. This can be a covert reaction such as blushing or looking modestly away, or the very opposite: looking directly at the person and all other techniques having to do with flirting and sexual come-on. An expert observer will quickly infer or know what our covert and/or overt desires are.

Also, when we don't like or even hate someone, we give ourselves away by certain signals. Often, we feign ostentatious disinterest when an enemy shows up. "To look right through someone" is a popular form of disdain and aggression. There are many variations on body language intended to convey to a foe the message to scram and be quick about it. Staring daggers and covert threatening gestures (arms akimbo) represent the next level of escalation. No matter what we do, the trained observer will quickly note what our real feelings are that lurk behind our emotional masquerade. Most people are not very good at hiding the animalistic and instinctive side of their feelings. Spouses and other people who know us well are frequently very good at "reading" our hidden feelings. Of course, the possibility of deception and mistake is always there, as we all know. We then speak, for example, of *projection*. Feelings (emotions – from Latin *movere*, to move) represent, in their immediacy, the link to our **animal**istic aspect. Now of course we aren't animals, but we undeniably have an animal side.

Pet owners swear to me that animals have a mixture of instinct and personal emotional life comparable to that of humans. You get the impression that many consider their pets to be morally superior to people. It is seldom noticed that they are thereby indirectly revealing something about themselves (and their subconscious shadow). For if the pet's good-heartedness and other traits supposedly make it superior to people, then it is, logically, superior to its owner as well – who has thereby given himself low marks. Since no one does that voluntarily, this is a case of suppressed, subconscious, and rejected parts of the pet owner's own character with which that person is uncomfortable.

One may ask oneself – for instance after one's first painfully unrequited love – what on earth emotions are good for. Feelings are the very "spice of life." Feelings make us authentic, lively, and real. They see to it that we are "approachable" and sensitive and that things can "get under our skin." Only they give life its depth and the hard-to-describe feeling of "real" reality. Without feelings, we'd lead a basically meaningless and monotonous life dominated by cold rationality.

Emotions are, like the yeast in bread dough, the crucial propellant that allows us to grow and develop personally. Without feelings, we would be indifferent to most everything happening around us. With feelings, on the other hand, every problem becomes real and highly charged. That which results when we grapple with conflicts and the feelings contained therein is called life experience, personal growth and maturation. We should therefore be enormously grateful to our emotional body, because it represents the actual source of our humanness. Without feelings, we could never develop an independent personality. It therefore doesn't matter whether we experience good or bad feelings – the main thing is having them! All feelings are valuable in the initial phase of emotional development. In time, we come to realize that we possess an inner treasure that we must tend and cultivate. The two magic words are *thoughtfulness* and *love*. As their personality develops, most people become emotionally more considerate of themselves and others. They become more and more aware of how important feelings of love are.

Unemotional rational types are often accused of being emotionally frigid, which is actually not true, since even emotional coldness is an emotion that is being generated – and behind which, by the way, many other feelings lie hidden. Emotions are the basis of all communication and, as Paul WATZLAWIK has famously pointed out, it is impossible not to communicate. Lack of emotion in the sense of genuine depression is in reality hell on earth, which is why every depressive yearns for nothing more than to once again feel emotionally alive.

Let's turn to the emotional coldness of reason – so-called *instrumental rationality*. Superficially, many people act like machines. These "robots" seem to have completely lost their emotional body. You see this in the stone-cold mass murderer, who seems to consist only of unfeeling intelligence. However, this impression is deceptive, as I have already pointed out, since we can never be without feelings. Acting like a machine is also a feeling, behind which true (and mostly unbearable) feelings lie hidden. We thus discover in the ice-cold killer enormous hate and rage, in turn concealing excruciating sorrow and rejection, and so on. "If you won't love me then I'll make myself dead inside, but I'll avenge myself by annihilating you!" – so goes the message. When we measure the emotional body of such people, we often find poor values as an expression of repressed feelings. On the other hand, I have never come across a case in which the emotional body was missing entirely.

When we take a closer look at the emotional body, the first things that strikes us is the almost total lack of a sense of time. As in the causal body, the emotional body is only aware of the "here and now." Still, we find in the emotional body the traces of a rudimentary time sense, such as we can recognize in a pet waiting patiently for its master's return. But it is also very hard for us humans to wait for something, which points to the animal and emotional parts of us. It usually has to do with things that really enthuse us and sensuously drive us "out of our mind." The reason for our impatience is the "all or nothing" attitude of the emotional body. Chocolate bars are seldom put down half eaten: the emotional body wants all of the chocolate, and now rather than later.

The other reason is the emotional body's extremely poor sense of time, which is conditioned by its tendency to mix everything together and its entropy. The lack of a time sense is a natural consequence of the playful dreaminess so typical of the emotional body (as GOETHE once said: "Every happiness wants to last forever."). To an animal, the time until our return seems endless. This changes only during the course of human evolution of a mental consciousness. The perception of a time axis gives rise to the feeling of Self. A woman can then swear eternal faithfulness to her betrothed and remain unmarried for years if he has to go off to war. Nevertheless, even the best-intentioned fiancée can weaken if the waiting time gets too long. Her emotional body then demands its pleasures of the flesh.

Musically, opera correlates best with the emotional body. Many operas typically alternate very quiet scenes with others where, suddenly, a loud primeval force breaks out. This abrupt change in volume dynamics corresponds to the nature of the emotional body, which likes to experience tragedy and hysteria to the fullest, and is drawn, as if by magic, from one extreme to the other. "That's enormously exciting!" says that within in us which corresponds to our emotional body. "Walking on air" and "down in the dumps" are typical extreme states that characterize the emotional body. Intermediate tones – i.e., moderately good or bad emotional states – are, surprisingly, much rarer than radical (extreme) states; mostly, these are fleeting negative feelings (disappointment or rancor) that block the Emotional Level for a while.

Therefore, if we measure the emotional body of a healthy, normally-reacting person with the REBA® Test Device, we will find either high values around 100% (if things are going well) or low values below 10–20% (if the person is in a negative emotional state). In the case of the mentally ill, who have been in an emotionally unfavorable situation for a long time, the emotional body begins to react differently; after a while, extreme excursions (up or down) are no longer present. The REBA® Test Device then measures values around 50%, such that the emotional body seems to be blocked. In our society, this correlates with widespread dissatisfaction and frustration.

These in-between emotional values can be designated as a neurotic condition of long-term frustration. This kind of situation plays itself out between heaven and earth, as it were, and people in it come across as sullen and irritable. They start swearing a blue streak the instant someone blocks their parking place – or, if their superego is in good working order, they seem to be always tired and pale. You can observe many people's poor emotional state most clearly when they think they no one is looking: one then sees, in their facial expression and body posture, all of the emotional sorrow plaguing them. This tortured unsatisfying condition is quite contrary to the essence of the emotional body, like a child who must be good and obedient. If we free the "inner child" of its neurosis, the liberated emotional body will go back to reacting according to the "all or nothing" principle.

The "inner child" hidden behind the mask of the rational adult is the topic of much discussion. At the bakery counter we observe a corpulent gentleman lasciviously licking his lips while checking out the cakes on display there. "Would you like a piece?" the saleslady asks him. She decoded the old man's signals at once and saw through to his real motives. "No thanks, I just ate!" he says, answering with his adult Self, which is remembering the message of his bathroom scale and his family doctor's dietary recommendations. The more we liberate our emotional body and become psychoenergetically more open, the easier it is for us – when the time is right – to let our inner child "come out and play," because we are able to show sincerely what it is we really want.

In the Indian tradition (and in Hawaiian shamanistic thought), the emotional system is like a child or an animal living within us. The Indian seeks his own hidden **soul or totem animal,** believing that it harbors a young animal soul maturing within him into an adult soul. This *totem animal* corresponds to his true essence. The kahunas (ancient Hawaiian shamans) thought similarly; their teachings are indeed very important to an understanding of energetic and spiritual phenomena. I made it a habit of mine for a while to evaluate people based on their inner animal. This often led to amazing (and humorous) discoveries, since it explained many otherwise puzzling actions as deriving from the behavior of the animal in question. Political caricatures take full advantage of the revealing, unmasking device of animal depiction in all its variations. At carnival time, we can let out our inner animal and drop the mask of the false Self.

Just as healthy children are either unhappy and stubborn or quite normally happy, so too does the essence of the emotional body react either with great openness or else with a lot of blocking. Our conduct with respect to the inner child or animal plays a large role in this. As long as we remain **loyal** to our inner emotional animal, our emotional body will be able to vibrate freely. In this context, loyalty means heeding our inner voice and not allowing ourselves to be led astray. Loyalty to our emotional animal or child is accompanied by a feeling of security, simplicity and strength. In a subsequent chapter on spiritual development, loyalty will once again come up as a topic – because it marks an important turning point in our personal development when we can look behind the mirror of our mask and look our own self in the emotional "face."

Feelings are our personal Heaven and Hell rolled into one, and (as we know) nothing is worse than an unbearable feeling! We'll do anything not to have to feel it any longer.

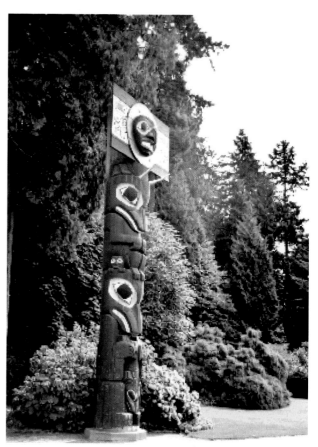

Totem pole in Stanley-Park, Vancouver/Canada

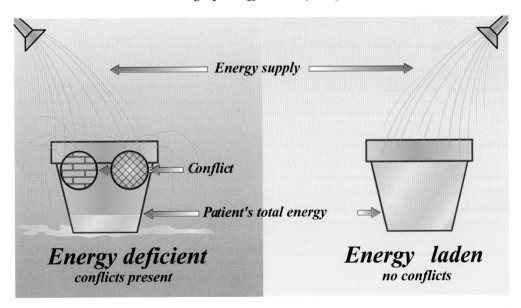

Intolerable feelings are often expressed as **pains**, or cached away (somatized) in the body in some other way. Great physical pain is easier to endure than the unbearable feelings that are often hidden underneath them. One can observe in many pain patients that the pain represents a protective mechanism against outsized menacing feelings that, in the event of a full-scale emotional discharge, would overwhelm and engulf the patient. Faced with this existential fear, the patient takes refuge in the pain.

From an energetic standpoint, the emotional body represents an opening through which vital energy flows into us, which means it can become a bottleneck. If we imagine the aforementioned "energy egg" as a circulatory system, then the emotional body and its emotional conflicts often acts as the primary energy thief:

Therefore, it's not lack of energy that is the main problem, but rather faulty uptake: thanks to the psychoenergetic blockages of the emotional conflicts, not enough life energy can be taken in. In principle, this is a problem that, to some extent, afflicts and affects all people. The situation is different for animals living in the wild, who do not yet have any conflicts. Migratory birds can cross oceans without sleeping or drinking. Animal herds cross hundreds of miles of endless steppes without showing the slightest signs of fatigue. Their enormous amounts of life energy are due to the fact that they are in no way blocked. Also, wild animals very rarely get cancer or other diseases characterized by energy deficiency. The situation with house pets is quite different: they must bear their share of conflicts, and so their situation often resembles that of their masters.

The Mental Body

No one is farther from the truth than he who has all the answers.
(Chuang-Tsu)

The mental body corresponds to everyday consciousness – but it also has a further significance: it relates to our awareness of having a Self and possessing a stable personality. The mental body creates in us an abstract representation of reality that encompasses both our inner world and the external universe. This leads, first of all, to a feedback process in the form of self-consciousness. Awareness of our own Self leads to improved control over our own body, since we can deliberately and consciously direct and control it. We can willfully perform movements. We can also recognize this self-control in such complex abilities as playing the piano. No animal can play a piano with the virtuosity of a concert pianist, because it lacks the supervisory possibilities afforded by self-consciousness.

But the mental body also portrays the outside world by producing a reality image of us and other people. What this means becomes clear when we find ourselves, as tourists, somewhere that is foreign to us. "When in Rome do as the Romans do!" we say, hoping to become accustomed to the strangeness. Yet at the same time, it shows us how very dependent we are on social feedback. Leaving others hanging, uncertain about the social situation, is a proven method for bewildering people and weakening their grip on reality. Taken to extremes, it leads to psychosis, because the Self is no longer able to manufacture a reasonable reality image. In the case of the *double bind* phenomenon, we see the contradictory behavior of close relatives of schizophrenics as being a significant predisposing factor in the origin of the disease. The schizophrenic keeps getting lectured by parents or siblings as to how much they care for him, but their body language and their actual emotional behavior convey rejection and remoteness.

In normal everyday life, the mental body correlates with the state of being in possession of one's mental faculties (i.e. sane) – meaning that we can "calculate" abstractly (as in solving a math problem) what it is we should do, after taking various factors into consideration. From the command center of our Self, we decide what is best and most logical. We are able to do this because we have in us a preformed reality of ourselves and the people around us. *Sense of reality* and *feeling of Self* are expressions of the mental body. The mental body is closely related to intelligence: the more intelligent we are, the more conscious we become of our Self. We understand – abstractly and theoretically, at least – the interactions between us and our environment much better.

But there is also emotional intelligence, far superior to the mental body in many areas, such as social communication. The mental body operates rationally and abstractly – but, in its self-infatuation, overlooks the importance of emotions; this is why intelligent persons can be appallingly stupid when it comes to feelings.

At a still higher level of abstraction, everyday consciousness creates an idea of the world. Amazingly often, we are not fully aware of our picture of reality, since it is shot through with numerous incongruities and emotional fractures. This can be seen very well in psychological tests, in which even experienced police officers give widely diverging descriptions of a perpetrator. In short, we mostly see what we want to see, editing out the unknown and the unpleasant. Our everyday consciousness is thus surrounded by all manner of dark spots of unawareness.

In the self-overestimation of early adulthood, many persons consider themselves to be intact and in perfect working order. This is known in psychology as **narcissism** – a mental state in which one feels invincible. In the self-image, one is an unbelievable good-looking and generally terrific person. Others are perceived as enemies and imperfect beings. In pubertal groups of kindred spirits, a group feeling develops in which one ascribes to oneself and the others in the group all positive traits and strengths, while weaknesses and negative traits are projected onto other, alien, groups. Normally, maturity and aging begin with the dawning recognition of our own inner limitations and imperfections. Our black/white mental categories begin to acquire shades of gray that include our own blemishes.

Unlike the emotional body, the mental body has a fully-developed **time sense**. It is through the mental body that we first become aware of our transience. We get a clear feeling of the frailty of earthly things. Awareness of one's own eventual death is part of a well-developed time sense. Children generally don't believe that they will someday die. But the situation changes at some point for adults – at the latest when our friends who are age peers begin to die off. I previously mentioned the medieval creed *memento mori* (Think of death), which back then summoned man to reflect and do penance. This relates to the awareness of one's own mortality.

To counter the fear of personal death, each individual produces a precisely opposed **Self** that is in love with itself and feels invincible and eternal. This Self turns up as the pathologically inflated ego of the narcissistic teenager, who has an unreal and extremely exaggerated self-image. This overdone narcissism is probably part of the normal development process. One encounters it in young children and puberty. But independently of excess, ultimately every healthy Self presents a similar structure, known in psychology as *intrinsic narcissism*. Anyone wholly lacking in self-love and self-respect usually has a severe personality disorder. We need, for our emotional health, a Self that is in a certain sense in love with itself and its body, and which considers itself somewhat invulnerable.

The cosmetics and fitness industries make a living catering to their customers' narcissism. In the USA, many sects carry the narcissistic belief in personal invulnerability to an extreme by claiming that death is purely an illusion, just an agreement of custom. According to this theory, you only die if you think you will. Now we know, of course, that every animal also dies, even though none of them know anything about the matter. Yet as unreal as this fundamental attitude is, it nevertheless holds a grain of truth: having to carry out an important task before dying can be a serious reason for not wanting to die before it has been accomplished. In Chinese culture, for example, grandmothers remarkably rarely die on the day of the Chinese New Year – for on this date, they are the center point of the family clan and have important representative tasks to fulfill. This was able to be worked out as a statistical trend in California by analyzing the ethnic groups individually.

The astonishing ability to influence the time of one's death was, incidentally, one of the reasons for the founding of psycho-oncology by physicians such as SIMONTON. Just as the ancient Chinese determined the time of their death, many long-term cancer survivors seem to have a meaningful task to perform which delays their dying. In psycho-oncology (the science of the relationship between the individual psyche and cancer), personal motivation plays a preeminent role. In my opinion, a strong and positive motivation evokes large quantities of life energy that would otherwise be inactivated. I have seen the same effect when eliminating large conflicts, which can also activate strong self-healing abilities.

The mental region is, as it were, a constant and solid island in the ocean of the changes that we have to go through in our life history. Basically, the *Self* can be defined as a personal continuity of consciousness that is extraordinarily crucial for our mental and physical integrity. Once that became clear to me, I had to modify my assessment of the *Self*. I had previously damned **egotism** as a negative character trait; it had not been clear to me that the Ego represented an immensely valuable treasure of personal existence. Without the mental body, we cannot develop a stable personality. So, psychologically speaking, egotism represents the exaggerated puffing up of a Self that is actually weak. Egotists defend their Self just as we all do; they just do it

more crudely and ruthlessly. Interestingly, gentle and reserved people who live in their own emotional niche often have amazingly high mental readings in an energetic test. Unlike the egotist, the strong Self of these gentle people evidently has no need to call attention to itself.

All in all, our Self is like a fragile island beset on all sides by life's storms. I observe low mental values of less than 50% as measured by the REBA® Test Device in cases of psychosis, long-term and grueling emotional or physical pain states and very large conflicts. But I also see low mental values in people with a very low IQ. Particularly for large conflicts, there arises a confining pressure on the Self that can lead to psychosis in extreme cases. In this context, there seems to be nothing more horrible to contemplate than the permanent loss of Self and being controlled by unknown forces. This is why psychosis sufferers are so enormously grateful for any relief – and why, on the other hand, they so strongly fear each new psychotic episode.

At some point in life, the developing awareness of the Self collides with narcissism, as the individual becomes aware of personal weakness and vulnerability. This does not at all imply inevitable psychosis, however: it is simply the fundamental human drama in which the victory of the Self at the same time automatically leads to the defeat of the Self. At the peak of our personality development, we become painfully aware of the fact that we'll someday have to give up this personality by dying. GOETHE's drama *Faust* is rooted in this topic, as are all the great heroic epics dealing with the tragic entanglement of victory and individual extinction (e.g., Achilles).

However, since my worldview is a positive one, I do not see the drama in such a desolate and pessimistic light. Later on, I'll more thoroughly substantiate my view, which is based on the idea of reincarnation and the constancy of important personality traits. In my opinion, the period of personal maturation that sets in after the heroic phase leads to a transformation in which the false, temporally limited self is dissolved. The underlying true Self, with its indestructible character, can then be recognized. This is a continuity of consciousness that outlasts the individual life, identical with our character type and our higher Self. As long as we – tragically and over long time periods – confuse our temporal self with our immortal soul, then the fact of individual death will obviously be a monstrous catastrophe. I suspect that, in a certain subconscious sense, we are all (whether religious or not) aware of our immortal soul, the loss of which would be the worst thing that could happen to us. It's just that we continue to confuse the false self with the true Self.

I'd like to supply a proof for my thesis that provides strong indications for a permanent personality. Amazingly, organic brain disorders, such as can be found in disease cases such as Alzheimer's, only lower the mental-body values, as measured by the REBA® Test Device, by a little bit. As the material organ "brain" is more and more destroyed, one would logically expect to see worse and worse energetic values. Yet oddly enough, they do not show up in cases of brain degradation such as Alzheimer's. How to explain this riddle? Evidently, the mental-body values reflect something other than mere organic brain function.

We need to keep in mind that the Aura of the mental body stores the individual's personality. If the Aura has the personality in storage, then material brain degradation understandably plays a secondary role. We know from hypnosis studies that, in a hypnotic trance, Alzheimer's patients are able to show their intact personality, only to fall back into semi-consciousness once the session is over. Evidently, in the trance state, their former personality can once again make an appearance, meaning that it has not been destroyed – which is explained by the intactness of the mental body. The renowned brain researcher and Nobel Laureate ECCLES comes to the same conclusion, namely that personality and brain function cannot be coterminous since, if they were, such phenomena would be inexplicable.[29]

Basically, the mental body cannot be influenced directly. We can affect the personality indirectly, but not influence the essential core of the personality. And no matter what so many educators and psychologists might think, all supposed personality changes are nothing but indirect phenomena. A person's character traits are, at bottom, unalterable – as we can see in sayings such as "a leopard can't change its spots." In later chapters, I will introduce four character types that represent the basic framework for personal growth and ego development. In this process, the maturation of the character types is reflected on the Mental Level, which explains why more mature personalities can have higher mental values than as yet undeveloped persons.

I'd like to cite yet another confirmation of my thesis of permanent personality structure: very young people with no life experience and no fully-developed personality can nevertheless have higher mental values than mature life-experienced persons. We do not come into this world as a blank slate (tabula rasa), but rather bring with us a personality from former lives. To be sure, only the main features of this personality are recognizable in the child, yet they are already present in such a manner that it can be measured energetically as a high mental value. I think that we can reach a logical understanding of psychoenergetic processes only by

accepting the existence of repeated rebirths (Karma). Otherwise, from where else would a newborn have acquired a fully-grown personality?

---

[29] **According to ECCLES, brain and consciousness are not identical.** As preparation for understanding the [upcoming] dialogue with the philosopher POPPER, one needs to know that ECCLES' Nobel Prize was in Medicine, and that he is considered to be one of the top brain researchers of the 20th century. Now, POPPER was the faithful guardian of the philosophical style (critical positivism) that was at that time quite popular in scientific circles. In the course of a conversation between the two scholars, ECCLES says to POPPER (the arch-rationalist), right to his face, that "brain and consciousness cannot be identical." The dialogue continues on as absurdly as it is fascinating, because POPPER, not being a neurologist, cannot for the life of him comprehend what ECCLES is actually saying there. POPPER withdraws "quite coolly" from the affair, pointing out how speculative this thesis is. I get the feeling that he simply interprets it as a figment of the doctor's imagination. At any rate, ECCLES deserves praise for his moral courage in putting his reputation on the line. By the way, the revolutionary dynamite contained in ECCLES' thesis been kept swept under the carpet as much as possible down to the present day (and likely for some time to come). For if matter and spirit are not one and the same, then this is a breach in the dyke of science that could of course flush the entire scientific worldview down the river.

The Causal Body

The *causal body* is often designated as the deep, collective, or archetypal unconscious (or subconscious). It is the subconscious common to all mankind. By contrast, our personal subconscious is located in the emotional body and vibrates at a relatively low frequency. We each have a personal emotional body, whereas all people share a common causal body. Thus, the collective unconscious of the causal body in a sense belongs to all mankind, and can be regarded as the collective property of the human race. The causal body vibrates markedly higher than the emotional body and, in terms of vibrational level, is even above that of the mental body. This higher vibrational level is an expression of the causal body's higher spiritual content.

The causal body's higher consciousness is ordered and structured in a way that clearly differentiates it from the personal subconscious. The personal subconscious on the other hand, situated in the emotional body, mostly resembles a moody, desire-driven, and downright childish creature. By contrast, the causal body's higher consciousness has very lofty spiritual qualities that are characterized by lucid orderliness, great love, and wisdom. Religious persons believe that it is of directly divine origin and has an eternal nature. The causal body is also known as *The Holy Ghost*.[12]

In terms of depth, the causal body is far below the personal subconscious that is normally accessible to us. Its depth has the feature that the unconscious contents of the causal body only become visible when one has left the personal subconscious behind and advanced further into these unknown regions. The contents of the causal body include collective consciousness elements such as the well-known archetypes, which have certain forms and contents. These forms include cross, pyramid, dagger, runic figures, and heart, whereas the collective contents include redemption, heroic journey, combating the dragon, and so on. The more a fairy tale or an emotional story (be it book or movie) appeals to us, the more likely it is to have archetypal content.

A closer look at the causal body reveals that it consists of two regions:

1. The personal region of the causal body contains some very important individual elements, including spiritual beings such as the personal guardian angel. Also, the deep and very large subconscious conflicts underlying our individual personality are stored here.

At a very deep level, the personal region of the causal body merges into the

2. Collective region of the causal body. Ultimately, it is via this collective region of the causal body that living beings have a permanent connection with each other, even though they are mostly unaware of it.

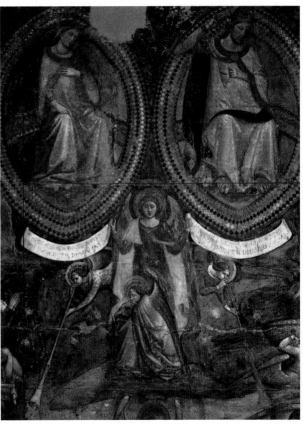

The order of creation with the creator parents Jesus and Mary and the guardian angel – Camposanto Monumentale, Pisa (unknown master ca. 1360 A.D.)

---

[30] I am grateful to Mr. Werner VOGEL for the information that the causal body level can be further subdivided into a still higher plane of cosmic and divine superconsciousness. The Indian wise man and teacher Sri AUROBINDO has grappled with these levels and their deep significance for the future of mankind.

In general, people speak of the *collective unconscious*. A better term would be **superconscious**, a term used by the great Indian sage Sri AUROBINDO – because the structures contained in the causal body are suffused with great order, beauty, and clarity, not at all like the chaotic, dark, and libidinal traits we commonly ascribe to the subconscious. Therefore, in what follows I'd like to refer to the causal body as the *superconscious*. The term also elucidates mankind's future task of raising the causal body more and more up into consciousness.

All people are linked together via the collective superconscious, which can be imagined as a kind of spiritual telephone exchange in which most of the communication takes place below the conscious level and so is not noticeable. Yet every now and then a message penetrates into our consciousness. The cosmic interconnectedness of the collective unconscious explains phenomena such as telepathy: you simply have to open the causal body's deep unconscious channels and develop a sensitivity for them in order to be able to receive these messages.

Many inexplicable phenomena of spiritual harmony between people can be understood when we understand the mode of action of the deep Causal Level. Baffling phenomena such as the pyramids in Egypt, South America, or Persia (Iran), in which far-apart continents and to some extent millennia separate the builders, can only be understood via the concept of the collective unconscious. Also supporting this thesis are the near-simultaneous patent-office registrations of certain world-shaking inventions, as has occurred more than once in modern history, even though the inventors were separated from one another by continents and language barriers. For instance, the American inventor Thomas EDISON turned in his patent application for the incandescent light bulb a scant hour ahead of a French inventor.

Since everything is connected with everything else in the vast unconscious sea of spirit and universal life force, both vital energy and the causal body permeate the entire universe. We conceive of vital energy as force and causal energy as spirit. Together, they generate a mutual field of life force and consciousness that the English biologist Rupert SHELDRAKE termed the *morphogenetic field*. Today we might conceive of it as a kind of Internet interconnecting everything. Part of this cosmic spirit/energy field contains preformed concepts and spirit-like structures that PLATO called *Ideas*. The basic idea of Platonism is the notion that fundamental forms such as star, spiral, seed, ball, and so on are pre-existing forms in the cosmic consciousness. Nature then makes its products such as plants, seeds, etc., on up to stars and galaxies, using these *ideal* forms much like a child makes houses and such with the pre-formed components of a Lego set. In the 20th century, it was the renowned biologist and philosopher Hans DRIESCH who coined the term **entelechy** for nature's repertoire of pre-formed ideas.

Now, in our normal daily life, we're not interested in building pyramids, nor tackling tricky philosophical questions. What we're most interested in is our own personal well-being and how to improve it. In this regard the causal body has an important function for our health and personal growth – **because the causal body corresponds to our true Self, our *higher spiritual identity***. The causal body is called *higher identity* because its characteristic traits are much more exemplary, benign and honest than our present self. It is the divine spark within us that represents our individual eternal spiritual core. Many people perceive the higher soul as a "still, small voice" that points the right way and gives us a genuine sense of right and wrong. Therefore, in the true Self we have an extremely valuable guide that enables us to tell right from wrong. We can call it our *true and honest **inner voice***.

Much confusion is generated by a misunderstanding of **conscience**. Conscience is known in psychology as the *superego*. However, the superego has absolutely nothing to do with the *inner voice*! The conscience sits between the *Ego* and the *Id* and acts as a regulatory censor of compulsive desires and lusts. Our personal subconscious holds our

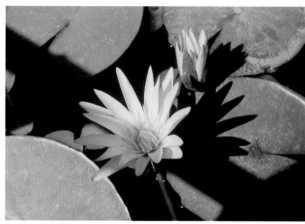

The lotus blossom symbolizes the awakening of the causal body (the Enlightenment) out of the sea of the subconscious into the brilliant light of knowledge of the true Self.

"inner beast" and wants to run free, satisfying all its desires and interests without let or hindrance. Fearing punishment and other imagined consequences, our conscience intervenes, admonishing and warning. Each of us knows that internal struggle when we have a fierce emotional craving for something that is, for whatever reason, forbidden. This wrestling match takes place in our conscience.

While children are growing up, their conscience is being organized as a permanent regulatory authority. Our conscience ensures that we obey certain social norms even when our parents are not present to personally monitor compliance. The conscience is thus also known as *parental surrogate* or, in psychological terminology, *introject*. In primitive societies, conscience or taboos see to it that people are law-abiding and decent members of the society. The superego is part of the infrastructure of a society in flux that at different times has different conceptions of what's right and proper.

For instance, it can be part of the moral code of a Stone Age tribe to slaughter on the spot any member of any other tribe. Conscience, or *taboo*, will activate with a warning when one meets a member of another tribe and does not immediately slay him. Yet the *inner voice* could also whisper to the caveman to let the person from the other tribe live, because murder is inhumane. The caveman then has a double problem, as conscience and the inner voice fight for supremacy. Modern stage plays that portray a scientist wrestling painfully in his soul because he is supposed to develop the atom bomb are based on the same problem.

Of course, one can also deliberately misinterpret conscience and inner voice. Many authoritarian religions and self-appointed moral guardians see themselves as the "long arm of the law" of a punitive god. They degrade the higher wisdom of the cosmos to a police state, and would have us believe that the earthly morality they preach flows directly to them from the divinity (their *inner voice*). It is actually nothing more than a personal, totalitarian power grab; these "Soldiers of the Lord" – as they often (revealingly) call themselves – are really interested, above all, in their own power. The history of the world is full of SAVONAROLAs, RASPUTINs, and totalitarian Mullahs.

Conscience lies on the borderline between the Self and the personal subconscious, where negotiations take place as to what is socially permissible and what not. This conscience region also includes the **character mask**, which presents our public self-image – prettied up and in a certain sense misleading – to the outside world. The character mask has an important role to play in the process of self-exploration, namely to burst the shell of the *false self* in order to bring out those parts of us that constitute our *true Self* (or *higher Self*). C.G. JUNG views the unification of the Ego and the Self as the true goal of our spiritual journey. All the great wisdom traditions proclaim the message that our true calling consists of the union of our temporal and our eternal personality. The current personality comes to resemble the eternal, true Self more and more, until they fuse together.

I'd like to sketch the true **Self** in rough outline. Our first approach to our true Self is often visualized in images of persons, first appearing to us as a parent pair with Yin/Yang polarity. The *Kahuna* religion of the Hawaiian medicine men speaks of parent *imagos*, who await us on our spiritual path. When we have advanced far enough in our spiritual journey, our inner spiritual parents are the first to meet us. These parental figures can be denoted as protective man/woman spirit beings or guardian angels, who are more advanced than we on the spiritual path. Presumably what we meet is our own androgynous being, which we – out of

habit – split into polar gender roles. We do this because it is hard for us, at first, to perceive in a non-dualistic manner.

C.G. JUNG calls the androgynous consciousness elements of the soul *anima* and *animus*. At the core of his being, the macho man is said to be soft and feminine, which corresponds to the feminine side of his soul (his *anima*). On the other hand, within the externally soft, dependent, and gentle woman, JUNG often found an inner spirit of uncompromising toughness and aggressiveness that is more suitable to a man (the *animus*). Based on these experiences, JUNG developed the concept of a polarly opposed spiritual side that a person needs in order to be whole and for the complete maturing of the soul's Self. In my opinion, the androgynous nature of the true Self is the clue to solving the riddle. Our personal maturing more and more reduces our sexual orientation, makes us more androgynous, as we become ever more like our true Self. One can often see, especially in older married couples, that they have each come to resemble the other, i.e., the man more feminine and the woman more masculine.

These interrelationships are graphically depicted in the illustration on the following page.

Our psychoenergetic existence as beings of different layered levels of consciousness is depicted above as a pyramid. The pyramid image (or stupa in Buddhist cultures) symbolically expresses the phenomenon of our consciousness and energy levels. The deeper truth that the pyramid allegorically represents exerts a strong psychic attraction that has a regular suction effect on us, for we sense intuitively the great and significant secret waiting for us in the pyramid. The pyramid corresponds to our consciousness and our spirit-like/energetic constitution, linked to the collective unconscious by means of our higher Self. The base of the pyramid here represents the collective unconscious.

In our conscious existence, i.e., our temporally limited personality with its ego consciousness, we project, as the pyramid's tip, out of the mist of the collective superconscious. Because we can no longer see the world below the mist, we gradually forget about it. Above all, we forget that the most important, eternal, and most valuable part of our being is hidden down there in the soup of mist. The mist corresponds to the Indian concept of Maya (illusion, pretense). We think we see the real world, whereas we have actually forgotten the most important part of it, needed for a full understanding of the encompassing reality: we have forgotten the true Self, hidden down there beneath the mist, in the subconscious.

When we want to understand the deep subconscious, we confront the wordless (non-linguistic) as its primary characteristic. People who contact this level, either through ecstatic states, deep hypnosis, or meditation, cease to speak and suddenly take on a very different, especially vivacious and authentic facial expression. Often, they also acquire a different, very natural and more upright posture that bespeaks

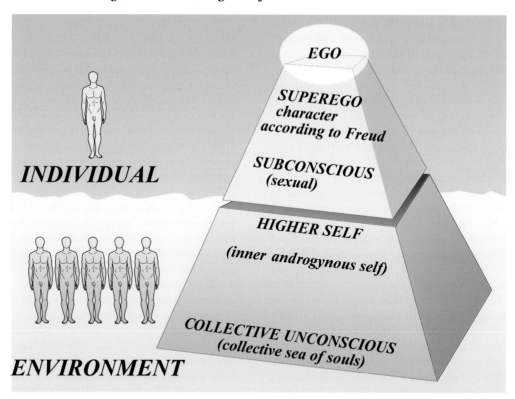

natural self-respect. Afterwards, such people seem to have been transformed in the depths of their soul. We are here on the level of the deep emotional body and the causal body, the realm of the holy and numinous.

On the deepest levels of the **superconscious**, the personal limitations of consciousness vanish. We then take leave of the true Self and find ourselves in an ocean of spiritual energy. This psychoenergetic ocean is generally referred to as the *collective unconscious*. In this ocean, all living beings are linked together in SHELDRAKE's morphogenetic field, which stores forms and images, and distributes them to all living beings. This level is the storage area for mankind's great symbols and every occurrence at the level of material reality. This universal or cosmic memory is known as the *Akasha chronicle*.

Turning to the psychological processes of the causal body, we find all the traits that we ascribe to the personal subconscious. The tendency to mix things up especially pertains to the **time sense**. To the emotional body's subconscious, there is no yesterday or tomorrow. This is especially clear in the chronological confusion of dreams, where we can meet our wife in kindergarten, or we can again run into old school chums that we haven't seen for decades, and they don't look a day older. The subconscious senses with a kind of simultaneity that predominantly deactivates the time sense.

For the causal body, the nullification of the time sense escalates to a continuum of **eternity**. For the personal subconscious, space and time are shifted in their dimensions, whereas for the causal body, these borders are completely transcended. We thus undergo in the causal body the experience of eternity. In states of religious ecstasy, besides the experience of eternity, a feeling of being as one with the cosmos, a feeling of supernal love and the unity of all life are all characteristics of causal body *Unio mystica* experience s. Besides mystics, the dying often report having such experiences.

Materialistically-oriented scientists ascribe these experiences (**religious trance**, **near-death experiences**) to the effects of endogenous endorphins. They interpret the experiences as befuddling inebriation, in which the organism puts itself in these dramatic situations as a protective measure. The brain self-narcotizes to spare itself the pain of the dying process, somewhat like a squid enveloping itself in ink. In my experience, endorphins (endogenous opiates) are a material expression of the causal body. The release of endorphins prepares the dying person for the entry into his causal body. Opiates generate all the characteristics ascribed to the causal body, e.g., great lightness, pleasant sense of well-being, peaceful and downright beatific mood, etc.

Another important point that bears directly on the causal

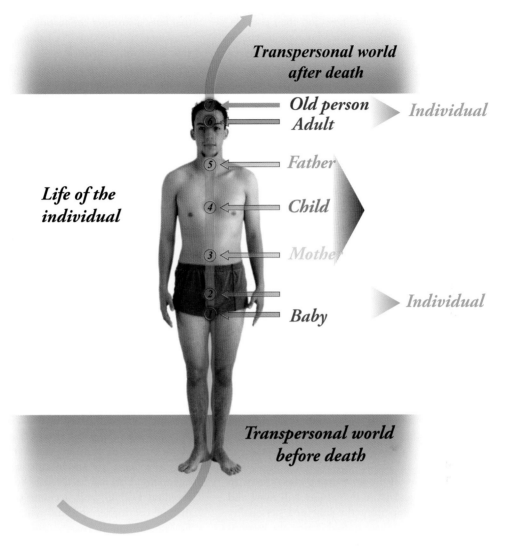

body is the enigmatic and remarkable phenomenon of **Karma**. According to the definition, Karma is "the consequence of a mental or physical act" – or, in another sense, "the chain of cause and effect on the moral plane." *Karma* is generally understood as the doctrine of reincarnation and requital of both good and bad deeds, in that Karma rebalances and makes justice in the sense of reparation possible. Linguistically, Karma means that something has *Causa* (causes, reasons) – that are stored in the causal body – that then generate Karma (consequences, effects). Thus the term *causal body* has directly to do with the doctrine of Karma. When I as physician deal with this topic, it is primarily because, in my opinion, Karma is enormously significant for our life and the resulting problems and diseases.

Now, exactly what more can we learn about **Karma**? Let's imagine the causal body as a big warehouse that can store all

our actions, wishes and thoughts. In a certain sense, thoughts are evaluated as anticipated actions and stored. Many spiritual guides believe that our thought-wishes and wishful thinking, charged up with vital primordial life force, are "processed" for our future in the causal body. Since, in principle, our future – thanks to human primordial freedom or free will – is not (**and must not be!**) predetermined, these thought-wishes can ultimately only "prestructure" our immediate future – i.e., in all likelihood only the next 2–3 days.

Because of human free will, it makes sense that Karma cannot be prestructured for any longer time. Very often, serious errors in reasoning are made at this point. Prophecies such as those of NOSTRADAMUS are thus, in my considered opinion, only worth (at most) the paper they're printed on, since everything beyond the predetermination of the near future is still open and undetermined. Therefore, only our very near future (i.e., days or hours) is so condensed that it can be altered slightly. With great effort, however, this is presumably now and then possible. We can read about the alteration of a seemingly inevitable fate in the Bible story of the inhabitants of the city of Jericho. Their eleventh-hour repentance of their sins prevented the city's destruction. So Karma is not predetermined in the sense that it tells us what to do and forces certain event sequences on us (determinism); rather, it supplies short-term set situations in which we can react one way or another.

In the later chapters on reincarnation, dying, and disease in the mirror of Karma, I will return to this topic and take it further. For now, we are concerned with the structure and the essential components. We must arrive at a more comprehensive picture of subtle-body energy, psyche, and soma, in order to understand, e.g., diseases that have a karmic cause. Admittedly, the causal body is, of all the levels, the hardest to come to grips with, because it so diametrically contradicts our accustomed ways of thinking and perceiving reality. We live in a dualistic world of *good* versus *evil*, *light* and *dark*, with everything taking place along the time axis. A world beyond opposites and time is thus very hard to conceive.

The basic idea – filtered out of working with thousands of patients – I have in mind is grounded quite fundamentally in the concept of reincarnation. At birth, the reincarnated person emerges from the primal ground of the transpersonal world, once again becoming an individual out of the causal body (the matrix of all preceding memories and the stored personality image). This individual possesses new vital, emotional and mental bodies, but brings along the spiritual inheritance of the pre-existing causal body. In the course of the life journey, a personality will more and more emerge and develop from the inherited personality components, which continue to unfold during the maturation process and to add new qualities.

The spiritual inheritance includes the respective character type and certain karmic memories. We can think of the cur-rent personality as a continuation of the personality inherited from earlier lives, which builds on and extends existing patterns. Near the end of our life, we develop those Chakras that have a stronger connection to the world beyond and to wholeness: the 6th and 7th Chakras – so that, after death, we sink down once again into the transpersonal world of the causal body, there to await reincarnation. We can detect, in the upward development of the Chakras, a process that runs through the individual as well as the group.

Now, a living being does not come alone and of itself – in an act of self-creation, as it were – into the world. It needs a father, who does his part by contributing sperm, and a mother, with her egg cell and womb in which the baby grows. We here see already, in depth-psychological terms, the primal pattern of the nuclear family, which is, interestingly, reflected in the Chakras of the individual. Within the triad of the inner Chakras, we find the mother in the 3rd Chakra, the father in the 5th Chakra, and the child itself (in its form as an "actual and true person" or soul in itself) in the 4th (Heart) Chakra, flanked by father and mother. At some point, we too will become, in the middle of our lives, again father or mother for another being. Thus does the generational *Rondo* continue. Ancestors remain as nurturing primal ground in the causal body, out of which the next new life will emerge.

In closing, I'd like to mention two more ways of looking at these things that can be helpful. One extraordinarily practical model comes from the indigenous shamans (*Kahunas*) of Hawaii. I have derived many valuable inspirations and concepts, which form the basis of my own system of *Psychosomatic Energetics*, from the *Huna* teachings. The *Huna* system of the indigenous Hawaiians is said to be traceable back to the occult wisdom of the ancient Egyptians. This has been researched by the American Max Freedom LONG, and it connects magic knowledge with that of the higher spiritual religions (Christianity, Islam, Buddhism, and Judaism). Although the *Kahunas* did not pay reverence to a specific monotheism, it nevertheless underlies their system in latent form.

The system of the *Kahunas* distinguishes between specif-

The Huna Tripartite Division of the Self

Forms of the Self	Energy Level	Chakra
Lower (inferior) Self	Material (physical) body Vital Level	1. – 2. Chakra
Middle Self	Emotional Level Mental Level	3. – 6. Chakra
Higher Self	Causal Level	7. Chakra

ic forms of the Self, and these can be matched up with energy centers (Chakras) and energy levels:

According to the *Kahunas*, three beings or forms of the Self reside and are active within us. We are normally only aware of the Middle Self. In the view of the *Kahunas*, we cannot reach the Higher Self directly, but only via the agency of the Lower Self, which is in a certain sense a communication channel with the Higher Self. The Lower Self corresponds to the totem animal of the Indian clans. We come into contact with the Higher Self via the Lower Self. We must communicate with the Higher Self if we wish to live in harmony with the divine life and change our future for the better (since our future is decided in the Higher Self). Negative, guilt-laden emotions (conflicts) in the Lower Self block the information channel to the Higher Self.

Yet another profound classification scheme originates with C. G. JUNG. He distinguishes four consciousness functions in all, which he calls *sensory qualities* and regards as preliminary stages of consciousness. It was, however, not clear to him that the causal body was an example of the superconscious. JUNG spoke of the collective or archetypal unconscious, interpreting the archetypes as image forms of animalistic instincts. I think, however, that we are here dealing with what PLATO termed "the ocean of preformed ideas"; archetypes are merely especially strong condensations of particularly momentous collective ideas.

C. G. JUNG proposed the following arrangement, which is not difficult to relate logically to the four vibrational levels (see table below).

At first, it's only in the rational region that we're "lord of the manor" as FREUD so aptly put it. Our Ego first develops on the Mental Level. Only here can we guide our reali-

ty ourselves and possess a consciousness. We think something with the aid of our conceptions (i.e., our Mental Level) and call this ability to have such ideas *free will*. In reality, free will ends in the realm of the subconscious, which surrounds us with a zone of un-freedom where we are helplessly at the mercy of other laws and rules, which naturally generates fear.

In the context of self-exploration, our mission consists of filling all the levels of being of our existence with life and sensation, of setting our True Self free and thereby becoming truly free of fear. The unknown and unredeemed levels of our existence that need to be liberated are the Vital, Emotional, and Causal Levels. Our goal is the knowledge of the True Self (which resides in the causal body), which we can only approach, according to *Huna* teachings, by dealing with our Lower Self (the Emotional Level). We first need to make the Vital and Emotional Levels conscious and redeem them, before we can turn to the Causal Level. We must learn to perceive and feel before we can attain intuitive ability. We must explore our emotional structure and our sensory perceptions before reaching the level of the archetypes. Above all, we must sweep away the barriers of the subconscious conflicts that block our vital and emotional energy, which is why we no longer have access to the True Self in the first place.

I'd next like to discuss the seven energy centers (Chakras). These are energy concentrations that have both storage and distribution functions. The most important thing about the Chakras is that they transform a person's entire feeling for life and consciousness in an evolutionary growth process. We can thus regard the Chakras as a quality that reflects the kind of life we live. Therefore, people whose Chakras are at the same developmental level understand one another

Vibrational Levels and Quality of Consciousness (Modified from C.G. JUNG)

Vibrational Level	Vital	Emotional	Mental	Causal
Associated entity	Plant	Animal	Human	Divine Level
Quality of consciousness (C.G. Jung)	Sensation	Emotion	Thought	Intuition
Consciousness	Unconscious	Unconscious	Consciousness	Unconscious
Psychological Category	Sensory organs	Emotional structure	Rational activity, everyday consciousness	Archetypes (instincts in image form)
Symbolic content/ Sensation	Strength/ Dynamism	Feeling/ Emotion	Thought	Law
Symbol	Plant	Heart	Human	Diamond

immediately. The Chakras are also closely related to character type, which is relatively independent of biological age. The amazing resonance phenomenon can also be found here: people of the same character type, regardless of age, get along with and understand one another right off the bat. Knowledge of the Chakras plays a key role in the process of personal growth and self-exploration, because only with the aid of the Chakras can we truly understand who we really are.

The Seven Energy Centers
(Chakras)

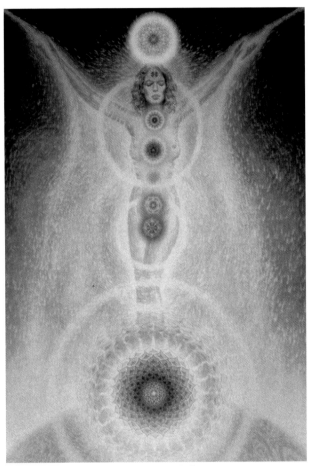

The Chakras and the Kundalini enlightenment experience

In the ancient Indian Sanskrit language, *Chakra* means *wheel* or *spoke*. This name probably has to do with clairvoyant Yogis having seen, in *Auras*, dish-shaped wheels or spokes extending from pelvis to head. There is some rudimentary knowledge of *Chakras* in the West and the snake force (Kundalini) that spirally connects the seven *Chakras*. In the mythological representation of the **Caduceus** (Mercury's staff), which became the symbol of Occidental medicine, we see the same energetic knowledge that is called **Kundalini** energy in India.

It is part of ancient human myths that healers would like to tame and control the life force in order to work with it. On a deeper level of understanding, however, the Caduceus also

expresses the intuitive insight that energetic healing and becoming hale and whole are intimately interrelated. Back in man's primeval beginnings, when priest and doctor were still one and the same, there stirred that intuitive knowledge that healing and redemption were closely related – in fact, at bottom identical – concepts.

In a depth-psychological sense, being sick has to do with sin and "falling out of the order," whereas health means living in harmony with oneself and the surrounding order. The fact that such simple similes are often incorrect does not mean that they are false in a mythological sense. We sense things in our heart differently, in a way that doesn't always match up with reality. Our heart thus reveals to us a deeper dimension of reality, described in the preceding chapter about the causal body. "Being healthy" can mean, for example, to a seriously ill person, that she knows, way down deep in her heart, that she is actually healthy. Her causal-body consciousness knows intuitively about the integrity and indestructibility of her soul.

According to Yoga, the size of the energy centers (Chakras) is related to the development of consciousness. The aforementioned sages of ancient India (*Rishis*) noticed that Chakra size reflected the degree of spiritual development. Chakras can be enlarged through meditation and right living (principles of Yoga and Buddhism). This is accompanied by an enlarged consciousness. Therefore, the size of the Chakras and a person's spiritual development are directly interrelated.

In ancient times, the king was the person who possessed the most developed seventh Chakra (Head or Crown Chakra). The 7th Chakra symbolized, for these early people, the overcoming of the individual ego. We therefore repeatedly re-encounter the 7th Chakra in the form of the nimbus (halo), the Indian chief's feather bonnet, and Jesus' crown of thorns. For the king's non-clairvoyant subjects, his high status was made explicit by his royal crown. Because of his dominant position, the king was the best informed and was able to think and decide synergistically in the tribe's best interests. That may have been true at some time in our distant past, and the myth of the wise and benevolent king continues to make the rounds. But at some point, ignorant power-mad kings ruined the ideal, so that the crown and its presumed spiritual properties no longer had anything to do with each other. Today, when someone wears a diadem at a ceremonial occasion, we don't think we're in the presence of an enlightened being. We're more likely to suspect a husband's or lover's fat wallet. On top of which, we'll likely suspect the person of having a strong need for attention and adulation.

Surprisingly, the diadem exerts an enormous fascination among more women than I would have thought possible before I started inquiring about secret desires to wear a diadem. The diadem is thus, like the crown or Indian chief's feather bonnet, a mythological symbol of the first rank, whose original meaning is still felt by many. I suspect that its secret significance is manifested in the general covetousness that diadems and crowns evoke. Beauty queens or royal sovereigns reflect the secret desire to belong to the nobility, as the *Cinderella* fairy tale makes clear. In my opinion, this reflects internally the intuitive knowledge of the causal body and the 7th Chakra.

In their totality, the size and shape of the Chakras correspond to a person's level of spiritual development at the time. This is not, however, a matter of outstanding talents and traits, but rather of the sum total of all psychoenergetic qualities. For example, someone might be a Nobel Laureate, thanks to a special talent such as an outstanding intellect, and yet still have small, underdeveloped Chakras. The clairvoyant American Lea SANDERS said that the most beautiful golden Aura she had ever seen in her life belonged to a mentally-handicapped girl, who radiated an angelic, downright beatific charisma. We can see from this example that, when it comes to the soul, different values apply than those of the everyday world, as Jesus' saying makes clear: *"For what is a man profited, if he shall gain the whole world, and have not love?"*

The Chakras guide our spiritual development in that, within the Chakras, we take part from childhood to old age in an upward development. Our current Chakra corresponds to the overall psychoenergetic level we have attained. A baby begins its development with the 1st Chakra, while we expect the attainment of higher Chakras in an older person. The wisdom of age is tied in with the energetic vibration of the 7th Chakra. Our overall energetic vibration and the spectrum of our personal freedom increase more with greater Chakra development. We see the same thing with expanding consciousness. Like ascending a tower, with increasing Chakra maturity, we look out over an ever greater spectrum of reality.

Parents can observe quite well the individual stages of **personal growth** in their children. With advancing age and more highly developed Chakras, the potentials in the individual rise enormously. Growth stages also involve the risk of failure: the increasing possibilities of the maturation process offer more opportunities for error. Often, too, our personal destiny confronts us with ever harder challenges – even if we are, in and of ourselves, not responsible for them. A kid can fall in with a gang of petty thieves, or cause an accident, or he and his parents can be tested by fate in some other way. This is the karmic dimension, which externally accompanies our personal development. One gets the impression that Karma matches the lessons to the individual's level of development. The Bible passage *"Whom the Lord loveth he chasteneth"* makes clear the instructive potential of **Karma**. Learning tasks come at us from the outside and influence personal growth and maturation.

The Chakras guide not only the personality development of the individual, but also the development of groups, on up to all of mankind. As Chakra development increases, the demands on the individual and on members of social groups rise to

Chakras, Associated Organs, and Functions

Chakra	Associated Organs	Endocrine Gland	Functional Systems
7. Chakra	Cerebrum	Pineal	Abstract thought, voluntary movements
6. Chakra	Cerebellum, midbrain	Pituitary	Autonomic nervous system, subconscious movement control
5. Chakra	Mouth, neck	Thyroid	Eating, drinking, communication
4. Chakra	Heart, lung	Thymus	Respiration, circulation, emotional center
3. Chakra	Liver, stomach, upper small intestine	Pancreas	"Positive" nutritional system, i.e., digestion
2. Chakra	Small and large intestine, anus	Adrenal	"Negative" nutritional system, i.e., excretion
1. Chakra	Minor pelvic organs	Testicles/ovaries	Reproduction

match. With increasing development, the dangers increase with the possibilities and freedoms. I will demonstrate later on, by means of an evolutionary model, that the psychoenergetic viewpoint shows human history in a new light that makes many hitherto incomprehensible correlations easier to understand. Understanding the Chakras as pace-setters of personal growth is, by the way, the indispensable tool for a correct understanding of the background factors.

The **seven energy centers (Chakras)** govern psychoenergetic body segments. These can be visualized as disks layered one atop the other, reaching from the pelvis to the head. The medical term is *segments*, in which a segment's Chakra governs the associated organs. In addition, each Chakra regulates complex functions such as digestion, reproduction, and other vegetative reactions. The Chakras may be viewed as central switching centers exercising a superordinate regulatory function, as in the chart on page 116.

For example, the Heart Chakra is responsible for supplying the thoracic organs (heart, lungs) with life force, and seeing to it that they function harmoniously. Long-term energetic blockage of the Heart Chakra leads to deficient energy supply and greater disease susceptibility, thereby favoring the development of pulmonary diseases such as asthma, or cardiac disorders such as arrhythmia. Speaking quite generally, one can say that the vast majority of diseases are a consequence of subtle-body energy and Chakra disturbances. Almost always, a specific Chakra disturbance is the first link in the causal chain by which a disease arises, which can manifest itself in a great variety of forms. Conversely, harmonizing a disturbed Chakra favorably influences the disease healing process.

This can be formulated with a pair of simple equations:
Chakra disturbed = Disease occurs
Chakra harmonized = Disease cured[31]

However, we should also beware of oversimplified equations of the sort: "A pulmonary patient must have a disturbance in the 4th Chakra." – since in many cases the cause-effect relationship can be inverted: someone with no Chakra disturbance in the lung region is infected with tuberculosis; the more the patient coughs, feels weak and feverish, the more life force is used up; at some point, the victim will wind up with a Heart Chakra blockage. If we examine a pulmonary patient with a recently-acquired disease, we will often find a very different energetic insufficiency than the one that corresponds to the pulmonary disease. For instance, the patient could have a pelvic Chakra blockage that weakens the life force so much that it increases susceptibility to infection. One could easily catch tuberculosis that

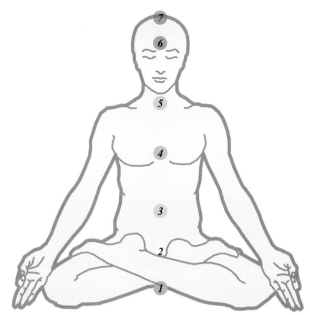

The seven Chakras in the typical Yoga representation

way. Therefore, in some of the cases, a Heart Chakra disturbance can occur during the course of the disease.

According to Indian Yoga, Chakras are considered to be relays, energetic transmitters via which the cosmic energy (the universal *Prana*) is filtered, distributed, and stored. **Chakras are like funnels through which life force can flow into the organism.** Large, open Chakras act as large funnels through which one can take in and process more energy. Large amounts of energy are needed for mental healing and more profound spiritual work. This is why I have observed, in many healers, large Chakras through which a great amount of healing energy can flow, which the healer passes on to the ailing person. Besides large stores of life force (vital energy), healers often have relatively open causal bodies. Both of these – a lot of life force and open causal bodies – seem to be extraordinarily important for spiritual healing, in which the causal body acts like a large "universal funnel" for the life force.

But large Chakras carry with them the disadvantage of being much more strongly threatened by negative energies. Being able to deal well with negative energies requires a stable personality. Many schizophrenics – including an astounding number of highly developed persons – therefore seem to me to have gone psychotic because they prematurely opened themselves up energetically, thus activating huge conflicts that had been acting as energetic barriers and sluices. The ego is then deluged by a huge tidal wave of subconscious negative content. I will return to this tragic circumstance, which underlies many psychoses, later on in the

---

[31] The disease will heal as long as the self-healing powers are strong enough, cell regeneration is possible, and pathogens or metabolic and genetic damages do not strongly predominate.

discussion of conflicts.

I'd like to illustrate this with a typical case involving psychoenergetic psychosis due to the activation of an enormous conflict. During the examination, the pale 16-year-old kid constantly looks to the side and doesn't say a word. He is an immensely talented teenager, but his schoolwork took a nosedive some time ago. At first, this was blamed on puberty. The youth's mother says that he hadn't been doing well for a long time. He began having more and more problems in school, as a result of which he had to repeat a grade. He became more and more withdrawn socially and increasingly agoraphobic. He thinks he is being watched, and he says that his thoughts are being drawn out of him by foreign powers. He had a nervous breakdown six weeks ago, the psychiatric diagnosis being schizophrenia.

The REBA® Test Device measures strikingly low readings at all energy levels. The life force charge is a mere 20%. The mental reading of 20% is shockingly low. The cause is found to be a huge Central Conflict in the Head Chakra with the theme Not wanting to face reality. *The conflict has an enormously high intrinsic charge of 100% Vital, 100% Emotional, 30% Mental, and 80% Causal. The conflict thus sucks up enormous quantities of the teenager's life force and hems in his ego almost completely. This can be seen in the low readings for his mental body, which has shrunk to a pitiful 20%. This makes normal thinking impossible, and the student can no longer understand what's being taught in class. It makes sense that he was not promoted. The conflict content* Not wanting to face reality *is a downright classically typical conflict content for psychoses.*

There's no need to go into further detail on this case, since the main point was to describe the cause of a psychosis. The boy is doing better now. In his case, treating just the conflict was not enough: the disrupted personality maturation processes also had to be encouraged. That was done in this case through supportive talks with a specialist, as well as a helping environment that has played a protective and supportive role.

Next, I'd like to present a brief overview of the seven Chakras, naming their most important functions and describing the typical disturbances and diseases associated with each Chakra. Virtually all esoteric traditions distinguish seven Chakras, arrayed from pelvis to head. Sometimes, the Chakras are classified or arranged differently. I have chosen a classification that conforms with traditional ancient Indian Yoga. It reflects, moreover, my decades of physician experience with thousands of patients. Since I have compared my results with other therapists, I believe I can say that these are reliable statements, which do not merely represent my ideas, but indeed possess universal validity.

The **1st** or **Pelvic Chakra** is situated at the end of the spinal column. This is the seat of the life force (Kundalini). The 1st Chakra corresponds to groundedness, *joie de vivre*, dancing and movement. The 1st Chakra is the most closely related to sexuality, as it has to do with personal desire(s). But the 1st Chakra also expresses a transpersonal survival instinct. This is reflected on the material level in the genetic code (DNA), by means of which our body is fashioned into a tool for passing on the genetic material (as in a relay race) to the next generation. When people sacrifice their lives for their children, as we see time and again in heroic situations, this is an example of the transpersonal survival instinct.

In many people, the sensual unfolding of the life force in the pelvis is severely blocked, thus sharply constraining the ability for sexual experiences. Somatic psychotherapy speaks here of a *pelvic blockage*. In this situation, the inner pelvic musculature is in a permanent state of high tension, recognizable by an indurated deep pelvic floor and restricted pelvic mobility. As soon as the indurated muscles loosen up, the previously blocked life force is released in the form of sensual feelings. Many people have reported on a *channel of desire* (which I mentioned earlier), said to be located deep in the genitals. It might be that the idea of Kundalini as a curled-up snake in the pelvis comes from the experience that is related to the *channel of desire*. The buttocks and legs also belong to the 1st Chakra, which is why we see, in many people with a blockage of the 1st Chakra, a tendency to lower-back pain and cold feet. Also, congested and swollen legs are often caused by a pelvic blockage.

The **2nd** or **Lower-abdomen Chakra** corresponds to the development of dynamics and strength. Very generally, it has to do with stress, aggression and the struggle for survival. The struggle for personal survival, with its associated stress, is reflected in the 2nd Chakra, which, from the standpoint of the hormonal glands, is associated with the adrenals, where the stress hormones cortisone and adrenaline help us deal with stressful situations. The *flight or fight* syndrome seen in tense social confrontations is reflected in the 2nd Chakra.

Since the 1st and 2nd Chakras are so close together, they have much in common. Blockages of the middle pelvis (which belongs to the 2nd Chakra) frequently affect the abdominal and lumbar musculature, as well as the muscles of the lower leg. In obese people, a flabby, protruding belly is often a sign of chronic stress that, via adrenal disorder and 2nd Chakra blockage, leads to overweight and weakening of the abdominal musculature. Many people with a disturbed 2nd Chakra also have static structural disorders in the lumbar spine that lead to lower-back pain.

The **3rd** or **Upper-abdomen Chakra** has to do with ingesting and digesting food, water and emotional energy. The upper abdomen (and the associated solar plexus) is the center of primal identity, which is related to the development of (spiritually enormously important) *basic trust*. We develop a basic trust in the nurturing/giving nature of our world. We find out that the world is drinkable and edible and that it means us well. So, at peace with the world, the just-suckled baby falls contentedly asleep. The umbilical cord as a symbol of the nurturing, mothering source of life likewise belongs to the 3rd Chakra. Many statues of Buddha show him with a big belly and a contented smile. The *Ch'i* life force is said to be quite strongly present in a big belly.

A 3rd Chakra disturbance can often be recognized by a blockage of the diaphragm that prevents proper breathing. I have learned from breathing and voice teachers how widespread breathing disorders are. Moreover, the diaphragm represents a psychoenergetic barrier with which we can prevent feelings from rising up and becoming conscious. We simply hold our breath, which then turns diaphragmatic tension into a permanent condition. For many people, sports, with their elevated respiratory activity, are (like singing) a way of getting rid of excess diaphragmatic tension. They feel better after this kind of activity because it has made them psychoenergetically more relaxed. Disturbances of the 3rd Chakra are often reflected in upper-abdominal complaints such as nausea, feeling of pressure, stomachache and digestive disorders. Diseases such as diabetes are also related to the 3rd Chakra.

The **4th** or **Chest Chakra** contains emotional qualities: compassion, love and all other good human qualities. Topographically, the 4th (Heart) Chakra corresponds to the thoracic cage, including the heart, lungs, and chest. The maternal breast symbolizes the nurturing, loving and protective quality of the Heart Chakra. Emotionally, the 4th Chakra corresponds to our emotional body, but also our true Self. Whenever something "moves us deep in our heart," the Heart Chakra is involved. The 4th Chakra also has to do with all our fears and everything that unpleasantly upsets us.

Patients with a blocked Heart Chakra often complain that they can't take a good deep breath. It can also lead to constricted and pressure feelings in the rib cage. Many people are tense and stiff in the region of the shoulder blades and the thoracic spine. The arms and hands are also part of the Heart Chakra. A hunched-over posture with drooping shoulders is often associated with the disturbed energy of the Heart Chakra.

The **5th** or **Neck Chakra** represents – besides the diaphragm – the second portal through which feelings have to pass on their ascent to consciousness. The Neck Chakra thus has an important function in the control of feelings, such as when we want to hold back weeping or sobbing. Psychoenergetically, the mental body corresponds to the Neck Chakra. Nowhere are we more "I" than in the Neck Chakra. The voice plays a key role in this, since human con-

sciousness is only possible through language. Recent research results in linguistics show that language is important not only as a communications medium but also as the basis for rational thought. The 5th Chakra has to do with intellectuality and control, the desire to communicate and the constancy of morality, precepts, laws, opinions.

The segment blockages of the Neck Chakra comprise the vocal folds, gullet, mouth and neck, as well as the lower jaw. People with stiffness in the Neck Chakra are known in the vernacular as "stiff-necked." One often finds stiff neck musculature when there are disturbances of the Neck Chakra. One also often observes deficient vocal function. In the lower jaw, there are frequently tensions, circulatory disorders and even dental problems. The tonsils are also closely related to the Heart Chakra.

The **6th** or **Brow Chakra** is designated as the Third Eye. It has been identified since time immemorial with intuition, the *sixth sense* and the awakening of insight. Basically, the 6th Chakra regulates the autonomous (vegetative) nervous system and hormonal balance. The Brow Chakra thus creates a higher order that brings many of the organism's subsidiary functions together into a higher whole. One can compare it to a conductor, who fuses the members of the orchestra into a higher-grade unity.

Brow Chakra blockages affect the upper jaw, temples and upper cheeks, and parts of the cervical spine. Suppressed tears and being irritated belong to the Brow Chakra and relate to the nasal mucosa and the upper throat. Sinus inflammations and many kinds of headaches have to do with a disturbed Brow Chakra.

The **7th** or **Crown** or **Head Chakra** is identified with the full unfolding of human potential. The Crown Chakra is associated with the cerebrum and, in its potential, corresponds to the infinity of potential interconnections among the cerebral synapses. From a purely arithmetical standpoint, the number of potential interconnection variations between the neurons of the cerebrum has been calculated to be vastly greater than the number of atoms in the universe. The Crown Chakra has to do with the self-chosen and reality-checked definition of law and meaning. Here is where the individual and the worldly order are harmonized with each other.

Segment blockage of the Crown Chakra primarily affects *eye blockage*. Many people either look around rigidly, lifelessly, and listlessly or else as if they were actually looking inward. Other spasmodic conditions relate to the upper temple or cranial muscles and the forehead; this includes headaches and brain diseases. Also, the Atlas (uppermost cervical vertebra) has a close relationship to the Crown Chakra. Deep within the cranium, the pulsating and resonating meninges form yet another locus for energy blocks that is used in craniosacral therapy as a healing quality.

Having described the seven Chakras and their significance for the individual, I'd now like to mention another way in which the Chakras are meaningful, one which I'll go into in more detail later on: the importance of the Chakras as pacesetters and graduated steps within an evolutionary process that mankind is part of. From this standpoint, the Chakras are the expression of a general maturity of consciousness. Each society thus has a particular, general evolutionary level of consciousness, shared by most of its members. This culture-historical evolutionary process is reminiscent of our organic development, in which – in the gray dawn of time – we were once single-celled creatures. The evolutionary program proceeds to the fetus, which (like fish) for a while has gills. Later on, we reach the mammalian stage, the terminus of this hierarchical development.

Mankind as a whole seems to have gone through a very comparable evolutionary transformational process that proceeds from the first to the seventh Chakra. I will present some commentaries and examples of this in the next (second) part of this book. This point of view has a number of advantages, since (for one) we find our experiences entangled in collective processes that we had taken to be individual. We thus learn something about ourselves from the behavior of the collective – but we also understand civilizational processes better.

I'd like to give an example of this. Certain collective actions can be viewed as an attempt to facilitate the next level of Chakra maturation. At the moment, we are living collectively in the Brow Chakra. Driving (automobiles) in our high-tech society confronts us with the necessity to think and perceive in terms of complex processes. In this manner, many people exercise the capabilities of the 6th Chakra. Our growing and expanding ecological consciousness also shows that more and more people are learning to think in terms of the categories of the Brow Chakra. Similarly, computer games and the Internet are preparations for a collective maturation of the Brow Chakra.

By its very nature, every evolutionary model of human development suffers from the unfortunate tendency to elevate man to a special developmental status as a "superman." It is not my intent to flatter human vanity. I have always been skeptical of illusory visions of a future "Age of Aquarius" populated entirely by happy people. Having personally gotten to know some of the leading prophets of the "Age of Aquarius" – some of whom were patients of mine (who must remain anonymous because of doctor-patient confidentiality) – I became aware of the deep inferiority complexes and subconscious delusions of grandeur that drive many of these authors and masterminds. But neither am I one of those pessimistic "professional grouches" who are always finding fault with the human race (because in their heart of hearts they can't stand themselves), as many cynical self-appointed critics do. As is so often the case, the truth lies somewhere in the middle.

Now that the seven Chakras' basic features have been described, the next chapter will deal with subconscious conflicts. It will present the "dark side" that works against our development into "superman." It is in these conflicts that we find the friction surfaces that crucially promote our personality development. It is from the struggles and privations, defeats and experiences that we learn what our real problems are. For the outer in a certain sense reflects the inner, such that the makeup of our external problems reveals (within limits) some things about our internal problems.

Demons,
Spiritual Conflicts and Disease

At all times and in the most diverse cultures, man has believed in spirits and demons. Modern man sees this as an expression of *animism*, an early form of naïve thought in which primitive cultures, like children, believe that everything is animated by a soul of some sort. We moderns, on the other hand, considers spirits to be a projection of emotional problems and conflicts. As a child converts his fear of darkness into a fear of ghosts and goblins, so also do primitives transform their fears into persons that they perceive as spirits or demons.

In short, psychologists believe that ghosts do not exist, that they are just figments of the imagination. And since people today assume that psychologists know what they are talking about, most of them believe the same. Whoever believes in spirits is accused of being superstitious. For instance, an amazingly high percentage of Britishers are convinced that ghosts really do exist. There are actual clubs promoting this belief, and ghost hunts where people stay overnight in haunted castles. These Brits are viewed by outsiders as eccentric kooks indulging in a harmless kind of collective insanity, which normal folk of sound mind cannot go along with.

The conviction that spirits and demons must be figments of the imagination is rooted in certain basic assumptions and prejudices. One could just as well ask why spirits cannot exist. In my opinion, is has to do with our subjective evaluation of what we can reconcile with logic and common sense. Our evaluation in no way corresponds to objective fact. It is my firm conviction that belief in spirits is indeed based on objective facts, but that it represents an antiquated, highly dangerous, and even destructive variety of magic. I've already explained at the beginning of this book why I condemn magic, even though I am convinced of its effectiveness. I believe in ghosts, but I also believe it is not good to think about them too much – because the more we think about them, the more active they become, under certain circumstances actually becoming dangerous to us.

Throughout human history, spirits have done an enormous amount of mischief. They have probably been worrying and terrifying people for a very long time, possibly for millions of years. In many parts of the world, people continue to this day to suffer the consequences of their belief in spirits. It makes them needlessly fearful and intimidated and causes much suffering and sorrow. On top of which, spirits are subject to a very subjective evaluation. Whether one

believes in them or not depends mainly on highly variable belief systems. In the Spiritism of Alen KARDEC and the Voodoo cult practiced in parts of the third world, one can still find remnants of the ancient spirit belief systems. Interestingly, when Spiritists or Voodoo cultists convert to Christianity, their spirits vanish. If these spirits were more real, they would presumably not be so easy to extinguish. In parts of the Caribbean, in Central and South America, and in Africa, one can trace the developmental process that led, first, to the mixing and then to the gradual disappearance of the belief in spirits when Christianity was introduced.

The Swiss depth psychologist C.G. JUNG was one of the few specialists who had the courage to stand by his belief in spirits. His doctoral dissertation dealt with spiritist experiences with a cousin of his who was a so-called *channeling medium*. JUNG reported having repeatedly heard spirit voices and observed the movement of objects with no ascertainable physical cause. On one occasion the aging JUNG received an important communication from a spirit which substantially inspired his work in the area of alchemy. JUNG suspected that the spirit might have been an old alchemist who used JUNG's interest as a resonance aid to passing on the important message to him. Spooky phenomena are usually found with greater frequency in the vicinity of people who are open to this sort of thing. JUNG certainly was, and it was also good for the development of parapsychology that, thanks to his undeniable fame, he was able to express such controversial opinions publicly without being considered crazy.

The annals of parapsychology are full of reports describing the unquestionable existence of ghosts and poltergeists. Amazingly, these phenomena often depend on the presence of particular persons. After looking through numerous cases, I am convinced that ghosts often target a particular person. Ghosts are said to be spirits of the dead who have some sort of problem with their death or the manner of it – it was unexpected or occurred under inhumane conditions. Here is a typical story from rural Barbados:

In the 18th century, after the owner of a plantation died, an uncle was supposed to take care of the owner's child until it was old enough to manage the plantation on its own. The mother had died years ago, and there were no other relatives. However, the uncle was an avaricious person. One day, the child and its nanny mysteriously disappeared. Later on, when the uncle died, the horses hitched up to the hearse refused to pull his coffin, so the uncle had to be buried on the plantation instead of the cemetery. After the uncle's death, it was said that the farmhouse was haunted. During a later renovation, a heavy wall was removed, revealing the skeletons of a child and an adult. Once these skeletons were properly laid to rest, the ghosts, it is said, were seen no more.

According to esoteric tradition and folk belief, ghosts are unhappy souls that wander about restlessly. Haunting is thus a kind of protest against an injustice, a way of calling attention to it – or a type of resistance, a way for the ghost to rebel against its premature passing. My personal experience, plus conversations I have had as doctor with thousands of patients, have very rarely brought me into contact with ghostly phenomena. Even open-minded colleagues report much the same, and the same goes for priests and psychologists whom I have queried about these things.

Ghosts seem to be a marginal phenomenon for which our modern society no longer has much use. Still, if one should, for whatever reason, get involved with a ghost, one can protect oneself from its influence with loving prayers, incense, and Christian symbols. In the Caribbean, where a great many animistically-sensitive people live, one recommendation is to strew grain in a threatened house. The spirits then spend the entire night counting the grain kernels instead of invading the house. The Indian *dreamcatcher* – a handmade spiderweblike affair in which the spirits are supposed to get ensnared – works in a similar manner. Trapping the previously visualized spirit in a container that is then burned is said to be another good option for transforming ghosts. Burning leads to a transformation in which the residual psychoenergetic structures are dissolved.

I'd also like to mention **nature spirits** in passing because my personal assessment is that they are similar to the ghosts of the deceased. Our receptivity, as well as our subconscious problems, play a crucial role in determining whether nature spirits will have a morbific effect on us. In certain regions of the world, nature spirits are said to have a hand in accidents and illnesses, if annoyed. In Iceland, the belief in nature spirits is widespread, being in fact grounded in the constitution, which stipulates that nature spirits must be protected to some extent. When, for example, a road was run through a meadow where trolls live, the accident rate went up there. Only after the road was rerouted around the meadow did things return to normal. In Thailand and in many parts of China, trouble with nature spirits is carefully avoided in a similar manner by building little pagoda-shaped surrogate houses next to one's own house. There, the nature spirits get offerings of fruits, cakes and joss sticks.

There's another form of spirit belief that has to do with **possession**. The spirit of the deceased possesses its victim, exploiting its life force and using its body and mind for its own purposes. In my experience, possession can only occur when the victim is emotionally weak and has subconscious conflicts that resonate with the spirit of the deceased and its character. For instance, if a child is particularly greedy, this character weakness provides an entry point for the spirit of a deceased alcoholic, which can then possess the child. The child's illness can manifest itself as epilepsy attacks, or a severe inexplicable personality change. If the child's greed-related subconscious conflict is treated, the possession will vanish.

Possession shows up in various forms and causes its victims to behave in ways that even their closest friends and family don't recognize. The feeling of strangeness is thus a typical characteristic of possession. Added to this is a predilection for unusual behavior patterns that have self-destructive aspects. Extreme cases include violent outbreaks and sudden changes in tone of voice, beating the head against the wall, and rabid, aggressive behavior. Many possession victims swear constantly, cursing all and sundry. Often, people with mental ailments are labeled possessed if the society recognizes possession as a disease type. A modern psychiatrist would diagnose such persons as schizophrenic or depressive, since possession is not a recognized disease form.

Despite the most careful observation and my own openness to such phenomena, I have observed very few cases of genuine possession in my patients. I am therefore quite sure that possession is a relatively rare occurrence in our society. I have observed cases of genuine possession in third-world countries. In Nepal, I once saw an older woman climb up into a tree and expose herself, all the while cutting herself with a knife and screaming in a harsh male voice. In the closed wards of psychiatric institutions, and in psychoses that break out abruptly, many patients act as if possessed. Amazingly, many of these people react more positively to gentle and friendly persuasion than to stern admonitions. They seem to be suffering the most from their ailment, and have pleasant memories of humane treatment, when their condition is in remission.

Possession seems to occur mainly when the victim is energetically open and/or weak. This is frequently the case with children, pregnant women, and people undergoing maturation crises (puberty, menopause, death of a close relative). From the standpoint of personality development, the main victims of possession are people whose personality structures are underdeveloped. The more stable and autonomous the personality, the more unattractive it is to a spirit.

The possession victim almost always has emotional problems that explain the appearance of the disease. If the subconscious conflict is healed, then the associated symptoms vanish as well. Cases of possession in the third world – such as resentful forebears or deceased enemies – can also be healed simply by breaking up the victim's subconscious conflicts. If the spirit can no longer resonate with the victim, then the possession will disappear. To this extent, I think that possession is an explanatory model that is largely out-moded.

However, there is a third type of spiritlike disease cause that occurs extraordinarily often, one that has a towering significance for modern man: the **subconscious conflicts** or **complexes** (C.G. JUNG). One can view them as spirits that one has conjured up, but they are actually split-off fragments of one's personality that, in a certain sense, lead a life of their own. In what follows, I'd like to present some sound arguments for why we can view conflicts as spiritlike structures that lead a psychoenergetically independent life. But before going into that in greater detail, I'd like first to outline the viewpoint of psychoanalysis and modern medicine.

The designation *complex* was introduced into psychoanalysis by C.G. JUNG. A complex is *"… the image of a particular psychological situation that is dynamically emotionally accentuated and which, moreover, proves to be irreconcilable with the normal state or attitude of consciousness. This image has a strong inner unity, its own totality, and has at its disposal a relatively high degree of autonomy, i.e., it is only minimally subject to conscious disposition and thus behaves like a foreign body within the realm of consciousness."* Although my own view of conflicts (which I will be presenting in the next chapter) includes JUNG's concepts, it goes far beyond them.

From now on, I'd like to use the term *conflict* rather than *complex*, because *complex* has become (somewhat negatively) associated with "inferiority complex." Thus, complexes can sometimes be the consequence of conflicts, but they are nonetheless not identical. *Conflict*, however, seems to me to be sufficiently neutral and comprehensive. I will describe in detail how conflicts arise in the next chapter. **Basically, inner emotional conflicts are based on irreconcilably opposed endeavors** – for example, having to remain calm even though one is terribly angry. Actions and feelings can be opposed just as contradictory feelings are, when it comes to triggering a conflict. A lover's exclamation – "I love you so much I could just eat you up!" – expresses this kind of ambivalence in its mildest form; of course, we do not (normally) assume that we're about to be put in the stewpot when we hear this expression. Still, the speaker **is** expressing, albeit subconsciously, an irreconcilable opposition in which strong feelings of love are mixed with strong aggressive feelings.

I'd like to point out, peripherally, that Sigmund FREUD was of the opinion that man's entire emotional life is ambivalent in nature – therefore, love is always bound up with aggression and death wishes. As strange as that may sound at first, I have come to believe that FREUD is essentially right: just take a look around at neurotic, conflict-plagued mankind. And yet, I think that the cause of this ambivalence lies in the conflicts and not the emotions themselves. It is very important to emphasize this difference, for otherwise there could ultimately be no rescue from the emo-

tional jungle – and I am convinced that such salvation is possible: it is based on becoming free of conflicts, whereupon the ambivalence of the fundamental feelings vanishes.

Let us turn once again to the phenomenon of the independent existence of conflicts. Surprisingly, JUNG was fully aware that conflicts can take on a life of their own. For a modern psychologist, this is a remarkable and highly unusual viewpoint. By way of guarding my reputation, I should point out that I first found out about JUNG's ideas long after I had come up with my own conception of the origin of conflicts – so I'd like to stress that I did not "copy off of" JUNG, and that I owe my insights purely to my observations in the energy fields of patients. I was of course delighted to learn that JUNG had come to the same conclusions.

In his autobiography, JUNG describes a number of cases in which his patient's conflicts actually materialized partially. This led to inexplicable incidents that suggested a symbolic link to the conflict content. For JUNG, therefore, spirits and conflicts were, in their essence, closely related phenomena. However, I'd like once more to make it quite clear that conflicts should never be confused with spirits. Spirits are souls of the deceased – i.e., the individual personalities of dead people – whereas conflicts are formed from parts of our own personality. The commonality of spirits and conflicts is that they are both spiritlike, invisible, and autonomous.

Another point in common is that spirits, like conflicts, frighten us and make us afraid. In general, they mean us no good, but rather have egotistical and even sadistic-destructive intentions. On New Year's Eve, we use firecrackers to try to gain the upper hand over dangerous spirits and drive away malevolent demons. When you take a closer look, an astonishingly large number of modern activities are still dedicated to driving away spirits and demons, even if we are no longer aware of it (such as: crossing oneself, murmuring protective mantras, or wearing amulets).

Skeptics usually dismiss belief in spirits as pure superstition, and this attitude has become so entrenched and widespread that anything having to do with spirits has largely disappeared from the conceptual world of modern rational man. Our current view of conflict reflects our general view of ourselves as modern, rationally-oriented people, so that conflicts no longer have anything to do with spirits. In this, the head, as a body region, plays a prominent role, since we locate the seat of thought there. We perceive our world with the head and think consciously with it. We are amazed to find out that not everybody in the world considers the head to be the site of thought. According to JUNG, primitives think either with the belly or the heart; they regard us modern folk as abnormal for claiming to think with our heads.

In my opinion, the location of the sensually perceived consciousness center depends on the level of development of the Chakras. Primitive cultures' highest developed Chakra is the Lower-abdomen (2nd) or Upper-abdomen (3rd) Chakra, which corresponds to the developmental level of the *lower Self*. The head is typically perceived as the seat of thought from the developmental level of the 5th Chakra, in which our civilization finds itself (development of the *middle Self*). We think with our head because our head has psychoenergetically become our active center; and because all members of the collective "think" this, it becomes a rock-solid certainty. Thus, the head has become the thought center because, from a historical developmental standpoint, it has attained a prominent position in our awareness.

Therefore, for us moderns, all psychosomatic symptoms and CNS phenomena originate in the head, be they
1. permanent neurotransmitter imbalances;
2. vegetative disorders with cold sweats, palpitations, diarrhea;
3. social functional disorders with diminished stress capacity, aggression inhibition or intensification;
4. mental problems with diminished self-esteem or disturbed self-image.

Our head orientation has limited our **perceptual capability** to localize our consciousness somewhere other than the head.

This has two serious drawbacks, which affect (in equal measure)

· the general consciousness of our overall personality and
· split-off fragments of consciousness in the form of conflicts.

With respect to consciousness in general, modern man must first arduously relearn that consciousness is not tied exclusively to waking consciousness. Techniques such as meditation, hypnosis, trance and such teach us that consciousness is by no means restricted to the head, that we can just as well learn to perceive with our belly or the soles of our feet, simply by shifting the focus of our consciousness to another part of the body. The BUDDHA advised his disciples to "think with the soles of the feet." Indian Yoga – and SCHULZ's derivative healing technique of *Autogenic Training* – expands consciousness in a similar manner. Ultimately, we learn from this (in the best case) that we actively "are" our Aura rather than that we passively "have" an Aura. By immersing our consciousness in the various Aura levels, we regain the feeling that energy levels are also consciousness bodies.

The second drawback of head-driven perception is that one sees conflicts from a limited perspective: one tends to view them (erroneously) as exclusively a head problem. This is so automatic that we don't notice it. At this point, I'd like to propose a new conceptual model, one that traces back to ancient shamanic wisdom. I mentioned earlier that shamans regard conflicts as **demons** that settle in the patient's Aura

or body. To shamans, conflicts are first and foremost energy thieves that steal life force from patients. Only secondarily are they spirits that mislead patients by altering their consciousness, redirecting it in their own interests. In this sense, they are like the spirits of the dead, who do the same thing more intensely. However, demons don't harm patients nearly as much as spirits do.

Demons and conflicts can be considered to be equivalent, since shamans view them as terrifying personified beings. In order to perceive disease demons, shamans need to enter into a distinctive state. The shamans of Siberia and North American Indians do this with songs, repeating them monotonously until they go into a trance. Hallucinogenic drugs are also used to make demons visible. In this altered state of consciousness, the shaman can make out malign beings that, like bloodsuckers, unleash their harmful effect either externally on the invalid's body or internally.

The shaman visualizes the conflict as an independent and malevolent being that harms the patient's health, causing disease. The hostile being is described variously as insect, vampire, demon, poisonous snake, or evil beast of prey. To my mind, these imaginative descriptions shouldn't stop us from appreciating the essential core of the shamanic descriptions. The significant and essential thing about viewing conflicts as "energy-robbing vampires" and suchlike is that they are describing universally valid psychoenergetic facts! The conflict is unmasked as an autonomous being that is stealing energy from the patient. The shaman is thus observing a real and present situation, which he clothes in ornate language simply because his state of consciousness leads him to do so. Plus, the shaman's cultural background of course favors these concepts, just as his patients prefer that their conflicts be described in vividly graphic terms.

I therefore impute to shamans the ability to perceive conflicts in a more realistic and comprehensive manner than conventional psychology can. Shamans see a psychoenergetic reality that encompasses the subtle-body essence of the conflict. They see that **conflicts steal energy from patients**! They thus grasp an elementally important issue. Second, shamans see (quite rightly) that **conflicts can settle anywhere in the body** – i.e., not just in the head, as modern psychology assumes. Even this represents a significant expansion of our knowledge, since segmental, locally-limited energy theft explains many diseases much better. If someone, say, has constant stomachaches because a *Rage* demon is sitting in the upper abdomen, stealing energy, that sounds logical and explains the upper abdominal pains comprehensibly.

The shamanic point of view has its limits, of course, which I will deal with later on, but I would first like to clarify this unusual viewpoint and promote the idea that conflicts are autonomous beings in our Aura. Psychology has a strong tendency to brand unusual viewpoints as "crazy" – because psychological orthodoxy defines normalcy and mental health are. Amazingly enough, I have noticed time and again, in discussions, that psychological laypersons are more favorably disposed and open to my thesis than specialists, who tend to skepticism and rejection.

And yet, there are psychological and psychiatric specialists who have arrived at conclusions not unlike mine. One of these is Gerda BOYESEN, a Norwegian psychotherapist and founder of *Biodynamic Therapy*, who – like the American Bioenergetics therapist John PIERRAKOS (developer of *Core Energetics*) – is convinced that the Aura does exist.

In her work, Gerda BOYESEN also realized that conflicts lead an independent energetic existence. Certain processes would otherwise be inexplicable – such as the fact that conflict contents can be activated by holding the palms of one's hands in the patient's Aura. At a very precise distance from the body – for instance 50cm (20") – relaxed supine patients re-experience conflict-filled scenes that they say is like watching a movie. In this process, odors and moods are also recalled. I have done this a number of times on various subjects and have been able to evoke very specific "movies" at specific locations in the Aura. What makes this all the more astonishing is that the subjects have their eyes closed and so don't know where my hands are. With a high degree of accuracy, at very specific locations in the Aura, the same inner "movie" would be described that had been evoked previously at that location.

The brain seems also to store a copy of the memory movie – so modern science is right to say that the conflict is associated with the brain! When the brain is surgically exposed, memory movies can likewise be triggered by stimulating the surface of the cerebral cortex with tweezers or an electrode. We know this from brain surgery in which the patient, having received only local anesthesia, is fully conscious during the operation. Like the observations I described above for the "Aura movies," the patient experiences very definite feelings and memories depending on which spot is stimulated. After World War II, observations of this kind were the occasion of mutilating brain operations – attempting, for example, to excise the "evil brain regions" of sexual offenders. Because the long-term consequences were not good, this kind of psycho-surgery was (thank God!) soon abandoned.

Deep relaxation exercises and drug experiences can also induce the recall of emotional conflict contents. The lowering of consciousness touches on deep layers of the subconscious. I have now and again heard from acupuncturists and neural therapists that patients will spontaneously mention emotionally burdensome ancient memories when the acupuncture needle is applied to a specific point, or certain vegetative ganglia are injected. Around 1940, the Italian CALLIGARIS claimed that gentle stimulation of certain skin points could evoke parapsychological abilities such as clairvoyance. Kneading certain muscle segments or massag-

ing certain organs can also bring emotional conflicts to the surface. We have all had the experience of recalling a long-forgotten event upon smelling a particular odor or hearing a certain melody.

We can here say with conviction that emotional conflicts cannot be reduced to a single object or function. Conflicts touch upon multiple facets of the *human body/mind* complex, from the subtle-body Aura to the substance of the coarse-materials body. Conflicts thus have numerous different deposition and activation points. It therefore seems an extreme oversimplification to assign conflicts only to the head, as is unfortunately so often done.

Conflicts reside in the material body at various locations:

1. the cerebrum and
2. the vegetative brain centers,
3. the vegetative plexus of the overall organism,
4. various muscles and muscular indurations (geloses),
5. muscle fasciæ and
6. periostea, as well as
7. specific organ parts.

Conflicts can be found in the Aura as well. Much evidence suggests that emotional conflicts are predominantly a mental-energetic phenomenon. For one thing, just touching the Aura – without touching the physical body – calls forth mental contents. Another argument is based on the possibility of the transmission of conflicts. In an earlier chapter, I related the example of an acquaintance who transferred her emotional conflicts to my wife and me. Phenomena such as possession also fall into this category. Other sound reasons are based on the fact that phenomena such as remote healing or intercessory prayer would otherwise be unthinkable. The reader might recall my previously-described attempt at remote healing[32] of an acquaintance, whom I tried to heal with magic. There's one more point that can help convince us of the spiritlike nature of emotional conflicts: the fact that at least large conflicts probably have karmic causes. When in a state of deep relaxation, an

---

[32] In a certain sense, intercessory prayer is also a kind of remote healing. In prayer, higher powers are asked to supply harmonic energy that then impinges on the ailing person's body. Meta-analyses by the American BENOR show that prayers are statistically efficacious at a rate above that of random chance, and can thus be considered, from a scientific standpoint, as established phenomena. In his books, the American internist Larry DOSSEY, who works exclusively with prayers and other parapsychological phenomena, gives a good overview of the numerous scientific investigations into this topic.

unusually large number of patients report recollecting traumatic experiences from former lives. If we accept the reality of Karma, then it would seem logical that such traumatic consciousness contents stem from previous lives. Evidently, they are stored as conflicts – but this only works if the conflicts had previously been stored in some nonmaterial manner. For how could conflicts be stored and transferred from one existence to another if, in the process, various material bodies die and new bodies are chosen? The whole thing is conceivable only if conflicts are spiritlike in nature.

Now, what does storing in a spiritlike manner actually mean? The preceding chapters help us answer the question as to how conflicts are stored. We need only recall that information can easily be stored in subtle-body energy. I'd like to summarize briefly the important points regarding the storage of conflict contents:

Energy has important qualities which can aid in storing conflicts:

1. Energy stores specific items of information (information carrier);
2. Energy moves about at will from one body to another (is nonlocal);
3. Energy stores information in a reliable and realistic manner in which feelings, odors, conscious contents and thoughts are stored like videoclips (reliable and accurate storage).

In the next chapter, I'll describe how we can visualize the structure and mode of operation of a conflict in detail. Here, I am primarily concerned with providing a basic overview of the numerous aspects of conflicts. The initially mysterious matter of the storage of conflict contents becomes more understandable if we think of modern inventions such as the computer. The Aura supplies our bio-computer with energy as information, so that we can make the comparison to both software and electrical current. The conflict then corresponds to a buggy program or computer virus that can alter our program or, in the extreme case, block it.

In the illustration below, I'd like to make it clear that, despite its originally energetic nature, the conflict does not hang out in a vacuum. On the contrary, the conflict shows up in the material body as well as in nonmaterial consciousness. The conflict thus leads a triple life that encompasses the Aura, the psyche, and the body (see chart below).

For this reason, a conflict can be designated as something that is *psychosomatically energized*. It is found at all energy levels of the Aura as well as in the material body and in consciousness. Therefore, to the question as to what, specifically, a conflict influences and harms, there can be no simply structured answer.

Conflicts change all levels of human beings
· By influencing the psyche subconsciously (and thereby behavior),
· By leaching out and blocking the energy system, and
· By weakening the body and making it sick over the long term.

As in the fable of the hare and the hedgehog, one can never say that a conflict is here only or there only. A conflict is situated in the body, in subtle-body energy *and* in the psyche. At the beginning of this chapter, I talked about shamans and their point of view. Shamans see conflicts as demons in the Aura, thereby bringing the energetic aspect into the foreground. Brain surgeons and psychiatrists interpret conflicts as material disturbances, inasmuch as they lead to neurotransmitter disorders or alteration of brain tissue. Psychoanalysts place the psyche and the subconscious in the foreground because, for them, conflicts are predominantly a personal-biographical and emotional problem.

One can of course ask what the consequences are for the patient of a tripartite conflict. In the final analysis, how a given specialist classifies a medical-psychological problem is of little concern to patients, as long as they are correctly diagnosed and properly treated. But it's precisely at this point that things get interesting for the patient – because it *does* matter what you think of a disease. After all, diagnosis determines therapy, which is why bad diagnosis results in bad therapy. So one can't just sit back and trust the experts to know what to do. Because of their ignorance of energetic relationships, the so-called experts are often as in the dark as the patient seeking their help. This is all the more regrettable because, in my experience, the energetic aspect in particular plays a key role in diagnosing and treating emotional conflicts!

I have named this method **Psychosomatic Energetics**, because of the triple stratification of conflicts into psyche, soma and energy, with the primary emphasis falling on the subtle-body aspect, in which I integrate soma and psyche in a way that is in line with current scientific knowledge. There are thus no individual truths; one must instead take all aspects of the conflict into account. The energetic aspect is empirically the most important because, in my experience, conflicts can only be correctly diagnosed via energetic diagnoses. No psychiatrist, brain surgeon, neurotransmitter researcher, psychoanalyst, or anybody else can arrive at such diagnoses with the same surety and rapidity as it is possible with energetic diagnostic methods, for the simple reason that *Rage* is nonmaterial. In fact, specialists with an overly biased view tend to arrive at completely erroneous conclusions. In the next chapter, I'll endeavor to substantiate in more detail why that is so, and what serious repercussions it has on therapy.

At this point, the problem is that we are dealing with various different truths. Therefore, when I so resolutely advocate an energetic point of view, I am speaking of a truth that I estimate applies to 95% of patients. For the rest, there are other truths. So, I am by no means trying to demolish entire professions and deny them their right to exist. Although the energetic aspect is the most important, there are patients who need other kinds of help. Some patients with depression can get excellent relief from chemical antidepressants. By the same token, a suicide-risk person might find his only genuine help in an understanding psychoanalyst who really listens and helps him along. A tumor patient needs a surgeon to operate to excise the tumor. In short, there is not just the one truth, but rather several, depending on the patient's initial situation.

Storage of the Conflict Information in Body, Psyche, Soma

SOMA → *Brain tissue* / *Muscle* **BODY FIELD**

Conflict Seat in Energy body → *Outside the body* = *Stored in the Aura* / *Inside the body* = *Stored in the Chakras* **ENERGY FIELD**

PSYCHE → *Consciousness* **PSYCHIC FIELD**

Conflict Origins
and Consequences

The most important causes of disease include subconscious conflicts. This has become one of the undisputed fundamental theses of modern psychoanalysis. Conflicts are the commonest (actual) cause of people not feeling well, as they thereby enter into an inner state of disharmony and low energy. Conflicts are also the at the bottom of most interpersonal strife and misunderstandings. The subconscious conflict is without a doubt the prime suspect, being chiefly responsible for our feeling unwell and ailing, for living in conflict with those around us, and even for missing out on happiness in life. No matter what the reason for something going wrong, a conflict is nearly always the culprit.

At first, I refused to believe such a drastically simple solution that reduced everything to a single cause – but the longer I deal with this issue, the more vehemently and resolutely I say: **"The conflict is guilty in (almost) every case!"** In what follows, I hope to be able to substantiate this one-sided charge against the conflict. In the process, I'll have to expand on the conventional psychoanalytic model, since the conflict doesn't just evoke emotional disturbances, it is also the actual starting point of personality formation.

The conflict exerts a crucial influence on our thoughts and actions as it subconsciously remote-controls us, altering

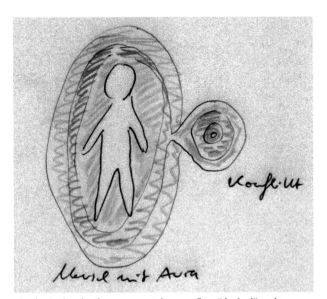

Author's sketch of a person with a conflict "docked" to his aura.

the scenario in its favor. I'll reveal the entire scope and dynamics in individual steps, even deriving from it an evolutionary model that has left its imprint on human development and dissected it into sequential steps. One can go so far as to say that the conflict, as the primal form of our fears, is the true germ cell of human consciousness. In this respect, it is what makes us human in the first place, corresponding to what is known in the biblical sense as *original sin*. Yet these dramatic repercussions start with what seem at first to be quite harmless inner emotional processes.

Therefore, I'd next like to describe how a conflict arises and what direct consequences to the individual can be derived from it. Basically, a conflict is a part of ourselves that has split off from us. This gradually becomes more and more independent and then acts like an inner foreign body. But what triggers the split? Where do conflicts come from in the first place? Since there were no satisfactory psychoenergetic models, I was forced to draw up a conflict model on my own. I am well aware that what I have brought together into an overall picture is a mélange of very different models, based on my own experiences and observation of patients. I would therefore like to ask the reader to regard what follows as a model whose key elements are firmly established, but which still needs further research and refinement.

Conflicts always arise when our life experience comes to an abrupt stop because we can no longer endure an emotionally felt situation. I need to describe in greater detail the quality of our life experience, so as to clarify what it is all about. The American social psychologist CSIK-SZENTMILHALY calls the continuity of our ever-changing state of feeling and consciousness *Flow*. The more harmonious the flow, the more contented and happy we feel. Keeping in mind that ideal state, I'd like to define a normal state situated between joy and sorrow that leads to a continuity of our emotional life experience. I call this normal state *emotional flow* because, in this state, our feelings flow evenly and smoothly. In this equable state I have in mind, we are not always as happy as in CSIKSZENTMILHALY's Flow, but we are above all in a state of emotional composure. If we take a careful look at ourselves, we'll note that we are in a state of *emotional flow* about 99% of the time. Being in harmony with one's feelings triggers a spontaneous feeling of normalcy and consonance. We need this normalcy in order to be able to remain emotionally balanced.

One might object that there are people who seem to live in a witch's cauldron of constantly changing feelings. One moment they're laughing and the next they seem mortally unhappy. Then there's others who live in a permanently chaotic environment – and yet, as turbulent as their situation might seem from the outside, these people likewise have an emotional flow about 99% of the time. It simply has more violent swings, but is still felt to be normal by the *chaotics* or *eccentrics* who live it. Similarly, many "southerners" come across to cooler "northerners" as eccentric and emotionally exaggerated. Nevertheless, they too live in an emotional flow. One can take it as a basic law that man tends to create a feeling of normalcy that corresponds to an emotional climate of uniformity and accustomed everydayness.

It seems to be a key aspect that the human organism needs uniformity of emotions with which to create a feeling of normalcy and security. People living with a constant feeling of threat and insecurity become sick in very short order. For instance, there were soldiers in World Wars I and II known as "war tremblers" whose emotional state was completely shattered by their front-line experiences. Comparably, one can find so-called *borderline disturbances* in the form of lifelong personality disorders: children who grow up in an environment of insecurity and threat. These kinds of emotional disorders arise from falling out of the **emotional flow of normalcy**. Yet this is nothing more than the consequences of disturbances to the emotional flow in the form of conflicts, as previously mentioned. Falling out of the emotional flow leads to split-off, emotion-laden consciousness fragments, which

are designated as conflicts.

However, conflicts often do not originate slowly in a pathological milieu of constant threat, but rather all of a sudden and spontaneously, in a type of fright reaction. The emotional flow of normalcy is interrupted by some event. Experiences that are particularly exciting and emotionally overwhelming overtax a person's psychological/emotional processing capabilities. Suddenly, we reach our limit, because our emotional reserves and regulatory capabilities have been used up. We become imbalanced, even if we had previously been able to cope for quite a while with the same stress factors. At some point, we break down. Suddenly, our emotional stability fails us and we say "I'm beside myself!" Others might say "I think I'm flipping out!" Excessively emotional states lead, at deeper emotional levels, to a shock-like choking and suffocating condition. These conditions are instinctively identified with the greatest existential threat and extreme fear.

One can view it as a protective mechanism similar to the gag reflex. It is precisely this horrible emergency mental state that becomes the actual starting point of conflict formation. Instinctively, the integrity of the organism is maintained. In a flash, the conflict arises in order to protect the organism as a whole by externalizing the threat, so that the emotional flow can continue to flow, albeit to a reduced degree. As in the mummification of extremities that have died off, a psychoenergetic material that is no longer digestible, that has become harmful and foreign, is exported as a foreign body to the body's energetic periphery (the Aura).

Strangled Emotional Flow and Conflict Origin

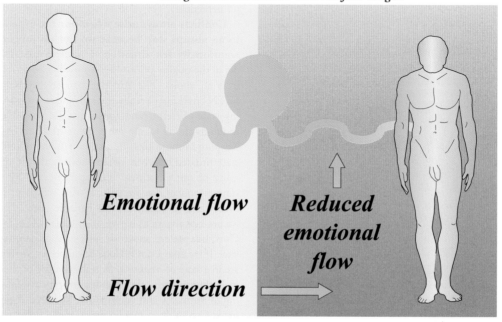

Emotional flow

Reduced emotional flow

Flow direction

We see similar processes for dealing with foreign bodies or toxic substances in the case of gout, in which excess uric acid is transported to the aching big toe, there to crystallize out far from the central part of the body. The skin rashes of infectious diseases also obey the archaic defensive measure of excreting, pushing aside, and displacing unpleasant and organism-threatening matter from the body. The viruses are enveloped in a measles or chickenpox rash, thereby rendering them harmless. In all these processes, we see the same protective principle at work: enclose and isolate that which is foreign to the body and dangerous, and thus render it harmless.

"If it can't be digested, it doesn't belong … so out with it!" Since energy can't just vanish, it condenses into a conflict. The conflict's indigestibility shows us that there is something like psychosomatic-energetic digestion that normally allows us to "digest" and integrate our experiences. Anyone who has watched children after an exciting experience has witnessed emotional processing. Initially, the damp little hands of the emotionally agitated child (and its palpitations and fidgetiness) tell us that something exciting and disquieting is going on. Later on, the young mind becomes calmer as it unburdens itself by talking about the experience, and the excitement is focused and recalled over and over again in the imagination and in dreams. There seems to be another processing option: abreaction and somatization. Involuntary excretory processes mediated by the autonomic nervous system, such as diarrhea or perspiration, or voluntary motor abreaction – such as drumming one's fingers or biting one's nails – are meant to lower high energetic conflict tension.

In conflict formation, all of these mechanisms fail. We wind up in an existential borderline situation characterized by a short-term state of emotional emergency. Our "knees turn to jelly," as the phrase so aptly has it. But instead of keeling over dead, our psychoenergetic system divides in two: the self and the other. The foreign emotional part, in the form of intolerable emotions, is split off in order to allow the overall organism to continue living. Here, it is of no consequence where the feelings come from, i.e., whether they come from inside or outside.

I'd here like to mention the depth-psychological basic rule that, at the deeper emotional levels, from a certain degree on, there is no distinction made between outer and inner worlds. It thus makes sense that one's own internal emotional states can be just as intolerable as external impinging events. In the case of torture, we have a typical mixed situation, in which the torturer seeks to make things <u>externally</u> intolerable for his victim in order to break down his <u>inner</u> resistance by violating his psychophysical integrity. The victim, to be sure, forms an ever-enlarging conflict meant to trap and externalize the frightful torture process. However, this often succeeds only partially, since the fright is way too great and it goes on and on. Similarly, the normal process of conflict formation can be interpreted as an unpleasant process that, emotionally, has some of the aspects of an intolerable torture situation. Although the torture usually only lasts a short time, it's still long enough in its intolerability to inflict emotional wounds that are externalized in the form of conflicts.

But the significant part seems to me to be less the "why" than the "how" of conflict origins – for in my opinion, the question of "how" takes us a lot farther than letting ourselves get tangled up in the "why," as traditional psychoanalysis tends to do. **Experience has shown that the "why" just leads to an endless chain of finger-pointing** that ultimately leads all the way back to Adam and Eve's *Original Sin*.

At a high level of insight into our deepest emotional layers, it becomes clear to many people in meditative contemplation that we – as a part of God – don't have to intend the good for ourselves in order to be able to nab a guilty party. We would to a certain extent be that part of God that hurts itself. We gladly yell "Stop, thief!" – and then see, to our great shock, that, at this deep level of insight, we have to pillory ourselves, that we are ourselves the scoundrel we have been on the trail of. The logic of duality with its accusations thus leads, in the kingdom of love and indivisibility, quite automatically to insanity and despair. Guilt and love are irreconcilable opposites.

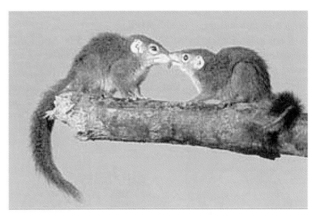

Tupayas are the only mammals whose stress level is made visible by their erected hair.

It makes much more sense to ask after the "how" of conflict origins, in the processes taking place in the individual. One can then also more clearly realize how to heal emotional wounds. The "how" leads to a position that actively includes the individual in the conflict origin rather than regarding him as a passive victim. It seems to me by far the better way, one which, moreover, enables one to more easily find solutions for conflict elimination. We ask, therefore, how an emotion can become something foreign to the organism, something which needs to be externalized by a protective reflex. In my opinion, it's because feeling content becomes so overpowering and indigestible that it at first completely bogs down the emotional flow. The emotional flow is blocked by the indigestibility of the feeling which has arisen.

Feelings condense into conflicts when emotional content cannot be integrated and digested. An indigestible feeling actually blocks not only our emotional flow but also, at a deeper level, our integrity. In a certain archaically-felt manner, the conflict threatens our existence! This happens in an inner emotional manner such that feeling content is subconscious equated with a threat to our life, all the way up to extinguishing it. When we get too angry or sad, we think we might die. **Our emotional body instinctively experiences feelings that are too big and too intense as life-threatening.**

It really is a matter of life and death. The existential distress of overwhelming feelings can be seen quite clearly in the well-known animal experiment which uses two male tupayas engaged in a territorial struggle. Normally, after the fight, the losing male runs away as quickly as possible, thereby settling the matter for all concerned. However, if the loser is caged up with the winner, separated by a glass partition, in a few weeks the loser will be dead. The tupaya males have no conflict formation as humans do, that could save their lives. They are the helpless victims of their emotions, which in fact kill them in short order!

Thank God that, in us humans, the terrible emotional situation is quickly improved by externalizing of the conflict, after which we can breathe easy again. In the experiment with the two contentious tupaya males, the losing adversary normally flees to a far corner of the cage, where he can no longer be seen. Fleeing into no-longer-being-seen

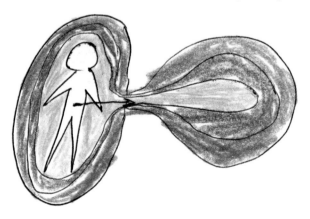

Big 3rd Chakra conflict

ensures the survival of the losing male (fight or flight). In our own conflict situation, the intolerable feeling similarly "flees" into the conflict, so that we need not die. **"Let's get outta here!" says the feeling, and in short order effects its own disappearance.**

Now, there are of course good feelings as well that can scarcely be endured. Why don't these especially fantastic feelings also become conflicts? Probably because, besides intolerability, there is another character trait – that of emotional emptiness: a kind of "black hole" into which our exclusively bad, destructive feelings threaten to drop us. This emotional emptiness corresponds to the hostility and threat that negative conflict contents trigger in us. Good feelings don't make emotional emptiness, don't generate emotional endangerment and distress in the way that negative, destructive feelings do. Bad feelings have a very important trait that has to do with emotional alienation and the loss of inner loyalty. Ultimately, it's a matter of the endangerment of our existence and integrity – because the tendency to conflict formation is greater when we can no longer be emotionally authentic with ourselves. When conflicts arise, we cannot digest something emotionally because it is foreign and does not agree with us. One is reminded of a pearl, which also begins with an object foreign to the oyster, i.e., a grain of sand that has penetrated inside the oyster, which is then enclosed and encapsulated as a pearl.

Conversely, the more authentic we remain in the depths of our mind, the less tendency we'll have to conflict formation. This context elucidates the nonviolence commandment of Christianity and Buddhism: "... turn the other cheek," Jesus commands his disciples, meaning (in modified form) that we should remain authentic. His commandment's primary goal is that a conflict not be escalated by retaliatory force. But retaliation also always means that we are torn out of our center and can create conflicts. Despite its seeming simplicity, the knowledge **that conflicts are evoked by inner alienation and non-authenticity**, carries within it the seed of far-reaching contemplations. Later chapters will deal with this in detail.

Of course, we all know from personal experience that it is very hard to be authentic and emotionally honest all the time. In daily life, there's always something upsetting and unbalancing us. Still, we can break out of the vicious cycle of violence and retaliation, of injury and revenge, if we block the mechanisms of conflict origins at their source. This will be discussed many times in the course of this book. In order better to understand the conflict in all its ramifications, I'd like to describe it in greater detail. The subtle-body aspect plays a big role here.

A conflict is a split-off part of our overall consciousness, as far as the level of the mental body is concerned. Yet the conflict also contains other subtle-body parts that originally come from our own energy system. Like a tied-off, miniaturized appendage of our own energy body, the conflict exhibits all the structural characteristics of our energy body. It forms something like a satellite system of our subtle-body energy system, attached to us like an embryo by an invisible umbilical cord. One can thus regard the conflict as an "energy thief" that feeds off our own energy.

Because the conflict takes energetic bodies from us, these removed components start to take on a life of their own. Our mental body, our emotions, our life force begin to be active in the conflict. They there develop an intrinsic dynamics that corresponds to the respective energy body. This means, concretely, that the conflict possesses life force just as we do, that it has feelings and even consciousness.

In particular, the conflict has the following attributes:

- It has its own **energy – on the Vital Level**, *though the conflict energy is above all morbific, since our own energy flow is throttled down by it. The conflict siphons off the energy that we then lack – although, strictly speaking, the harmful aspect is not really energy removal per se, but rather the blockage of energy flow (like a boulder on a streambed blocking water flow). In truth, the conflict doesn't really steal as much energy as it might seem from the outside; rather, it disrupts our energy flow. The bigger the conflict gets, the more energy flow is throttled. This subtle distinction is important because large conflicts can survive for a long time without draining off substantial amounts of energy; it is then "hibernating," so to speak. If it becomes active, it will then begin to block energy flow.*

- It has **feelings – on the Emotional Level**. *Unfortunately, the feeling contents just simple-mindedly orbit the conflict contents, like the monotonous recitation of some formulaic phrase that has been programmed into a none-too-bright robot. The emotions in a conflict feel extremely strong, basically foreign to our nature and thus extremely uncomfortable.*

- It has **intelligence** (in the sense of consciousness) – **on the Mental Level**. *Its awareness is at bottom a reflection of how aware we have become of the conflict – so that its consciousness is actually our consciousness. The conflict itself is nearly completely senseless and trapped in its own narcissistic world! Although the conflict's intelligence (like a robot's) is initially limited to the execution of the program that the conflict needs for its realization, the conflict does have, like any living being, a kind of survival instinct, which leads it to use its intelligence to influence its host and the world around it in its own interests.*

- It has a **deep subconscious – on the Causal Level**. *This is an automated goal-seeking mechanism for the realization of its needs and desires. Everything here revolves around deep convictions of an unqualified will to live, that exhibit typical traits. It is this power-hungry egotism that makes the conflict essentially evil and destructive.*

I have called the totality of conflict content and its energetic stratification simply ***conflict***. In traditional psychology, it is a purely mental structure in its host's subconscious. I, on the other hand, view the conflict as a subtle-body energy-charged, largely autonomous entity. It is a type of island, heavily walled off from the rest of the organism. One could also call the conflict a "feelings/consciousness island." Another synonymous concept is C.G. JUNG's *complex*, the description of which strongly resembles my *conflict*. Had I been familiar with JUNG's views at an earlier date, I would have adopted a good deal of JUNG's terminology. I instead developed, fortunately, an independent system of conflicts, whose primary accent is much more in the energetic area. This has considerably improved the healing prospects, just as one can only properly recognize the conflict at all by means of its energetic structure.

C.G. JUNG, by the way, was the first modern explorer of the psyche to regard the emotional conflict as being, in a certain manner, an autonomous entity separate from us. He realized that the *complexes* (C.G. JUNG's term for conflicts) are entities split off from us. They normally attach themselves to us, but they can also detach themselves. JUNG believes he also recognized the complex in phenomena such as synchronicity (i.e., unlikely coincidences), in which the conflict content brings together incredible incidents (*coincidences*). It does that, according to JUNG, by mysteriously manipulating the fateful interplay of events. I will return later to this far-reaching interpretation of conflict, which goes far beyond the manipulation of the individual subcon-

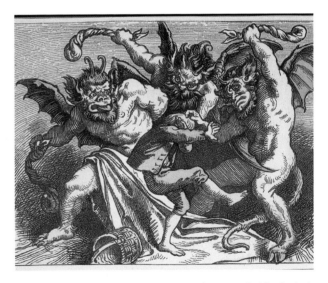

Demons thrashing a "bad boy." Actually, it's probably the boy's inner emotional conflicts attacking him in the form of demons in a nightmare. The painter is here depicting a seemingly just punishment. In the real world, unfortunately, we usually first attack those nearest us, forcing them into the scapegoat role. Woodcut by Moritz von Schwind, ca. 1860

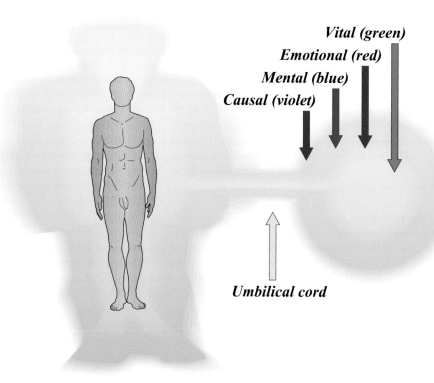

Vital (green)
Emotional (red)
Mental (blue)
Causal (violet)

Umbilical cord

scious. We find, in this eerie power of destiny an important principle of our personal life (i.e., *Karma*).

Next, I'd like to describe the conflict in greater detail. Later on, I'll go more deeply into how I came to investigate and was able to describe the conflict in such detail in the first place. Basically, my knowledge of conflict structure is based on subtle-body measurement methods that make the conflict visible. If we take a closer look at the conflict with these measurement methods, we make an astounding discovery: the structure of a conflict bears a surprising resemblance to our own four energy levels. **The conflict is thus a type of *homunculus*!** Just as one can measure a person's Aura (which I will describe in detail later on), so can the conflict's Aura be measured. I already mentioned that humans possess four Aura levels. Amazingly, the conflict has exactly the same Aura levels we do, just somewhat differently constituted and with different contents. I have already made reference to some aspects (e.g., the conflict's rather obtuse and stubborn – somewhat childish-mulish – nature).

In the fairy tale about the *homunculus*, and in the depictions of demons, the conflict can be identified as an independent entity. It lives in its own world and has its own reality. Basically, it is a small man-child that inhabits a special world of its own. Of course, this special world also exists in our subconscious – but it is also active on entirely different levels of reality that have nothing to do with our subconscious! Consider the Vital and Causal Levels, which are totally inaccessible and unknown to our consciousness. This special hidden world seems to me to be the main reason why conventional psychotherapy has so much trouble recognizing and healing conflicts. Like a bar of soap in the bathtub, which we try in vain to grab hold of, the conflict always eludes the searching consciousness because of its sheer otherness.

Now, what happens when we have created a conflict? Like the male tupaya fleeing his superior rival, we also believe we have escaped from the horror of the full-blown horrible feeling. The externalization of the conflict leads to a kind of *permanent flight*. We erroneously comfort ourselves with the delusory assurance that we can pick up our daily life where we left off, since we are no longer in pain. But we are fooling ourselves to the extent that the conflict prevents us from resuming our normal existence. Like the gouty big toe in which the body crystallizes out excess uric

---

[33] The coloration of the conflict accords with a simple color logic that, by tradition, assigns the color green to the life force at the vitality level, red to feelings, blue to the mental region, and violet to the spiritual-causal region – or, as a mixture of all colors, white. Yet I must admit that other classification schemes are also valid, and that the one I am proposing does have its subjective and arbitrary aspects.

acid, the externalization of split-off emotional content does not take place without repercussions for us. In the case of gout, the consequence is a painful attack. As we know, getting rid of an unpleasant matter has its price.

The conflict host thus pays double – first, by having to supply the conflict with energy and, second, by losing some emotional independence. The rest of this book deals predominantly with the far-reaching psychological consequences of the conflict. I shall endeavor to explicate the most essential aspects of the incalculably complex consequences of the conflict and its resulting manifold manifestations, symptoms, and aberrations. For reasons of sheer space, I cannot go into every aspect in full detail, because the conflict involves many more consequences that far transcend the psychological. In what follows, I shall therefore limit myself to the most vital processes.

What is most fascinating is that the conflict host is influenced by the conflict so weirdly and so strongly that we are tempted to think that sorcery and magical powers must be involved. Nothing frightens and fascinates us at the same

> **Basically, the conflict has two important verifiable and extremely unpleasant consequences for its host:**
> 1. **The victim is energetically throttled down,** because of also having to supply the conflict with energy and because the conflict blocks energy (and the "energy block" siphons off the strongest energy the most);
> 2. **The conflict host is also subtly and subconscious manipulated and influenced by the conflict content.**

time more than **enchantment**; it stands at the beginning of the entire process. *Black magic* possesses the vital character trait that most aptly describes the conflict. In the dramatic story of Lot's wife or the Medusa, the hypnotic, downright bewitching power of the conflict contents is made clear. In ancient times, the evil petrifying gaze of the Medusa was considered the cause of emotional affliction. Her gaze could only be endured in mirror reflection. The snakes writhing about the Medusa's head simply reinforce the dreadful feeling of horror.

Almost no fairy tale leaves out the difficult phase of enchantment and curse, as the hero or heroine is put to the test. Then there's the evil witch or the nasty magician who casts a spell on the prince or princess. Symbolically, freeing the poor victim means vanquishing the conflict and breaking the spell. But before deliverance can take place, the victim first falls into a deathlike sleep. In this unproductive spectral slumber, the victim becomes a rigid, remote-controlled, evilly enchanted zombie.

The eerie part of the conflict is, of course, the fact that it has a hypnotic, cryptic and bold-tyrannical effect on us. In so doing, it subjects us in part to its own will. All of these processes are reflected in fairy tales and myths, when the sorcerer gains power over his defenseless victim. It is precisely the victim's defenselessness that both excites and outrages us. Basically, our reaction is so churned up and intense because we recognize in it our own story, since in a way we are all spellbound princes and princesses! Each of us harbors unconscious components that make us unresponsive and inflexible because they are not appropriate for us. Evil enchantment is thus our common destiny, not just that of noble princes and princesses.

To my mind, fairy tales understand the true nature of conflicts far better than psychotherapy does. This applies above all to the individual and personal aspects of the conflict itself. In the fairy tale, the conflict makes its appearance as Rumpelstiltskin or a goblin. The conflict is something external that no longer has much in common with our center and our Self. It becomes an unfamiliar entity that one can still vaguely remember, to be sure, but normally the conflict is a split-off part of us that has become foreign to us, that is located "out there."

It is at this point that I draw heavy criticism from psychology experts: they accuse me of too much separating the conflict and its indwelling magic from its victim. According to psychoanalysis, the evil sorcerer in the fairy tale is somehow supposed to be a hidden part of ourselves that shoves all unpleasant and strange emotions and drives into the subconscious, where all the suppressed drives and censored feelings are stored. In my opinion, psychoanalysis is here guilty of wildly overestimating the willful part that we bring to conflict formation. I believe that the fairy tale's helpless victim role is a much more accurate depiction than psychoanalysis cares to admit. In my experience, nobody freely admits being plagued by conflicts – unless they already have conflicts that are giving rise to new ones. This is why the resistance to healing originates in fact in the victim role, which has its genesis in the hypnotized remote-control exerted by the conflict itself.

On the other hand, psychoanalysis' basic premise is correct: that the conflict consists of split-off rejected personality parts. At some point in life, people can get so sad, so angry or in some other type of extreme negative mood, that they just cannot stand it. The intolerable emotional state corresponds to a part of the personality that from now on will be displaced into the subconscious in the course of conflict formation. For example, if at the time of the conflict origin one is too enraged, a rage conflict is created that from then on lives a subconscious shadow existence. The aggressive and destructive aspect of the rage is externalized and "defused." Psychology speaks of the ***shadow***, the dark, subconscious and hidden forces of our personality.

Yet we continue to have secret longings to look at and touch this dark side of our personality. The puritanical prude exhibits this same mixture of abhorrence and fascination, looking at pornography with a mixture of ostentatious revulsion and surreptitious lasciviousness, or vicariously indulging his furtive killer impulses by reading crime thrillers, thereby avoiding having to become violent and evil. Thus, the conflict contains many parts of our being that subconsciously infect us[34] and influence us psychoenergetically. Still, these personality parts have become so foreign that one can think of them as being another person. I am firmly convinced that the conflict has truly become a second person that manipulates and directs us behind the scenes.

All kinds of variations are possible, ranging from subtle indirect influences noticeable only to one's closest friends and family (but usually not oneself) all the way to major permanent character changes. In this process, we always change, not for the better, but rather in a way that is harmful and detrimental both to us and those around us. No one becomes a better person by creating conflicts. I remind the reader of the battered child who grows up to beat his own children. Virtually all murderers, violent criminals, and sex offenders had horrible childhoods that explain their crimes as re-enactments and the consequences of conflicts. In so doing, the criminal represents an extreme form of something normal and everyday, something all too human that befalls each and every one of us. Since no one is conflict-free, the only thing separating us from the criminal is the intensity of the conflict, and a lack of strength to resist the conflict's pernicious influence. The chapters that follow will deal with this comprehensively.

At the other extreme, the conflict's evil and its demonic power lead not to criminal acts but to full-blown obsession and mental illness. In these tragic cases, the victim has fallen under the nearly total dominion of the conflict. The evil abreacts against the victim, which is why the mentally ill (contrary to widespread prejudice) have only minor criminal tendencies. As proof of this, I'd like to point out that empirically, schizophrenics commit few criminal acts.

Basically, evil and sin is evoked by the conflict, even though the conflict contents do not initially seem all that bad and destructive. Thus, a conflict full of sadness can trigger an eruption of frustrated anger because the victim is briefly driven beyond the limits of self-control. We can all recall everyday experiences in which we tell ourselves to "stay cool, don't get upset" – only to fly off the handle suddenly because something rubs us the wrong way. At such times, the conflict has gained short-term control and is running the show. This is an instance of a spur-of-the-moment, quickly subsiding conflict activation.

Most frequently, however, the conflict generates a character deformation, so that the harmful, bad and evil aspects of the conflict develop rather slowly, in a downright sneaky manner that quite often goes unnoticed by its host. The conflict gives rise to a lopsided and distorted view of the world based on false premises. We become fixed personalities, exhibiting specific peculiarities, shortcomings, and faults. Most of the following chapter deals with various kinds of conflicts and the resultant character types. Yet the fundamental topic is always grounded in the knowledge that we can ascribe our primeval human foibles and inadequacies to the conflict. Without conflicts we would be as angels, with nothing human about us.

But the bad part comes from the fact that conflicts weaken us energeticall, diminishing our life force and *joie de vivre*, making us energy impoverished, emotionally embittered, and hurtful. We envy others their energy and become demons, hurting others. Although the suppressed Good is always there behind the Bad – i.e., the yearning for the soul's lost homeland – this depth-psychological knowledge does the poor victim no good at first. Normally, an injured party has a hard time breaking the karmic chain and forgiving the offender – much less going so far as to (in Jesus' words) "turn the other cheek." Inflicted harm usually leads to self-perpetuating chain reactions. Consider revenge, say in the form of the Sicilian *vendetta* that turns entire families into sworn enemies in feuds lasting for centuries. And yet the starting point for evil is not the conflict contents, as one might first suppose, but rather (and above all) the resulting energy poverty. Nothing makes us more peaceable and amicable than being energetically satiated and contented – and nothing makes us more dangerous than being energetically discontented and hungry.

The creation of the conflict has given rise to an autonomous living entity. Of course, we ask ourselves how far this autonomy goes and whether it can travel. Contrary to widespread assumptions, it does this relatively seldom. Spiritual tradition has it that, in dreams, the conflict can migrate from one being to another (so-called *astral journeys*). Presumably, the conflict accomplishes this by establishing contact through resonance with other conflict hosts. They then exchange conflicts, since they have similar conflicts. Like the phenomenon of telepathy, which takes place in broad daylight and with a clear mind, and in which resonance is established via thoughts (i.e., the Mental Level). Still, I am quite certain, after all my observations and experiences, that conflicts doggedly remain with their creators, despite this separation and *wanderlust*. Our primeval human fear of roving demons thus seems unfounded.

The potential ability to roam about also explains the possibility of conflict transfer from one being to another. Everything we knows suggests that this occurs very rarely,

---

[34] In this context, esoteric writing often refers to "astral poison." The Astral Level corresponds to the emotional body, which can be poisoned by the emotional toxins of repressed feelings exactly like the material body can be by toxic substances.

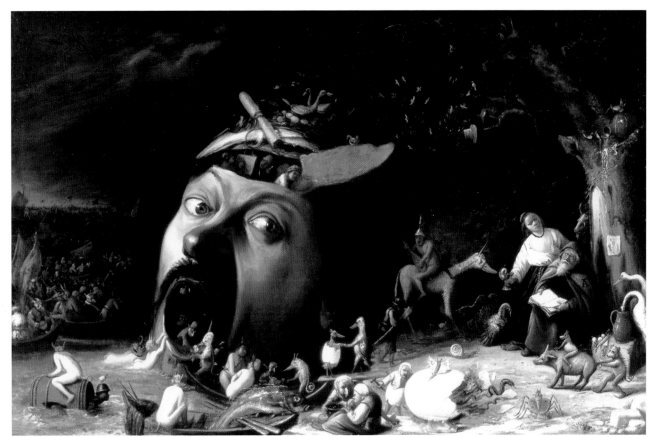

In the Temptation of St. Anthony, horrific nightmarish creatures emerge from the skull pan and mouth. The saint's subconscious is frantically unloading its conflicts. We see here a full-blown obsession in which consciousness is completely *overwhelmed by the conflict contents. In the lower right corner of the painting, we see a conflict represented as a cracked-open egg full of snakes and insects (typical symbols of conflict contents).*

being more the exception than the rule. One such exception would be an externally provoked **possession**, which is to a certain degree generated artificially and willfully. This leads to foreign conflicts and spirits attaching to the victim's psychoenergetic system, to the detriment of the victim's emotional stability. It seems to me that a precondition for a foreign conflict being able to hook up is that the victim have a similar conflict. If the inner conflict that resembles the transmitted conflict vanishes, then the possession breaks off at once. Another rare special case of possession involves an inner void that enables the foreign spirit to invade a body. This seems to be the case for children or the mentally handicapped. And yet, energetic voids are almost always due to conflicts! Nothing external can threaten us unless we are internally inclined to let it do so.

The next question is what becomes of the conflict and its host. To better understand all stages and dimensions of conflict formation and processing, let us recall the four energy levels. In these four energy levels, we see a layered model of the subconscious reminiscent of a multistory dwelling (the metaphor of the subconscious as a house with a cellar can

be traced back to C.G. JUNG, who was the first to use it). Inside this house, conflicts are stored according to size and significance. Everyday consciousness (ego) corresponds to the ground floor, below which are two dark cellars known as the subconscious (Emotional Level) and, lower still, the deep subconscious (Causal Level).

The stability and proportions of the house are impaired by the fact that the house walls include the amorphousness of the conflicts. In the case of big conflicts, we wind up with a quite cockeyed and wobbly structure. The largest conflict (Central Conflict) thus understandably has the most significance for the stability and proportions of our "house" (which actually represents our personality, of course). This leads to shifts and instabilities that have both internal and external repercussions. Outwardly, we develop a character that exhibits specific peculiarities, Achilles' heels, perceptual distortions, and emotional imbalances. This also leads to consequential internal personality flaws that express themselves as emotional instability, dissatisfaction, and so on.

Finally, I'd like to emphasize the *energy thief* effect, which is often neglected in psychology reference books. In traditional medicine and psychology, **fatigue** is erroneously viewed as a purely subjective phenomenon. It is in fact an objective phenomenon that is almost always based on an energy deficiency. People who are very fatigued come across to those around them as lazy and lethargic, as in CICERO's biting aphorism: "Laziness is the fear of impending work." Based on what I've observed in thousands of patients, I venture to declare that laziness and fatigue can almost always be traced back to energy deficiencies that are in turn a consequence of energy-sapping conflicts.

Since we must thenceforth feed the conflict as well as ourselves, we become exhausted, worn out, and energy-deprived. Moreover, the conflict distorts our energy field, which also weakens our energy flow. Later on, we usually get used to the reduced energy level and think it normal. The conflict gradually integrates better into our energy system, so that its impact gradually diminishes. For large conflicts, especially if the emotional content is quite painful, the habituation phase often lasts quite a long time. Eventually, we get used to the conflict and integrate it into our organism. We are, to be sure, no longer as vital and life-affirming as before, but we get used to that as well, and no longer notice the conflict. It is only when we rid ourselves of the conflict that we realize – thanks to the resulting enormous increase in energy – how severely we had been burdened. As when putting down a heavy backpack after a long hike, we feel relieved – and amazed that we've been able to get used to such a heavy load.

The Subconscious,
its Conflicts and Therapy

For most people, emotions are the most intimate and central part of their being – but at the same time the remotest and most unfamiliar. Why is this corner of creation so paradoxical, peculiar and just plain weird? Before trying to explicate the mystery of our emotional mind, I'd first like to describe its structure. The simplest way to gain access to the emotional part of our mind (which psychology calls the subconscious) is to observe ourselves during normal everyday experiences that usually take place unnoticed and unconsciously.

Our most familiar experience with the subconscious is during sleep. We are all aware of different levels of our subconscious, whose significance we know from the common experience of restless nights – for instance, our annoyance at the bothersome condition of being hung up in the upper levels of our subconscious and therefore only sleeping fitfully. We encounter all kinds of thoughts and worries that would otherwise not so easily get into our heads. Crazy ideas and downright childish fears torment us. We feel absolutely whacked out because we cannot fully sink down into our subconscious. It sometimes seems as though we're not going to get any sleep at all – and then, astonishingly, we do after all. "You looked like you were fast asleep!" our partner then says, who (unlike us) was awake and had been watching us. Our own perception of "not having slept a wink" seems to be wrong; our sense of having been awake or asleep can be unreliable. In deep sleep, we normally lose consciousness totally, such that everything would actually have to be unconscious to us. Yet that isn't always the case, because it can happen that we remember specific dreams.

In some particularly deep dreams, an additional remarkable circumstance comes into play that has to do with our feeling of self-esteem. These deep dreams affect us way inside and preoccupy us for days. In these deep, very intensely felt dreams, we seem to experience an especially strong feeling of self-esteem, and we get the impression of being "in the middle of our own self." I think that, in these intense dreams, we encounter the deep and authentic parts of our so-called "higher Self." The previous chapter on the causal body mentioned that our higher Self resides in the deep emotional layers of the causal body. It is called the **_higher Self_** because it corresponds to the part of our personality in which our spiritual, angelic and mentally superior character traits are to be found – as opposed to the **_lower Self_**, which resides in the emotional body and houses our lower drives and passions.

The Huna religion of the indigenous Hawaiiand differentiates between the *higher Self* and the *lower Self*. The classification of the energy centers and the personality components of the *Kahunas* (Hawaiian medicine men) is based on the essential main features of the superstructure of *Psychosomatic Energetics*. Instead of conflicts, the *Kahunas* speak of fixations and spirit beings that, in their view, block the vital contact to the higher Self. Deep, intense and beneficial dreams seem to be a particularly good sign that one has established contact with one's higher Self. Patients with big conflicts often report not having had such nice deep dreams for a long time – or never having had them in their lives. Their contact to the higher Self has been cut off by the big conflicts. This bars them from an important inner source of mental strength – which of course changes once the conflict is resolved: the source of strength that deep dreams bestow on them are then once again at their disposal.

There's a heresy (even an arrogance) that represents another error in our relationship to the subconscious, which one runs across time and again. Instead of sensing very little from their subconscious, many claim to know their subconscious exceedingly well. Many people with years of experience in encounter-group and conversation psychotherapies are convinced that they are familiar with their subconscious and its contained hidden emotional components. Once in a hypnotic trance or an ecstatic state, they then get an unexpected shock, since they experience areas of their subconscious that they had never been to before.

I have been present a number of times when psychoanalysts with years of professional experience underwent borderline experiences – triggered, for example, by ecstatic breathing (so-called *hyperventilation*). The depths of their subconscious that they then experienced were totally unfamiliar to them. They include reincarnation experiences and journeys in the microworld, such as the miniature world of atomic structures, or unsuspected and fascinating experiences in the macroworld, such as the universe of galaxies. With the aid of hallucinogenic drugs, or via meditation, many artists and scientists have had experiences similar to those reported by the mystics of all the world religions. These occult worlds are generally accessible via our subconscious, which is why it would be presumptuous and foolish – considering the immense individually perceived depths and cosmic variety – to presume to already be familiar with everything in one's subconscious.

If we liken the subconscious to the floors of a house, then there are, time and again, surprising discoveries as previously unknown cellars and dark corners come into view. I recall an interview with the psychoanalyst Erich FROMM near the end of his life, in which he expressed, with a mixture of fascination and resignation, still being able to discover, on a daily basis, new aspects of his own subconscious. *It doesn't seem to ever end!*" was his modest summary, with overtones of adventurousness and enthusiasm. The subconscious is thus an enormously large universe that can never really be plumbed to its ultimate depths. We are always confronting the subconscious as rank beginners, having to start from the very beginning.

The more modestly and openly we are in our dealings with the subconscious, the greater (paradoxically) the insights and secrets we will gain access to. A childlike innocence and a positive unconditional impartiality open our causal body and enable us to be open to our subconscious. I have learned the most from precisely those of my patients whose personality development was the most simply structured. One is tempted to agree with SOCRATES, who said: *"Only he is wise who knows that he is not."* Just as children can sometimes remember back to earlier incarnations, so can simply structured adults often have terrific insights that allow them to partake of a greater wisdom.

Yet there are other consciousness states that are not directly related to the personal subconscious. These states depend above all on an altered energy situation of our emotional body. Being in love and other ecstatic states of being, it can seem to us as though we catch a glimpse of another world. This bewitching, enigmatic reality (of the archetypal subconscious, i.e. the causal body) is linked to a changed and much higher energy situation. We then feel much better than usual and can thus afford to risk being much more open and relaxed. If we observe ourselves carefully in such states, we become aware that our perception of reality is crucially influenced by energetic forces. **Therefore, the world largely seems to be what it is in accordance with the way we feel.** We normally don't think about this, since it seems to be so self-evident.

Of course, our perception of reality is constricted not only by our energy state, but also by our subconscious. We humans don't see reality as it actually is, but as we believe it ought to be. We no longer fully perceive the customary and familiar, since it has become a part of our subconscious. One can get a good impression of these processes when returning to an old familiar location after a long absence. Everything looks both strangely different and yet so familiar. Psychological investigations have shown that our perception is much more subjectively limited and hazy than we'd like to admit. It takes a lot of open-mindedness to acknowledge this subjective weakness and see through our own limitations.

Above all, our energy system plays a larger role than we are normally aware in our perceptions. Energy tests make it easy to determine that energetically similarly vibrating people perceive their surroundings amazingly alike. **We perceive the world as we feel!** We can see this very clearly in children. Their energetic openness makes it clear why children can perceive the world around them so openly and undistortedly. As, with increasing age, a fixed personality emerges, this is often accompanied by a shrinking and diminution of the energy values. As adults, we wall ourselves inside a *mental fortress*, and feel generally worse than we did in our childhood. We decorate our inner world with habits and preconceived ideas of "how the world has to be."

Perception and the subconscious are so closely related primarily because the subconscious can simply be defined as that which is not perceived. All the attention exercises of Eastern contemplative methods uncover subconscious processes by training perception. This can be taken so far that Yogis gain control of body functions that are not normally subject to the conscious will, usually proceeding fully unconsciously. It has been documented that they can stop their heart artificially for a while, and survive this completely unharmed. Moreover, descriptions of deep meditation experiences permit the assumption that the attention-focusing part of the meditation makes some parts of the subconscious conscious. I say "parts of the subconscious" deliberately, because one can conclude, from many varied experiences, that meditation cannot replace psychotherapy.

Much remains subconscious no matter how long one meditates. I'd like to elucidate this with a typical case history:

Mr. W. is a psychoanalyst with a lifetime of professional experience. He has also been practicing meditation for a number of years, as taught him by a Zen Buddhist master. He comes to me for treatment because, despite many intensive attempts with various other methods such as Gestalt Therapy, Rolfing and Reincarnation Therapy, he has been unable to get rid of his stubborn neck stiffness and migraine headaches. This annoys him on the one hand, but it also makes him curious about what there might be to energetic blocks. The energy test finds a geopathic stress zone in the head and neck region (geo-radiation in the form of morbific stationary disturbance zones). A dowser is called in, who confirms this and recommend shifting the bed location. I also find an enormous conflict in the pelvic region with the conflict theme In control. *The subconscious motto of this conflict theme is to subconsciously enter into rivalry with authority figures and always to try to dominate every situation. This has made it impossible for Mr. W. to let go and open himself up, so that his softer and weaker aspects can surface. Only after the* In control *conflict has been resolved is he able to make significant progress in his self-analysis and meditation. For the first time, he can feel that his migraine has something to do with his permanent self-control.*

Categorically, **the psychotherapeutic basic rule applies: self-awareness** (in the sense of attentive awareness) **can make the unconscious conscious.** This is why it is so important to deal with the role of perception if you want to get more closely involved with the subconscious. Yet FREUD's assumption, that self-awareness automatically resolves conflicts, is only partly correct. The case history just described is representative of hundreds of analysts and patients who have undergone years of analysis, who have not begun to be rid of their conflicts, as *Psychosomatic Energetics* measurements have shown. Still, these people can provide excellent information about their emotional problems. Becoming aware of one's emotional problems is a far cry from overcoming them and getting rid of them.

Because the subconscious is so centrally important to our overall topic, I'd like to say a few words about **psycho-analysis**. It has lately become part of the standard repertoire of critical authors to disparage traditional psychoanalysis. These authors' message, summarized, is that the old analysis is no good, but that some new form of analysis has the answer. In fact, none of the current psychotherapy methods I have become acquainted with actually has a greater probability of being able to resolve and heal conflicts. To this extent, there is little significant difference between modern therapeutic methods and those of classical Freudian analysis.

Amazingly, the rediscovery of the subconscious in the West began only about 100 years ago, i.e. relatively late in mankind's development. At this time, FREUD discovered that otherwise inexplicable consciousness phenomena pointed to the existence of a subconscious. Originally, FREUD had derived his insights from hypnosis. The physician Franz Anton MESMER, the forefather of modern **hyp-nosis**, had made use of the tight relationship between life force and the subconscious in his healing séances. This was 100 years before FREUD, when mass hypnoses were all the rage in 18th century Paris. MESMER used his own life force as *Fluidum* to heal people in an altered, lowered state of consciousness. Later on, he made use of magnets, which can attract, amplify and direct the life force. In my experience, however, magnets can only help and heal over the short term: after a short while, the positive effect turns into its opposite, probably because the life force is too strongly violated and thereby blocked in the long run.

I expect that, in hypnosis, the center of consciousness is temporarily shifted to the emotional body, thereby circumventing the resistance of the mental body and its endless critical indecision, its "Yes, but …" objections. The patient becomes psychologically open and relaxed, making it easier to take in external life force, which the hypnotist, with his "magnetic strokes" can now supply with less effort.

The essential healing principle of classical hypnosis as developed by MESMER, is based on …

1. both the healing principles associated with the "healing sleep" in the form of a hypnotic state (a principle closely associated with the famous ancient "healing sleep")
2. as well the transfer of life force, as can be observed today in the laying on of hands and faith healing.

Yet modern hypnosis, a few exceptions aside, hardly uses the transfer of life force any more. I thus think that modern hypnosis' effectiveness is much weaker than it was during MESMER's time.

FREUD banished all the mystical and scientifically suspicious elements from psychoanalysis that one can still find in hypnosis. This particularly includes the life force, which was a pain in the neck for the ascendant science of the 19th century. We thus find psychoanalysis presenting a sober, rational and enlightened face that includes a minimal version of the original hypnosis, one presentable enough to be allowed into the universities. In a private conversation, FREUD had once expressed his lifelong hope of being able someday to scientifically validate the life force in the form of the *Libido*, in order to re-integrate it into his system through the back door, as it were. That would have been a major triumph for psychoanalysis, for it would then have had a universal healing principle. Wilhelm REICH, a disciple of FREUD's, tried in vain to fulfill his master's long-cherished desire with his *Orgone* theory.

To this day, REICH's theory exudes the ingenious but unworldly and at times curious aroma of the eccentric, which REICH certainly was. REICH's contribution was his emphasis on the life force, whose universal and elemental significance he recognized with a much surer instinct than did FREUD, and to which he paid appropriate tribute in his writings. REICH's tragedy lay in too little appreciating religion, its wisdom and transcendent greatness, as well as the traditions of subtle energy. He was too much of a rationalist lone wolf, a child of the utterly materialistic Enlightenment. Added to this, I regard him (like FREUD) as a victim of his own character type. REICH was most likely a schizoid whose innate flaws included the tendency to allow himself to be crucified for the sake of fanatically held ideologies, and to mutate into an crank – qualities that have not helped his theories at all.

Numerous modern forms of psychotherapy, from Artur JANOV's Primary Therapy to Alexander LOWEN's Bioenergetics, John PIERRAKOS' Core Energetic and Gerda BOYESEN's Biodynamic Psychology invoke REICH as their progenitor. They all share a fetishistic adoration of streaming life force and sexual desire, whose advancement they turned into a kind of Golden Calf. The sexual revolution of the '70s carried its imprint, but the hoped-for rescue of the world by sexuality failed to materialize. Happily, in the last few years, PIERRAKOS and BOYESEN have been developing in the direction of subtle energy and religiosity, which can point the promising way to a new spirituality and greater sensibility (attentiveness in the Buddhist sense). It is thus worth the effort of getting to know more about their methods. I'll return to Gerda BOYESEN's work a number of times later on.

FREUD's most important insight was, without a doubt, that there must be a subconscious hidden behind everyday consciousness. It makes itself known in veiled form through dreams, slips of the tongue and secret wishes. The most revolutionary aspect of FREUD is having recognized that the subconscious is the secret conductor of our entire personality. This makes psychoanalysis an extraordinarily attractive doctrine whose fascination continues unbroken to this day. According to psychoanalysis, the subconscious and its conflicts are the cause of hidden rationales in a person's life, which, viewed from the outside, look like fateful entanglements whose deeper meaning is only revealed gradually. The old saying "Know thyself!" thus becomes once again a motto for modern man. To this extent, we seem to be significantly closer to the solution, by means of psychoanalysis, of mankind's greatest riddle, which is: "Who am I really?"

theory but rather the *what* of the actual interpersonal setting, for another person's esteem is evidently one of those basic emotional needs that we need all our lives.

One big problem that psychoanalysis has to this day is its subjectivity. This leads to numerous problems affecting both daily practice and the theory itself. In particular, conflicts and their evaluation present the greatest difficulties. One can easily trace in the annals of psychoanalysis how this has led to the origin of numerous new schools of analysis. The arguments with Sigmund FREUD that ADLER, C.G. JUNG, REICH and many other analysts had at one time or another were based on divergent evaluations of the subconscious and its conflicts. The fact that none of these analysts knew precisely which conflicts were present in individual patients explains the resulting Babylonian confusion in this area. Psychoanalysts quarreled over the problems of how detect conflicts in the obscurity of the subconscious and how to heal them. The body-mind puzzle got sharper, moreover, because no one knew exactly where these conflicts were stored. Many psychoanalytic schools sprang up,

Subconscious Levels and the Conflicts As Well As Time of Conflict Origin

Subconscious Levels	Conflict Size and Number	Time of Conflict Origin	Meaning of Conflict	Psychosomatic Expression
Superficial level (upper Emotional Level)	Small = current conflict (very many conflicts)	Youth/ adulthood	Situational conflicts (verbal)	Current organ talking (cardiac pain)
Middle level (lower Emotional Level)	Medium = side conflict (usually 4-8)	Early childhood/ childhood	Varied and rounds out the character type (preverbal)	Organ disease
Deep level (Causal Level)	Large = Central Conflict (usually one)	Karmic pattern (a "past life")	Forms the character type (nonverbal)	Mimicry, posture, metabolism

Unfortunately, many people have made the disappointing discovery that psychoanalysis is not a universal solution. I know legions of patients for whom analysis has been little or no help at all – but who are nevertheless exceedingly grateful to their analyst because s/he was the first person in their entire life to have listened to them sincerely and nonjudgmentally. There are now scientific studies that confirm that it is not the analytic method, but rather the analyst himself who is the key factor, even as regards therapeutic effects. This brings into the foreground not the *how* of a certain

with widely divergent conceptions. To this day, each school claims be the one to have found the truth. The outsider who belongs to none of these schools of thought may well ask who then is right.

But the bewildering situation becomes easily comprehensible the moment that conflicts become energetically measurable. Whereas before we were forced to rely on speculation and guess, we can now, for the first time, recognize the conflicts' true significance and size. With *Psychosomatic Energetics* we can very quickly determine which conflict is present, what its dimensions are and what psychoenergetic repercussions it has had. If we think of the darkness up to now as the dark cellar of a house, *Psychosomatic Energetics* shines a light for the first time. We have taken a decisive step toward recognizing and classifying the true state of affairs.

After the many investigations that have been performed using *Psychosomatic Energetics*, we can fundamentally distinguish between three levels and three conflict sizes – namely the surface and middle subconscious that correspond to the emotional body, and the deep subconscious that is associated with the causal body. Now, the larger a conflict, the deeper it sinks into the subconscious. The largest conflicts are thus found in the causal body, while the smaller and medium-sized ones are stored in the emotional body.

This tripartite division of the subconscious gives us an initial orientation as to which level we find ourselves on. The deeper one descends into the subconscious, the larger the conflicts stored there. As with gravity, the subconscious also has conflicts of differing weightiness. The subconscious perceives the conflicts' varying weights as ever heavier and stores them away accordingly. Thus, from the storage location alone, we can deduce how large and weighty a conflict is. The ages-old *Central Conflict* appears to be quite large and weighty, while a half-dozen medium-sized conflicts are located in the middle subconscious and numerous small conflicts in the upper subconscious.

Many a reader might be wondering at this point how I ever found out which conflicts there are and how large they are. *Large* and *weighty* are concepts that make sense because, with the aid of *Psychosomatic Energetics*, we can truly measure and quantify conflicts along these lines. In a sense, we place conflicts on a kind of energy balance. I'll explain later on more precisely how that is done. In addition, certain energy measurements make it possible to identify conflict contents, so that one then knows what kind of themes the conflict is concealing. There is also the option of measuring the energy levels accurately.

Thus, the subdivision of the subconscious and its conflicts that I am presenting here is a system I have developed in conjunction with numerous therapeutic colleagues over the course of many years. Basically, I am simply describing what we have identified in the energy measurements performed on many hundreds of patients. Although there have been slight variations, but never serious qualitative differences, I'd like to be so bold as to declare that this represents the clearest and most true-to-life representation of the subconscious that has yet been drawn up. To use a cartographic metaphor, I like to think of it as an Atlas that helps us decipher the *terra incognita* of our subconscious.

From the table above, we can already tell how a conflict's contents might be expressed in language and thereby brought into conscious awareness. When it comes to the really big conflict, it seems to "leave us speechless." The so-called **Central Conflict**, of which there is always only one, is the largest conflict of all. Its frightening terribleness so silences us that it can only be identified by means of a "wordless" language – primarily mimicry, body posture and metabolism.

Only the medium and smaller conflicts can be expressed in words and thus made conscious. For example, if someone has a small or medium *Rage* conflict, then relaxation exercises and similar techniques can be used to determine that it must be the rage from the time that a toy was taken away when the person was three years old. All the details of the enraging scene can be described and put into words. The rage of a Central Conflict, on the other hand, seems to me (after all I have learned so far) to be impossible to put into words. As a rule, the infuriating experience is seldom consciously remembered, but rather remains, with constant regularity, in the subconscious.

For this reason, large conflicts are inaccessible to speech-oriented therapies. All talk-based psychotherapeutic techniques break down at the latest in the deep subconscious. The actual reason for this incapacity is the speechlessness that surrounds the Central Conflict. At this point in fairy tales, enchanted heroes are turned into animals who can no longer talk, but just look at one mutely and sadly. Or, if the enchantment is particularly dreadful, the victim turns to stone (becomes hard-hearted). The tragedy of calamitous emotional rigidity is paraphrased thus in the Gospel according to Mark: *"For what shall it profit a man, if he shall gain the whole world, and lose his own soul?"* The loss consists primarily of the total inability to talk about what happened. The damage escalates to the point that emotional petrification sets in to wall off the emotional pain and prevent it from rising into consciousness. We all know people who became coldhearted and embittered after suffering a cruel blow of fate. We can see clearly in them that which plays out in the innermost recesses of all people – ourselves included because, since everyone has a Central Conflict, a greater or lesser part of our being is speechless and embittered, even if we are normally no longer aware of it.

The Hero's Adventurous Journey Begins

If you wish to understand life, stop believing what people say and write.
Instead, observe yourself and come up with your own thoughts.
(Anton Chekhov)

Before turning to the great psychic themes that underlie conflicts, I'd like to depict the structure of the subconscious from yet another angle. We can better understand the actual essence of the subconscious with the aid of a primordial mythic image: the subconscious is like an ocean in which the conflicts swim about like sea monsters intent on destroying the Hero. The picture of the psyche as a vast ocean of unplumbed depths whose horizon fades into the hazy mists of infinity is based on ancient mythic images. This picture's various elements are fused together in a curious manner into a unit, typical of the subconscious. Remarkably, the subconscious transforms itself into both the ocean and the Hero himself, the sailor journeying across the ocean.

The Ocean of the Subconscious and Its Conflicts

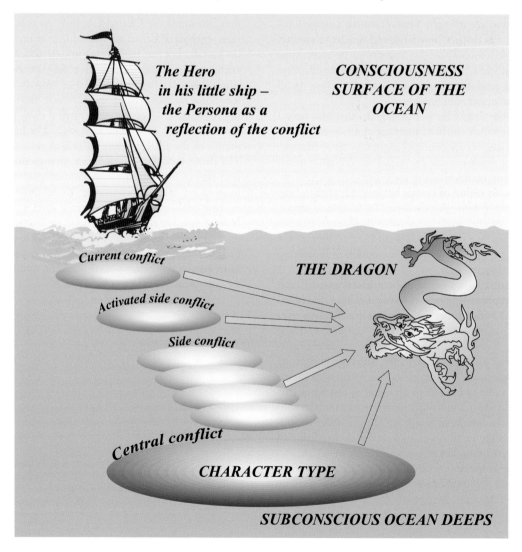

The mystic identification of the Hero and an adventure to be overcome is a profound universal riddle, as the Greek hero Odysseus discovered on his Odyssey. In reality, Odysseus symbolically voyages across his own psychic ocean. In this heroic psychic journey, consciousness becomes a tiny, endangered nutshell of a ship traversing the ocean of the subconscious, threatened by storms and reefs. To the horror of the terrified spectator, the success of the journey is threatened by all manner of danger in the form of violent and devouring monsters that lurk about, intent on annihilating the Hero.

We call the dangers that block the Hero's path *conflicts*. They are the dragons and demons in the depths of the psyche that threaten the Hero's life, well-being, and victory. He must fight them, vanquish them, and put them behind him in order to resume his spiritual journey. Just as the Hero encounters foes of different sizes, there are small, medium, and large conflicts. There is an interesting and instructive interrelationship between the Hero and his foes – for a Hero without a foe is absurd. He would just be a loudmouth, trumpeting his imagined strength. But he can only harm us, since he was adjudged by destiny unworthy of having proper foes. A real Hero needs strong and dangerous foes in order to be a Hero. The greater the malevolence and size of the foes, the more dragon's blood will flow and eventually make our Hero's fame immortal.

We and our spiritual journey are not in a Hollywood spectacle in which we help some bored gods pass the time. Frightening and seemingly senseless catastrophes and challenges of all kinds can give the impression that the world is a "ship of fools," but we may suppose that these are just the projections of the paranoid desperation that sometimes overcomes us. If we think about massacres, atrocities, and natural catastrophes, the world looks like a fearsome chaos, as if a crazy person were trying to make nightmares come true.

Since a part of emotional health is the confident conviction that our world is based on an underlying sensible order, we should not let ourselves be infected by the pessimism of many of our contemporaries. As a doctor, I have frequently been able to uncover latent depressions in these cynics, who paint everything in the dreariest colors. At some point, this cynicism tips over into a psychic gloom that belittles, devalues, and sees everything through grime-covered glasses. I am convinced that, in spite of all the horrible things that happen, we should never lose faith in our destiny and our self-esteem. Emotional health does not seem possible to me without a minimum of religious belief. No matter how little it might be – just the belief, say, that one's life has meaning – experience has shown that this is enough to maintain emotional health.

Turning back to the Hero, we can only fervently hope that, on his spiritual journey, he will prevail over all dangers and ordeals – for failure, as we know, means despera-

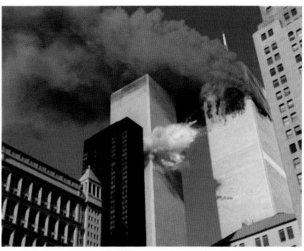

Manmade terror and awful horror have increasingly accompanied humankind as civilization has developed. Pacific and martial aspects have thus developed equally in our civilization – which of course also has consequences for our overall psychic well-being.

tion, dementia, disease, and death. In this respect, cynicism and world-weariness are just another form of personal failure. The victorious Hero, on the other hand, wins an extraordinarily valuable prize. Because each of us goes on a spiritual journey, it is probably in order to acquire experience and maturity. Our life goal seems to be to develop a stable, self-confident, and full-grown personality that has plumbed its psychic depths and learned what it truly feels and really wants.

Conflicts are distortions and falsifications of that which we actually are in the depths of our soul and what we really want. Yet it takes us a very long time to grasp this simple truth and apply it intelligently. At first, we know nothing of the secrets of our soul, confidently assuming that we are dealing with external hostile attacks. It is at this point that the entire process becomes enormously stimulating and is deserving of our undivided attention – since, because our Hero's struggles represent an internal psychic process, the Hero is actually fighting foes inside of himself. The craziest part of the whole thing is the absurd circumstance that, at the beginning, the Hero just doesn't get what it is really all about. In a certain sense, the Hero truly is "crazy," since his paranoia is based on a mistaken belief: the Hero at first thinks that the actual foes are situated in the external world.

Unlike the clueless Hero, we onlookers already know that the true dangers of the journey do not come from a hostile external world, but rather from the Hero himself. But we are not so wise at the beginning of our own self-exploration: we first see our own problems as difficulties that have villainously been inflicted on us from outside. The outside world seems evil to us, while we have absolute-

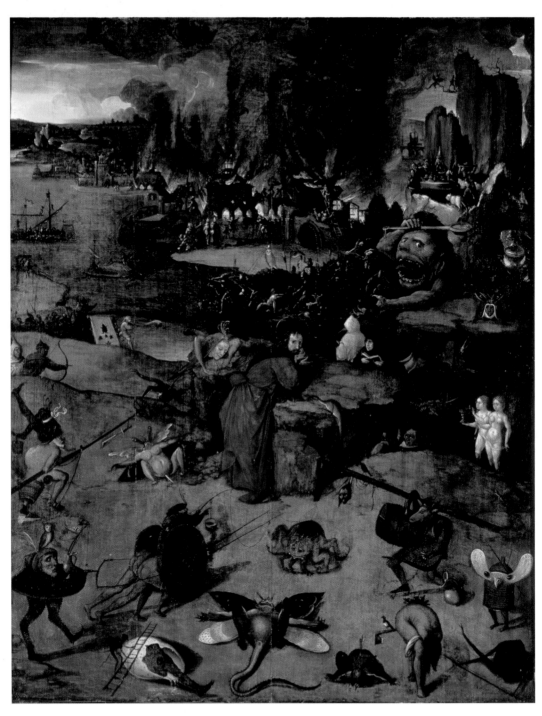

The Temptation of St. Anthony, depicted by Hieronmus Bosch, shows in nightmarish clarity the world of the subconscious, populated by conflicts (symbolized by the insectoid horror figures in the lower half of the painting). War and one of its causes, the lust for destruction, are shown in the upper parts of the picture, with burning cities and gruesome tortures. In the lower part, we encounter all humen sins—from gluttony and lust all the way to sadomasochism. Educated noblemen mutate into donkeys (lower left), as soon as, seen from the subconscious perspective, their mask is torn off. Human creatures are writhing with pain in bizarre postures (lower right). St. Anthony can only hold on tightly to a rock and pray—just as humans cling desparately to the shreds of their Egos when possessed by their Central Conflict (as in a psychosis).

ly nothing to do with the problems that crop up. We know nothing about the psychic ocean in which our worst foes lurk. We are still living completely at the surface of our Persona (character mask). At this point in our spiritual journey, we are like simple-minded clowns, putting on an unbelievably conceited and fraudulent show, not at all realizing that we are playing – and thus lying – to no one but ourselves.

And yet the show results in the development of a stable self-image that serves the Hero as the reliable foundation of his perception of reality. Personal vanity is an important transitional phase, known in psychology as narcissism. Every Hero seems to go through this phase, thinking himself ever so marvelous and basking in the admiration of his fellows. We know from infantile psychology that all children go through this narcissistic phase in more or less the same way.[35] This phase is also observed in adolescents. These narcissistic processes create a mask that C.G. JUNG designated as the Persona.

On the developmental level of the Persona, it is very important what other people think of us. We only become aware of the fragility of our self-image when we lose the emotional support of others. The Persona (character mask) undergoes strong alteration and alignment from its environment, be it occupational group, race or ethnicity, or other ideological and religious reinforcements that give a person's self-image additional impetus. We originally come into the world with no Persona mask and then, as children, go through a repolarization that, as part of our upbringing, reprograms us away from true Self to Persona.

We sometimes as adults meet old childhood friends again, and on these occasions we can examine the changes to their Persona mask. When you know how people were as children, you're often disappointed or even appalled at what drastic changes adulthood has wrought. If we were honest with ourselves, we could also apply these shocking insights to ourselves. We normally don't do this, out of fear that the awareness of how far away we have moved from our true Self might prove to be too agonizing. The false and true selves lead to painful antipodal positions that are, in the worst case, part of growing up.

---

[35] The view of psychoanalyst Alice MILLER is that a mother who withholds love and appreciation causes a very elemental disruption in the formation of a child's personality structure, leading to irreparable disorders in the feeling of self-esteem. Such people then become long-term depressives or try to conceal their depression behind a grandiose façade. Mothers with disturbed self-esteem pass on their disability to their children, triggering a generational chain-reaction of lovelessness. I'd like to add to this surely correct observation of MILLER's that a large active Central Conflict is frequently the actual reason for a mother's coldness. I'll go into more background on this – e.g., the role of Karma – in subsequent chapters. Why would one choose such an unloving mother? Because, pre-birth, one brings to the decision a certain lovelessness oneself, when deciding on reincarnation. Since like attracts like, cause and effect are much harder to keep apart than it might seem from the outside.

The more adult and uptight a person is, the farther the Persona will be from the true Self. The social order is not pleased when we let our mask slip. The people around us want us to stay the way they've got used to, the way we work best for them. In this, the opportunity for manipulation plays a leading role, since repressed and phony people are much easier to manipulate. "I simply had to function" is how this condition is paraphrased, in which remote control overshadows self-control. Carnival time is one of the few times we drop our mask – by putting on fabricated masks behind whose cover we let ourselves act out our otherwise carefully concealed childish foolishness.

From the Persona level, one next dips into the ocean of the subconscious. The **upper stories of the subconscious** house our animalistic aspects. Here lurks the furtive child with all its emotions and urges. The Persona is a fig leaf covering this volcanic cauldron of unruly emotions, and here is where the Freudian *Superego* exercises an important control function. To my mind, Persona and Superego are closely related structures that usually begin to break up pretty much at the same time – in Alzheimer sufferers, for example. These victims don't really care if they are caught stealing or (embarrassing scene!) exposing themselves. What others should think of us (Persona) and which moral precepts we should obey (Superego) are thus directly interrelated.

In the upper level of the subconscious, we encounter strong feelings such as jealousy, envy, avarice, and erotic lustfulness. The strong eroticism of this level seems to me to be the main reason why FREUD so totally equated the subconscious with erotic urges. This of course sets in motion a chain reaction of follow-on errors, since the other deeper segments of the subconscious are by no means eroticized. What's more, this viewpoint is forced to confine itself to the superficial layers of the subconscious, or else misjudge the deeper layers. C.G. JUNG was one of the first of FREUD's disciples to speak out against the dominance of the erotic aspect, which FREUD had so conspicuously and excessively emphasized. JUNG's more comprehensive view also took in the deep subconscious, in which the non-erotic areas of the archetypal and transcendental are located. The subconscious encompasses substantially more than the lustfulness of the surface-layer subconscious.

I'd first like to describe the surface layers of the subconscious, which are located in the upper **emotional body**. Because this part of the subconscious has been so overemphasized in psychoanalysis, many people mistakenly equate this region with the entire subconscious. The upper region of the emotional body has been so emphasized and centralized in Freudian psychoanalysis that its attributes have become a downright folksy part of everyday thinking. Nowadays everyone knows that camouflaged erotic intent, repressed complexes, and unconscious carnal agendas put their stamp on all human behavior – i.e., jealousy, competitiveness, concealed hostility, and traumatic childhood memories.

And yet the levels of the Persona and the moralistic Superego are quite thin. Each of the many moral missteps and countless other daily transgressions of moral precepts – even if it's just running a red light when nobody's looking – bears witness to the fundamental fragility of everyday morality. Surprisingly, even a slight disinhibition is often enough to completely demolish the façade of moral probity. Every strong emotion represents a breaking loose from this level, whether it's another driver flipping the finger or someone casting a furtive erotic or envious glance. The animalistic feelings thus released seem so impulsive and powerful because they are instinctively hardwired. They are what is known as the "beast in man." Authors such as Desmond MORRIS discern in these atavistic behavioral patterns the ape in man, defending its territorial boundaries. As soon as you see the apelike primate behind your neighbor's façade, a lot of things become more understandable.

These preset **instinctive** and survival-oriented behavioral patterns can be found in animals in very similar form. "My dog gets up on our bed, all insulted and pouty, if we haven't come back at the appointed time," a dog owner tells me. This is a particularly wicked example of vengeance on the unfaithful master, since the dog is arrogating to itself the privilege of crawling onto the alpha animal's bed: "That's what you get, it's all your fault I'm behaving so badly!" Once in the bed, he enjoys all the perks of the affronted diva, who gets to relax in broad daylight if someone disrespects her: "When I have been sooo insulted and ignored, then I just have to be nice to myself to make up for it!" At the same time, we see the small child in the dog's behavior, regressing by taking refuge in the parent's cozy bed: "Nobody loves me, I'm abysmally unhappy and need the consolation that only my masters' bed can give me!" We can here very well see the different **emotional facets** that virtually every conflict displays: various divergent emotional contents blending together into an overall feeling.

As long as we can maintain our Persona façade, we will try in a positive way to win people over to our side. Strife is the last and least suitable way to come out a winner. When you take off your Persona mask because you have lost control, the game tends to escalate, and at some point you'll no longer give a damn what others think. The animal in us tries beforehand – with all kinds of strategies – to come out on top every time. Animal "language" is often made use of here, for example dominating and impressing behavior. Thus, a department head whose reputation has taken a beating will try to show his staff who's really the boss by adopting a conspicuously blasé attitude. In animal language terms, the department head is behaving like the pack's actual alpha animal. He takes for granted the privilege of parking in the slot right next to the office's front door, or having underlings hold the door open for him.

The discreetly (barely) concealed intent becomes even clearer when it comes to flirtation and seduction. Thus, behind his seductive wiles, we clearly see the affectations of the "Italian Romeo" who, with every fiber of his sensual body and his eroticizing behavior, pursues a specific (dead easy to guess) goal with respect to the opposite sex, namely to get his quarry in bed. Behavioral researchers see, in the perpetual presence of erotic drives in the human species, one of the main reasons why we react in such a permanently eroticized manner, which animals tend to do only during mating season. Eros is thus one of our most important drives, as FREUD so correctly realized.

It always revolves around the two poles of **power and sexuality**, which the subconscious pursues as cryptic goals:
- **Power** is anything that influences our reputation and status with other people.
- **Sexuality**, on the other hand, is anything that furthers our personal pleasure and reproductive instinct.

In his Individual Psychology, the psychoanalyst Alfred ADLER identified the power drive (besides Eros) as the primary driving force behind our subconscious motives. When we observe people more closely to see whether and to what degree they exercise power, we discover, in the power drive, an enormously strong, widespread, and frequently unrecognized driving force. Whether it's a fancy car or putting on airs in public, we will always find the power drive as the hidden background motive. A good deal of subconscious energy is expended to secure our hierarchical power position vis-à-vis other people and bumping it up a notch or two whenever possible. Ludwig BÖRNE identified the secret recipe: *"The secret of power consists of knowing that other people are even more cowardly than you are."*

Sigmund FREUD, on the other hand, thought otherwise: he viewed sexuality, not power, as humankind's most significant subconscious driving force. Solid proof of this can be found everywhere. An old widower once revealed to me, while I was examining him, that male potency is a big deal even in the retirement home: "You wouldn't believe what those old folks are up to! Tea and cookies? No way! It's all about you-know-what." We find indications everywhere that FREUD's assertion of the omnipresence of sexuality must be correct. Giacomo CASANOVA, the world's most famous lover, summarized his numerous escapades thusly: *"Love is three-quarters curiosity."*

Naturally, the driving forces of power and sexuality don't involve just us humans. **Power and sexuality** are the primary activities in nature. In a sense, we can view them as two sides of the same coin. Every living being is constantly trying to extract maximum power and sexuality for itself. One can thus regard the powerful billionaire with a huge harem as a clear winner, although mostly it's the villains in James Bond movies to whom these criteria apply – presumably because the viewer wouldn't be able to stand watching the film otherwise, out of sheer envy. Not just villains, but rather every living creature makes every effort to reproduce and lead its genes to success in the evolutionary Indy 500. In the struggle for survival, the most powerful have the best chance of success, which is why power and sexuality are closely related. Former American Secretary of State Henry KISSINGER asserts that *"Power is the strongest aphrodisiac."* That seems to be true for men at least – and for those women who find powerful men irresistible.

The recently founded very topical system of *Psycho-Darwinism* uncovers surprising parallels between the behavioristic discoveries of animal ethology and FREUD's psychological models. Originally, psychoanalysis and Darwinism were considered to be totally irreconcilable theories. In particular, FREUD viewed the incest taboo (in the form of the Oedipus Complex) as mankind's highest cultural achievement – while animals were believed to copulate with anything that comes their way, even including their own parents. A few decades ago, the Finnish ethologist WESTERMARCK was able to prove that the incest taboo is not an exclusive human cultural achievement. Quite the contrary: it is a genetically predetermined behavior found in the animal kingdom as well, presumably to avoid the drawbacks of inbreeding. Despite widespread assertions, therefore, incest is vanishingly rare in the animal kingdom. Thus, although the mightiest ape in a pack can mount any female he wants, he always stays away from his mother.

An infallible sign of common ancestry of man and beast is their common instinct. I like to describe instincts **as preset behavior sequences that are associated with intense feelings**. Instincts are thus precursors to feelings. The uncoupling of instinct and feeling that can be observed in humans corresponds psychologically to the expulsion from Paradise. During childhood, we exist (as animals do) mostly in the emotional body, where our feelings and instincts are largely coextensive – which is why we experience the indescribable blessedness of youthful paradise in those years. But eventually we are expelled from paradise. In the pain of this expulsion, the hero experiences his first defeat, as he is catapulted out of the parental nest and out of the protective cocoon of childhood. He must now take his first unaided steps in the cold, hard world.

As we grow up, we pass through the usual cultural upbringing and develop a Persona. We are then "someone" and represent something to ourselves and our fellow humans. The thorny path to adulthood represents the spiritual exercises of our upbringing. Feelings and instincts are partially separated from each other by the socialization process. Although they may be hungry, well-raised children must not touch anything until all the others have taken their places at the table. As children we have to learn, at great effort, to control our impulses and suppress unpleasant feelings – for instance that we'd like to haul off and slug our dumb Aunt Agnes because she gave us such a boring present. Suppressing urges is one of the subliminal forces that, according to FREUD, promote cultural achievements – and in fact, make them possible in the first place. But here I think that FREUD underestimated the human playful element *(Homo ludens)* and joy in creativeness. Experience has shown that erotically arresting people are especially creative, as we can observe in such erotomanic artists as PICASSO.

On the plus side, the separation of feeling and instinct gives us an enormous amount of extra freedom. We are no longer slaves to our drives, as is the case with animals, but rather can (up to a point) lead and control ourselves. We know, of course, that this doesn't go as well as we might wish. Virtue and vice are known to be often just as mutually opposed as upbringing and freedom. Somerset MAUGHAM comes to the following sobering conclusion regarding human *dressage* and its outlook for success: *"Most people only renounce their vices once they have become bothersome."* This sounds very pessimistic and is only partly true, for upbringing is of course not without its positive results. Taking a short-sighted view, our upbringing may indeed make us less free – because, for example, we can no longer play like children whenever we feel like it.

But, over the long run, the ability to exercise self-control is what makes us socially tolerable and cultivated members of the fellowship of man – and this is a gain in personal freedom. Anyone who has had to endure the crude and aggressive behavior of uncivilized persons will immediately bemoan the lack of freedom that an uncouth person forces on one with his deficient demeanor. If you observe these uncivilized roughnecks more closely, you discover in them the unwilling victims of circumstance that such ill-bred people have spawned. Such crude people are in fact extraordinarily unfree. Abusing others and being impolite is actually a sign of inner emotional tension. Thus, asocial behavior usually covers up considerable emotional damage that makes the offender (not to mention his victims!) unfree and unhappy.

The anti-authoritarian movement thus founders on the necessity for children to learn limits, in order later to become friendly, socially acceptable, and emotionally free adults. The other extreme – turning children into emotional invalids by means of a sadistically strict upbringing – is the other pedagogical mistake that can often be observed in the lower socioeconomic strata. Properly dosed education leads to stepwise acquisition of personal freedom. The crucial element of good pedagogy seems to be the appropriate admixture of love, strictness, and rationality. Love means the basic feeling of wanting the best for children and, for example, being able to forgive them. Strictness means drawing definite boundaries that a child can adjust to. Finally, rationality means following an overall pedagogical plan that best furthers the child's abilities.

Let us take a closer look at the separation of feeling and instinct that characterizes our humanity and distinguishes us from animals. The feelings thus set free generate a consciousness space that is a necessary prerequisite for the development of the *Self*. Along with greater brain capacity, the **mental body**, which houses our understanding, develops the capacity for rational thought and powers of recollection. The mental body is thus in part a tool that expresses intelligence and combinatorial ability, but also (and above all) is the seat of personality and selfhood. If we think back to the first time we had a feeling of selfness, that was the initial awakening of the power of the mental body. As soon as feelings are decoupled from instinct – aided and accelerated by educational processes – the Self begins to emerge.

An anecdote related by the American anthropologist Gregory BATESON vividly illustrates how the unexpected evolutionary advance, when prehistoric man began to think, may have come to pass at some time in the distant past. Dolphin trainers often see their pupils make up imaginative leap sequences that break up the repetitive training routine. Afterwards, the bewildered dolphins try to recapture their trainer's affection with especially creative leaps. In like manner, it's conceivable that man needs creative flights of fancy to survive – because, compared to animals, the human species is much less well adapted to environmental rigors than animals, having neither fur, sharp claws, nor any other native accessories. It is a great challenge – especially with an unpredictable environment – to "come up with something really special." Like irritated dolphins, humans are challenged by nature to compensate with cleverness for their lack of tools and weapons.

Just like a confused animal, we develop (through trial and error, good and painful experiences) the knowledge of how we can reinforce good experiences and avoid bad ones. This gives rise to operational thinking, which invents useful survival strategies, develops a sense of time, and structures reality ever more strongly. Modern developmental psychology can explain these processes in great detail. In the end, we acquire a consciousness that can think about itself and says "me" to itself. If we put ourselves in the hero's place, who (in mythology) lives out the average person's life journey, the feeling of self is associated with a first feeling of triumph. Theodor FONTANE's saying, *"Many a rooster believes that the sun rises every morning at its behest,"* gives a good impression of the self-enamored magnificence that is associated with the emergence of the Ego. A teenager is totally in love with his first car, and the self-

confidence it gives him has such irresistible force that over-confidence ends up costing him his life, since it makes him feel invulnerable.

Later on, the hero – assuming he survives his heroic martial deeds – will be able to gather his first experiences with love and the feeling of individuality. We are here in the middle emotional region, in which the basic experience meanders from erotic "storm and stress" to the humane feeling of love, yearning, and individuality. At this level of the subconscious, the separation of instinct and feeling is already far advanced. Individually tinged feeling themes arise that, although they still bear the instinctive stamp of the upper subconscious, already have strongly individualized features and reach far into early childhood. Erotic fantasies, feelings of power, and other *Ego* themes are lived out here: "Who will be the victor and spend a passionate night of love with the princess?" asks the Ego. All great novelistic themes circle this level's topics, populated by Romeo and Juliet and other heroic figures.

One can first see that polarity is amplified and the consciousness of Self increases equally as the feeling for one's own subconscious does. This applies both to the evolution of mankind and to the life history of the individual. The more clearly we sense that we possess an Ego, the more sharply and clearly the subconscious moves into the foreground. That may sound contradictory, yet it's quite logical when you consider it more closely. Just as light and shadow are conditional on each other, so does human Ego formation lead to activation of the deeper subconscious. However, this entire process comes to a strange end at some point. As the personality continues to develop, something quite unexpected happens: the hero succumbs to an evil sorcerer who wipes out his memory. Suddenly, the subconscious seems to have disappeared!

At some point, the hero in our spiritual tale forgets that he is supposed to be seeking the princess (who represents the subconscious). This is precisely what happens to so many people, who have completely lost any memory of their subconscious – or, in mythological terms, of paradise itself. The subconscious paradise symbolizes mother's lap, early childhood, and the True Self. All of that gradually fades from memory. The **Ego** and its delegates in the outside world – be they possessions or instrumentalized fellow humans who are dependent on one and have been degraded to mere objects – must make do as miserable replacement figures who are expected to provide a modicum of satisfaction. The spiritual thirst of these people is, experience has shown, unquenchable, once they have been spiritually uprooted.

The Ego can even turn into a fortress in which the world outside the walls seems more and more unreal. Egomaniacs of this kind live from then on in their snail shell. At this stage of the spiritual journey, the hero goes through the "dark night of the soul." The hero has seemingly lost everything, and therefore sinks into the deepest despair. This stage of the spiritual journey runs straight through an inferno characterized by egomaniacal seclusion and severe loss of emotional naturalness.

This eventually leads to a dramatic transformation and a new beginning – what is known in Greek tragedy as *catharsis*. For the hero, the worst is behind him, and he begins a fresh contemplation which takes him back to a deeper level of the subconscious, where instincts dealing with power and sexuality are now largely irrelevant. FREUD's and ADLER's psychoanalytic theories are invalid here. On this deepest level of personal consciousness, the mind is concerned only with itself and its relationship with others. Deep religious and emotional feelings surface, sacral and primordial. We are now in the **causal body**, corresponding to our deep, completely preverbal subconscious. At the same time, we recover our True Self, which we had thought irretrievably lost.

The True Self (the **superconscious**) encompasses the highest, most quintessential part of true being (what Sri AUROBINDO calls the *supramental*). This is the purest, most honest and authentic part of us. One is surprised, at first, suddenly to find the superconscious element at the deepest subconscious level. Yet what initially seems a contradiction is really easy to understand. Because we remain completely unaware of our true being for so long, we can call the deep subconscious "subconscious" only for as long as we have not yet become aware of our True Self. To my mind, working on becoming self-aware is one of life's all-important tasks. We transform our True Self from the subconscious to the conscious, and it then helps us attain to a clarity of consciousness, which from that point on feels hyperconscious. In this process of becoming self-aware, emotional conflicts play a crucial role (that I will get more into later on): they are, as it were, the striking surfaces on which the self-awareness process "ignites."

We encounter **character type** for the first time in the causal body. This is the strongest, most long-lived, and fully individualized shaping of mental feeling contents in the sense of a clearly delineated structure. To some degree, one can designate the character type as our "hard-core essence." If we mentally picture once again our hero's spiritual journey – which is basically a universally-valid sequence of spiritual transformations applicable to every person – then the hero transforms himself in the final stage of his journey into a mature adult exhibiting clearly-delineated character traits. From the shy youngster via the foolhardy lover and brave warrior to the mature adult who has taken the measure of all the highs and lows of his life, we discover in the hero the matured character who has plumbed his own depths. The character type spells out what we carry around with us in terms of individual preferences, attitudes, habits, and basic viewpoints – and what will presumably persist over the course of numerous incarnations.

It now becomes gradually clear that our hero's journey is like the metamorphosis of a butterfly, that first pupates in order to shed its skin and emerge with ever clearer character traits. The first pupation consists of putting on the Persona mask, behind which the vulnerable soul ensconces itself, like a knight in armor protected from hostile surroundings. Just like armor, the Persona has a primitive mechanical aspect that enormously restricts the degree of mobility and individual freedom of its wearer. Still, it's better to swelter in rigid, clumsy armor than be slain by savage enemies. After a while, most people no longer notice their armor because wearing it has become second nature. In fact, in most cases they mistake it for their True Self.

In this fearful phase of first pupation, in which the Persona mask is still prominent, caution is in order. The anxious mood of the Persona mask wearer is well summarized in an epigram of the American journalist Ambrose BIERCE, who commented on the cowardice of Civil-War soldiers with indulgent irony: *"A coward is a person in whom the sense of self-preservation is in good working order."* Saving face and surviving is for many people the same thing, even when based on such crazy principles. In Asian societies, the Persona mask is supremely significant, and committing suicide because of poor grades or one's company's bankruptcy is based on the equation *existence = Persona*.

Even though such extremes may surprise us, every normal person does have a Persona mask. Generally speaking, it can be said that it functions as an emotional protective mechanism as long as the emotional self-preservation drive operates normally. Usually, there are only two extreme types who can afford to go through life without a Persona mask: fools and criminals. With fools, it's a lack of foresight, but mostly of course a pitiable inability to take timely precautions in the service of emotional protection, while the unscrupulous psychopath and career criminal finds himself in the advantageous position of having others be afraid of him as gets the long end of the stick through his fear tactics.

When people learn from life experience and personal development that the Persona is based on social rules and dogmas, they begin to discover their own emotional components and their actual drive and desires. This often happens in puberty or the so-called *midlife crisis*. But revolts against social norms can also take place in entire population groups, when people infect one another with the wanna-change virus. For instance, one can regard the sexual revolution of the '70s as a collective outbreak from the then socially predominant Persona mask. Young people had simply had enough of the "normal" person's hypocritical double standard. These people were "uptight" and unhappy inside; they fantasized about sex but didn't do anything; they built atom bombs or killed Vietnamese, but they knew nothing about tolerance and peace. Youth, on the other hand, longed for fun and personal self-actualization – i.e., the levels behind the Persona mask (behind the façade of pretend respectability, double standards, uptight false front).

Since social rules and emotional structures are so tightly interwoven at the level of the Persona, rebelling against the Persona is of necessity a social revolution – whether a frustrated wife leaves her husband and children, thus shocking the entire town, or revolutionaries rise up against the rigid structures of the state; the pattern remains the same. The ensuing fiasco is well known since everyone has a Persona mask, and not even the revolutionary can run away from it. On the contrary, the situation often gets worse, and the revolution gives way to an even worse dictatorship.

The thing is, the more people act as if they no longer have a Persona, the falser their attitudes become. Then, the emotional shadows hidden behind the half-off Persona emerge, that had hitherto been held in check by Persona structures. Destructive urges, hatred, envy, and jealousy break out – because a development was forced prematurely. Unfettered urges are about the moral pressure that conservative types like to exert whenever liberalization threatens, true to the motto: "If we relax the rules, all hell will break loose." Of course, dangerous chaos breaks out only if people, due to inadequate emotional progress, have not yet developed any self-control.

The Persona mask protects individuals from their own emotional abysses and dangers in exactly the same way as laws and moral precepts within the society do, as long as self-control is not yet advanced enough. Just as driving students should only drive in traffic with the instructor at their side, the Persona mask plays the role of the driving instructor. However, the time comes when one can make one's own way in traffic and "steer" one's own life unaided. One could even go so far as to say that, from a certain stage of personal development on, it becomes urgently necessary to let the Persona mask gradually fall in order to make room for individuality and to reestablish contact with the subconscious.

At this stage there arises a hybrid mixture of Persona mask and character type: the **personality**. It can be viewed as an interim stage between Persona mask and conflict theme, one that the individual needs to pass through as a maturation step; there is likewise a collective developmental phase. It is my experience that, these days, personality is the most widespread and normal expression form of the average adult. It represents an expansion of the Persona mask that corresponds to individual desires, traits, and drives, and that which is called *individuality*.

The **character type**, the next level, exhibits a broader spectrum of possibilities, in that we can more clearly discern what kind of distinctive and unique entity we really are. We become unmistakable "originals" who can live out and realize both our social roles and our deep subconscious parts in equal manner. This is why grandparents are often so popular with children, because they too can let out the inner child and express the undistorted humanity of their deep emotional components, which the parents cannot or dare not do, because they need to function in society and are still strongly attached to the Persona mask. Adults continue to play their fixed roles and exhibit fairly static personality structures. Grandparents, on the other hand, have reclaimed the freedom to be themselves once again, i.e., to live out their true essence.

Character type corresponds to the mature phase of the older person who has gradually become worldly-wise and experienced. However, one often notices that older people cannot fulfill these expectations because their emotional development does not permit it. Many people simply do not become wise and clever as they get older, but instead get opinionated and narrow-minded. Therefore, calendar age cannot be equated with emotional maturity stages. When even children show more wisdom and emotional maturity than their grandparents, my guess is that it has to do with previous karmic experiences. Children who have amassed more life experience in former lives can thus be emotionally more mature than their grandparents.

With the development of the character type, the spiritual journey slowly nears its end; at its conclusion, the hero rediscovers his **True Self**. Many mythological tales tell of a secret yet deeply true foundational basis of our existence. The renowned mythologist Joseph CAMPBELL sees in Parsifal's quest for the Holy Grail a coded message that is actually about the search for the True Self. C.G. JUNG interprets the alchemist's efforts to turn base metal into gold as a purely spiritual process meant to bring out the true and indestructible Self. In many fairy tales, the princess and the treasure are ciphers for that true happiness that the Hero is actually seeking. Thus, the Hero is not hoping to find foreign faraway treasures, but rather longs to return to his own spiritual center, his True Self.

Just as personality is an intermediate stage between the Persona mask and character type, so too can character type be viewed as an intermediate stage between personality and the True Self. Even though in the character type we already reveal much of our spiritual bandwidth, many parts of the Self still remain hidden. Only the True Self is able to manifest all the facets of our being. It is often depicted as a "large rectangle" symbolizing the four character types. In difficult situations that challenge their whole being, many people sense that there is a lot more in them than they had thought. In these difficult situations, many outdo themselves as they come into contact with their higher Self. Artists create great works that give us an idea of the enormous possibilities that lie dormant in all of us. People in enraptured, holy, and transcendent states exhibit the superhuman nature of their True Self, which expresses itself in a godlike, ecstatic, and beatific emotional state. All this tells us that we carry about with us significantly more potential than we can normally live with. We express just a fraction of the being that is actually within us.

The illustration on page 154 depicts the assignments of the various emotional structures.

Besides the spiritual journey, there is another way, quite true-to-life and everyday, to get to know the various layers of the individual and the subconscious. For this, let us visualize the stages of intimacy that connect us to a specific person. The beginning of every relationship consists of strangeness, which is why, at first, another person seems to us strange and unknown. We encounter this strangeness quite strikingly when the other person really is a stranger. This cancels all sullying influences that can crop up due to resemblances to other people one knows, projections, and so on.

Strangers first present us with their mask, the Persona. This is in line with the superficial level on which we communicate with one another. Yet when we want to get to know people better, we get to know their personality, which reveals the basic traits of their character type. We get to know the more intimate characteristics of their being. We can here divide people into two groups, depending on whether we are dealing, spiritually, with a masculine or feminine soul. Basically, this classification is relatively independent of gender role, and it divides people into polar types having a harder or a softer soul. The Chinese call this *Yin* and *Yang*. Psychologists speak of **introversion** and **extroversion**, according to which there are those who turn inward, are soft and yielding, and others who are outwardly oriented, hard and demanding.

On closer inspection, one finds a remarkable discovery, one which amazed even C.G. JUNG: the extroverted type's inner soul corresponds, illogically, to the female Yin polarity, whereas the introvert exhibits a masculine Yang. This is succinctly expressed in the vernacular phrase "hard shell, soft center." Many a hard male harbors a soft, yielding female spirit. On the other hand, many a soft female really has a very hard core being. As a physician, I have had this confirmed many times when, in times of crisis, the true core of being is revealed. A serious accident turns the tough guy into a wailing, miserable bundle of nerves, wallowing in self-pity, whereas the formerly soft woman in the same situation displays unexpected self-discipline. Numerous psychological studies have meanwhile confirmed that women are more stress-resistant than men – which ultimately means simply that, spiritually, women have a harder core than men. Of course, one shouldn't overgeneralize here; this is a relatively rough general rule.

As intimacy increases, we encounter ever more candidly what lies behind the stranger's mask. Privately, we sooner or later drop the mask and reveal our true core of being.

Inside the family, a pecking order often forms that one would not have expected from the outside. For instance, a worldly-wise pastor is said to have once posed the question in his fully-packed church, as to which of the men "wore the pants in the family." Not a single one of the men present raised his hand. But all the hands went up when the question was in which households the woman decided what was what. Emotionally, extroversion means "wearing the pants." Thus, the vernacular knows that, in a patriarchy, there is often a Big Woman behind the Big Man, pulling the strings in the background.

At this point, I'd like to return to a controversial issue that's already been raised in this book. It has to do with whether power or sexuality is to be regarded as the dominant element in the subconscious. According to C.G. JUNG, power is the main theme of the introverted mentality, while sexuality is the leading theme of the extrovert. There is thus no one universally valid answer, since there are two truths for two polar mental types. FREUD would then be a therapist for extroverts and ADLER for introverts. Keeping this in mind, emotionally weak, introverted men indeed seem to be seeking sexual satisfaction, yet are actually fighting for power and dominance. Power, for example, includes football, politics, computers, cars, and other symbols.

For emotionally strong, dominant, and extroverted women, power is basically uninteresting in their heart of hearts, since they already have power. In this viewpoint, women are interested in sexuality – not necessarily the purely mechanical sex act, but rather (in an expanded understanding of sexuality) dealing with questions such as "who is the fairest in the land," who has the lead reproduction-wise, and who is copping the largest portion of the big "love cookie." Anyone who takes a look at men's and women's magazines will quickly realize that there's a lot of truth in this classification scheme. If one defines sexuality as a superordinate concept of sensuality and quality of life, then experience has shown that essentially all women are concerned primarily with more sensuality and sexuality.

Now, this extroversion/introversion classification scheme sounds quite simple at first – but things are actually much more complicated: to be sure, the division into introversion and extroversion can very nicely explain the "battle of the sexes," but it tells us too little about individuals and their characteristics. The real problem is that biological and emotional sexual affiliation can turn out to be different, so that there are emotionally masculine and feminine women, just as one can identify men who are more masculine or feminine.[36]

What I said about women who "wear the pants" and are emotionally strong is of course still valid and doesn't need to be taken back, since it involves instinctive processes of the Persona and the upper subconscious. The battle of the sexes takes place in the upper stories of the subconscious, where-

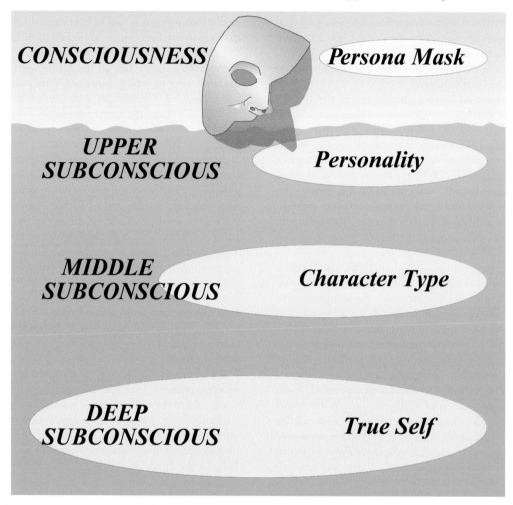

as emotional gender polarity resides in the deep subconscious. At a certain level of the subconscious, therefore, emotional and gender polarity are retransformed and, oftentimes, a soft essential nature (corresponding to her actual Yin type) will become visible behind the inner-emotionally hard woman after all. Other women will exhibit a Yang character type, on the other hand. Extroversion and introversion therefore vary in significance, depending on which levels of the subconscious one is dealing with.

And now I'd like to describe yet another kind of approach to the subconscious, one that best agrees with the personal experience of the individual. It is also the viewpoint adopted by fairy tales and myths, in which the subjective comes very much to the fore. Our Hero on his spiritual journey first encounters the violent beast in himself, popularly symbolized as a dragon. This is the suspenseful key scene that has us holding our breath. The next thing the Hero must do is free himself from the dragon's clutches. This is not an actual occurrence, but rather an encrypted representation of inner emotional processes.

We recognize the encryption because the dragon-slayer motif is a quite archetypal and universal one. As so often in subconscious processes, the actual depth-psychological significance becomes visible if one relates all the motifs to a

---

[36] My conception of prenatal gender selection is that, in the origin of an individual soul, we instinctively decide on a more feminine or masculine orientation – from which I'd like to derive (based on certain experiences in reincarnation therapy) that, sometime thousands of years ago, we had something like freedom of choice as we decided, before the first reincarnation, to slip into a particular soul. We presumably said instinctively "That's how I want to be! I sense that I'll feel good in there!" – and thus become, from then on, a particular character type with clearly delineated characteristics. From that point on, one keeps the same character type from one incarnation to the next. Viewed this way, homosexuality is nothing other than living out the primevally determined spirit gender – just that, this time around one had the bad luck to end up in the sexually wrong body type. Another issue is the theory that homosexuality is a latent tendency concealed in every one of us. However, this doesn't seem to apply in all cases, since I have observed latent homosexuality only in those men who had a mentally feminine character type (i.e., were hysterics or depressives). They thus are merely expressing that which is concealed in their inner souls.

single person. The Dragon and the Maiden are just as much a part of the person as the Hero. All the figures in the dragon-slayer mythos reveal something of the antithetical dynamics in the soul of an individual – in our own selves, that is.

All that I have said serves to show that the Dragon represents the violent drives of the upper subconscious. The Dragon is the "inner brute" that wants to indulge its impulses without let or hindrance. His greed makes him a voracious monster. The Princess is presumably the True Self hiding behind the character type. Like the Princess, our Self is the prisoner of evil powers. The Princess is threatened by the Persona's phoniness, its shadowy conflicts and meanness, as well as (above all) its animalistic violence and evil. The Hero must thus rescue himself by allying himself with his good drives and resisting the temptation to exploit the situation and becoming a scoundrel himself.

The dragon-slayer motif grabs our attention because it deals (like all major myths) with the entire subconscious, including the conscious. It has a universal character and evokes very deep feelings and moods in every listener. The dragon-slayer motif represents one of the deepest wisdoms of human life. In this respect, such myths encompass the **causal body**, as we (on our spiritual journey) approach that which is mysterious, meaningful, and truly important, namely the True Self. C.G. JUNG speaks of the "numinous" which is so difficult to capture in words. A famous Zen Buddhist saying summarizes the impossibility of describing the holy, here in the form of a short poem (Japanese *Koan*):

He who knows speaks not,
He who speaks knows not.

It is on this level of the subconscious that the great archetypal symbols first surface, that circle about the Cross, Salvation, and the great myth of the all-devouring Snake. It is the beginning of deep existential feelings from the Self: "Who am I really?" asks our Hero. Sex and power, the great themes of the personal subconscious, play ever diminishing roles, which the spirit themes now surfacing can no longer describe at all. The Hero confronts the Almighty and the infinitude of the Cosmos. The deeper his desperation and his hopeless journey into the depths of the soul, the more the Hero finds himself in transpersonal regions belonging to the collective unconscious. The character type disappears more and more, and the Self rises up as the divine, beatific core of being. In these deep regions of the causal body, the polarities and problems of the world are transcended and overcome. According to the promises of religious texts, the end of all this is the glorious victory that reconciles our Hero with all the preceding battles and deprivations, and an eternal peace that makes future battles unnecessary.

Finally, I'd like to turn to yet another kind of self-awareness having to do with the **feeling of self**. This is the feel-

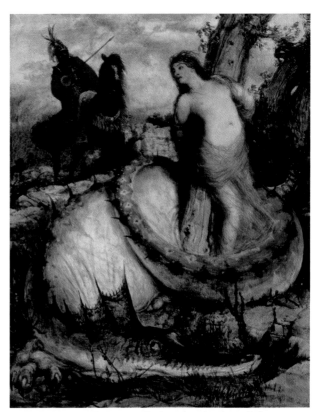

The dragon's ambiguity embodies the gluttony of the pent-up drives in the subconscious, as well as the dangerousness and destructiveness of the conflicts stored there. The hero rescues the maiden not only from her (and his) own destructive lustfulness, but also from their helplessness vis-à-vis the conflicts.

ing we have when we sense how much we are "in the middle of ourselves." If we imagine the subconscious as an ocean whose depths we plumb more and more as our spiritual maturity increases, then the question that occupies us most is where we are "at," like a deep-sea diver repeatedly checking his depth gauge – for our "diving depth" corresponds quite precisely to our level of spiritual development. It is part of the basic conception of spiritually oriented psychology (of which I am here the advocate) that our soul is considered to be more and more advanced the more open we become vis-à-vis our own subconscious. This opening up to our subconscious leads to a feeling of self that is ever more authentic and centered.

In my opinion, a stronger feeling of self is also the secret reason why spiritually advanced persons have such a generally warm-hearted and familiar effect on those around them. Because the more we open ourselves to our subconscious, the stronger our feeling of self will be, since it is ultimately a feeling of being loved and accepted. Virtually all who have gone on deep expeditions into the border regions of the subconscious report having found themselves once again in very familiar home territory. "When is the last time I felt like this?" one asks oneself involuntarily, and senses that the last time one had such a strong feeling of deep familiarity was in early childhood.

From this standpoint, it is clear why the idea of a lost paradise sounds so familiar: it is our own Self that we lost. Nature's wisdom has seen to it that we are permitted to live in the cocoon of a deep feeling of self as long as we are babies needing to be protected. One can often measure very high causal body charges in babies. Evidently, babies are enfolded in a blanket of cozy well-being, a kind of psychoenergetic womb in the form of the causal body. As one gets older, the memory of that original condition remains, which is designated depth-psychologically as *Ouroboros* or *Oceanic Bliss*. Of course, the perfect is the enemy of the good, and therefore we cannot rest until we once again have it as good as we did back then when we felt entirely "at home."

And with that, I'd like to conclude this chapter on the layers of the subconscious ocean of the soul. Even if we can now better understand many things, there remains an unsatisfying suspicion that there is still something essential missing in our understanding. The missing puzzle parts are the conflicts that, like the walls of a house, give the subconscious its structure in the first place. If we don't take the conflicts into account, we wander around aimlessly in the building of the subconscious. The conflicts are the subject of the next chapter. Conflicts, the "salt in the soup," provide frictional resistance against which our soul can develop.

The Conflict Orchestra

*People like so much to be talked about that even
a conversation about their faults delights them.*
(André Maurois)

Anyone who has acquired enough experience about himself and others will at some point realize that every person "carries a lot of baggage around" – i.e., a highly personalized collection of problems, fears, and the most varied human weaknesses. So "nobody's perfect." My experience as a physician has made it clear that, in more than a few cases, it's precisely those whom at first we most envy who are most to be pitied. The façade can often be deceptive, because we have forgotten how to look behind the curtain.

Now, we doctors are prone to adopt the extreme position of seeing disease everywhere and finding disorders in everyone. This attitude quickly turns human society into a gigantic untreated sickroom whose inhabitants have to be made aware that they urgently need help. And who gets to play rescuer? Why the doctor, of course, who (like *Superman*) needs to be everywhere at once to save suffering humanity. The derisive undercurrent of those last sentences should make it clear that I consider such an extreme attitude to be 100% wrong, even though I am myself a physician. Naturally everybody needs help at some point. But to pronounce all fellow human beings to be by their very nature sick and in need of treatment was one of the most fateful mistakes of psychoanalysis, one from which it has never fully recovered, in my opinion.

Therefore, in order to avoid misunderstandings, I'd like to start by clarifying my position on mental health and illness. In this context, I do not take my cue from some sort of "homemade" edifice of ideas, but from reality, which I as physician have been able to observe in my fellow man and measure with energetic methods. In fact, in a randomly chosen group of ordinary people taken off the street, I expect to find about 60–70% of them to be moderately to very healthy – precisely the ones who, when asked in a survey, say that they feel well and healthy. Naturally, these people seldom visit the doctor because they have no reason to. Yet if you examine these people closely enough, you will indeed find some unresolved emotional conflicts. But if these people feel healthy, their conflicts remain dormant and they don't need any treatment.

In my experience, in fact, activating these dormant conflicts in order to treat them is often extraordinarily risky. I have seen patients whose suffering can be traced back to the very moment some conflicts were artificially aroused. This can also happen in aggressive encounter groups, overly intensive meditation, and other psychoactive techniques.

Many people who have been harmed by sects also fall in this category. Careful questioning reveals that these people often accurately sensed that the therapy in question was not going to be good for them. An inner voice warned them to move on, but some self-appointed Guru or therapist thought he knew better, or the person was too timid to break it off, and so began the whole problem. If, on the other hand, you have the sure inner feeling that you need to be treated, because you feel unbalanced and unwell and sick, that's a very different matter. Yet my feeling is that the percentage of those who start out relatively healthy and then come to harm from various psychoactive techniques is significantly higher than we think.

In my opinion, the best course is a gentle non-provoking examination in which one checks the organism with energetic measurement methods for blockages or other disturbances. I allow myself to be guided by the wisdom of the patient's organism, so I don't assume the role of the "omniscient" and "omnipotent" therapist, but rather remain modestly in the background as the questioner. Nature then reveals on its own what it prefers, as corresponding disturbances in the subtle-body field become discernible. If no disturbances are found, then I perform no treatment.

Based on my experiences described here, therefore, I'd like to recommend emphatically not waking up dormant conflicts. One can tell quite clearly when conflicts become active and need to be treated. In the chapters that follow, I'll describe the signs of conflict activation in greater detail. Basically, one may say that conflicts don't need to be treated as long as one feels tolerably well and healthy. I'll deal later with some exceptions to this rule, i.e., in cases of purely physical disorders in which the feeling of apparent health can be deceptive. Fortunately, that is relatively rare, such that for most people their feeling of needing help or not is generally reliable.

I'd like to turn next to the description of the conflicts, in particular with respect to their size, significance, and interplay. The previous chapter spoke of the ocean of the subconscious. It is in this gigantic ocean that we store our memories, feelings, and thoughts, and conflicts are a part of this. I'll admit that, for many readers, the concept of "conflict" takes some getting used to, either because they find it too psychological or they associate it exclusively with interpersonal strife. Yet I think the history of psychoanalysis has shown that technical terms can take on more general colloquial meaning

Organ or Disease	Symptoms	Meaning (some examples only, i.e., more meanings are possible)	Associated Chakra
Sinuses	Chronic colds	Suppressed crying or disapproval	Chakra 6
Cervical spine	Neck stiffness	Stubborn, unyielding	Chakra 5
Thoracic spine	Pain between the shoulder blades	Hidden sorrow	Chakra 4
Lumbar spine	Lower back pain, sciatica	Sadness	Chakras 1 & 2
Tension headache	Annular headache	Anger, tension	Chakras 5, 6, & 7
Globus hystericus	Lump in throat	Anxiety, fear	Chakra 5
Lungs	Shortness of breath, chest complaint	Anxiety, fear	Chakra 4
Heart	Cardiac pain, palpitation	Fear, grief	Chakra 4
Upper abdomen	Stomach ache	Rage, anger	Chakra 3
Bladder	Strangury	Anxiety, fear	Chakras 1 & 2
Intestines	Diarrhea	Angst	Chakras 1, 2, & 3
Intestines	Constipation	Anger, tension, wrath	Chakra 1, 2, & 3
Knee	Knee pain	Lack of self-esteem	Chakras 1 & 3
Varicose veins	Heaviness in the legs	Feeling of not being grounded	Chakras 1 & 2
Warts	Skin itching	Inability to demarcate	Chakras 4, 5, & 6

amazingly quickly. It is thus my hope that the technical terms I have chosen will likewise soon find wider acceptance.

I described earlier how it is that conflicts arise. They can be regarded as unprocessed emotional memories that derive from particularly painful emotional situations. Trauma thus represents the basal situation of conflict formation – even when events, as viewed from the outside, might not seem at all traumatic. The crucial point is that overwhelming emotional pain represents the primeval trauma in conflict formation. Basically, conflicts can be active or dormant. As a rule, dormant conflicts don't generate symptoms, and when they harm us, it's over the very long term and in a way that is extremely hard to notice. Normally, dormant conflicts cannot be measured by energy testing, and even then only by means of special short-term activating substance mixtures. In what follows, I'll be talking about active conflicts, whose presence one is aware of – say, by feeling tired or unwell more often, reacting more irritably than usual, or by just not feeling emotionally centered. Conflicts inhibit normal energy flow, making us feel tired and unwell, for example.

Also, conflicts provoke long-lasting changes in the way we experience events, in that we internally "stumble," time and time again, over the same emotional contents. The painful emotional contents within the conflict have not been processed, which alters and distorts our internal perception. Now, the tragic thing about this perceptual distortion is the peculiar paradox that the largest conflicts are the ones we are least conscious of – for the greater the conflict, the deeper it tends to be buried in the subconscious; the greater the conflict, the harder it is for the victim to become conscious of it. And yet, astonishingly, even deep-rooted conflicts can be consciously present – but they are strangely situated in the fringes of one's "field of view": one sees them and yet does not. Psychoanalysis terms this process repression. The reason is that large conflicts harbor particularly painful emotional contents, so that the person does not want to notice such extremely unpleasant emotional contents and thus quite logically tunes them out.

Basically, we can distinguish between small, medium and large conflicts. Conflicts get larger the more painful the unprocessed emotional event was and the farther back in the past it lies. A small "current" conflict is normally very close to conscious level, and its origin is relatively recent. Thus, when people are asked how they feel, they just need to reflect briefly before finding the responsible *current conflict* in the surface layers of their subconscious. In the case of these near-conscious conflicts, people know at once what the matter is. "My, but you look tense!" you say sympathetically. "Yeah, a few weeks ago I got real ticked off at my neighbor for making a racket in the middle of the night." We thus see in their poor appearance how the anger is eating them up. This kind of anger can give rise to many kinds of symptoms and ailments; it can "eat a hole in your stomach" or be "a pain in the neck" (because, in a quarrel, one doesn't want to be the one to give in). Characteristics of a current conflict include instinctive feelings such as jealousy, wanting to hold on to power, sexual desire, envy, or resentment.

A current conflict generates direct and unmediated symptoms known medically as **organ language**. This leads to a conflict idiom, including such colloquial phrases as: "his heart fell" or "she was heartbroken." Thus the lovelorn get heart pangs and moist hands, people react to disheartening family situations with breathing problems, students fearing an upcoming exam suffer an attack of diarrhea. Organ language is almost always a sure sign of a small, superficial, and near-conscious conflict. Still, one shouldn't overrate organ language; although it points to non-trivial conflict contents, they are nevertheless basically harmless.

Organ language's significance is often overrated: not everyone with an upset stomach is "fed up"; not everyone with a sinus inflammation is suppressing secret weeping. Organ language can only provide meaningful assistance if one relates it to recent ailments that have in some way strongly upset the person emotionally. If someone gets a stiff neck right after an argument has been settled, it could indicate suppressed emotion arising from a subconscious unwillingness to give in. One can very often see organ language in emotionally open persons such as children or naturally-reacting adults. In primitive cultures and in the case of the hysterical character type (about which more later), one sees organ language unusually frequently, even in larger conflicts. Therefore, organ language often reveals something about emotional openness and the underlying expressed emotional intensity.

The next issue relates to healing the emotions involved, which are often perceived at this emotional level as *insults*. The best course is to persuade these people to let go of their suppressed feelings, just to let loose and roar, or cry, or pour out their soul in a long heart-to-heart. In cases like these, a Best Friend is the best therapy. Yet this kind of talk is not always enough to loosen up the emotions. This might be because a person simply isn't ready yet ("too stubborn, too mad") or the feelings are too strong ("can't forgive that quite yet"). Anyone who has ever tried to quell a student's test anxiety or comfort the lovelorn can write a book about how hard this is. The psychotherapeutic procedure on this level is called "supportive conversation," in which we try to give emotionally groggy people some helpful support. "Keep your chin up!" is the colloquial variation, as we comfort and encourage these people.

Especially for people to whom *psyche* is a dirty word and who take any sign of uncertainty as a personal failure (commonly adult males, macho types not exactly in touch with their feelings, nor wanting to be), energetically calming naturopathic remedies[37] are a great help. After all, you wouldn't get very far with them just with words. Children also respond particularly well to psychoenergetic tranquilizers, without having to address the upsetting conflict theme. Of course, the best route to healing is direct dissolution of the affected feelings. In most cases, the victims of painful emotional attacks turn to alcohol and other drugs as their means of running away from them. That they thereby betray themselves is common knowledge, but it is, after all, the "easiest" way. It is a comfort to know that these small emotional conflicts eventually "burn out" on their own.

Those wishing to do something for themselves and to find out what current conflicts are behind their ailments can

---

[37] It seems to me that classical homeopathy is an outstanding healing method for curing these current conflicts. Their symptoms listed in the medication picture very often correspond to current conflicts. The blossom agents of the British homeopath Dr. Edward BACH can also treat such conflicts quite rapidly and gently. The proper agent is best ascertained with an energetic testing procedure. Since segmental vegetative dysfunctions are often encountered, one can use the appropriate Chakra remedy (Chavita) to re-loosen up the *Vegetativum* and get it vibrating again. There is a reference in the appendices of this book regarding availability of the remedies mentioned.

best do this in a state of deep relaxation. One directs one's consciousness to the affected organ or disease region and tries, very carefully, to approach the hidden feeling, all the while thinking with loving and tender care about the ailment. "How're you feeling? What's bothering you?" one asks gently, as if talking to a small child. Just as a bashful and injured person will, sobbing, suddenly give free rein to his feelings when enfolded in a loving embrace, so is it with the disease. I recommend having a trustworthy and understanding person nearby who can help out in the event of an intense emotional outbreak.

At a deeper layer of the subconscious, we come upon the medium-sized conflicts that are fairly inaccessible to everyday consciousness. We find ourselves in the middle of the emotional body, where we often encounter emotional themes from childhood. This is the domain of psychoanalysis. The organ language of the upper layers no longer applies because the emotional causes have become too uniform and unconscious. Many errors are often committed in this context, and much confusion and needless suffering is generated through erroneous backgrounds to such diseases.[38]

In the worst case, simplistic psychologizing creates new emotional "knots" instead of recognizing the existing conflicts – to say nothing of dissolving them. Unfortunately, uncounted psychological counselors and thousands of printed pages in illustrated magazines belong in this category. I won't take this any further, leaving it to the reader to evaluate these pseudo solutions that can be found on every street corner. Although they are offered up so often, they are nevertheless totally false in their basic approach and, regrettably, often lead to secondary damage.

The conflicts of the middle subconscious are especially hard to put into words. They are grasped indirectly, raised into daylight via dreams, associations, and hypnotic states. We thus know empirically that very few people can say directly which medium-sized and large conflicts they are hauling around – although, interestingly enough, spouses and close friends almost always know. For instance, a woman told me, after I had examined her husband: "That spiritual theme you found in my husband? I've known about it for a long time now." So we usually find out things about ourselves when we have our subconscious problems reflected through other people, since in our conflicts sits our Shadow; this is what psychotherapy calls the rejected and repressed feelings that cast a sort of shadow of the personality, as our body does in the late afternoon sun.

I'd like to designate the middle-level conflicts as **side conflicts**, because they appear "beside" the Central Conflict (which I'll get to next). This doesn't mean they are negligible; like the Central Conflict, they have an important emotional function. In the emotional maturation process, side conflicts supply missing character traits, like an interpreter who translates a foreign language into our native tongue. A person of a certain character type has trouble understanding other character types. By developing emotional conflicts that belong to other (foreign) character types, a person's understanding is forced to expand. Side conflicts thus lead to a gradual broadening of our personality. Through side conflicts, we mature emotionally and can thereby attain to a better understanding of other people.

Side conflicts arise frequently during early childhood development. When we ask hypnotized patients what is behind a side conflict, they tell us childhood memories. They report having felt horribly abandoned, and this has now become a basic feeling. Or that they had an uncomfortable feeling that their siblings were favored over them. Unlike a current conflict, these deep-seated side conflicts are never forgotten. Yet they lie in storage in complete silence, detectable only by the fact that they alter the affected person's personality, like a magnet that attracts iron filings. This generates distortions of self-image and perception of reality. Conflicts deform normal personality. Specialists designate such people as neurotic. People think, for example, that others always get preferential treatment, or that they've been cruelly abandoned – ignoring the fact that these are outdated childhood experiences.

The larger conflicts get, the more a person suffers – and not just that person, but the people around him as well. The side conflicts – along with the largest conflict we have, the **Central Conflict** – provoke all manner of social repercussions. Although a small current conflict can be regarded as each person's private affair that (unlike the larger conflicts) doesn't tend to lead to social problems, in the case of side conflicts, the social impact comes much more to the fore. Since larger conflicts are significantly more subconscious, their unnoticed hidden influence on feelings and actions increases much more strongly. The most severe repercussions – with respect to both the conflict host and friends, family, and associates – are those deriving from the side conflicts and the largest conflict a person possesses: the Central Conflict. I'd next like to sketch out the most significant consequences in rough outline, then elucidate them more comprehensively and in greater detail in subsequent chapters.

The first impression one gets from hosts of larger active conflicts is a feeling of unease and a sense of rejection. This is because each distortion of our *persona* mask makes us

---

[38] The hysterical character type is an exception — which can, amazingly, clothe even deep subconscious conflicts in an ostensible organ language. In the initial stages of psychoanalysis, this led FREUD to the discovery of the subconscious. The French psychiatrist CHARCOT drew FREUD's attention to the sexual significance of the *Arc de circle* among his female patients. These hysterics, frantically arching their bodies about, under hypnosis, without exception had sexual wishful dreams that were explicitly depicted through spastic flexing and bending of the body. This led psychosomatic theory to adopt a very biased position, as it derived from these observations a universality that continues to this day. Just as many conflicts have no subconscious sexual content whatever, many organ ailments are not so superficially symbolic (nor have they anything meaningful to say) as is so often claimed.

unattractive, at least with respect to emotionally healthy fellow humans. Conflicts are a largely ignored cause of social inequality, and their impact is far greater in an open democratic society than in the Middle Ages, for instance. Back then, the emotionally disturbed king's son continued to be the undisputed heir to the throne despite his unpleasant personality traits. Nowadays, a child with a large active conflict becomes a hyperkinetic "Fidgety Frank" whose progress in school is hampered from the very beginning. Later on in life, large conflicts (as soon as they become active) are often the true causes of career downturns, divorces, and all manner of other social problems.

I'd like to illustrate this with a typical example from my clinical practice:

Seven-year-old Michael comes with his mother and his younger sister (who is completely healthy and normal) because he has been a problem all his life. Even pregnancy and birth were a total fiasco. During pregnancy, his mother suffered from itching skin eruptions, and during the birthing process, both mother and child fought for their lives. His mother is at her wits' end and is seriously considering giving up Michael, even though she loves him no end. But she can no longer endure the ceaseless power struggles, the sleepless nights due to his nocturnal wanderings and the extremely stressful constant tension, because Michael turns every activity – be it ever so trivial – into a dramatic occasion. He has trouble concentrating at school. He is unpopular with his fellow students, and he only laughs when all around him are crying. In the energy test, I ascertain extremely low emotional and mental readings, as is common in hyperkinetic children. I also find an enormous Central Conflict that is the true cause of Michael's problems, and which has to do with restlessness and tenseness. The mother confirms that this outlines Michael's basic problem perfectly, since he never calms down and cannot relax. The energy readings of Michael's conflict in the energy test are in fact greater than his own! Basically, then, Michael doesn't live his own life at all, but rather that of his conflict – which, like all conflicts, exhibits self-destructive and socially harmful characteristics.

Amazingly enough, there are many people with large conflicts who are able to lead socially acceptable lives. How can this be? In my experience, the reason is that conflicts often do not attract attention because all the members of a social group have them in common, i.e., each of these people has similarly stored-up subconscious problems. This gives rise to a uniformity of neurotic equality, which can at times put its stamp on an entire society. Ethnically related populations often have very similar **character masks**. "Character mask" is psychoanalyst Wilhelm REICH's designation for the totality of a particular neurotic structure, for instance the authoritarian character type who "tramples on those below and bows to those above." Thus, any unprejudiced and liberal-minded person visiting the witch's cauldron that was

Nazi Germany in 1933 would be appalled by the uniformity of the prevailing neurosis and would find the "ugly German" repellent. And yet, there were also many totally enthusiastic foreigners who were fascinated by this up-and-coming fascism. There was a feeling of something big in the air, and great enthusiasm, which many found infectious, and they got swept up in it, as numerous older patients have described it to me.

Which "strings can be made to sound" seems to be crucial to the basic feeling that such pan-social phenomena can trigger in us. For example, if some people are carrying around a large conflict consisting of subconscious resentment and great frustration, they will be magically attracted by the fascist's promises of liberation, because it holds out to them the prospect of finally obtaining comprehensive satisfaction of their feelings of frustration. On top of that, they are promised the secretly longed-for opportunity to vent their rage, which they had so agonizingly been missing.

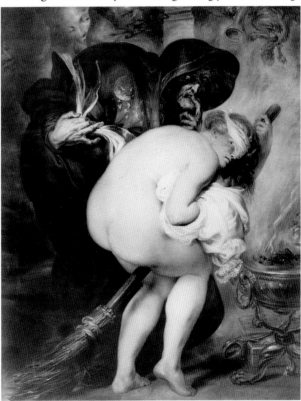

The witch is the ideal projection figure of evil, forbidden sex and the secretl yearning for sexual debauchery. Yet, as one who knows about the supernatural and the subconscious, about magic and hallucinogenic plants, the witch's significance is far greater – for the witch has passed on the shamans' ancient wisdom that was suppressed by Christianity and which we are only now rediscovering at great effort.
The Young Witch *painting by A. Wiertz, 1850*

What beckons, ultimately, is not just individual happiness, but rather collective contentment with their own kind. And, as an added extra free bonus, they get the opportunity, as fascists, to take out their deep-seated frustration on scapegoats such as of Jews or gypsies, without being punished for it.

It goes without saying that such horrible events as the extermination of Jews in concentration camps are not merely a matter of simple neurosis. That would trivialize and individualize the tragedy far too much, and would, moreover, fail to take into account adequately the extreme nature of the phenomenon that underlies such horrors. Psychology is helpless in the face of such phenomena and, in my opinion, has no persuasive explanation as to why civilized people turn into such horrific beasts. My suggestion to explain such things is based on the destructive force of the Central Conflict. Psychodynamically speaking, we are dealing with actual externalized **character wars**. We are faced with deep-seated feelings that come into contact with our Central Conflict. This is why issues between ethnic groups and political systems are life-and-death matters, and the entire problem complex takes on extremely tragic aspects. We can't begin to grasp the monstrous dynamism that arises when incompatible ethnic groups collide until we become aware of the subconscious existential motif. At bottom, such people are fighting an existential battle that, despite its internal emotional roots, they project outward. These collective neuroses then lead to civil wars and on up to the extreme case of genocide.

I must admit that it took me a long time to realize what was actually going on here. Why do Catholics and Protestants bash each other's heads in? What is truly behind the enormous hatred that drives many fundamentalist Muslims? It was only after I had identified the character types and realized their significance that the scope of the fundamental incompatibility of certain character types became clear to me. We say, colloquially and quite correctly, that we "hate [a certain person] to death." Anyone who senses the aggression and hatred behind "ethnic" jokes (in which cultures ridicule each other) is experiencing a similar, universal phenomenon. Fights between persons and wars between nations are very similar processes once we understand the subconscious dynamics.

Many movie directors, like political demagogues, are experts at working with the character types of the "good, brave, sympathetic" hero and the "wicked, nasty, mean, evil" villain. Nazi propaganda films depicted the ugly, emotionally unstable, and deceitful dark-haired Jew versus the morally upstanding, handsome, and noble blonde Aryan. Actually, this represents the subtle ideological exploitation of antithetical character traits. People are by nature oppositional, and this disparity is exploited politically to agitate groups against each other.

But these behaviors can be found everywhere in everyday life. In the smallest social venue of all, many families have their mini-wars and sibling rivalries stemming from the dissonance between differing character types. To bring it down to a simple formulation: some people cannot understand each other because they are far too different. Of course, the lack of understanding is not by itself a sufficient explanation, since the debilitating frustration of the Central Conflict needs to be added to the mix in order to ignite the bomb of hatred. Together, these two elements create a highly explosive mixture.

Turning again to individuals and their problems, we find that many character disorders are hard to detect. This is because many individuals have learned how to hide their dark side from others. In fact, repulsive and socially proscribed character traits are concealed with particular subtlety, so much so that the person can even become convinced of his own innocence. This is why the dark side of other persons is often hard to spot at first.

"Boy, was I wrong about him!" we exclaim, greatly disappointed, when we have overlooked a person's dark side for a long time. We ask ourselves whether the person was too clever or we were too gullible. Often our entire life experience is not enough to anticipate the snares and traps of our life together that will eventually lead to problems. It is only in the close interaction of marriage that we have the opportunity to get to know another person's "quirks." Experienced marriage counselors recommend trial marriage, since we can only get to know the other person properly once life's everyday problems begin.

Speaking of which, I keep hearing the most amazing things from my patients. Surprisingly, many divorced patients confess to having sensed their marital difficulties quite early in the relationship. They knew, right from the beginning, what was coming. Their problem was actually somewhere else entirely. Realistically, therefore, one should ask oneself, in the early stages of a relationship, whether one would still love the other person even if he or she were to keep his or her worst "quirks."

I already mentioned that married couples are reliable indicators for the themes of the big subconscious conflicts. "My husband always feels unfairly discriminated against, that's deeply anchored in him," says the wife when, in the energy test on her husband, I ascertain an enormous Central Conflict with the theme *Mistrust*. It doesn't take much imagination to picture how it would be for us to have someone as a next-door neighbor or office co-worker whom everyone basically mistrusted. In the case of a husband with the *Mistrust* theme, if he is a tax examiner or police detective, then that is clearly a different matter: it takes little thought to come up with the reason for it, since, in an environment that is already saturated with deep suspicion, the emotional problem of a co-worker is hardly going to stand out, since it is a desirable professional trait.

Emotional dark sides can thus be hard to detect when

their content is masked by socially desirable features. In fact, in most cases the person in question does his job especially well, since he "takes it to heart," living out his conflict contents in his work: as a vice-squad detective, say, with the theme *Mistrust*, to suspect everyone of being a "perp" until proven otherwise. Or to pursue every injustice with particular passion because it accords with his basic mood to see to it that (like a type of Robin Hood) justice prevails, because deep frustration cries out for compensation.

Often, one cannot recognize conflicts when they totally contradict reality. In such cases, no one would come up with such a "crazy idea." This category includes absurd beliefs such as the distorted self-image of the lovely Marilyn MONROE, who considered herself to be abysmally ugly. After her suicide, one can surmise that her secret confession to friends that she considered herself to be an outwardly repulsive person sprang from her years of depression. I'd like to give a typical example of how external appearance can often be deceptive in the case of inner emotional themes as well. External behavior is then intended, paradoxically, to conceal inner feelings, thus serving to maintain social and opposite-sex roles.

We project an image so as to make a good impression on other people. No woman is attracted to a "Caspar Milquetoast" and no beauty queen dares let an inferiority complex show. You can see how widespread the problem is in the increasing popularity of cosmetic surgery. No one suspects a softie behind the especially tough-looking man who seeks to compensate his character weakness with muscular strength. Time and again, the gentle nature of (outwardly daunting) bodybuilders never fails to surprise me, their friendliness and warmth being in such sharp contrast to their bellicose bodies.

Psychology calls it *compensation*. The vernacular puts it this way: "Older men with impaired sexual potency like to drive sporty cars" and comes to the conclusion that every overstatement signals an inferiority complex ("… he must really need it!"). Therefore, outward appearance can be the very opposite of an inner feeling, especially when dealing with subconscious themes. The psychoanalyst ADLER built up his entire theory of the subconscious (*Individual Psychology*) from the concept of *striving for recognition/superiority/power*. ADLER viewed the feeling of inferiority as the beginning of all emotional disorders. To my mind, he has thereby erroneously turned a symptom (a consequence of conflict formation) into the actual cause – since inferiority feelings disappear quickly once the underlying conflicts have been dissolved.

Still, ADLER's inferiority concept is to a certain degree correct. Famous men have very often been shorter than average, as if their greater fame were meant to compensate their lesser frame. ADLER speaks of substandard organs, inasmuch as such physical weaknesses bring about emotional disturbances. The example of the celebrated orator DEMOSTHENES is often cited, who overcame his speech impediment with pebbles, which he stuffed in his mouth and then attempted to speak in a loud, clear voice over the sound of the roaring surf. One can thus become enamored of the idea that ADLER's theory of bodily-conditioned inferiority is correct.

Despite these seemingly sound arguments, I maintain that the feeling of inferiority can only result from a correlative inner emotional frustration. Thus, there are short men and ugly women who are indifferent to their physical appearance, because they are internally satisfied with themselves. Inner contentment is conditioned on feeling well inside and being in harmony with oneself, which ultimately means being conflict-free. Moreover, the example of Marilyn MONROE has also shown that even an outwardly flawless woman is not immune to emotional problems. Therefore, the important thing with respect to inferiority feelings is emotional conflict themes, which seek out physical weak points in order to attach their *raison d'etre* to them. As has been said, the most convincing argument is that when emotional conflicts are healed, the associated feelings of inferiority vanish as well.

Basically, we assume that everyone tries to make the best possible impression and to conceal personal conflicts from others as much as possible. But there are behavioral disorders that contradict these basic rules, such as when an undesired impression is deliberately provoked. Why do people do such silly things? One asks oneself what kinds of subconscious motivating factors might be at play when people behave in a totally improper manner, so that others turn against them. I'd like to present a particularly drastic example to illuminate the emotional background with particular clarity. We all know, for example, the role of the genuine "SOB" (sonofabitch). Everyone knows these annoying dramatic talents that cut a swath of social havoc and cause "God and the world" to rise up against them – and people exclaim "Thank God!" when such people leave the stage.

Amazingly enough, conflict healing in children leads quickly to dramatic improvements of their behavioral disorders (I'll have more to say on this later on in some case histories). When these children show up for their second appointment, I sometimes can't believe my eyes as I watch how polite and well-behaved these previously difficult children can be. We see from this how devastating can be the effects of conflicts on behavior and conduct, especially in children, and how beneficial the consequences of healing their conflicts and energy blocks.

In this context, the situation with children is special because their social interaction abilities are even less developed. They abreact their internal tensions and frustrations directly and unfiltered, as they let everyone in the vicinity in on them. In my experience, subconscious themes do not play the leading role they do in adults, although they do have some significance. The following account thus applies primarily to adults with behavioral disorders. This category encompasses innocuous variations on up to grumblers, psychopaths, and other sorts of people who generate terror. Ultimately, I'm convinced that even terrorism can be understood as far as its subconscious dynamics and origins are concerned. I'd here like to leave out social and religious motifs in order not to exceed the bounds of the topic. As I see it, in most cases they are of secondary importance, which becomes clear when one considers that most terrorists come from affluent social circles. In terrorism, the conflict's resulting inner emotional frustration is very often the true driving force.

Also, too little attention is paid to the fact that terrorists play an overall social role that transcends the scapegoat phenomenon, and whose function can be compared to that of a catalyst. The phenomenon of terrorism thus also has to encompass the psychodynamic order of events in the society, if we wish to understand it. In a sense, the frustrated terrorist is not conceivable without a frustrated society. If the members of a society were to behave more calmly, more liberally – and at the same time stronger emotionally, this would represent real progress. The terrorist's emotional strength feeds on the emotional weakness of the people he terrorizes, long before any terrorist act is carried out.

But before we drift any farther into the realm of therapy, I'd like to investigate the unique phenomenon of antisocial behavior more intensively. When we study the intrapsychic processes involved in ostentatiously antisocial behavior, I'd like to assert that the malefactor gains the inner emotional upper hand when he gets others to rise up against him. More than likely, there will be a large conflict behind it all, which has taken control over thoughts and actions. The "SOB" has a conflict theme that evokes antisocial and emotionally nasty behavior, such as "secretly being inferior." The feeling of inferiority is then anticipated as he tries to show off in a particularly annoying manner in an effort to conceal his own feeling of inferiority and, ultimately, to evoke it eventually in the other person! For it is well known that the truly superior and strong person has no need of such emotionally nasty behavior. So, when someone takes on the role of "Mr. Icky," he often feels inferior inside. The message being sent is: "You may think I'm a repulsive person whom you can look down your nose at, but I don't give a damn what you think of me!"

At this point, we have arrived at a most unusual place, that of **_emotional transference_**. In psychoanalysis, this is the phenomenon whereby others evoke emotions in us that are actually their own. Just as enthusiasm can be contagious, another person's sadness, rancor, restlessness, and such can infect us. In the patient dialogue, the analyst pays attention to the feelings and thoughts that the patient evokes in the analyst's own mind, and calls the process _transference_. Generally speaking, neurotics tend to evoke an unpleasant mood of discontent, of feeling hassled and coerced. One

sometimes senses a vast emotional emptiness and a pasty viscosity that can be greatly reinforced by the monotonous vocal style of many patients. Experienced doctors usually sense what is emotionally depressing the patient, and can observe quite a bit of this depression and emotional distress reflected in their own perceptions. With transference, they learn something about the patient's subconscious problems that is otherwise not explicitly vocalized.

In addition, transference has a general social impact, in that nobody can conceal forever what is wrong inside emotionally. Eventually, it comes out and, usually, the feeling "I don't like him," when put into words is nothing other than "He brings out feelings in me that I don't like." When we take a closer look at the source of this antipathy, we almost always discover conflicts dealing with rejection, discomfort, and the like. If we then look into the person who said "I don't like him," we will in most cases find conflicts that have been induced to express themselves. Therefore, there can be no objectivity when it comes to transference because the participants' emotional distortions build up and reinforce themselves.

The great difficulty in differentiating cause and effect (victimizer and victim) becomes particularly clear in those situations in which it would seem that guilt can be assigned rather quickly. In therapy groups intended to cure wife-beating husbands, it is striking how often victim and victimizer get interchanged. During a therapy session, strong wife-beaters turn into whimpering little heaps of misery behind which the child can be seen who was beaten in childhood (and who, inevitably, arouses the pity of the abused wife, who thereupon almost always forgives her abuser!).

The battered child internalizes the horrible message: "I am worthless and that's why I am being beaten like a piece of filth." Eventually, the battered child becomes an adult and begins to project his feeling of worthlessness onto his wife, transforming himself from victim to victimizer – which is a morally reprehensible, but an emotionally understandable, type of reparation. Ultimately, the abused wife's contempt leads to the re-establishment of the abusing husband's "I am worthless" feeling, since, after a beating, his wife despises him all the more and considers him worthless as a husband.

Reincarnation therapists and depth psychologists have made yet another interesting discovery, namely that the child has by no means entered into this situation innocently, but rather sought out its parents before birth with the firm intention of entering this situation. The (pre-birth) child says to itself: "I want parents who will beat me" and thus seeks out parents who fit this pattern. We know about these event sequences from countless therapy sessions in which patients in deep contemplative states have relived pre-birth situations. In these sessions, submerged recollections surface frequently, with a certain regularity.

Interestingly, self-injury and self-punishment desires in later sessions can often be traced back to still further situations in even earlier lives.

Before getting tangled up in interminable chains of repercussions that some traumatic experience has triggered in some former life, I'd like to suggest looking at the entire progression from the viewpoint of the conflict. In the chapter on the origin of conflicts, I mentioned that the conflict can be viewed as a kind of autonomous life form. Living creatures are characterized by the will to survive, and they do everything they can to ensure their continued existence. If one looks at the entire issue of victimizer and victim as an aspect of a conflict, which as an independent being wants to be fed and to survive, most of the fateful sequences of events can be understood and classified with no problem whatsoever. From the standpoint of the conflict with the theme *Worthlessness*, things are going well when the husband beats his wife because, after all, he is then keeping the conflict alive by supplying it with fresh energy (the wife's contempt)!

There are basically two ways that conflict hosts can make sure that – in a type of self-fulfilling prophecy – conflict themes are fulfilled and validated: by either passively-introvertedly or actively-extrovertedly seeing to their fulfillment. If they do it passively, then they'll make sure always to get the role of the one discriminated against, e.g., either through exaggerated obsequiousness or shyness in their dealings with others. If the active route is chosen, they'll play the braggart who always interrupts others, or the SOB who uses extreme measures to get others to unite against him. Such people need to be taught a lesson – and they are, e.g., when they are skipped over for promotion, for example. Braggarts get exactly that feeling of being discriminated against that they had subconsciously (deliberately) provoked in their associates.

The crucial factor that decides whether or not we react actively or passively is the **Central Conflict**, which strongly dominates our subconscious realm. At this point, we have gone down a level in the subconscious and find ourselves in a completely nonverbal and extremely subconscious region. The Central Conflict is the character scaffolding that most strongly influences our thoughts and feelings, and which (necessarily so) resides in the deepest subconscious. On the somatic level, this subconscious dynamism manifests itself in posture, ingrained movement patterns, and personal facial expressions – all traits of which we are deeply unaware, and which are therefore extremely difficult to change.

On the interpersonal level, the Central Conflict regulates behavior by making us act either passively or actively. The numerous themes that it can contain will be discussed thoroughly in subsequent chapters; for now, we are concerned with the Central Conflict's structure and mode of action – which we can only fully understand, in my opinion, if we accept the concept of reincarnation. Everything points to the character scaffolding, with its underlying Central Conflict, being kept alive and conveyed through numerous reincarnations.

Whoever thinks reincarnation unlikely can for now just as well imagine the set character types as being nonverbal molds that crucially shape the infantile mind. For myself, I am firmly convinced that reincarnation exists, if only because of the logical conclusiveness of the theories presented here. The model of (Central Conflict) character types, as well as the strong prenatal preformation of personality and many intrapsychic contents, cannot, in my opinion, be explained exclusively in the here and now – through genetics, for instance. We need reincarnation to make any progress and to decipher the greater underlying contextual framework.

So let's assume, for the time being, that reincarnation exists as an actual phenomenon. Much then becomes understandable and can effortlessly be integrated into a comprehensive contextual explanatory system. Thus, we as individual souls can "stay in character" from reincarnation to reincarnation. We can then view the Central Conflict as the true starting point of a permanent personality. Like a sturdy anchor, the Central Conflict sees to it that, at the deepest levels of the subconscious, we can determine how we perceive ourselves and the world around us – as well as how we will act in certain situations. Therefore, we most likely keep the same Central Conflict as we pass through our many lives.

That sounds rather pessimistic at first, as if our fate were to have gone astray and been deformed by the Central Conflict. But this overlooks the positive and life-affirming aspects linked to its surfacing, because it is an indispensable support of our entire existence! One may even go so far as to declare that the Central Conflict is the fundamental framework of Self-consciousness. As the largest component of our spiritual shadow, it forms the indispensable precondition for the light of the origin of consciousness and maturation of the Self – for without the Central Conflict we would not know who we really are. In the next chapter, I'll endeavor to substantiate this sweeping thesis.

The Central Conflict is found in four variations that result in four different character types. I will describe these four character types in the following chapters, and attempt to flesh them out with concrete examples. Essentially, to recognize them, we need to follow some basic rules having to do with emotional maturity and the level of character development. The Central Conflict has fairly little effect in the early phases of a personality, so that in a weakly developed personality, the underlying character type can scarcely be made out. This applies during childhood as well as to relatively undifferentiated adults.

The more clearly our personality is cultivated – as we continue to develop emotionally – the more vigorously our associated character type comes to the fore. The highpoint

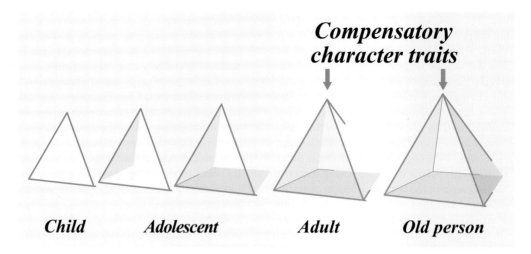

Compensatory character traits

Child   **Adolescent**   **Adult**   **Old person**

of individual uniqueness is likewise the Central Conflict's acme. As our psyche continues to mature, our character traits begin to re-coalesce because personal maturity leads to the development of compensatory character traits. This is why it is much harder to classify the character type of people who have done a lot of work on themselves and are therefore mentally mature. Nevertheless, you can almost always make a clear assignment once you get to know a person better. The structures of the underlying character type are clearly discernible for every person.

The illustration on this page represents the processes involved in the maturation of character type. Character is symbolized as a triangle, and its maturation (through compensatory characteristics) as a pyramidal quadrilateral (symbol of wholeness).

There are four discernible maturation stages that can be related to the most significant biological phases of our lives, namely childhood, youth, adulthood, and old age. The older we get, the more mature and balanced our Character should have become.

I'd like now to address the character types themselves, of which there are four variants:

· The schizoid type (element: Earth, melancholy – "sad and withdrawn")
· The depressive type (element: Fire, choleric – "furious and irascible")
· The obsessive-compulsive type (element: Water, phlegmatic – "quiet and hesitant")
· The hysterical type (element: Air, sanguine – "mood swings and quick to enthuse")

It isn't hard to recognize the four elements discussed in earlier chapters. They reflect an emotional affinity for the coarse-material, which is equivalent to a very profound

blend of emotional mood and metabolic "mood." Thus each person has a fundamental feeling that is anchored quite deeply in metabolism and is affiliated with one of the four elements. Since this element correlates with character type, a choleric type (for example) is to some extent choleric due to a choleric metabolism. Psyche and Soma thereby form a seamless union, and the body collaborates perfectly with fundamental mental efforts.

I will touch later on the precise origin and far-reaching significance of the Central Conflict; right now, I'd like to touch on the relationship of the side conflicts to the Central Conflict – for one may well ask: what's the point of this pandemonium of differing conflicts? What's the benefit for the individual and his or her developmental possibilities? The easiest way to understand why we have this inner emotional layering of different conflicts is to picture an orchestra.

Within this "Conflict Orchestra," the Central Conflict is the master melody, played by the most important instrument. Now, a character with only a single master melody is fairly intolerable, both for the individual and for others, as hard to take as a single instrument playing monotonously to itself. Yet our mood determines more than just the emotional effect we have on our fellow humans: personal development and individual happiness are determined over the long term by our fundamental "mood." All this is dependent on our characterological *bandwidth*: the greater the bandwidth, the happier and more socially successful we can be, because our mood becomes ever more harmonious and satisfied.

The side conflicts represent the accompaniment to the solitary figure of the Central Conflict, helping to enlarge the mind's "Conflict Orchestra" bandwidth. It is only through side conflicts that we learn to empathize with people of different character typologies, since we sense – as a personal experience – how it looks emotionally in the other person's interior space. True empathy is thus only possible given a great deal of previous experience with numerous conflicts extending over different emotional regions. People with this prior experience are felt to be especially life-experienced and congenial. Side conflicts are thus a valuable treasure that serves as a mental supporting beam, to grow inside the process of emotional maturation, in which the characteristics and feelings of all four character types have been integrated. "Fourness" or quadrinity (represented as a quadrilateral) as the goal of our emotional maturation is thus only possible with the aid of the side conflicts.

The illustration on page 168 shows the connection between the Central Conflict and side conflicts.

How did this model come about? When patients are examined psychoenergetically for the first time, we find, in many cases, either no conflicts at all or else only current conflicts. The longer a patient is treated, the deeper the conflicts that rise to the surface. Like an onion, very often the first thing encountered is a current conflict. Later on, a number of side conflicts appear – usually five or six at the most – only to disappear once more and then reappear. It is reminiscent of a theatrical performance in which only one Act can be onstage at a time. Watching several scenes being staged simultaneously would in all probability totally confuse us, which is why this is an extremely rare occurrence. Evidently, the psyche feels the same way, so its prudent direction sees to it that there is usually only one conflict in the foreground. The other conflicts are passive or (in theatrical terminology) "behind the scenes," concealed in the subconscious and evoking few symptoms.[39]

Every side conflict can be regarded as a specific scene of a stage play. These different scenes are staged in order to vary the conflict themes of other character types so as to round us out and stabilize us emotionally. This can be seen in that healing side conflicts makes people more relaxed in their surroundings, and internally more whole and emotionally open; they generally pay more attention and are more understanding. Eliminating side conflicts also brings greater psychoenergetic harmony. Because of this, a person penetrates deeper into the subconscious and often dreams a lot, dreams that are more profound and more clearly perceived. Moreover, the dreams are often much more meaningful and helpful. In terms of the overall state, energy readings improve greatly once the side conflicts are eliminated, so that more life force is available, which in turn initiates a period of emotional maturation, simply because the person feels fresher and more vigorous.

Sometimes, though, the process comes to an abrupt end. People then tell me that they had been doing well – even great – for a long time, until all at once they found themselves in a crisis for which they often could find no explanation. Apparently, there had been too much life force available, so that, given time, conflicts were able to fully "ripen,"

like overripe fruits that then fall off the tree. That is the point in the spiritual journey at which the large Central Conflict rises up. Also, this often has to do with biological transformation related to the surfacing of the Central Conflict, such as puberty, emotional trauma, or the hormonal changes associated with childbirth – or, similarly, the "taking inventory" crises at the beginning of menopause. At such times, a woman might ask herself: "What have I actually gotten out of life so far?" If she can't come up with a satisfactory answer, this often gives rise to a depressive basic mood that goes unnoticed on the outside for a long time.

Such people often complain of lower-back pain or headaches, with no long-term improvement. Then, when an X-ray reveals a worn-out intervertebral disk, experience has shown that the search for deeper underlying causes stops right there. The patient has presumably identified the broken-down disk as the somatic cause – without having the slightest idea that there are much more important emotional problems lurking in the background which underlie the lower-back pain. It is not until intervertebral disk surgery fails to bring any lasting improvement that many therapists (and even patients) reconsider, and wonder whether there might not be more to it after all. Also, doctors who deal with exhaustion states are told about all kinds of feelings of ill health (dizziness, ringing in the ears, intestinal ailments, and the like) by patients for whom the actual underlying problem is a depressive mental crisis. There are countless ailments that could have an emotional background. One could even argue that there are few ailments and diseases that do *not* have an emotional background.

Next, the dramatic case of a young woman whose Central Conflict became active at the beginning of menopause, remaining untreated for decades:

She is an older woman, very down-to-earth, of modest background. She does not in the least come across as emotionally disturbed, but "normal" through and through. This now 74-year-old woman first suffered, at age 42, a crippling and horrifically strong attack of asthenia that came on suddenly out of nowhere. This debility has persisted without letup ever since, without the slightest trace of improvement. No doctor has ever been able to find anything. She has tried all kinds of healing methods and

---

[39] Experience has shown that patients with several simultaneously active conflicts are usually psychosomatically disturbed and exhibit strikingly conspicuous behavior. If such a condition persists over a longer time span, it gives rise to severe, frequently 100% therapy-resistant clinical pictures. The victims are literally inner-emotionally paralyzed – surrounded, as it were, and under attack from all sides. A step in any one direction immediately weakens the opposite defensive position and therefore cannot be taken. In extreme cases, such people wait their entire lives for their inner inferno to pass away and let them wake up from their nightmare. All experience points to them having to wait forever for their salvation if a beginning is not made to melt away their conflicts (more on this in the therapy chapter).

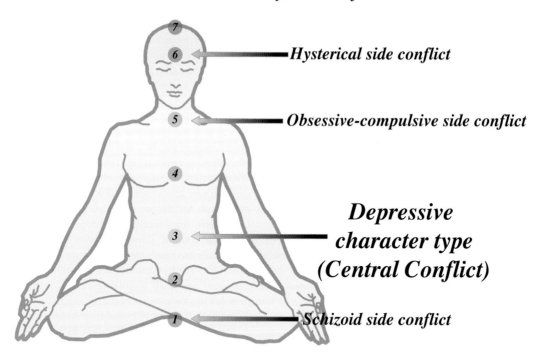

Hysterical side conflict

Obsessive-compulsive side conflict

Depressive character type (Central Conflict)

Schizoid side conflict

has seen hundreds of physicians and naturopaths. She also went to university clinics, but to date nothing has helped. In the beginning, she lay, powerless, in bed for two years; the least little effort tired her out terribly. Then, pulling herself together with all her strength, she got out of bed, but this made her so weak that she could only keep it up for a few hours at a time. She got heart spasms just from wiping off the table. The sickness has changed her life. Her greatest happiness is, she says, that her husband is so considerate and solicitous, and has always been very understanding because he knows her so well, so he knows that her complaints must be real.

The conflict theme found is Uneasy, mentally hyperactive in the 6th Chakra, with extremely high conflict readings that point to a Central Conflict. In all likelihood, it is medically a "generalized anxiety disease" which emerged in this simple, externally completely calm-seeming woman as a physical exhaustion state which none of my medical colleagues saw as an anxiety disease. When I ask her about it, she immediately admits to feeling horribly uneasy inside. Up to now, no one but her husband had known about her uneasiness, and no other doctor had asked her about it. She herself never thought that it had anything to do with her illness, passing it off as a purely personal problem that didn't bother her much because she'd gotten used to it.

It was therefore possible for no one to notice her leading symptom, namely the inner uneasiness so typical of anxiety diseases. These cases of overlooked psychosomatic diagnoses are by no means rare, occurring again and again – but this is understqandable: in my experience, anxiety ailments could only have been detected with psychoenergetic testing. After all, no one noticed any trace of her inner uneasiness. That the active conflict must be viewed as responsible for her decades-long disease history becomes evident when, just days after treating the Central Conflict (with specific homeopathic compound remedies) her condition improved markedly, and has continued to improve until she was able once more to live a normal life.

It is all too easy, in these descriptions, to fall prey to pessimism, as if the Central Conflict were exclusively bad.

But one mustn't think that! For the Central Conflict confronts us with the largest dark side of our personality, and this represents an enormous learning task and challenge.

Thus, the Central Conflict can be regarded not only as our worst enemy, but also as our best friend. Through no other circumstance can we make such a thorough mess of our life, piling up problems, as we can through the Central Conflict. Yet at the same time, there is no other growth factor that allows us to mature emotionally so strongly and effortlessly. "Whom the Lord loveth, he punisheth" is the appropriate biblical passage in this context. This is why all spiritual traditions teach that great problems represent a great gift to the soul, helping it to grow and mature.

Central Conflict and Character Types

'Character' is nothing more than a resilient habit.
(Plutarch)

This chapter deals with the Central Conflict, the largest conflict of all, which undetectably dominates the subconscious. Because of its central importance within the subconscious, it occupies a key position and, because of this, it is the most important starting point of individual personality growth. I put this forth as a pure assertion, to unveil gradually the true significance of the Central Conflict. Basically, one can think of the Central Conflict as a kind of "hypnotic continuous magic," like a curse that someone has without knowing it, although they constantly confront its consequences.

Actually, any person should get suspicious if things in one's personal life start to go wrong for no apparent reason. In this situation, the environment, parents, unfavorable social situations, and suchlike are blamed for personal adversity, because people never suspect that the problems might have something to do with themselves. So it's natural to blame difficulties on other people or sheer "bad luck." The real dilemma is grounded in the fact that most people have no idea what kind of Central Conflict they have in the first place. They are guided and influenced very deeply by unknown forces of which they are unaware, The psychoanalytic term *repression* refers to the process of blanking out from one's consciousness the uncomfortable and painful dark sides of one's psyche. One is therefore dependent on external help to illuminate the Central Conflict and bring it up into consciousness.

Despite its "secret life," the Central Conflict's impact is unexpectedly strong and pervades all of human life. A person's entire character is determined by the Central Conflict. One can say (with some exaggeration): "Tell me which Central Conflict you have and I'll tell you what kind of person you are." Using the methods of *Psychosomatic Energetics*, the Central Conflict can be ascertained in just a few minutes (see a later chapter), after which, knowing the kind of Central Conflict, one can predict which personality traits and character attributes a person has.

For instance, I constantly amaze mothers who bring their children in for an examination. Children are much harder to characterize than adults – and yet, after a few minutes' inspection, I can tell mothers details about their children's likes and dislikes, things that one normally would know only after becoming well acquainted with them. Thus, one can confidently predict that a child with

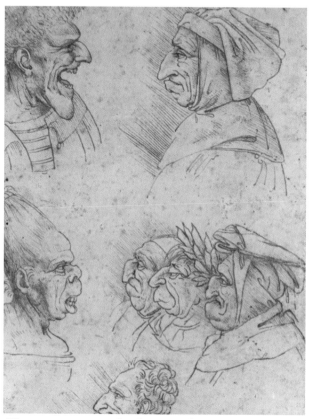

These seven grotesque heads are graphic caricatures, through which Leonardo da Vinci depicts various character heads and exaggerates their features to grotesque dimensions.

a *Hysteric* Central Conflict likes to be the center of attention. Or an obsessively structured child will insist on precise instructions, so that everything in the course of its day follows strictly prescribed rules.

Therefore, character type guides a person's elementary personality attributes and characteristic behavior patterns, which can reliably be predicted. Of course, this applies much more to adults, whose character is more developed; and spouses virtually always confirm the correctness of my predictions. Now, this is no guessing game; it is, rather, a matter of dependable laws that can be derived quite logically and inevitably from the person's character type. The correctness of the diagnosis arrived at is nearly always confirmed, as the Central Conflict's theme is recognized by the patient as his dominant and subconsciously resonating life motto.

Knowing one's own (or another person's) Central Conflict is of inestimable value, because only by uncovering those subconscious attributes that make up our own Central Conflict can we learn how almost grotesquely our life is predetermined by it – and in a manner totally unnoticed by us. The main difficulty in this is apprehending one's own Central Conflict. Astonishingly, this is true not just of patients, but also experts such as physicians and psychoanalysts! Experience shows that it is far easier to recognize another person's Central Conflict: we have much more trouble with our own weaknesses and subconscious dark sides.

So none should reproach themselves for not being able to see their own weaknesses. Nothing is more human than being blind to one's failings. Discovering one's Central Conflict takes help and support, someone else holding up the "mirror" for us. In the next few chapters, I hope to provide some useful support by describing the most important character types clearly and expressively enough that anyone can recognize themselves in the descriptions. What is needed, above all, is a good deal of honesty and courage, if one is to find out to which type one belongs.

Before describing the most important character types and their associated Central Conflicts, I need to clear up some fundamental questions with respect to the nature of emotional conflicts – questions which, if not answered, will lead to misunderstanding everything that follows. The simple question is: why do we create conflicts? Without a comprehensive medical-psychological worldview that includes spiritual and religious dimensions, the true nature of the Central Conflict cannot be properly understood at all. A purely mechanical and one-dimensional approach will get us nowhere. We must understand the deeper meaning of the Central Conflict, if we are properly to comprehend the processes – where "properly" means to ascertain the hidden meaning of life that underlies our emotional disequilibrium.

My concepts, based on a conjunction of Eastern wisdom, Christian spirituality and modern science, go far beyond the usual boundaries of conventional medicine and psychology. The core idea is centered on the notion that life is a spiritual journey that we experience like a stage play with different scenes and acts. The meaning of life by no means consists of just having fun and "passing the time." Our task is to develop a self-aware character with an individuated consciousness. This might also be paraphrased as the "School of Life" – that painful thorn-strewn path along which we become personally mature. In this context, the Central Conflict represents the most important "driving force" of emotional growth, like the baker's yeast that causes dough to expand and grow.

The question as to why we humans create conflicts in the first place is hard to answer from the standpoint of conventional understanding. I have already mentioned that a moralistic outlook – of the kind that haunts many a conservative mind (and from which many patients suffer, because they feel misunderstood or even mistreated!) – will not get us anywhere. Why does something as illogical as the formation of emotional conflicts happen, unnecessarily complicating people's lives? Is someone who does this a bad person who needs to be "read the riot act"? We need to look for deeper answers that are fairer to those affected and that indicate better approaches than simply (and for the most part ineffectively) wagging an accusing finger.

It is at first hard to understand why, for no discernible reason, people make their life harder than it needs to be. Why, for example, do people succumb to crippling sorrow; behave ever more oddly as they get older; develop unattractive character traits and antisocial behavior patterns – all changes having to do with emotional conflicts? Why do people make all manner of mistakes that make them or others sick, and are accompanied by suspicion, revenge, malicious glee at other's problems, inferiority complexes, unprocessed grief, anxieties and fears, *idées fixes*, narrow-mindedness, and similar feelings and characteristics? Why is there so much grief and evil in the world?

As we know, science can come up with a rational explanation for most processes and events. For instance, biology says that our hands are <u>for</u> taking hold of food and <u>for</u> defending ourselves; the head, with eyes and ears, is <u>for</u> conscious orientation; the stomach is <u>for</u> digestion. Everything in the world makes some kind of rational sense. The primary question "What is it good for?" can almost always be answered satisfactorily, after some thought – especially in the case of biological functions. To be sure, there are blind alleys in nature, also errors and setbacks, but these are exceptions, normally quickly corrected by nature, simply because they are contrary to survival. Emotional conflicts, on the other hand, are much harder to come up with an explanation for. After all, why should there be emotional conflicts in the first place? What purpose do they serve? Our rational need for a rational, logically understandable explanation founders on this question: "Why (are there conflicts)?"

The "why" of emotional distress and the characterological misbehavior of our fellow man has preoccupied us from time immemorial. In earlier times, evil spirits and sinful lapses were blamed; we moderns adopt a considerably more mundane viewpoint. Psychoanalysis and modern brain research consider human emotional disorders to be a kind of "workplace accident" – because we humans, in this view, are presumably some kind of degenerate animal. Humans are hominid mutants that, at some point in the dim past, split off from the apes. According to this

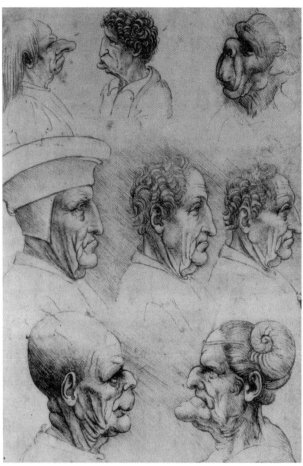

Leonardo da Vinci's character studies of grotesque heads give a good idea of the psychoenergetic distortions that characterological traits are capable of triggering in a person's outward appearance. Of course, this makes it easy to arrive at the mistaken conclusion that ugly people are emotionally ugly but beautiful people have beautiful minds. Yet life's experience teaches that the exterior façade is often misleading, and that such simple similes can lead to serious mistakes. Still, we fall for the superficial façade time and again!

animals, since instinct and behavior are quite directly linked in them. Besides, wild animals can't afford the luxury of emotional disorders, since it would threaten their survival in the most drastic and direct manner. Animals that start behaving strangely – i.e., due to rabies or some other disease – are, as a rule, expelled by their fellows from the pack rather quickly, to live precarious (and generally brief) lives as hermits.

This drama – the uncoupling of instinct and behavior that results in the human species' drift away from instinct – begins, however, with domestic animals. Sigmund FREUD understands emotional disorder to be the inevitable price that *Homo sapiens* must pay for its having become human. Modern Freudian psychoanalysis is pervaded by a pessimistic philosophical attitude, the true cause of which is that it can conceive no rational reason for emotional disorders. Modern science takes a similar attitude. This point of view holds that man is a type of "half crazy" being, driven by its unnatural nature out of nature's paradise, in which instincts and behavior (in the gray mists of time) had once been identical.

I'd like to make it clear that it is by no means my intention to poke fun at modern science or disparage its theories. Still, it is increasingly evident that many traditional opinions regarding genetics need to be supplemented and expanded – something I'll get into in more detail in the Karma chapter. Fundamentally, it's becoming apparent to more and more people that modern science's knowledge is, regrettably, too limited to be able to provide satisfactory answers to our urgent human questions. No scientist can rationally to explain what the meaning of life is.

When we seek answers as to the true significance of emotional conflicts, we need a larger contextual frame than that offered by conventional science. And yet the solution is quite simple! It lies within, as we look for the true answer inside ourselves. **The most important step in the direction of a new worldview that can unite spirituality and the sciences is grounded in the unconditional confidence that our life, in all its facets, is undergirt with a deeper meaning.** That is the first step – which by all means has to do with religious belief

view, we can be considered to be neurotic "human animals" locked into a permanent antagonism between morals and instinct, brought about by the fact that the precautionary and protective guiding hand of instinct mostly fell away during the course of our evolution.[40]

This concept characterizes the modern scientific worldview, according to which all of man's primordial emotional and behavioral problems are rooted in the fact that we no longer possess a firmly-rooted instinctive guidance mechanism, and so we behave (in the worst case) like a speeding car with no one at the wheel. The antagonism between morality and instinct sees to it that we humans are always stuck with one leg in emotional disturbances – which can never happen to wild

---

[40] Critics have argued – correctly, I think – that the modern concept of instinctive inhibition in contemporary man tends to adopt the same moral stance which religious authorities have taken for centuries to intimidate sinful mankind and make it dependent on their benedictions. One can even say that modern science – as critical thinkers such as FOUCAULT have correctly noted – is steering a far more unrestrictedly misanthropic, remorseless course than any religious dogmatist has ever managed to do. "Ethical" science (fig-leaf and protective shield), held up as the theory of humaneness, can in my opinion accomplish but little, simply because the modern view of man has become despiritualized and coldhearted. Whereas in earlier times the religious sinner only fell temporarily from God's grace, modern ideology leads to a terrifying and terrible conclusion that views the perverse sex offender, concentration-camp guard or terrorist as a worthless "workplace accident," on whom morality is wasted and who therefore must be mercilessly banned from human society – like a rabid dog that can be killed with a clear conscience.

– if one is to succeed in arriving at another, new point of view.

Here I'd like to mention that, time and time again in my energy-medicine clinical practice, I see people finding their way back to religious belief as soon as they make progress energetically – and this happens best and most easily via the dissolution of conflicts! People with partially or fully opened-up Brow Chakras and relatively high causal body energy readings almost always tell me that they believe in something higher than daily material life – calling it either "God" or "higher consciousness" or "life's meaning." By means of my measurements with subtle-body examination methods, I'll demonstrate that emotional development obeys specific laws and evolutionary principles that are completely harmonizable with religious conceptions of a spiritual journey and a deeper meaning to life.

Let's begin with the fact that we assume a (to be sure, often concealed) logical sense behind emotional disorders. (I ask skeptical readers to play along for the time being; otherwise what follows will not be understandable.) By having a meaning assigned to them in our lives – that of catalysts and growth facilitators – emotional disorders attain to the noblest purpose: allowing the individual soul to mature into an independent personality. In spiritual traditions, life has always been compared to being in school, where we are expected to develop an autonomous personality. Mainstream psychology was for a long time totally unaware of this esoteric viewpoint.

The depth-psychologist C.G. JUNG was the first to notice, from his experience as a physician, that emotional disturbances (and only they) help us to enter into the entire process of individuation. With this, he adopted a religious and mystically oriented stance that his medical colleagues found unusual. Many readers might be suspicious of this religious viewpoint, and think it all untrue. The trouble is, this is in the long run an insuperable obstacle because, in my opinion, we can only understand the true nature of emotional conflicts if we assume that they have a fundamental purpose. I hope, moreover, to be able to persuade the skeptical reader in the following chapters, using case histories from daily practice, that these successes prove this approach to be correct – because it makes possible such fantastic healing successes.

Comparing life to a journey or a school also implies making mistakes. This is actually desirable! For **we get to know ourselves as humans best by making mistakes!** Without mistakes, we slumber on, unconscious "pupated larva" out of which someday a beautiful butterfly will emerge. Making mistakes means developing emotional conflicts out of which our consciousness arises. If we made no mistakes, we wouldn't be able to learn, and thus we would not develop a consciousness. We would not become unique individuals, but rather interchangeable, anonymous creatures, like wild animals which all exhibit similar behavioral patterns, and who are still in the pupated and unconscious "larval stage."

The Scottish writer Thomas CARLYLE supplies the following thought-provoking bon mot on the topic of human fallibility: "*The greatest of faults, I should say, is to be conscious of none.*" This is not just a moral insight that applies to know-it-alls and dictators, it also expresses something fundamental about human nature. When we make mistakes (which we are sure to whenever we do something), we have to accept and deal with them. Notorious know-it-alls and dictators absolutely refuse to accept responsibility for their mistakes because (of course!) they have never made, nor ever could make, any. In their own eyes, they are infallible: mistakes are made by others, not by them![41]

If we are to become fully realized human beings, we know that we'll have to go through the painful stage of learning to admit and accept our mistakes – and not just on the outside. Among supposedly enlightened persons ("sensitive new-age guys"), an increasingly popular pose is to act externally vulnerable, humane, contrite, and so on, while maintaining an inner life that is often the opposite. Those who know people like this eventually learn to see through them. One speaks (quite rightly) in terms of a double standard whenever appearance and reality diverge so blatantly. Many fake gurus and charlatans belong to this category, having perfected their showmanship to a captivating degree that at first beguiles their disciples, but eventually leads to much confusion and growing disenchantment, to say nothing of physical and emotional harm.

Among fans of modern psychotherapy, one can find a third group of supposedly "better" persons. They believe they have freed themselves of error by giving free rein to their emotional conflicts and "letting it all hang out" – rather like throwing a garbage dump's rubbish around in order to get rid of one's own filth. This has to do with the naïve and delusional idea that one can improve the situation by simply acting out and parading one's emotional problems ("shout it out, pummel pillows to let the rage out, weep unabashedly, and so on"). I have often seen the exact opposite happen, as a conflict got more psychoenergetic attention and thus power, unfortunately and, from the standpoint of the basic intention, undesirably!

Next, I'd like to talk a bit about the beginning **development** of human **consciousness**. In order to grasp the full extent of our humanity, we need a reasonable idea of when and how human consciousness arose. The problem of consciousness and the subconscious can most simply be derived from the principle of opposites: "Where there is much light, there is also much shadow." Man's emerging consciousness can be compared to a light that "rises up" in oneself. From this viewpoint, emotional disorders are the dark, subconscious aspect in the shadows, which must arise when individual consciousness develops. Just as we cannot be aware of

---

[41] I very often find, in dictatorial types, enormously large conflicts that have psychotically taken control of the Self, in a kind of "possession." The dictatorial type can be regarded as a kind of "puppet on a string" who is incapable of acting in a responsible and rational manner!

bright daylight without darkest night as a contrast, so do emotional conflicts arise automatically and inevitably during the course of the evolution of human consciousness, because shadow is part of light.

I'd like to say something about *sympathy*. I don't mean to sound "cold" when I say that "Emotional conflicts are important for our spiritual maturation." I am painfully aware that human suffering – as a consequence of emotional conflicts – is in many cases virtually intolerable, both for the victims and their friends and relatives. The consequences of emotional conflicts include all the gradations of human troubles that are triggered thereby – from small forgivable lapses such as a "little white lie" (but which can indeed have serious repercussions) on up to the extremes of hatred, murder, and war.

Emotional conflicts underlie all human error. Therefore, the idea of regarding emotional disorders as something meaningful automatically winds up at the belief that everything bad, contemptible and evil about ourselves and our fellow man is somehow meaningful. Yet this has nothing to do with callousness and cold-bloodedness; rather, it pertains to a hidden meaning which at first seems incomprehensible. In this understanding, *meaningful* by no means signifies *good* or *pardonable*, but rather *necessary*. Necessary so that, in the (happy) end, a unique individual emerges. Between here and that goal there lies, admittedly, a struggle that is often characterized by pain, desperation, and bitterness, and which, from the outside, can seem like utter failure. However, it is the only possible process that allows human actualization and individuation.

If we penetrate deeper into the mystery of the development of human consciousness, we encounter some primitive looking processes, based primarily on the reward/punishment principle. **The beginning of consciousness is based on the pursuit of pleasure and the avoidance of pain.** This insight is one of the fundamental axioms of modern psychology and behavioral research. The actual background formative dynamics are based on something as simple as pure fear! Fear represents the anticipated perception of pain and is thus a prototype of consciousness. The antiquated *"spare the rod and spoil the child"* pedagogy is based on the principle of the fear of punishment. Even if they don't learn better, fear at least makes students more attentive.

Everyday life threatens us with the "rod" all the time. We learn to be alert when crossing the street, so as not to be run over – which already evokes subconscious fears, since we can imagine how much it would hurt to be hit by a car. We therefore look around carefully before stepping off the curb. As we know, only unconscious beings such as young children, drunks, and idiots know no fear as they blithely cross the street without looking around first! The entire development of consciousness ultimately springs from the feeling of fear. Fear is the attempt to avoid pain, which requires skill and alertness. Later, this turns into an individual consciousness that grows up into a personality. But in order for that to hap-

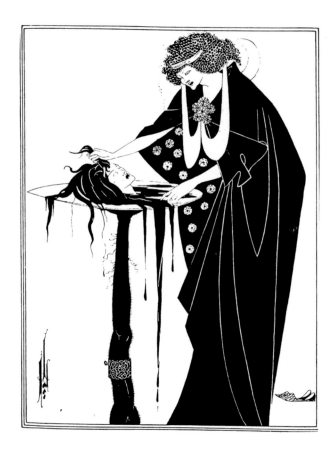

The story of the lovely Salome, triumphantly looking at the severed head of St. John lying on a platter, is our first confrontation with the dreadful fear of decapitation and mutilation, which immediately gets mixed up in our subconscious with salacious fascination. Because Salome's sexual desires fell on the saint's deaf ears, the spurned woman asked King Herod that she be granted a wish that he cannot deny her if her seductive dance delights him: the saint's lopped-off head. It is crucial to understand that the subconscious dynamics of this picture (which represents the conflict dynamics as an allegory) is based on the admixture of fear and sensual energy, which contributes decisively to conflicts being so doggedly retained, and why they are so hard to resolve (because, in a very strange way, they "feel so good," are so "scarily beautiful" etc.).

pen – i.e., developing a personality – we must first be afraid!

Fear as the only basic precondition for the formation of consciousness doesn't seem enough, since any animal knows fear, and even a great big strong lion fears for its life in a thunderstorm or earthquake. However, lions don't go on to develop any sort of consciousness comparable with human consciousness. What distinguishes us from animals is a long-lasting memory of fear along with a type of mental processing in which we begin to think about our fear, as well as how to avoid it. For instance, stone-age man prayed to a thunder god when it stormed, which represents a practical approach to seeking a favorable outcome from higher authorities – provided that one believes in the efficacy of magic, as well as the existence of thunder gods. Animals don't do this, because they lack the necessary consciousness.

Keep in mind that formation of consciousness does not inevitably lead to rational decisions. We are also capable of doing irrational things like running around unprotected in thunderstorms. However, if we insist on making dumb decisions, we will most likely wind up paying a price sooner or later. This means that, like it or not, we humans must learn to find sensible solutions, and the more rational our efforts, the less fear we need have.

Modern man of course makes other serious errors, related to the fact that we enlist insurance companies, local police forces, and the like as assistants in our fear-avoidance strategies – but we fail to realize that the real dangers that beset us are thereby, at best, only slightly diminished. If our house is on fire, our insurance isn't going to save us from a fiery death. Yet wishful thinking seduces us into thinking that insurance provides some mysterious kind of "protective shield" because we have paid our premiums on time. This widespread misbelief, which has its origin in subconscious mechanisms, is of course the subliminal theme of many commercials and ads. In a certain sense, all these fear-avoidance institutions – insurance, armies and police, and so on – are the modern "thunder gods," which modern man builds up and overloads with magical powers just as primitive man tended to do with his nature gods.

With respect to the difference between human and animal fears, the most significant difference is memory – a kind of condensed consciousness. As humans, we remember past fears, but animals can do this only to a very limited degree. Ultimately, this is a psycho-energetic phenomenon I touched upon in an earlier chapter on conflict formation. On the purely emotional level, we encapsulate our fears in conflicts, thereby banning them to the subconscious. That is the psychological aspect of the process – but subtle-body processes are involved as well, since fears also become autonomous objects in the subtle energy field, where our memories of fearful events are stored.

In the memory storage process, the energetic aspect plays a crucial role – which not many, even in energy medicine, fully appreciate in its full scope. Some day, people will realize that subtle-body energy plays an enormously important part in memory formation. In this, the emotional body is much less important than the mental or the causal body – components that only humans possess and animals do not have. The mental body corresponds to everyday consciousness and the causal body to the deep archetypal subconscious. Both of these energy bodies vibrate at extremely high frequencies, which presumably plays a big role in memory storage, like the high-frequency structures of quartz crystals that make digital clocks so accurate, since the quartz crystal's high frequency is extraordinarily stable.

Of course, animals can also think back, so human memory does not seem to be a unique prerequisite for consciousness formation. Elephants are famous for remembering events that took place decades ago. In my opinion, the surprising memory of many animal species is based on a particularly large storage capacity in the respective emotional body. This capacity seems to be very large in elephants, but it has nothing to do with a mental or causal body, since energy measurements on animals have failed to detect either one, so that the emotional body must be regarded as the sole storage location of animal memory.

With domesticated animals, we have the beginnings of a new process, in that they begin to develop certain human characteristics having to do with neurotic behavior patterns and conflict formation. All of this is deeply related to the decoupling of instinct and emotion, better known as "conditioning" or "socialization." The altered emotional body increases the domesticated animal's susceptibility to disease – a process that has reached its culmination in man. Yet all this does not yet have anything to do with the origin of animal consciousness, which to some extent might be viewed as equivalent to that of humans.

What makes us different from animals, in a subtle-body sense, is most importantly the mental and the causal body. Causal energy enables storing conflicts' contents over extremely long spans of time, presumably because it vibrates the highest – far higher than the frequency spectrum of mental energy. Unpleasant memories are thereby stored in a way that is almost impossible to erase. As incredible as that might sound, I have come to the conclusion that the Central Conflict can be stored over many reincarnations, and for millennia! Numerous hypnotic processes would not otherwise be convincingly explicable. One is thus dealing here, when it comes to the Central Conflict, with long time spans that extend back into past lives. This is why, in the deep trance states of hypnosis, one can recall events that had to have taken place in past lives. I will delve deeper into this in the chapter on Karma.

I'd like to get back to the topic of fear, because it is central to the development of an independent consciousness. **The Central Conflict contains our greatest feelings of fear.** These fears solidify into a fateful decision that permanently influences life and personality once it has come into being. One draws, as it were, some elementary conclusions from one's worst fears, which thereupon lead to entrenched basic convictions and behavior patterns. These lead, in turn, to similar human types that share these traits and correspond to a particular **character type**.

How might we picture the formation of these fundamental fears? For instance, you tell yourself, based on the extremely painful fears that must at some point have played a role in the formation of the Central Conflict, "I must make myself internally rigid so as not to feel anything any more." Let's assume an initial situation in which a person was forced to stand by helplessly and watch family members be massacred by marauding soldiers. The scene might have taken place in the gray mists of time in a previous incarnation. I find these initial situations among schizoids with the corresponding experiences very often deeply buried in the subconscious, and they underlie the actual trauma of the Central Conflict. (Other character types have different triggering scenes.) One can now see that the feelings evoked in the observer by the massacre threaten to drive him insane, which is why he makes himself internally rigid and unfeeling.

Becoming unfeeling represents a perfect solution, one that immediately alleviates the tragedy and makes it emotionally bearable, even if it's ultimately just a pseudo-solution. But a bad solution is still better than none, and the victim was unable at the time to come up with a better one. This kind of internally rigid person will in time develop into a schizoid character type, for whom any and every stirred-up emotion will be walled off from the rest of the organism by the entrenched paradigm of emotional (f)rigidity. The rule set up to tune out unbearable feelings by being rigid and lifeless will one day turn into a universal essential element that for the victim has become a deeply anchored basic pattern with the force of law.

To illustrate this, I'd like to cite the typical example of a schizoid patient in whom the Central Conflict is very likely traceable to a war situation in a former life:

The 40-year-old man suffered his first total breakdown 2 years ago. He is an extraordinarily gentle person with a friendly demeanor. He was unable to come up with any good reason for the breakdown, except to say that he had been using an energy device at the time, one with which the subtle-body energy system could be altered (according to the manufacturer's claims) by means of light quanta and certain healing geometric patterns. He's still not sure if his changes at that time could have something to do with it, but he suspects it strongly (Note: I'd like to point out that, in my opinion, the acute damage and triggering of the illness could have been caused by a magical procedure!).

Since the breakdown, everything seems unreal to him. He sometimes hears voices. He feels constantly broken down, exhausted in the morning, can't concentrate, so he has been on sick leave for two years. His psychiatrist diagnosed incipient schizophrenia, so he has been taking pharmaceuticals prescribed by the psychiatrist that, while they do make his clinical picture tolerable, are not really healing him. He came to me because he is hoping for long-term help from Psychosomatic Energetics.

An energetic examination with the REBA® Test Device turns up a very good charge of 80% in the vital body. On the other hand, the 30% energy reading for the emotional body and (above all) the 10% mental reading are low. In partic-

ular, the extremely low mental reading may be regarded as very typical of a psychotic ailment. The mental body corresponds to the conscious Self and the feeling of being oneself. When the mental body has very low energy readings, one understandably often feels unreal, as if the entire world were some kind of sham. This case excellently confirms my basic thesis, according to which the current energetic constitution conditions the corresponding fundamental feeling.

For a Central Conflict, the conflict Wrong thinking *in the 7th Chakra responds. The conflict itself has readings of 100% vital, 80% emotional, 30% mental and 90% causal (typical values for a Central Conflict) – in particular, the high causal reading of over 80% is considered a signpost, because experience has shown that such high readings are often triggered by a karmic scenario. Thus, the higher the causal reading, the older karmically – but at the same time the more automatic and entrenched – are the conflicts in question! After I tell him what kind of Central Conflict he has, the patient confirms my diagnosis – in fact had already suspected, before the examination as he was reading my book, that he would have this conflict as primary theme (but without having told me before the examination).*

In a free-association session, the highly intuitive patient (his causal reading is 80%!) and I try to find out what the situation might be with respect to the Central Conflict and its origin. In my experience, Wrong thinking *often involves a conflict theme having to do with strongly ideologically infected and heavily fraught situations, in which one thinks something up and then believes it to be completely true. One becomes a fanatical radical activist fighting for an ideology. One often winds up "buying the farm" for this belief, in that the entire situation – both existentially as well as emotionally – often comes to a dramatic and (very often) fatal end. What lessons can be drawn from this? In future, the organism associates (for example) being a "crusader" or a "Moslem" – i.e., ideologically fraught fighting situations, with the frighteningly emotional consequence of having to die an agonizing death. "When I believe devoutly in something that I feel to be correct and true, I will have to die for it," is the subconscious conclusion that underlies the origin of the Central Conflict as a paradigm.*

The patient confirms that, while in a trance during previous reincarnation therapies – as well as on the occasion of nocturnal nightmares – many times finding himself in war situations taking place in Mesopotamia or some similar ancient time and place, in which he, as General, was helplessly cut down in the midst of his troops, while the blazingly hot sun above and the circling avaricious vultures accompanied his death scene.

One is immediately surprised when it comes to interpreting the overall case. Although the patient was at that time a high-ranking officer and feared for his warlike demeanor, in his current incarnation the patient had developed a totally antithetical nature. He had, as it were, shoved his entire

aggressivity (along with the fears that accompanied the for-
mation of the Central Conflict) into his subconscious and
thus turned it into a subconscious shadow. None of his fam-
ily or friends was remotely able to conceive, he said in an
amused tone, that he might harbor, deeply buried and cov-
ered over, some very hard, warlike, and merciless character
traits belonging to his emotional dark side, which he has
completely suppressed. He, on the other hand, was quite
aware that he harbored these masculine and warlike charac-
ter components. I advise him to (very carefully) reawaken
this warrior in himself and gradually integrate the useful
masculine components into his current life.

In the epilogue to this patient's story, I'd like to add
that, since the melting away of his most of his Central
Conflict with appropriate homeopathic compound
agents, he is doing markedly better. He is again able to
work and feels once more emotionally "centered." Yet his
healing process was not without problems at the outset.
The first examination revealed a large conflict with
Uneasiness in the Brow Chakra, the healing of which (over
a period of 2 months) did very little to improve his overall condition. To make matters worse, there was initially
geo-radiation in the head region. One can see from this
that these difficult cases can very often be rather "clogged
up" in an energetic sense as well, like a heavily fortified
castle with multiple, heavy, locked gates. It took over a
year before the patient's condition showed lasting
improvement.

At this point, it's natural to ask how many basic kinds
of Central Conflicts there might be, especially when we
imagine the endless variety of all possible emotional
traumatization. Added to this are the countless different
ways that people perceive and react to experiences and
events. Surprisingly, the range of variation of Central
Conflict types turns out to be relatively comprehensible
and modest in scope. There are just over two dozen
Central Conflict basic variations, namely 28. These 28
Central Conflicts do not generate an unforeseeably vast
multiplicity of character types, but quite the contrary: an
unusually small number (4) of sharply delineated fundamental fears produce four character types. One can thus
classify all people, in the deep essential core of their being,
within a clear and ordered system of four clearly differentiated groups.

The **four character variations** are:

- **Schizoid**
- **Depressive**
- **Obsessive-compulsive**
- **Hysterical**

These four character types are based on fundamental convictions derivable from the respective Central Conflict.
However, before describing these character types and the
associated fundamental convictions, I'd like to first present
a few considerations regarding the **Central Conflict**. We
know that every person possesses a Central Conflict that
dominates the subconscious. Experience with thousands of
people seems to confirm that there is likely no one without
a Central Conflict. Whether a Central Conflict is active
(generating complaints and symptoms) or passive (dormant
and present in the background) has little significance with
respect to the Central Conflict's impact on character development. It's not its momentary activity that makes the
Central Conflict so significant, but rather its mere existence.
Everyone has a Central Conflict and is permanently shaped
by it.

The Central Conflict shapes our thoughts and actions in
predictable ways, just as it influences perception in a particularly intense and lasting manner. As a magnet under a plate
sprinkled with iron filings forces them to line up in specific
orientations, so does the Central Conflict lead to a predetermined orientation of our entire life. All my experience to
date indicates that the Central Conflict is the essential
shaper of a person's character. Of course, we want to find
out which character type we belong to, and what kind of
Central Conflict we have. But since the point here is not
just satisfying the reader's fleeting curiosity – like psychological questionnaires in popular magazines – I must ask the
reader to be patient.

In what follows, I'd like to reward the reader's patience by
pointing out that, although the topic of *character type* might
seem a bit abstract at a casual glance, a more careful look
yields novel insights that are extraordinarily rewarding and
fascinating – because, ultimately, it's all about why individuals are "the way they are." A side benefit of this approach
is that it makes comprehensible the entire history of the
healing arts and psychology, starting with the energy medicine of ancient India and China and the theory of the elements of ancient medicine on up to present-day psychiatry
and psychoanalysis. I'd like to re-emphasize that these are
not utopian theories; this view culminates in the very real
and currently highly important issue of how the body, its
metabolism and subtle-body energy system, successfully
work together with the mind.[42]

Such issues include curiosity as to what physique might
have in common with a person's underlying emotional constitution. A thousand questions are raised, such as: Do our
facial features and idiosyncrasies of movement reveal anything about basic emotional constitution – as we (correctly)
assume? Where does the mind's sphere of influence end?
Another important question is: To what extent do our
symptoms and illnesses link to specific unknown emotional
themes – and, if they do (one asks), with which ones? In
particular, how do our body and mind cohere? What does

physique reveal of our inmost nature, and can this revelation be reliable?

Why, for example, are fat people often naturally peaceable and jovial, even though they sometimes tend to unexpected choleric eruptions? Strikingly often, overweight persons dream and fantasize about concealed aggressions, but they usually keep a lid on such eruptions; ancient medicine refers in this context to *cholerics*. Yet another question is: What does the disrupted metabolism in an overweight body evoke? Could "overweight" be an emotional theme having to do with suppressed aggression? These and similar questions all deal with the concept of *character type* and the underlying Central Conflict. If we want exhaustive answers to these gripping questions, in order to derive practical solutions therefrom, we are going to have to take a much closer look (than we have so far) at the associated phenomena.

We first need to clarify what we mean by **character**. Every psychological human classification scheme attempts to bring order to the chaos of phenomena by groupings. At the beginning of the 20th century, the psychiatrist KRETSCHMER proposed dividing psychiatric patients into two groups based on physique: corpulent pyknics (more frequently depressive) and slim-bodied leptosomes (said to be more often schizophrenic). KRETSCHMER thus reasoned from physique back to specific inner emotional behavioral patterns that an examining psychiatrist could use as a preliminary orientation aid. KRETSCHMER's division into pyknics and leptosomes was the first psychosomatic model developed since ancient times to gain widespread medical recognition.

The coarseness of the underlying matrix must understandably lead to numerous errors. "You're skinny, so you must be schizo!" would be an overly simple and often misleading generalization. And yet, astonishingly, KRETSCHMER's division in many cases is right enough to permit an initial diagnosis. Plus, the model can also aid in tracking progress, since, e.g., a schizophrenic putting on weight can be taken as a sign of healing. The opposite is true of depression, where losing weight often goes hand in hand with a more cheerful mood. "He's eating again now, because he's doing better!" is a rule of thumb that applies to the schizophrenic but not the depressive who, in his hour of emotional need, has turned to the soothing relief of overeating to anesthetize his unbearable emotional condition. Eating then takes on an existential aspect whose withdrawal is equated on a subconscious level with the withholding of love. When depressives improve, they often spontaneously stop overeating. Moreover, many antidepressants are also appetite suppressants, which also reflects the logic of "depression equals overweight."

Another classification scheme that mostly ignores physique, putting the main emphasis on a disturbed early childhood psychosexual developmental stage, originates with the discoverer of psychoanalysis, Sigmund FREUD. It uses a classification that has been popularized and is now part of general knowledge.

FREUD identifies the following (fixation) types:
- **Anal** – Subjected to overly strict early-childhood toilet training; goes on to develop a parsimonious and pedantic character.
- **Urethral** – A special type for whom toilet training led to power struggles with sadistic overtones.
- **Oral** – Not breast-fed (enough) and is thus, as an adult, forced to anesthetize himself through excess eating in order to numb a gnawing and depressing frustration. Oral types thus tend to overweight.
- **Hysteric** – Emotionally seduced into a clandestine liaison with the opposite-sex parent and therefore has delusions of grandeur throughout life.
- **Schizoid** – As a small child lived through an emotional roller coaster, and so was unable to build up a stable basic trust. The schizoid will be a life-long shy and mistrustful person.
- **Borderline** (on the brink of psychosis) – Like the multiple-personality type, a special form of severe early-childhood disturbance in which trust and rejection have traded places in an unforeseeable manner – or in which basic trust (as with the schizoid type) is almost totally lacking.

If we take a closer, in-depth look at the classification scheme developed by FREUD, it will eventually come to an abrupt end. Therapists who fail to notice this tend, in my experience, to start going in circles, at which point the therapy no longer makes any real progress – often with neither therapist nor patient realizing it. The psychosexual drive model thus turns all too easily into a blind alley, which is no surprise, since it seems to apply only to the superficial subconscious. C.G. JUNG realized that, beyond a certain subconscious depth, characters make the transition to broader contexts of meaning. Drives, in the Freudian sense, no longer have meaning there. Thousands of experiences with

[42] Modern psychosomatics, as officially taught in the universities, has lately almost totally abandoned the effort to derive psychological traits from biological data. None of the leading psychosomatics exponents has any objection to this abandonment of an idea that had once begun so promisingly with LAVATER's physiognomy. There is virtually nothing left of the euphoria of the years around 1930 to 1950. Thus, the official theory of the interaction of mind and body (i.e., psychosomatics) finds itself, in my opinion, in a severe crisis, explainable above all by the fact that real-world psychosomatic interactions are more complex and difficult to apprehend than the conventional model is capable of coping with. What is needed are innovative test procedures (such as Psychosomatic Energetics) that do justice to the complexity. Also needed, as a second pillar, is subtle-body thinking and appropriate energetic investigations, without whose aid no sensible diagnostic model can be developed – and from which then (and only then), sensible and practicable theoretical conclusions can be drawn.

patients in deep hypnotic trances have shown that the deep subconscious harbors totally different themes with altered weightings – ultimately those having to do with the Central Conflict, which cannot adequately be explicated with the Freudian model.

Still, FREUD's character classification, based on insufficiently-traversed psychosexual developmental stages, should by no means be considered incorrect. In my opinion, it simply needs to be supplemented with a larger contextual frame as soon as one gets into deeper subconscious levels. The question arises as to which of the numerous depth-psychology models is best, especially with respect to subtle-body connections. After extensive checkout of various systems, it seems to me that the best character classification scheme is the one described by the German psychiatrist SCHULZ-HENCKE and his apprentice RIEMANN. In terms of depth psychology, this classification is the most profound and widest ranging, and is – intriguingly – one into which all the other models (including those of energy medicine) can be effortlessly integrated, as I'd like to show below.

RIEMANN distinguishes **four basic types of fear** that represent variations of fundamental fears, which I will get into individually later on. From mankind's four fundamental fears there arise four character types, designated as follows:

· Schizoid
· Depressive
· Obsessive-compulsive
· Hysteric

Taking a closer look at RIEMANN's typology, we once again find, to our astonishment, the familiar four types from element theory. These, as we know, represent an ancient, millennial classification of the human body into various metabolic and typological groups which have been thoroughly discussed in previous chapters.

By way of preface, I need first to clear up a terminological misunderstanding. The designations *schizoid, depressive,* and so on come from the specialized jargon of psychiatry. They have a different meaning when applied to healthy persons, since it is only pathological exaggeration of a character type that leads to the corresponding illnesses such as genuine obsessive-compulsive neurosis, depression, schizophrenia, or hysteria (manic depression). In the case of emotionally healthy persons, this designation expresses a normal character type unique to each person in its gradation. Thus, the original psychiatric designation has no pathological sinificance here.

From these four types, one can also extract a hit-parade of emotional disturbances of varying severity. Because every character type basically exhibits the same faults, even though they show up in differing shadings and accents, there is no *better* or *worse* in a moral sense. I suggest that the reader simply accept these concepts as designations of primeval human weaknesses to which no one is immune.

In depth psychology, moreover, the terms have become so established that they are used to classify universal basic human attributes or idiosyncrasies of personality that come in all gradations. An orderly, neatly dressed, and well put-together man (obsessive character type) will be esteemed, while the amplification of these character traits on up to pedantry will occasion derision – e.g., the punctilious bureaucrat of comedy – or sheer desperation (if one is forced to live in a close relationship with a tyrannical pedant). Thus, from each character type rises a range of variations, from the completely harmless to the extreme forms.

RIEMANN's four character types can be smoothly and effortlessly integrated into the system of classical element theory, so that we have untied the Gordian Knot of psychosomatics in an ingeniously simple manner. Ultimately, it couldn't be any other way, since our emotional sensations and our associated bodily reactions must as a rule match up perfectly. "A leopard can't change its spots!" as the old saying expresses the well-known phenomenon in which a person's reactions tend to follow predetermined courses laid out by metabolism and physique. Physique and basic personality must accordingly be coterminous! Everyone recognizes the bull-necked choleric whose irritability and outbursts of temper can be seen from far off. Or the slender, obsessive, and genteel *grande dame* whose affectations and stolidity drive the others waiting behind her in line at the post office up the wall as she laboriously cross-examines the clerk with stubborn pedantry about every minute detail.

As I've said, the four character types match up precisely with the concepts of classical element theory. The first thing about the four character types is their division into the polar groups *Yin introversion* and *Yang extroversion*. Basically, each two pairs of the four character types correspond to one of the two groups, i.e., either more toward the masculine or feminine pole. The obsessive-compulsive and schizoid types are associated with the masculine character type, while the depressive and hysteric types exhibit more feminine character traits. I have already mentioned that **biological sex and the associated character type do not have to be the same!** Of course, this can have quite serious repercussions, especially when sex deviates from character type. One is then stuck, for instance, with a feminine mind in a masculine body – or a male soul in a biological female. My experience tells me that sex and character type differ in about half of all cases. The resulting imbalance understandably gives rise to serious identification problems.

Most men with feminine character traits (hysteric or depressive character types) go to great lengths throughout their lives to conceal their feminine nature from themselves and others. After all, "wuss" and "wimp" are not exactly popular male types – though these are, to my mind, offensive labels that (from an evolutionary standpoint) belong to the era of instinct-driven tribal apes. The last thing our high civilization needs today is more (physical or mental) *Tarzan* types. Unfortunately, these asinine prejudices continue to dominate the thinking of surprisingly many people – particularly in the female subconscious – and are the source of much needless human suffering.

Gender-role prejudices are amazingly hard to root out, primarily due to the fact that emotional weakness is projected onto others. In my experience, the dissolution of emotional conflicts invariably makes people more tolerant in dealing with others. In this case, their approach toward their own gender roles and those of others may be reasonably viewed as an important measure of how liberal and mature a society is. This applies not just to societies, but to each individual member as well.

Often, men with feminine characters (hysteric or depressive type) exhibit classic compensatory behavior by trying to act conspicuously masculine. This can include bodybuilding to counterbalance diminished self-confidence with a muscle-bound body. I'd like to describe two contemporary prototypes that can be found in any number of variations. We meet the classic depressive type in the form of the good-humored fatty – with a tendency to eruptions of rage (choleric), but all in all a very gentle, compliant, and friendly creature who thrives in social gatherings and exhibits a striking propensity for sensual oral delights. The other variant of a male with a female soul is the hysteric, who often is exceptionally good looking, likes to wear jewelry, centers his life on wine, women, and song, and, thanks to his charming manner, is the center of attention at social events.

I have had quite contrary experiences with men who have a masculine character (schizoid and obsessive types). Because they don't need to prove their manliness to anyone, they are often remarkably casual about their gender role. These masculine men tend by nature to be stand-offish and unapproachable. Ultimately, they don't much care what others think of them. This type tends to present an unfavorable external appearance, i.e., droopy shoulders, bald head, and/or potbelly don't seem to bother them much. In social situations, men with masculine souls are usually little interested in coming on like the "strong man." Just as we know that every exaggeration indicates an underlying inferiority complex, here we have its opposite: an excess of self-confidence leads to sloppiness and understatement with respect to gender-role display. In short, one finds it to be "not necessary."

I'd now like to turn to the distaff side, for which, basically, the same applies with reversed polarity. If we ask ourselves what the concept "feminine" makes us think of, the emotional domain should spring to the foreground. When the emotional aspect dominates character type, that automatically leads to a strong overemphasis of feelings, as we

expect from women. We assume that women will possess either a depressive or hysteric character structure. Classical female roles are thus the depressive "crybaby" who tries to please everybody, or the sophisticated, ravishingly beautiful seductress (hysteric) whose charms turn all men's heads and who expects everybody to please her.

But this doesn't apply to about half of all women, simply because the biological and emotional gender roles are not the same for them. Then, fatefully, a masculine soul winds up trapped in a woman's body. As long as such women have not learned – or don't think it necessary – to conceal their true nature, women with overtly schizoid or obsessive-compulsive character structures often come across as "mannish" or "hard-hearted Hannahs." And yet these women's only misfortune is having a masculine character type.

One can often observe compensatory behavior as well, which tends to show up as exaggerated femininity. We can observe behavior patterns that correspond (with sign reversed) to the examples cited of effeminate men. Here too, a façade is erected, in order not to attract unpleasant attention. Nevertheless, both variants lead to inner rancor and various pent-up feelings of frustration, which amounts to the same thing in the end. Those who are forced to put up such a warped, sham facade feel, deep in their soul, misunderstood and exploited by those around them.

It goes without saying that a discrepancy between biological and emotional gender roles puts the affected person in an awkward predicament. The issue is often a problem precisely in the case of gender selection, since the "mis-sexed" person, in a strange paradoxical reaction that at first seems incomprehensible to outsiders, often does the opposite of what the outside world expects him/her to. The person becomes grouchy, and often subconsciously provokes the very relationship problem that s/he secretly fears by living out the gender role in a destructive manner. Simply put, the person feels unlovable and behaves accordingly, so that nobody can possibly like him/her.

Somewhat overstated, one can speak, in these mixed-up situations, of a kind of emotional "hermaphroditism" (a medical term indicating bisexuality, as when a female equipped with a vagina has a penis as well). Of course, this applies in the current context in a figurative sense, to express the emotional balancing act made necessary by the discrepancy between the biological and emotional gender role. The whole thing can also be viewed as a balancing act between the outer and inner worlds, in which the actual problem does not lie exclusively with the affected person, but rather in the interrelationship with the environment – for experience has shown that the problem escalates into full-blown drama when an intolerant world collides with a person unwilling or unable to compromise, to adapt and comply with the environment's guidelines.

Often, the difficult task of being forced to play one's biologically expected role in a sexual relationship – even though one's internal emotions shy away from it – eventually leads to *decompensation*, the pervasiveness of which drives the high divorce rate and other relationship problems. At the same time, I don't want to overdramatize the gender-role problem; although it is certainly significant in some cases of difficult gender identification, the actual basic problem has its roots in the untreated Central Conflict. Its pathological subconscious influences are the real triggering factor. Thus, if the Central Conflict is cured, the gender role problems often disappear as well. I will get more deeply into the gender role of character type in the discussion of individual character types in the next chapter.

There is, first, a distinction made between a feminine (depressive/hysteric) and a masculine (schizoid/obsessive-compulsive) variant of character types. The two genders form harmonic pairs, just as in real life. These harmonic pairs form "primary groups" because they naturally get along well together:

⟨ the schizoid/depressive primary group
⟨ the hysteric/obsessive-compulsive primary group

Next I'd like to present an overview of the four character types. To make it easier to get into, I'll first present their important attributes – a kind of "wanted poster" as an initial overview.

These pairings involve character types that share essential traits, mirror-inverted, with each other. Why the pairs *must* fit into each other like a lock and key will become clear later. At this point, the aim is an initial orientation. Understanding the character pairs is made easier once one has grasped that these pairs which belong to each other relate to the conflict's time of origin.

Thus, schizoid and depressive types make up a rather wild, primitive character form. Such forms are often widespread in primitive societies as a primary type; here, one encounters archetypal figures of the classic role models of the maternal/nurturing woman (depressive type) and the warlike/lone-wolf man (schizoid type). By their nature, depressive/schizoid pairs correspond much more to the primitive emotional state of prehistoric man, whereas hysteric and obsessive character types come across as much more differentiated and civilized.

One thus encounters obsessive/hysterical types much more frequently in more developed civilizations. This sometimes goes so far as to appear affected and unnatural, for instance the pompous bureaucrat (obsessive-compulsive type) or the mischievous Don Juan (hysteric type). This kind of affected and unnatural-seeming behavior is hardly ever found in depressive and schizoid types. This permits the generalization that schizoid/depressive people by nature seem wild and natural, while obsessive/hysteric people often exhibit a somewhat domestic, civilized, and even affected nature. Apparently, there is something like an evolutionary hierarchy of character types that correlates with their time

of origin. In a later chapter about evolution and emotional development, I'll return to this in greater detail.

The next table gives an overview of fundamental fears, typical characteristics and classifications of the four character types. The first row (with the arrows) shows the character pairs, whose character traits most favorably supplement each other. These are the harmonic pairs we were just talking about, interacting in a kind of *elective affinity* (German: *Wahlverwandtschaft*) to borrow Goethe's title phrase. These related types understand each other very well and constitute a harmonic pairing. Later on, I'll discuss other, more difficult (even antithetical) constellations. The Chinese Yin/Yang polarities, as well as the Element types of ancient Greek/Arabic medicine reveal, moreover, in the table below, how the respective Depth-psychology character types relate to the temperaments (humoral types) of ancient medicine.

(See table on following page.)

	Character Type	Schizoid ⟷ Depressive		Obsessive ⟷ Hysterical	
Character Type		Schizoid	Depressive	Obsessive	Hysterical
Chinese Polarity		Yang	Yin	Yang	Yin
Element type		Melancholic	Choleric	Phlegmatic	Sanguine
Polarity (actual emotional trait)		Extroversion	Introversion	Extroversion	Introversion
Jungian Polarity (compensatory, acting "as if")		Introversion	Extroversion	Introversion	Extroversion
Type or anxiety (Riemann)		Existential (fear of commitment exaggerated self-preservation)	Separation (fear of self-development, overdone commitment)	Change (fear of transitoriness, overdone safeguards)	Finality (fear of the inevitable, overdone desire to be free)
Fundamental fear and appropriate depth-psychological compensation		Fear of losing oneself = "Don't want to be here/leave me alone/must always be strong	Fear of isolation = "always want to fit in and be nice/ want to always be by your side	Fear of the new = "If I'm good, nothing will change/always be organized"	Fear of being tied down = "If I tie myself down, I'm a goner/always be free and unattached"
Primary psychological/ fine-energetic accentuation		Overvalued mental domain	Overvalued emotional domain	Overvalued mental domain	Overvalued emotional domain

In the table, the fourth and fifth rows present C.G. JUNG's famous character classification scheme of introversion (emotionally "turned inward") and extroversion (emotionally "externally oriented"). I had to use two extra rows to represent correctly JUNG's flawed conception. In his character typology, JUNG made use of another schema based on a different viewpoint – one, however, whose essential ascriptions also fit into my schema. Still, one notes with astonishment that JUNG felt that certain types belonged to exactly the opposite essence from the one that they actually possess.

In my opinion, JUNG misclassified the character types. Presumably, he was taken in by a "show" of the respective types, which had to do with compensatory efforts and cover-ups – as when totally harmless animals in the wild put on a fearsome show in order to impress rivals in combat or sexual partners being courted. That seems clumsy and easy to see through at first glance, but at the actual depth-psychological essential core, it is extremely hard to make out.

In this context, I would cite as an example the warlike schizoid that I described a few pages back. None of the people near him ever suspected – inside this gentle and friendly man who seemed so introverted and shy – an extroverted person with the toughness of a warrior, which was his true essential core (and which he had suppressed remarkably well).

The bottom three rows of the table contain RIEMANN's fundamental fears, which can be related to the corresponding character type; plus the deeply-engraved basic convictions derived therefrom; and finally the corresponding predominant subtle-body energy domain in which each character type feels most at home – i.e., whether it senses the emotional or rational domain as feeling more "right" and consistent. Masculine schizoid and obsessive types prefer the rational domain and tend to belittle the emotional arena or – in the extreme case – even to denigrate it, whereas depressive and hysteric types (the feminine pole) place the emotional aspect at the center of their lives.

The fundamental fears are crucial to an understanding of character types, since they constitute the type's essential core. According to RIEMANN, the fundamental fears orbit the following themes:

- Fear of personal annihilation (schizoid type)
- Fear of permanent separation from others (depressive type)
- Fear of change (obsessive-compulsive type)
- Fear of finality (hysterical type)

One can picture the fundamental fear as a *leitmotif* or banner headline, superordinate to the Central Conflict, that has, over time – presumably many reincarnations – formed and firmed itself up. It corresponds to the emotional essential core that seeks totally to protect and conceal the respective type from itself and others, because it is the central (yet vulnerable) core of the soul.

The origin of each fundamental fear, along with the convictions derived therefrom, is most likely based on extraordinarily painful emotional experiences linked to existentially fateful consequences such as one's own death. The Death theme is associated, especially for schizoids, with overblown fears, which often leads compensatorily to a devil-may-care indifference to personal death – although this attitude does not correspond to actual experiences, but should be construed as a defensive posture. Subconsciously, the future avoidance strategy leads (in schizoids) to the mentioned convictions, as per the motto "Just leave me alone!" ("… or else I'll probably have to die again.") or "I've always got to be strong!" ("… otherwise someone else will come along who's stronger and kill me.")

Similar considerations apply analogically to the other three types, although the existential threat does not always have to do with death, as it does with schizoids. It is much worse for the depressive, for instance, to have the ominous premonition of being permanently cut off from other people. This gives rise to the subconscious tendency to act especially nice and accommodating. In relationships in which "making nice" is not a desirable character trait, all kinds of other behavioral patterns can be used to cement the relationship – e.g., putting on an especially diligent and strict façade when one is courting a potential partner who values highly those particular traits . Depressives always try hard to adapt their behavior to the other person in order to receive emotional affection and warmth. For obsessives, it is change that is deeply threatening and fearful. They will therefore be especially orderly and "good" in order not to trigger any potential change. The exact opposite applies to the hysteric, for whom finality and irreversible stability trigger the deepest fears. Hysterics – like schizoids – often display an uncontrollable need for freedom in order to avoid anything becoming permanent. Very often, the hysteric also evades decisions, becoming capricious and indecisive but rationalizing it with excuses.

Because the fundamental fears of the four character types are deeply subconscious emotions, it is, experientially, unusually difficult for most people to learn much about them without outside help. With respect to self-discovery, it is extremely rare to find people who know their spiritual

Character Types and Depth-Psychology Parent Representation

Character types	Depressive/Hysteric	Schizoid/Obsessive
Parent representation	Mother	Father
Consciousness level	Emotions	Self (Reason)
Expansion pattern	Introversion	Extroversion
Existential significance	Passive taking "I am one with my mother"	Active giving "I am one with myself"
Sexual affiliation	Feminine	Masculine
Archaically experienced body region	Stomach/heart	Pelvis/head/neck/throat
Primary pleasure organ	Oral	Anal-urethral
Secondarily developed pleasure organ (assigned to both character pairs together)	Genitals	

theme – and this often includes specialists in the subconscious (such as psychoanalysts). Therefore, regarding the question "Who am I?", one needs to pick another access route that leads more easily to the goal. First of all, one needs to know if one has a more feminine or more masculine soul. As a rule, this is relatively easy to answer as soon as one has become better acquainted with one's deeper essential core.

There are some tips that can be helpful in answering the question regarding which main group one belongs to. Fundamentally, people with the, in principle, hard, rigid characteristic traits of the schizoid or obsessive-compulsive attempt to defend the Self like a fortified castle. The Self can be compared emotionally with principles such as *father* and *authority*. Schizoids and obsessive-compulsives subconsciously try to get closer to the father and to related emotional symbols such as ideals, laws, and the eternal typically masculine quest for the "Why?". Unpleasant traits, such as standing on principle and an authoritarian demeanor, can be taken as typical behavioral patterns of schizoid and obsessive-compulsive types. The notorious refusal in and of itself (defiance, persistence) and defense at all costs (conservative, upholder of traditional values) are, for such persons, typical basic mechanisms that often harden into an impression of general immobility and relentlessness – in the extreme case even senseless-seeming obstinacy and unrelenting severity.

The second group, that of feminine character types, looks quite different. The softer depressives/hysterics, tending toward Yin, generally would like to find the yearned-for redemption from their emotional need in a commitment to a person they experience as liberating and protecting. Other people are supposed to help them feel good again – either with a flattering/servile attitude (as one often finds in depressives) or in an emotionally distant, strategically calculating manner (as often observed in hysterics). Fundamentally, other people become the emotional focus, since the feminine character types inherently don't know how to deal with themselves very well. Emotionally, safety and security are associated with the role of the mother, unlike the schizoid and obsessive-compulsive who tends more toward the father principle. In a remarkable analogy, the emotional body corresponds in depth psychology to the maternal source, in whose warmth and shelter one would like to remain, like a baby. This dissolution into an encompassing safety and security is one of the basic tendencies of such persons, which explains the generalized and deeply-felt yearnings, the search for protection and human warmth, which originate in the innermost basic experiences of the depressive and the hysteric.

This all gets confusing because there are often **compensatory attitudes** that cloud the issue, making a clear assignment difficult. As an illustrative example, I'd like to refer back to the schizoid client whose case I described in detail. In his case, nobody would have thought him a schizoid,

Embryonic Emotional State

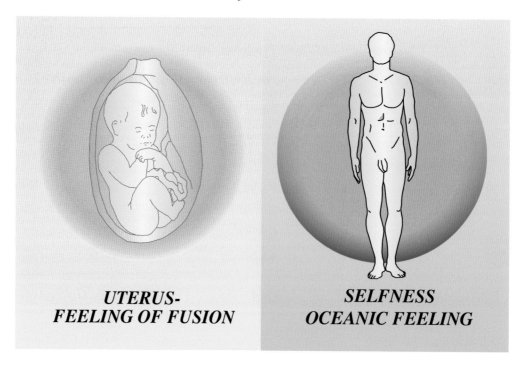

UTERUS-
FEELING OF FUSION

SELFNESS
OCEANIC FEELING

with the associated toughness and the often unrelenting essential nature. The Central Conflict, along with the underlying trauma, had in this patient's case drawn the masculine-hard characteristic traits to itself and turned them into shadowy anti-images. At a superficial glance, the patient seemed outright feminine and soft. Interestingly, though, the patient was well aware of himself and his true nature during my questioning. He knew that, way down deep, he was "a tough guy" structured along the lines of "soft on the outside, hard on the inside."

Self-discovery ultimately succeeds well, despite confusing compensatory attitudes, provided that one adopts an absolutely honest and neutral attitude toward oneself. There are some other useful classifications associated with the corresponding character types that can make self-discovery easier. The details are listed in the table on page 183. First off, one can select the attitude toward the biological parents as a distinguishing characteristic. The feminine-oriented hysteric and depressive character types often have a close emotional bond with the mother, whereas masculine-dominated schizoid and obsessive-compulsive types tend to choose the father as an emotional model. However, the relationship with the father can be replaced by an autistic (extremely self-centered) relationship with oneself, in which the person completely renounces relating to any other person. These are often the people who brag about having "done it on my own" and "with nobody else's help."

Our emotional fundamental fear will determine where we feel better and more at home – either with ourselves (Ego) or with the environment (mother/fellow human). "I feel safe and secure when I crawl deep into myself!" is what the schizoid and obsessive-compulsive will say. On the other hand, depressives and hysterics will say: "I feel safe and secure in mother's arms!" Now of course, when it comes to the fundamental feelings, there is no *right* or *wrong*, because each of the character pairs has the impression, based on its inner emotional needs, that it is acting logically and consistently. Depressives and hysterics thus seek their happiness in contact with fellow humans, whereas obsessive-compulsives and schizoids believe to their core that happiness can only come from within themselves. Each of the two character pairs thus seeks the solution path that works for them.

As regards the classification of psychosexual drive development, also listed in the *Parent Representation* table, I'd like to touch on it only peripherally, since it is, in my opinion, of secondary importance. I'd just like to say that the primary erogenous organ of the feminine character pairs is often the mouth, since it is through the mouth that the exchange with the first contact person takes place, i.e., the mother. For the masculine character pairs, on the other hand, it is the excretory organs that, in the alternation of resistance and commitment, develop as pleasure sources. In the later, more mature genital phase, one can hardly differentiate the types any more, since the adult drives have a very universal

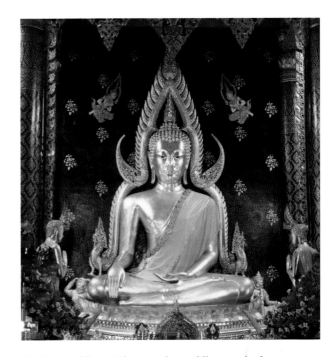

Golden Buddha in Thai temple. Buddha was the first person to have developed consciousness of the causal body to such an extent that an immortal "golden" enlightenment form was able to develop.

essence that functionally serves the goal of reproduction.

We get a much easier access to character formation than with FREUD's aforementioned drive model if we put ourselves in the place of the fetus during its intrauterine development. In this situation, the essential inner emotional cycles of either the masculine or feminine character pairs become very clear to us. We thus encounter, in the fetus in the womb, the key scene already present, which gives expression to our most important characteristic traits. As a tiny fetus, we evidently already confront the basic dilemma of our existence: "Should I run away or stand firm?"

As soon as the uterus begins to contract, or other stressors act on the growing child in the womb, the fetus gets a horrible feeling of threat. If strong enough, this kind of intrauterine stress would certainly be strong enough for the fetus to feel existentially threatened, above all because its dependent minuteness puts it at the mercy of the entire process. We cannot of course question a fetus, but we can, through empathic observation of ultrasound images, and other inspections of prenatal psychology, get an idea of what is going on in the fetus' inner emotions. Moreover, one can derive generally valid stress indicators from heart rate and hormonal levels, as well as recognize the fetus' mimicry in high-resolution ultrasound images – for instance, when the fetus' face spasms in a typical distortion of pain.

In addition, there are hypnotic and drug experiences, in which a person, in a deep trance, can regress to the embryonic state. Questioning a mother about intrauterine experiences, in which something dramatic like a car crash is described (from the fetus' point of view, which experiences a sudden loud noise or shock, and then the mother's pain), confirms the reality of such experiences. However, the emotional experience seems to be much more significant. The fetus is thus by no means an eternally slumbering, unconscious homunculus, but rather a fully-sentient being – at least during the later months of pregnancy. The Greek hallucinogen researcher KAFKLIDES' patients reported numerous intrauterine key scenes that bore a remarkable resemblance to the adults' later emotional problems.

These hypnotic states dealing with intrauterine key scenes lead to elementary decisions that are drawn as conclusions from such anguishing emotional states, i.e.: "Should I run away or stand firm?" And the person thereafter assumes a basic stance that is never abandoned in later adult life. Basically, these descriptions have to do with dramatic fundamental fears. Of course, the fetus' emotional language is very simple and contains no conversational communication along the lines of "You're a bad mother because I feel bad here inside you." The fetus is largely incapable of such dialogical emotions. Instead, a very simple either-or feeling arises: "I am threatened – so I'm going to focus on survival in order to protect myself" or, as soon as the danger is past, "blissful continued dreams in the cozy warmth."

In the '70s, the Czech psychiatrist Stanislaf GROF noticed, in LSD psychotherapy sessions, that many patients described birth experiences in their visions that were in striking accordance with the basic format of how these people as adults saw themselves and the world around them. GROF was the first to observe and evaluate this along a broad front. For example, those of GROF's patients who described a gruesome, horrible birth perceived as torture, later on often experienced the world similarly. GROF believed he could reconstruct this especially often in the case of violent people. To these people, the world is a threatening, instrumental, and manipulative place and wants to swindle them of their freedom and most important life contents. It goes without saying that a basic attitude this distorted has severe repercussions, since one has been defrauded of basic trust and is a deeply mistrustful person. From these kinds of observations, GROF drew the obvious conclusion that his patients' large emotional problems issue from a traumatic intrauterine/birth experience.

To my mind this is only partly true. Based on my experiences to date, pregnancy and birth reflect particularly good future spiritual themes. That presumably has to do with conflicts that are already active in the fetus, vibrating along on the resonance of the child-mother interaction, since large conflicts act like psychoenergetic blocks that block the mother energetically during birth. This makes the birth process much more traumatic. Birth and pregnancy often mirror the child's energetic constitution. At birth, the characters and their karmic fundamental conflicts reflect each other particularly well.

Particularly in children with large active conflicts, who have been so-called "problem" children all their lives because they exhibit many kinds of behavioral and developmental disorders, one hears very often of a problematic birth and a difficult time in the womb, e.g., during pregnancy the mother had often felt unusually sick, or the it was a breech birth, or the umbilical cord got tangled up, and so on. The example of little Michael in the previous chapter (Conflict Orchestra) illustrates this particularly well. Yet the entire process needn't take such a dramatic course. Even if children seem externally inconspicuous, important inner emotional themes can already be activated in this early phase – for instance due to experiences in the womb or during birth of which the mother and others would be unaware.

The situation in the womb leads to a fundamental feeling that has universal significance for all people. The psychoanalyst Erich NEUMANN calls it the paradisiacal state, experienced as a sensual fusion with the world, the Ouroboros state. In the blissful maternal cocoon, one experiences the primary feeling of perfection. The eternal circling of this perfect state about itself is depicted archetypically as a snake eating its own tail and spitting itself out as it constantly gives birth to itself. This is an ancient image of self-unfolding nature that we encounter time and again in all cultures in the most varied representations.

This blissful state of perfection comes to an end at birth. The birth of the individual marks the decisive turning point that now leads to suffering, as BUDDHA explains in the first proclamation of his teachings at the Gazelle Grove in Benares.

Buddha distinguishes three types of suffering:[43]
1. **Birth, old age, sickness, and death (symptoms of physical suffering)**
2. **To be united with unloved ones, to be separated from loved ones, not to get what one desires (symptoms of emotional and mental suffering)**
3. **The five grasped-at groups or aggregates of suffering (body, feeling, perception, mental formation, coordinated consciousness)**

In BUDDHA's view, the wheel of rebirth begins to turn because we spiritual beings decide to leave the original world of blessed unity. We desire to take on human form in the material world and be reincarnated as human beings.

---

[43] The three stages of suffering refer to the transitoriness of the Material/Vital (Level 1), the Emotional (Level 2), and the Mental (Level 3). Only attaining to the immortality of the Causal Level brings redemption and release.

Life in the material world is inseparably bound up with suffering, however – no matter how much we might enjoy life, the great suffering of death and parting waits for us inexorably. Eventually the party is over and the suffering of separation begins. We often fall prey to the illusion that we are beings separate from the universe and its cosmic consciousness. It is precisely this egotism (this "ignorance") that is, according to BUDDHA, the true reason why we must be reincarnated over and over. Even if we do not at all wish to be reincarnated, the illusion of the Self leads to reincarnation, in the Buddhist view.

One can recognize in egotism the aforementioned feeling of Self, which the fetus experiences, since it is forced to have painful experiences. Fear as the primordial beginning of consciousness surfaces here once again. On the other hand, the *in utero* feeling of "fusion" signifies, from the depth-psychology viewpoint, a spiritual sense of the return home and enlightenment. In this context (returning), enlightenment does not mean merging with the Void (*Nirvana*) but rather Self-consciousness becoming one with the eternal causal body. BUDDHA's shimmering gold body expresses the immortality and true nature of his sublime causal body.

Getting back to understanding the character types, I'd like to bring up an important point that is often the source of much misunderstanding. For example, one could resent someone for having a certain character, as if there were evil intent or a personal weakness involved. Yet when it comes to the four character types, it is not a matter of personal quirks and individual predilections. It's not that a person has a certain character because, to put it informally, he or she likes that type, as one might like a certain shirt or blouse. On the other hand, one also doesn't get a certain character as a punishment from fate to teach one a lesson, as it were, because a higher justice deemed one to be a particularly good or bad person. That too is a totally false approach! It is rather that, for each of us, character type is based on an enormously strong distress and dynamism that has to do with **fear of death**.

One's spiritual theme becomes the starting point of an inner spiritual landscape that exhibits certain regularities for each character type. All external influencing factors are processed in a monotonous and orderly manner. "Can't he see that any other way?", we ask. But we each have our own unique way of seeing the world, which becomes so much a part of us (incarnated) that, with time, we simply cannot perceive it any other way or react differently. It is important to know this, because these are the true essential roots of **fanaticism** and **egotism**. We defend our country or religion along with our possessions and ideology rigidly, intolerantly, and violently because we subconsciously equate it with ourself. But that is not enough for a truly satisfying understanding. What is the real reason people react so fanatically in civil wars, terror attacks, mobbing attacks in the workplace, or inheritance squabbles? What is driving them emotionally?

In dealing with this important question, it's necessary to understand that the deep-rooted fears of each character grow into fundamental existential questions of the first rank – like giants with appalling destructive power. Mythologically, violent giants and one-eyed (simple-minded) Cyclops are equated with such tremendous emotions. Character thereby becomes highly explosive. It becomes in the subconscious a life-preserving defensive bastion against everything that threatens existence at an elementary level. Thus one can also understand at once, from this point of view, why we react so intolerantly and exaggeratedly, when the foundations of our character are called into question. We then say: "That goes against every fiber of my being!" There's Wilhelm BUSCH's well-known description of Böck, the compulsive tailor: *"Böck could take it all in stride, keep it nicely tucked inside; but when he got the news of this, poor Böck began to fume and hiss."*

What was it that made the tailor so angry when he was teased by sassy kids like Max and Moritz (the original Katzenjammer Kids)? They compared the compulsive tailor to a clumsy and uncivilized beast (a Bock, or goat – his namesake) – which, in the language of the subconscious, takes aim at the repressed and taboo shadow side of the compulsive character. For the tailor, this is as detestable and infuriating as calling a fine, cultivated lady a "cheap slut." This is precisely what the fine lady does not want to be under any circumstances! Such an injurious attack aims right at the heart, because one is unfairly equated with that which one most vigorously rejects and renounces. Our inner nature is based on these fundamental fears, and existential distress leads to our "not being able to take a joke" and to our getting really nasty when we're "rubbed the wrong way" or our feelings are hurt.

Another approach to understanding character type is its relationship to life's phases. We cannot avoid dealing with each of the four fundamental fears at some point in our lives, so we can also assign them to **life phases**:

1. **Birth and old age – being faced with the fear of losing oneself** – dissolving away into nothing and having to die (schizoid)
2. **Childhood – fear (due to individuation) of being expelled by family and/or society** – thereby being isolated, no longer loved and having to die (depressive)
3. **Puberty and growing up – fear of the need to commit** – excluding other possibilities by making decisions, thus depriving oneself of other life possibilities, and the fear (in the worst case) of falling into a deadly trap (hysteric)
4. **Adulthood – fear of transitoriness** – of the decay of order into chaos, and the fact that there are no enduring values and everything invariably dies (obsessive-compulsive)

Each character type thus traverses all life phases – i.e., its own type's phase as well as that of the other types. The reason this is so can be viewed as the first learning assignment for the maturing soul. One learns thereby how to deal better with the fundamental fears that are foreign to one's essential nature. One is also challenged to master certain tasks associated with the corresponding maturation phases of the other types – e.g., as an aging depressive, to be confronted with earthly transitoriness (obsessive-compulsive theme), as one becomes more and more alone (one's own depressive theme sounding again). At this point, people ask themselves which life phase is likely to be the one they do best in. In my opinion, people feel most at home in that phase which has the most to do with their own character type. This is understandable, since they are best acquainted with and have best mastered their type-specific material. They know their way around it best because it is where their own spiritual theme expresses itself.

When I give lectures, I always get critical objections from audience members who question emotional conflicts and character types either in part or as a whole. These people's questions usually center on three core issues:

- Is there such a thing as character (types) at all, or isn't it just a matter of a categorical generalization of traits that we all latently possess?
- What do these character types do? What is the deeper meaning here?
- Is it true that, according to the theory of emotional conflicts and character type, all people are sick? Or are there emotionally healthy people as well? Does the healthy person have a character (type) too?

I'd like to answer these questions in sequence, but I'd like to postpone the third question until the end of the book. First, a personal confession: as a young student, and later as a physician, I was for a long time of the opinion that there was no such thing as character type of the kind described in textbooks, and that the whole classification scheme in fact arose from the need of psychiatrists and psychoanalysts to impose order on a chaotic situation. Instead of butterflies, they "collected" their patient's characteristic traits, storing them, in crude oversimplification, in one of four boxes. In short, I viewed the entire process as a hobby for specialists who, in their passion to pigeonhole, were being unfair to the individuals in question because they were over-generalizing. Evidently, many medical colleagues felt the same, so they invented hybrid types, describing in their medical correspondence, e.g., the "rigid-hysteric" character for someone who exhibited both compulsive and hysteric characteristic traits.

It came as quite a surprise to me then, as I performed more and more energy tests and began to understand the four character types better, that my earlier objections were no longer applicable. I realized that one of these four char-

acter types was verifiable in each and every person, and indeed never mixed, but always clearly identifiable! They also turned out to be extremely valuable (and logically consistent) in clearing up other difficult questions. The deeper I penetrated into depth-psychology levels, the more clearly aware I became of the universality of character types. The thing that is confusing at first, when making the classification, is mainly the compensatory attempts and the varying conformation of the types. I have already alluded to this a number of times in earlier chapters.

By compensation I mean that each character type is somewhat unstable. Character can be compared to a car rolling around on just a single wheel, unstable and wobbly, weaving about hither and yon. Compensatory efforts are initiated, with the aid of the other character types, to restore stability and emotional centeredness. Through the compensatory efforts, one acquires foreign character traits, which makes initial type determination much more difficult. It takes some tricks and background knowledge – which I'll be revealing in subsequent chapters – to see behind the façade, despite complications, and correctly identify the character type in each case.

The other confusion in classifying character types arises from evolutionary emotional processes and biological life phases – because, depending on the developmental stage of the individual at that moment, energetically and emotionally, one will encounter different varieties of the character type. This applies to children and adults, intellectuals and unlettered folk. All of these influences modify the "phenotype" of the respective character type. In the discussion of the spiritual states of emotional remedies and karmic upward development, I will get into this in more detail. The crucial thing here, too, is to have an eye for what's important and essential – because the more we look behind the scenes in a person, the more clearly the respective character type emerges without any admixture of other types.

The next question is why there are character types in the first place. The point of character types can be explained in a great number of ways. There is evidence all around that "the dear Lord had something in mind" when he invented character types. This includes the opportunity for maturation of the individual soul within an evolutionary program . The simplest and most obvious reason for character formation seems to be that individual consciousness is formed thereby. As with favorite musical themes, one has a *leitmotif* that serves as a guide to the world's multifaceted complexity. Externally, one acquires a predictable behavioral pattern, so that, in social situations, one is a known quantity.

The character types give therapists the invaluable ability to categorize patients' behavior and feelings[44]. The concept of *categorization* has a negative undertone for many people. With respect to *classification*, I'd like to describe some personal misinterpretations I was guilty of at the beginning of my encounter with character types, as cautionary examples of how not to do it. Like many a beginner, I fell into a nasty trap, that of thinking that identifying character type was some variety of athletic competition.

At first, it was quite amusing and informative to compartmentalize people unknown to me along the lines of "That's definitely a hysteric!" when, for instance a woman is strikingly attired to call attention to herself. It's all sport and amusing puzzle-solving, and it has, moreover, the great advantage of keeping people at a distance and placing oneself on the pedestal of the superior spectator. This kind of sneering observer's role is a popular pose among teenagers. Behind this one often finds the emotional function of keeping unattractive feelings at arm's length, in that projection is the most convenient and certain way to puff up one's ego and belittle others. Making fun of and judging others is a quick and dirty way to make oneself larger and more invulnerable. Not even academic titles and trophies protect one from such primeval human weaknesses.

But of course it's different when you're the victim. So it was a shock that shook me to my toes when I became aware of the far-reaching consequences of confronting my own emotional problem complex. The taboo-laden repression mechanisms function so well that you see certain parts of yourself only in brief glimpses; you think you've finally got a hold of it at some point, only to watch in bewilderment as it fades away like a mirage. This applies most to your emotional center, in the middle of which the Central Conflict's fundamental fears are stored. If you then stand facing the towering emotional mountain in its cumulative size, it hits you like a ton of bricks. To my mind there is no greater occurrence that conveys such deeply moving and beautiful experiences as it simultaneously brings to light such monstrously dreadful and frightening emotional contents.

The Central Conflict feels strangely familiar and at the same time extremely foreign, like a small child that, after a long separation, sees its mother again. Most children at first react to such overpowering emotional experiences by looking away or (depending on age) pouting, running away, or crying. Adults, confronting their own "horrible and hateful" side often provokes existential crises that can lead to psychoses, severe organ ailments (cancer, stroke), suicide, and

serious mental crises (that can manifest themselves in many ways, including socially conditioned ones). Nothing like that happened to me, thank God, but a residue of beneficial humility stays with you after you've confronted your deepest dark side. The fun turns serious when you realize that you need to be extremely cautious and careful in categorizing and judging others, because a single false move can inflict enormous harm and grief.

You ask yourself, of course, how you can recognize your own Central Conflict. I'll be giving advice and suggestions originating from my experiences with thousands of patients. But you should be clear about certain fundamental difficulties. Due to the strategy learned in earliest childhood of concealing one's character type and being as inconspicuous as possible in the social environment, many character types are at first unusually hard to recognize. This problem arises when a person represents the kind of kook who doesn't at first fit into the family and social environment. This person must then fake a sham character in order not to attract unpleasant attention. I'll cover the attendant repercussions of this tactic in a later chapter on the meaning of conflict and family.

If one grows up in a society that is the polar opposite of one's character type, then it is of course very hard to develop one's essential character traits. In a hysteric society that loves pathos and in which people go about melodramatically airing their problems – for example, in tropical countries – a schizoid, depressive, or obsessive-compulsive type will only appear in public with persona mask firmly in place. If one is not versed in the mentality of a society, then one will of course have a great deal more trouble recognizing a masked character type. For obvious reasons, people who grow up in an environment foreign to their character long for a spiritual homeland in which they can relax and let it all hang out. They want, at long last, to be truly themselves. For these people, the continuing foreignness understandably leads to yearnings, problems, and illnesses. Many seek refuge in addiction and sickness, because they feel spiritually displaced and unloved, or they dream of emigrating.

Identifying character type depends crucially on how well acquainted one is with a person's social and familial environment. We can much more easily recognize the different character type variants when we are familiar with the basic characteristics of a social group. Another aid is emotional maturity. The more developed the personality, the more clearly visible the true character type. Of course, this can be viewed as a detachment process in which one finds the way back to one's true center, because the more that social conventions and learned familial behavior patterns retreat into the background, the more clearly delineated the individual becomes in the foreground.

---

[44] I consider unlikely, based on my experience, the conjecture that there are better typologies . The Sufi Enneagram tradition, for instance, distinguishes 9 types that, when examined closely, correspond to the four types introduced here: the schizoid to Enneagram types 1,5, and 8; the depressive to 2 and 6; the obsessive-compulsive to 9; and the hysteric to 3, 4, and 7. Since into every typology goes the self-knowledge of its developer (one cannot help but discern one's own type, and only one's own, since everything else is deep subconscious), one can draw some conclusions (based on the large number of schizoid and hysteric Enneagram types) about the character types of those who developed the Enneagram concept. What's more, the Enneagram has many characterizations belonging to the shallow subconscious persona level. These provisos apply to other typologies as well.

The most impressive way to identify our own character type is to answer four basic questions: What are we most (subconsciously) afraid of?

1. ... losing ourselves? (schizoid)
2. ... losing others? (depressive)
3. ... surprising and large changes? (obsessive-compulsive)
4. ... loss of freedom and final commitment? (hysteric)

We're all familiar with the themes of these four fears in one form or another – but which fear is predominant in the subconscious is often not so easy to discern. The problem is the subconscious. Because we normally deal with deep subconscious fears, we can often identify other people's character types better than we can our own. Experience shows that it takes a lot of observation and appraisal before we can better recognize the types of the people around us, and develop a way to recognize their recurring patterns and prominent characteristics.

With that, I'd like to wrap up the theoretical introduction to the depth psychology of the Central Conflict. The next chapter deals with the everyday external characteristics of the character types as we encounter them in actual people. I have tried to present as vivid a description as possible by introducing the four character types via typical patient histories. Still, the reader should understand that the character traits of the individual types cannot apply point for point in each individual case. For example, not all hysterics are gamblers, just as not all schizoids are loners. It's more accurate, actually, to invert the logic: enthusiastic and passionate gamblers are statistically very likely to be hysterics, just as notorious lone wolves are to be schizoids. Still, because relatively few people exhibit such striking characteristics as are encountered in eccentrics and the like, when it comes to average people, one will be dealing, rather, with evidentiary chains. One must therefore develop a "sixth sense" for each particular nature, which, in most people, is a composite mosaic of individual images and some useful clues that form the overall picture of the true character type.

The Four Character Types

If one has character, then one also has one's typical, ever recurring, experience.

(Nietzsche)

In this chapter, descriptions of the four character types introduce their most important attributes as I have observed them in my studies of thousands of people. In the interest of clarity, I have selected, for each type, an exemplary case that represents it particularly well. The advantage to my method of character type assignment is that I, as physician, am less likely to be deceived by psychoenergetic testing than by any other kind of diagnostic approach. For example, when first meeting a person, one is sometimes misled by the outward appearance or demeanor, as well as by other sources of error, such as the subtle compensatory processes with which a certain character type camouflages itself. At times, even an uncommon ethnicity can give the wrong impression – i.e., the tendency to ascribe hysteric character traits to people from tropical countries, since they are so lively and exuberant.

But thanks to the inestimably valuable energy testing, I know quickly where I am with each patient, and which character type I'm really dealing with. Unlike other psychotherapeutic methods for studying character type, it's like a crime novel in which I learn who the murderer is right at the beginning, thanks to the procedure I use. By energy testing the Central Conflict, I get a much clearer and more accurate picture.

I'd like to start off with the **schizoid** type. The term derives from the fact that people with markedly schizoid character traits display a split between their emotional and intellectual aspects, such as is found to a pronounced degree in schizophrenia cases. Schizoids basically have a cool and aloof nature; cordiality and emotional warmth are not their strong suits. This is because schizoids by nature have masculine character traits. Thus schizoids have a forceful and often unyielding nature, although one might not think so at first, because they often cleverly behave outwardly as if they were quite different – i.e., soft and yielding.

The true cause of the well-known phenomenon of "soft on the outside, hard on the inside" is the fact that the repressed conflict cultivates a make-believe gentle nature, like a magic cape confers invisibility. In this manner, the schizoid tries to avoid the same sort of painful situation that led to the formation of the Central Conflict in the first place. Of course, this is a foolish hide-and-seek ploy that has nothing to do with the schizoid's true nature – and is usually pointless, since the time of the existential threat (and

the conditions that prevailed back then) is long since past. We are thus dealing, for all character types, with historical relics of personality traits that have outlived their usefulness. They hang around, however, because they have got lost in the deep subconscious.

Schizoids are incapable of understanding why we reproach them for their character masquerades, because their defensive moves, such as gentleness and exaggerated friendliness, have become second nature to them. "I am how I am," they think to themselves. Schizoids at first defend their gentleness by adopting an emphatically pacifist pose. They come up with all sorts of excuses to praise and defend their presumably worthwhile (but put-on) personality traits. But at some point the tables are turned, since the closer schizoids get to their emotional center, due to healing of their Central Conflict, the more their original masculine characteristic traits resurface. The same applies, by the way, when being put to the test, which can lead to startling surprises that one had not reckoned with: supposedly gentle and yielding schizoids suddenly confront you with their true hardness. In these trying situations, schizoids by no means outdo themselves, as is often erroneously claimed, but simply reveal their true nature.

Classic schizoid natures include the unemotional philosopher and the notorious lone wolf. The lonesome cowboy has likewise become a classic image, as he rides off into the sunset at the end of the movie to the accompaniment of mournful music, usually leaving behind a heartbroken woman yearning for him. The woman is an indispensable part of the drama, and in fact its contextual meaning would be incomplete without her! The archetypal image of the *lonesome cowboy* is a very good portrayal of the schizoid's emotional loneliness.

Deep inside, schizoids have a deeply buried melancholy that seems downright maudlin and endlessly wistful. This is why the schizoid is classified as a melancholic in the ancient temperament theory. The depth-psychological reading is that the melancholy thread corresponds to the longing for the lost maternal center. Schizoids crave emotional warmth, and they seek it wistfully even as they run away from it, yet they never understand that they make life hard on themselves with their stand-offish and unapproachable nature. "Ride on back to your sweetheart!" you feel like shouting to the departing cowboy – but you know that his decision, once made, is unalterable and irreversible. Schizoids are tough *hombres* who don't change course so easily.

Pathological escalations of the schizoid nature include the crank and the outsider, the epitome of which we encounter, ultimately, in the asocial, criminal, and unfeeling psychopath. The tragic thing about such extreme schizoid character types is their excessive warding off of any and all impulses to commit, which are equated with personal destruction. Emotional and maternal impulses are, on the one hand, urgently craved and, on the other, forcefully (if ambivalently) rejected. "Tough guys don't cry!" is what these hard cases claim, even though they may feel like doing so. Fending off emotions turns into a rigid defensive front that eventually leads to emotional frigidity. As we know, many emotional cripples had a harrowing childhood whose emotional suffering is nearly incomprehensible to those who haven't experienced it first hand, and which has (understandably) led to the formation of a psychopathic character structure.

The defenses of the emotional side are so overdone in psychopaths that such people at times seem downright machinelike – like intelligent robots who track down anything emotional in their fellow humans, as if it were something horrible needing to be destroyed. In fact, they are naturally terribly afraid that the powder keg of their emotions could be blown sky-high by the tiniest spark. Psychopaths therefore fight every external source of emotional infection, preferring most of all to turn positive feelings into their opposite, e.g., by using sadistic schemes to guarantee coming out on top.

Now of course (thank God!) very, very few schizoids become extreme psychopaths. Most schizoids are friendly, normal people. And yet, the healthy façade often conceals a tragic trauma whose theme is the total destruction of the individual's own life. Schizoids are thus always fighting the unceasing struggle of "to be or not to be." Their insane-seeming basic emotional situation resembles that of a fetus whose umbilical cord has been severed, even though it is not yet viable. The fetus feels existentially threatened by what it feels to be a hostile world. Schizoids thus have a fundamental fear that bears some very existential features.

The story continues on from here in a logical manner. Like a dying man with a thousand thoughts buzzing around in his head, the schizoid – driven by his fundamental fear – begins to inquire into the actual cause of his misery. As he does, he encounters the archetypal Indian goddess KALI who, after giving birth to them, barbarously devours her own children. This archetype of the bloodthirsty maternal godhead has its origin in the circumstance that our mother brings us into the world, which means that, basically, our end is also in her hands. "If you hadn't given birth to me, I wouldn't have had to go through all this!" complains the soul (with impeccable logic). The schizoid gazes into the horrific countenance of the maternal KALI, in which love

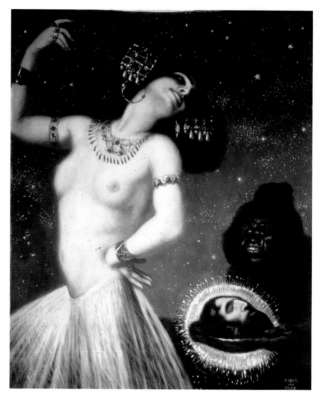

The painting depicts, from the viewpoint of the beheaded John the Baptist, the origin of his schizoid Central Conflict. Following this logic, the dancing Salome is presented with the bloody head of the saint by an apelike monster, which itself symbolizes the demon or conflict that Salome serves. I think that, behind the horrific decapitation there is, psychodynamically, a second drama, namely the collision of two incompatible character types, that of Salome as the seductive hysteric and the pious schizoid saint.

has metamorphosed into sheer hate and murderous delight in destruction.

The stalemated situation of the schizoid manner of experiencing life has aspects of a diabolical paradox, because life and death, being born and having to die, seem to shade into each other seamlessly and inescapably. In its extreme form, the schizoid's loving impulses take on destructive attributes, as can be seen in the example of the sunset-bound cowboy, who not only leaves behind his sorrowful sweetheart, but also destroys his own longing as he flees into the lonesome wilderness. And yet the schizoid has an enormous yearning for love and warm-heartedness – which he also subconsciously fears. One senses, even so, that it would take only a little push for the schizoid to overcome his inner inhibitions. This little push often comes from a depressive type, whose emotional structure perfectly complements that of the schizoid. Which brings us to the relationships variations arising out of the four character types. In the depressive, the schizoid finds, as mentioned, the ideal mate. In a sense, the depressive represents the missing emotional component that the schizoid needs to be whole. Here are the emotional warmth and the strong bonding desire that offset the schizoid's deficits.

In the hysteric disposition, the schizoid encounters his greatest conceivable characterological antithesis. By their very nature, schizoids and hysterics live in totally different worlds. The essential drives and emotional motives of the hysteric are thus totally unfathomable to the schizoid. The schizoid's inability to understand the hysteric is easy to comprehend once you understand the elemental differences in the natures of the two types. While the schizoid's basic feeling always has a tragic undertone, the hysteric has a fundamentally comic and playful nature, as if life were a gigantic amusement park. The schizoid can not only not understand this attitude, he finds the hysteric's behavior disgusting and repellent (his admiration is clearly tinged with contempt). Compounding this are other unfortunate aberrations, such as that the hysteric's rivalizing and playful-pugnacious attitude is sensed by the schizoid as an existentially threatening challenge. Thus, the hysteric's comedy quickly becomes a tragedy for the schizoid.

The schizoid's relationship with obsessive-compulsives is much more temperate. The obsessive-compulsive, also a masculine character type, is much easier to understand. Often, a schizoid's best friend – to the extent he even needs one! – is either another schizoid or else an obsessive-compulsive. The schizoid's restless and chaotic tendencies are cooled off (at least superficially) by the obsessive-compulsive. The schizoid's anarchistic aspect is gentled and moderated by obsessive-compulsive elements, so that obsessive-compulsive influences do the schizoid at least a little good – but too much is bad, because, for the schizoid, the obsessive-compulsive represents an ultimately morbid attitude that goes against his true nature. Thus, for him, obsessive-compulsive character traits always have a neurotic, pathological undertone. Obsessiveness represents, namely, a pathological surrogate action, as if the schizoid were to have chosen the wrong exit in trying to escape from his emotional prison. Thus, compulsive washing and cleaning, or collecting stamps or coins, are to the schizoid neurotic actions that cannot lead to any genuine solution of his emotional problems.

The schizoid's primary questions center on *existence* (topic of Chakra 1) and *meaning* (topic of Chakra 7). The schizoid can thus be understood as that character type which marks the beginning and end of every journey of spiritual development – if one relates the spiritual journey with the Chakras. This journey then begins at the first Chakra and ends at the seventh, the two energy centers that

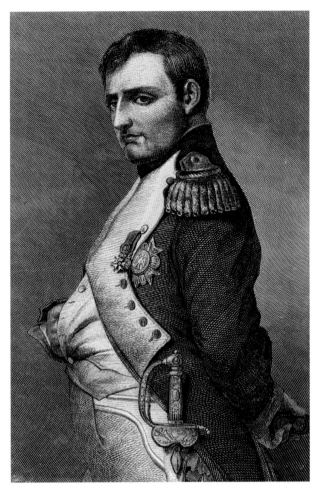

Napoleon as the self-crowned autocrat of his world represents the classic schizoid, an autocrat par excellence. The schizoid's pride and self-representation differs from that of the hysteric in that, way down deep, the schizoid doesn't care a bit what others think of him. The schizoid is completely sure of himself, which is why all yes-men and sycophants are to him superfluous freeloaders trying to ride the coattails of his magnificence.

are most strongly occupied with the problem complex of the schizoid and have the associated schizoid Central Conflicts. Pelvis and head – the regions of the first and seventh Chakras – are thus problematic body regions for the schizoid, the likely areas of illnesses and disorders, since they are the schizoid's energetic weak spots.

The case described below, that of a businessman, illuminates the entire problem complex of the schizoid's emotional world:

John, 51, a large good-looking man, semi-bald, who looks at first glance like the eternal student type, wears grubby jeans and an open shirt, and has a stressed expression on his pale face, as if he had not been out in the sun for months. John has come to the "Health Center" to learn more about our naturopathic healing methods. He had attended our lecture the evening before and heard that we were giving a practical demonstration of Psychosomatic Energetics, testing patients the next day. Although John is a therapist, he didn't bring any of his patients along, as many of his colleagues are wont to do; instead, he wanted to be tested himself. This is fairly common, since more than a few therapists have enormous health problems and emotional disturbances of their own – but this didn't seem to be the case with John. John sells alternative medicine devices and is always on the lookout for new and interesting products. He is of course interested in "what's up with him," but it's not his main priority; he mainly wants to know whether there's anything to the method. To my standard opening question as to what symptoms he has, he answers (quite unexpectedly and non-standardly) that he doesn't want to tell me, since I would then know everything in advance. I'm speechless at first; with a patient, I'd usually terminate the session at this point – but since John was not a patient, and he was actually putting the method to the test, I decide to go along with the (to me) extremely unappealing situation. Energy testing has to do with emotional intimacy and friendliness, and to start off by turning it into a game of chance or a validity test often leads to poor results. I tell John this, but he's OK with it.

Confounding my expectation that I was dealing with a reasonably healthy person, the REBA® Test Device readings were 30% vital, 60% emotional, 70% mental, and 40% causal (The Rebatest values indicate what percentage charge the respective energy level has, i.e., how healthy it is.). I find that Chakra 1 (pelvic region) is disturbed with the conflict Emvita® 4 (Self-controlled, emotions not allowed…). The conflict has above-average readings of 80% vital, 70% emotional, 10% conscious, and 50% causal. I explain my tentative diagnosis to him: that he is probably feeling fairly exhausted (vital 30%) and listless (60%) and might have problems, moreover, in the lower abdomen such as lower-back pain, since there is a vegetative block there (Chakra 1). In addition, he has trouble showing emotion and constantly keeps way too tight a grip on himself.

After a longish pause, during which he doesn't move a muscle, he tells me – in a monotone voice and with expressionless face – that I had hit the nail right on the head on all counts. The method really works well. Everything I said applied to him 100%. He feels constantly drained of energy and exhausted, even though he takes a lot of mountain-bike trips in the nearby mountains, paddles his canoe, and recently even took a long vacation that didn't do anything about his exhaustion. He thinks he misses his girlfriend, with whom he is hopelessly in love. When I ask him, flabbergasted, what on earth the problem is, he mentions the enormous distance between them,

because she lives on another continent.

I point out that that's not a problem in this jet age, since neither he nor his girlfriend are joined together in a formal relationship. No, he replies hesitantly, he really can't expect her to come and live with him, he loves her far too much to do that to her. When I ask him what he means by that – does he maybe have AIDS or something – he answers, somewhat evasively, that he and another woman had lived happily together for a number of years – but she had left him nonetheless. He was so disappointed and upset that he has since then lived alone. There's also another woman who lives nearby and pays him a lot of attention, but he simply isn't interested in a close relationship. When I suggest that he ought to try the emotional and Chakra remedies, he becomes dismissive and says he doesn't want to take anything for his situation. His problem is just the way things are, he says. I haven't heard from John since then.

Evaluation:

The façade of grubby philosopher and loner conceals a shy man battered by fate who is apparently unable to get past an earlier parting from a woman he loved. His continued extreme dramatization of this long-ago separation corresponds to the schizoid feeling of basically not being loved and not daring to show any weakness. Any opening up emotionally, such as committing to a relationship, is anxiously avoided – even though, deep inside, that is precisely what he secretly longs for. The sadistic aspect of this character type is revealed in the refusal to name symptoms (admitting weaknesses) – a move intended to put me as therapist under his control. Sadism (rejecting other people before they can do it to you) also involves the refusal to accept help from others, i.e., to use my prescription – but also, of course, rebuffing the amorous advances of his two current female companions.

I'd like to turn next to the **hysteric**, since this type is the polar opposite of the schizoid. In the hysteric personality structure, the primary fear is of being permanently forced into any situation; reality is viewed as consisting of immobilizing necessities and binding obligations. This antipathy to any kind of being "tied down" leads to an exaggerated desire for freedom that tends to devalue things and experience them all simplistically as equivalent. This one-dimensional world is a rosy Disneyland in which one can enjoy the indulgent freedom granted to a child whose every wish is granted.

For hysterics, happiness is always just around the corner. Everything is always beginning anew from zero – which applies above all to hysterics' own transgressions, for which they (acting as their own indulgent judges) forgive themselves forever without further ado. Anything negative and limiting is blanked out and repressed, which leads in extreme cases to living a lie and projecting everything bad out into the environment. This calls to mind an entertainer who, with charm and trickery, entices those around him to allow him, time and again, just a little more freedom and wish-fulfillment. Most intolerable for hysterics is having to wait, and postpone gratification. Everything must be enjoyed at once, in full, with intoxicating ecstasy. Children going through a particular infantile phase tend toward hysterical characteristic traits, wanting to experience everything to excess, not wanting their birthday party to end, playing and laughing until they collapse.

The image is that of a light-hearted, childlike, joyful Dionysian nature, somewhat like the Greek god Pan – but which, upon closer inspection, morphs into an immoderate and insatiable glutton. This is why some hysterics' body structure turns into a shapeless colossus of fat, since eating doesn't satisfy them either, so they can't stop. This was easy to see in Elvis Presley near the end of his career, a classical hysteric through and through. In this process, short-term satisfaction tips over into renewed frustration, a hydra-headed wish-fulfillment monster that, when one head is lopped off, grows three new ones in its place. Hysterics know very well how to have fun, which distinguishes them fundamentally from schizoids. You don't have to show a hysteric how to "grab the gusto" and what to enjoy in life: he has known it "from the crib" – unlike the schizoid, who often has to learn (at great effort) how to have fun and enjoy life.

From a developmental standpoint, one can make out an Œdipal rivalry complex behind the hysteric personality structure. Often, the father was inaccessible as a role model – which is in my opinion just a consequence and not a cause. Either the father was too strict and unapproachable or else was a pompous blowhard. Of course, this is mainly the hysteric's fault, because his adversarial nature and occasionally undisciplined, provocative, and coercive attitude is a problem for authority figures. Because the hysteric's behavioral strategy can shift about like a chameleon's colors, he is an irritant to those in authority, whom he loves to tease until they're boiling mad. In this respect, the hysteric and the schizoid have something in common, namely a sadistic note that can escalate to barbaric cruelty. In hysterics, the sadistic streak originates in their sense of pleasure, which is why perverse sex offenders are not infrequently hysterics. The schizoid, on the other hand, is more likely to be the insensitive castigator who feels little or no pleasure, and for whom the motivation to punish issues from specific notions, such that he believes himself to be acting in the name of a higher moral authority.

Now, extreme cases such as sex offenders should not tempt the reader to jump to conclusions, since they play a minor role in everyday life. Moreover, these pathological cases represent extremely distorted versions of a particular character type, and as such have no general applicability. Indeed, the great majority of both schizoids and hysterics are normal people with a great many downright likable personality traits. Most hysterics have strongly toned-down characteristic traits that enable them to live a normal life in society. Still, even a normal hysteric exhibits certain idio-

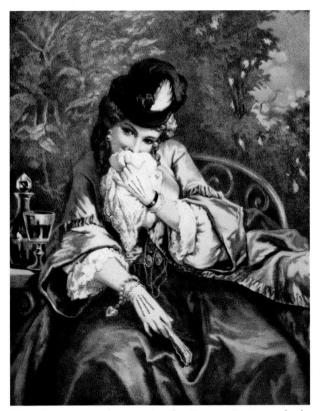

The Coquette – *this painting by Gustave Dorè reveals the unmistakable attributes of the hysteric, especially the seductive-playful basic attitude, the beautiful jewelry and the appealing clothing as an opportunity for representation and sensuous joy, as well as the wineglass as expression of the love of physical pleasure.*

syncrasies that have something contradictory about them. Thus, hysterics' tendency to annoy others and make themselves hugely unpopular is balanced out by their touching readiness to make amends and by the fact that they seldom hold a grudge. Also, the empathetic warmth of their feminine polarity and the tendency of coquettishly wanting to please help make it easier for the offended party to forgive and forget.

One can make out, in all these descriptions, opposing characteristic traits that very often impart to those who know hysterics a contrasted "heaven and hell" experience. Sometimes you feel jubilant at the hysteric's likable manner, only to wind up shortly thereafter cursing him vehemently and even hating him. All the contradictory feelings that hysterics provoke in those around them have a profoundly inconstant quality about them – which of course issues from the hysteric's fear of being tied down. Hysterics project their characteristic traits (as do all character types) onto those around them, whereby these others then perceive the true feelings of the respective type and, moreover, "pay for it."

Fickle and disparate character traits that are hard to reconcile are popularly associated with the female character in a patriarchal society. The hysteric temperament was thus long considered to be a purely feminine character trait – which of course scrupulously ignored that fact that half of all hysterics were men. In a patriarchy, hysteric men are, due to their basic talent for play-acting, very often disguised. They play the unapproachable and authoritarian schizoid (boss), the warm-hearted and obedient depressive (servant), or the faithful and tidy obsessive-compulsive (bureaucrat) – but, once they get home, they reveal their true colors behind closed doors as the tyrannical "master of the house." The expression "bowing to superiors and treading inferiors underfoot" captures and censures the lamentable character flaws associated with this kind of hide-and-seek behavior. Because the play-acting character suffers from a permanent feeling of frustration – which he is all too ready to work off with temperamental outbursts and the like – it often leads to domestic violence.

As for hysteric depressives, there is a compensatory tendency to effusive adoration of fatherly authority figures, who are affably, naively believed, trusted unreservedly, and served with great idealism. Hysterics are thus frequently great idealists – which, however, stems from childlike adoration and emotional enthusiasm and not from rational and abstract deliberation. When such enthusiastically held ideals are questioned and threatened from the outside, they are defended and protected in a paranoid manner. Hysterics often create an artificial counterpoise to their fear of being tied down by grotesquely glorifying and mummifying certain ideals. One is then dealing with emotional islands that have absolutely nothing to do with the rest of the hysteric's feelings.

Unsuspected chasms open up behind the façade of hysteric gaiety, which usually conceals a deep-seated, profoundly panicky fear. There is, first, the hysteric's fear of being immobilized, which is, in a sense, the cultural medium for all derivative fears such as agoraphobia, fear of insects, and the like. No other character type is so dominated by fear as the hysteric – but it would be a mistake to assume that all anxiety disease sufferers are hysterics. Fear is a profoundly human phenomenon underlying all the character types as a primary emotion. Still, no other character type, it seems to me, is so subjugated by fear as the hysteric.

The classic hysteric type is *Don Juan* who, with his charming and extroverted manner, quickly becomes the darling of the ladies and of society, loves to be the center of attention and is always forcing his way into the social foreground, lives life to the fullest, and fritters away his money and belongings in ecstatic enjoyment. In any social circle, the "life of the party" who's always in the thick of things will be a hysteric. At the beach, everyone turns to look when Don Juan calls out to some Eve with his loud, laughing

voice. The hysteric's days are one big exciting game, a magnificent intoxicating party. Looking back, the aging hysteric tends to recall his earlier life as a kind of transfiguring dream. When unlovely, naked reality makes this dream world impossible, the hysteric's old age can take on a tragic note, often becoming a nightmare that often ends in suicide, e.g., via excessive drinking or eating (severe obesity), which amounts to suicide on the installment plan. The aging hysteric struggles against being terminally branded and immobilized by old age and death.

"*Praise not youth but well-lived age.*" Thus spake the Greek philosopher Epicurus. This statement could never be uttered by a hysteric, to whom the "here and now" is so important. The past has low priority for the hysteric; what counts most of all is the present. There is also the fact that, for the aging hysteric, the façade of youthful beauty crumbles progressively. He or she often fights back with cosmetic surgery and an illusory self-image. In everyone's life, aging and death eventually become undeniable realities, which the hysteric fears profoundly because of his fear of fixity. The hysteric's present-orientedness is shown in his attitude not only toward transitoriness, but also toward the future. Having to await future uncertainties is, for the hysteric, the worst possible punishment, as is the uncertainty of upcoming events. As soon as he is told precise details on future plans, he calms down. Therefore, clairvoyants and such are inordinately important to the hysteric, since they presumably spare him the uncertainty that the future inevitably involves.

Regarding relationships with other character types, hysterics' ideal partners are obsessive-compulsive character types. Because of their chaotic and unstructured lifestyle, hysterics need them as an essential counterpoise; they need compulsives' order and strictness to provide a clearly-defined framework for their wild and anarchistic temperament. Just as wild, misbehaved children can only be brought to their senses and find their emotional center through a strict yet loving upbringing, so also do hysterics explicitly long for the strictness that obsessive-compulsives embody, like drowning people clinging fiercely to the lifeguard. Hysterics thus need "the carrot and the stick" because, without externally imposed guidelines and precepts, they drift about aimlessly, needing to be led back to the right path with strictness and admonitions – with the "stick," so to speak – but without overly frustrating their desire for enjoyment (the "carrot"). Once one has grasped these elementary mechanisms, the otherwise notoriously difficult hysterics are very easy to guide.

Hysterics get along least well with schizoids, who live at the opposite end of the universe from hysterics, automatically making them strange and incomprehensible to the hysteric nature. Hysterics ask "What's the point of wasting time with serious stuff like 'the meaning of life' like schizoids do? After all, life's a party to be celebrated!" Or: "Why on earth does the silly schizoid cowboy ride away into the setting desert sun – and, as if that weren't loony enough, leaving his sweetheart behind to boot?" asks the hysteric Don Juan, to whom schizoid behavioral peculiarities such as "renunciation" and "moral austerity" or "lone-wolf lifestyle" are totally incomprehensible. Hysterics consider schizoids to be completely off the beam and out of their minds.

Hysterics find in depressives a neurotically-tinged emotional affinity, since they're attracted to depressives as kindred types. At first, depressives' tragically fixed and final aspect seems to be good for inconstant hysterics, but the depressive attitude is very dangerous for them (I'll go into this in more detail later on) because depressives can't give hysterics the stability they need, nor put up enough resistance, which is necessary so that hysterics take note of limits and don't do the wrong thing. In fact, the depressive attitude is extremely dangerous for hysterics because it de-inhibits them emotionally, leading in the extreme case to self-destruction.

The disturbed Chakra is the 2nd (lower abdomen), associated with the intestinal tract and urogenital control and supplying the kidneys (anxiety organ) with energy. The adrenals, along with the sympathetic nervous system, are likewise affected organs. The 6th Chakra also belongs to the hysteric expression type (brow region in the vegetative centers) in which the intuitive, chaotic, and dysregulated aspects of hypothalamic dysfunction find expression. Lower abdomen and brow region are important segmental weak points at which hysteric organ ailments develop strikingly often.

Next, I'd like to describe a hysteric female patient, in whom one can recognize many of the traits of this character type:

Ms. M., a 31-year-old slim and very erotically attractive artist, has been separated from her husband for a while. She has a 2-year-old extremely spoiled and querulous son who, during the entire session, kept everyone in the waiting room and all my assistants hopping, even though his grandmother was there to watch him (but who proved to be useless at this). The patient shows up in my consulting room in purple dungarees and pigtails that make her look like Pippi Longstocking. Sitting still and concentrating long enough to tell me her problem doesn't seem to be her long suit. She smiles at me, embarrassed and flirtatious, as she bounces around in her story from one topic to the next, all the time swaying restlessly to and fro. Several minutes pass in this manner, without making any significant progress with the anamnesis.

We skip from one point to another. She says she has always had trouble settling down. This is followed by an incoherent enumeration of various biographical details. At this point, I suggest that we (break with my customary procedure and) begin with her family history, in the hope that such an emotionally binding topic might help her give her tale some structure. She

agrees, and recounts the most important dates in her life. Everything has its upside and downside of course, she says, and this is why she constantly changes partners, apartments, and part-time jobs. As an artist, she is considered highly talented, but she doesn't want to be tied down in this area either, so she vacillates between photography and painting – or maybe graphic design might be just the thing for her....

She grew up without a father and had an especially good relationship with her mother, who takes care of her son when she wants to go to the disco, balances her checkbook (because money is just <u>not</u> her thing, you see), and is otherwise indispensable. You need men now and then, she says, as any healthy woman does – but, other than that, the "guys" are optional. So she lives with a girlfriend, which is much more practical.

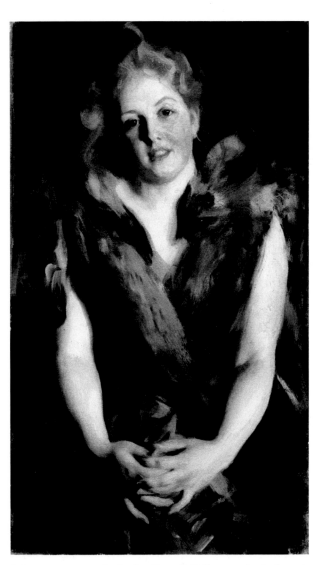

Maja – *a painting by Anders Zorn (1900) unmasks the hysteric via the clearly recognizable sensuous-seductive pose.*

197

I interrupt the patient's stream-of-consciousness narrative and point out that she had come late to this first consultation, that I had another urgent appointment, and that a half hour had already elapsed. For completeness' sake, though, I ask her why she happened to have chosen to come see me. She said she didn't really have anything like a real illness, her body was way too healthy for that and she was, by the way, still as perky as a twenty-year-old (casually casting a brief coy glance at me as she said this). The symptoms that brought her to me are just a bothersome tension headache and, every now and then, terrible thoracic tension just before her period. As for breasts, mother nature had indeed been very good to her, but she knew from other women that they really didn't have to hurt so much, and that I had healed an acquaintance of hers, who had a similar problem, using acupuncture. With this we say goodbye and set up another appointment.

Surprisingly, she doesn't show up for the second consultation, nor does she pay the bill for the first one – because (as she told my assistant who had called her up to find out what was wrong and why the bill hadn't been paid) I had not, after all, done any healing. You wouldn't expect a real doctor to run off, as I did, when we had just barely gotten started. Maybe the truth is that I simply had the hots for her and that this confused me. After all, we had only been talking a couple of minutes and, anyway, it had been more like a casual get-acquainted chat. When my assistant asked her whether she thought she was being fair about the whole matter, she replied that doctors make way too much money anyway, and that, besides, they're insured for this kind of thing, aren't they, and if I sued her, the insurance company would just deal with me.

Evaluation:

In Ms. M.'s case, the hysteric's fear of making decisions is visible in nearly every detail: in her young son, on whom she places no limits; her inability to stay with any career or companion; her tardiness at the first appointment and non-appearance at the second. The erotic undertone in her speech and body language is impossible to overlook: when I first entered the consulting room, she flirted with me charmingly with her eyes. She put her body on display – at least verbally, by mentioning the large breasts and sexy figure that mother nature had bestowed on her. The indulgent mother and absent paternal identification figure also fit this picture seamlessly, as does her inability to manage money. The hysteric's restlessly driven style often leads to vegetative dysregulation, as the constantly whipped-up body, forever being spurred on to new activity, at some point disregards the first warning signs. In her case, the signs were hormonal dysfunction in the 6th Chakra (mastopathy) and tension headaches, although the breasts of course are also related to the 4th Chakra. Basically, hysterics are more susceptible to hormonal imbalances than the other character types.

With this patient, I didn't have a chance to measure emotional conflicts with emotional remedies nor obtain other results, but I can hypothesize, based on similar cases, that there would have to be a considerable vital weakness. With regard to

conflicts, one often finds in hysterics the anxiety remedies of Chakra 4, as well as all the themes of Chakra 6 that are related to tension and timidity. Chakra 2 themes also appear, likewise associated with the hysteric character type. The latently aggressive and petulant know-it-all attitude of the hysteric came out in the refusal to pay the bill and the legal-protection insurance threat.

I'd next like to introduce the depressive type, which (like the hysteric) has a feminine psyche. For the **depressive** character, emotions are uppermost, and as long as her feelings aren't right, nothing can be right with the world. The depressive's feelings focus conspicuously on those around her, who become the center of the depressive's world, as a moon orbits its planet. Whereas other people and the immediate surroundings come across as hostile and evil to the schizoid, the depressive tends, in naïve self-deception and clueless minimization, to trust those around her unhesitatingly, and to give them far too much credit.

Depressives are characterized by their pronounced social orientation, as if they were not viable on their own. Like an infant who looks at its mother with great big trustful eyes while nursing, a depressive's entire happiness depends on commitment to others. A depressive's biggest fear is losing the nurturing mother. There are, of course, surrogate mothers and surrogate nourishment – but this never seems to occur to the depressive. Loss of the "reference person" thus feels like the end of the world, which will automatically also terminate the depressive's own existence – this is the dreaded Armageddon fantasy.

In depressives' early childhood, disturbances in the mother-child relationship become the basis for their fear of losing the mother. Drive-oriented developmental psychology claims that this is due to the mother having been either too easy or too hard on the child – which seems totally wrong to me. Psychoanalysis is famous for making mothers responsible for a multitude of ills – if not indeed *all* the world's miseries, at least as far as emotional problems are concerned. If you take a look at depressive people's mothers, you'll find neither pampering nor cold-hearted women, but rather very often warm-hearted, ordinary, and normally-reacting mothers. Because depressives come into the world with a correlative Central Conflict "pre-installed," their emotional orientation can lead to serious problems with their primary reference person (the mother) – which they then, of course, later on relate to their psychoanalyst, who in turns takes it at face value. But the patient doesn't learn that the root of the evil lies within. This interpretation all too easily turns mothers into scapegoats, and thereby completely misses the crucial point.

Yet the mother figure has an ambivalent symbolic significance for depressives, as depicted in the archetype of the "evil mother." There is a parallel here to the Indian goddess KALI, whom I mentioned in the context of the schizoid character type. Evil mothers are also found in fairy tales as the "evil stepmother." In *Cinderella*, one can see both variations: the mother outrageously pampers her arrogant, lazy daughters while also playing the ultra-severe stepmother to Cinderella – who plays the classic depressive.

Depressives very much want to please, much like hysterics. The actual motivation for being accommodating is the secret hope that doing so will bind others more tightly to them. Depressives thus keep a secret scorecard, never revealed to anyone – unless they lose control and get so angry at someone that they blurt out the entire detailed list of meticulously registered affronts over the years, of which the accused didn't have the slightest inkling – or else they enumerate all the plus points with which they meant to gain advantage over the other person.

Depressives' desire to please nearly always lands them in roles that include socially desirable traits. Depressives are charming and witty when their environment calls for it. They can just as well be quiet and humble if that scores extra points. Most depressives are more kindly and well adapted than the average, and are liked by all and sundry. However, when laziness and arrogance become socially desirable traits (which is fairly rarely) – for instance, in the case of a lazy, arrogant mother who belongs to another character type and needs an ally (i.e., her daughter) as an alibi – then the depressive character type's other-directedness can induce laziness and arrogance. This is not genuine, of course, merely a pose. Poor Cinderella's attributes, on the other hand, are found much more often: serving others and adopting a subservient position in their rivalries and power struggles.

Cinderella types tend, sacrificially, to derive their happiness from that of others, like a faithful family dog that gets the dinner-table leftovers ("I'm happy for you when you're happy! The important thing is your happiness!"). Cinderella types thus seem to be extraordinarily unassuming creatures who can be satisfied with the slightest reward – a hearty hug, say, or a simple thank-you – after having worked all day helping one move or taking care of kids. Or they can be bought off with a fancy certificate and some words of appreciation for decades of self-sacrificing toil on behalf of some charitable organization.

We all know these warm-hearted people: always ready to lend a helping hand and all too easily shamelessly exploited. In fact, many people firmly believe that they are doing depressives a favor by exploiting them. These ideas occur easily to hysterics, for example, whose egotistical self-centeredness leads to the erroneous (but logical) assumption that other people are just as egotistical as they are. In their opinion, nobody does anything voluntarily, that they wouldn't feel like doing, unless they derive some benefit from it. Any other interpretation is totally foreign to hysterics, who logically assume the existence of secret egotistical motives (the ample reward) behind every altruistic act –

along the lines of: "The truth is, even Albert SCHWEITZER and Mother TERESA were only looking to score points in heaven by helping others."

Yet these Cinderellas are not really as meek and ingenuous as they put on. Anyone who can get a depressive, in a moment of weakness, to admit and confess honestly what really motivates her at the bottom of her heart, is in for a big surprise – because Cinderellas actually have a (concealed, very pronounced and haughty) feeling of superiority, and know very well how marvelous they truly are. Cinderellas are of course well camouflaged princesses, much like the ugly frogs (the male version) who are actually handsome princes. Plus, Cinderella has some other surprising emotional stirrings hidden away, such as the same deep-seated – often murderous – vengefulness as schizoids, who also let themselves be too easily exploited. Of course, these hateful and murderous feelings are kept strictly hidden (from themselves as well as others) since they totally contradict the depressive's own self-image.

Previously unremarkable persons who go on killing sprees can belong to this character type: for years they store up aggressive feelings that, ultimately, discharge explosively. Ambrose BIERCE defines the pre-planned revenge as follows: *Meekness: uncommon patience in planning a revenge that is worth while.* One often gets the impression that the depressive has all the time in the world, i.e., the long-suffering wife of an abusive husband who, without warning and in an ice cold manner, exacts her revenge. Film themes such as "The Revenge of the Disinherited" or the well-known "Robin Hood" motif are immensely popular because in their daily lives so many people carry an incredible burden of frustration that they can seldom, if ever, unload. Moreover, everyone in an unjust world wants to see justice done. From the standpoint of depth-psychology, these themes correspond to the socially adapted behavior of the depressive. No other character type is so willing to make sacrifices. This, understandably, leads to the buildup of enormous emotional pressure.

In the choleric temperament, this undisclosed side of the depressive becomes particularly clear. Understandably, not all cholerics are mystery mongers concealing their true nature; among the millions of representatives of the depressive character, there are also openly aggressive types who allow their explosive temperament to erupt in fury at any suitable opportunity (of which there can be many). It should be clearly understood that a depressive's character formation is very dependent on his social and emotional surroundings. If the depressive lives in an environment that tolerates aggressive outbursts, or even encourages them by rewarding them with increased attention and care (calming, much soothing conversation, and so on), then the depressive will give free rein to choleric outbursts.

Because depressives depend on healthy relationships much more than other types, social ostracism is an extreme-

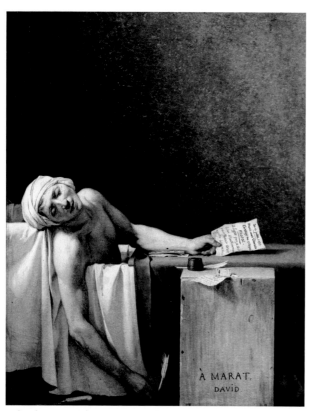

The depressive's basic emotional mood is comparable to that of the schizoid, characterized by deep seriousness and tragic destiny. In the death scene of the revolutionary Jean-Paul Marat – who quite logically had the typical depressive profession of doctor (serving one's fellow man) – the depressive's basic feeling is abundantly explicit. (The Murder of Marat, painting by David, 1793)

ly powerful lever with them – you just need to know that, in this respect, you have a powerful instrument. Particularly with men, often the most reliable prophylactic against rowdiness and temper tantrums is to threaten total social ostracism. It might take the form, for instance, of threatening to withhold sexual favors, as was famously used successfully by women in ancient Greece to scare some sense into their bellicose husbands (cf. *Lysistrata* by Aristophanes).

Turning now to possible partners, the depressive Cinderella's ideal rescuer is the schizoid knight in shining armor. The schizoid embodies exemplary freedom from all attachments, and it is precisely this behavior that seems to be, for the depressive, the fulfillment of her inmost secret dreams, since she can thereby escape the quandary of social dependency. Obsessive-compulsives, on the other hand, are deeply despised by the depressive, because they represent the largest characterological dark side. Forcing her to be a bean-

counter is simply the worst thing anyone could impose on a Cinderella type. Cinderellas have, above all, an emotionally devoted and pathetic attitude that completely opposes the narrow-minded spirit of the obsessive-compulsive.

Things are quite different when a Cinderella is wooed by a Don Juan. The ease and playful merriment of the hysteric Don Juan at first exerts an absolutely magical attraction on the depressive Cinderella. But the hysteric's character neurotically accentuates attributes that are not good for the depressive. The hysteric's flighty, free-as-a-bird and, in the extreme case, phony nature wind up profoundly disappointing the depressive, because the depressive most needs a reliable partner with whom to bond. As soon as the depressive begins to develop hysteric character traits, a neurotically inappropriate attitude arises. The depressive then begins (for example) to play-act and stage-manage interest in a relationship which runs totally counter to her true nature.

The energetic weak points of the depressive are located in the upper abdomen (3rd Chakra). The upper abdomen is also known as the "maternal" Chakra, in which orality, passivity, and emotionality are most pronounced.

The following case history of a patient with a depressive character structure contains all the indicative typical character traits on up to the choleric aspect:

Ms. L., 68-year-old retiree, trained as a social worker and currently a Yoga instructor, has a gentle motherly air about her, and a rounded yet seriously overweight figure. What I find striking in a woman her age is her short haircut and sandals, which would be more suitable for a child. She comes to the appointment on a bicycle, although she lives far away, because she gave her car to some poor people. The feeling of having made some poor souls happy is reward enough, she says. She had recently been in Africa, doing unpaid volunteer work at a Christian mission. She had also gone to India and bought food for beggars, so that they could, now and then, eat to satiety.

Ms. L.'s main interests are attending meditation seminars and making her own house available for the seminars of an esoteric association. When the 20–30 attendees emptied out her refrigerator, that was too much even for her, so she put out a bowl for donations. It upsets her that, even though she is known to be a retiree with a low monthly income, the people have only put a few dollars into the bowl. Now, she simply makes sure the refrigerator isn't so full before a seminar. She came to see me because of chronic exhaustion and bothersome diarrhea. She has also had lower-back pain for years, which meant having to walk her bike for a good part of the long way to my practice.

The REBA® Test Device readings of 20% vitality and 10% emotional indicate a chronic exhaustion state which, along with her "morning low" and sleeplessness, has a decidedly depressive tinge. Yet her life (she says) is by no means listless and unhappy; rather, she feels great joy and gratefulness because, in the seminars with Buddhist Lamas, she is able to realize so many spiritual truths. It also makes her happy to be able to do so much good for other people in their daily lives. It sometimes makes her very sad that there is so much suffering in the world. The conflict found is emotional remedy 9 ("Pent-up rage, wanting to explode") with a blocked 3rd Chakra. I prescribe a preparation of St. John's Wort for this.

After a few months – with intervening consults to monitor treatment progress – Ms. L. surprises me with the information that she had come this time in a new car. She now simply thinks more of herself and realizes that she needs to learn to "use her elbows" more (i.e., be more assertive). This may not be so good for her Karma, but she no longer cares so much about that. The first step was to stop making her house available for seminars, and not donating so much money that she only has enough left over to buy "bread and water" for herself. That's how she was able to afford the car. Her diarrhea is gone, as is the exhaustion. Her orthopedist told her that her broken-down intervertebral disks were due to obesity and recommended an operation. She has already made an appointment for the operation and is confident that this is the best way to go.

Evaluation:

This patient is a prime example of the self-sacrificing Cinderella type who lives only for others; there's a reason why she learned and worked in two pedagogical occupations. This woman has always lived for the well-being of others, and her recognition and love of other people is the gift that the patient actually craves for herself, and needs most desperately. The desire for power is well concealed: to be able to dominate others, via the detour of self-sacrifice, as a teacher, telling them which way to go and what to do. The masochistic aspect is seen in the ongoing tendency to allow herself to be exploited by seminar attendees, and living a rapturous religiosity that has about it an element of flight from the world – as well as in letting an authority figure such as the praised-to-the-skies orthopedist operate on her disks.

The depressive's high ideals are also seen in her strict vegetarianism and Spartan lifestyle, in order to have money left over for people in the Third World. Orality and regressive needs are seen in the compulsive snacking that led to her obesity – and all-day sessions in bed when her lower-back pain "keeps her chained to her bed." Although she wants to play down the lower-back pain with me, she keeps finding ways to mention it indirectly in our talks – for instance, in the context of the bicycle that she had to walk because of the unbearable pain. Typically, the pain has, in her description, to my mind something of the idealized object – and a chance to feel a sublime satisfaction and a feeling of reality. In the context of the tested emotional remedies, this is a classic emotion concealed behind the depressive façade, namely Rage. These patients often seem particularly well-adapted, friendly, their aggression reined in. They seem to sense that everything could come tumbling down if they were to explode and really let out their pent-up rage.

The **obsessive-compulsive** character type resembles the schizoid in many respects, since they are both male-oriented. In both types, logic and reason are obsessively overvalued, which makes the emotional life of many obsessive-compulsives and schizoids undervalued and disparaged. Reason based decisions seem more valuable and obvious to schizoid and compulsive types than "gut" feelings, even though feelings exert a great influence on human life. The male oriented type simply cannot grasp this, which often leads to irritation and disappointment when there are differences of opinion. Male oriented types are always surprised by the reaction of those around them when their logical decisions are rejected for emotional reasons. Taken to extreme, the excessive logicality and suppression of the emotional aspect take on a pathological tone. One speaks in such cases of *Alexithymia* – the inability to experience and express feelings.

From the standpoint of developmental psychology, the obsessive-compulsive type has some association with toilet training issues, with training usually beginning in the second year. According to Freudian libido theory, the obsessive-compulsive is said to suffer permanent developmental damage if "put on the potty" too early and too strictly, which impairs the subsequent stages of psychosexual development. Adherents of the libido theory like to illustrate the sequence of events with the image of a jacket that cannot be properly and completely buttoned up if the first button is matched with the wrong buttonhole: the anal disturbance inhibits all remaining psychosexual development, so that the following levels are also disturbed.

I think this "libido buttons" image is wrong, even though it sounds so temptingly logical. In my opinion, equating compulsive character and overly strict toilet training interchanges cause and effect. Since the Central Conflict is present long before the anal phase – even in the mother's womb – the anal phase itself has nothing to do with the primary cause of the obsessive-compulsive disturbance. One erroneously unites the process, via the subconscious dynamics in the patient's fantasies, with a disturbed toilet training phase.

Because *money* and *feces* have, in the formal language of the subconscious, an enigmatic deep affinity, the most precious (money) and the most disgusting (feces) can develop a cryptic kinship. This essential affinity can only be explained in that the antithetical and irreconcilable aspects of certain emotional contents motivate the subconscious to construct a secret symbolic equality. Thus, no audacious contortions are needed to get at the true roots of the process. The extremely orderly obsessive-compulsive types are thus, by nature, in opposition to everything dirty and fecal, like an elegantly dressed lady's pained disgust at having to walk down a filthy alley strewn with dog excrement. And yet it's clear that the lady's *noblesse* has nothing to do with the dog doo. This is exactly the situation with the obsessive-compulsive's presumably anal problem complex.

The compulsive is plagued by an excessive fear of transitoriness. In this, he is like a fetus, having to remain still in the womb, controlling the least movement, so that nothing disastrous happens, especially anything unforeseen, such as birth, for instance, with its threat of annihilation. Any change can mean the end of personal existence for the obsessive-compulsive. The compulsive shares this existential fundamental fear with the schizoid, who likewise feels permanently threatened to the foundations of his existence. The obsessive-compulsive wants everything to remain the way it is, since this seems like the best way to ensure his continued existence.

We confront the ancient image of the obsessive-compulsive in stuffy bureaucrats who exhibit all manner of grumpy, hesitant, and, at times, overambitious characteristic traits. The obsessive-compulsive is generally found around those with an inordinate love of orderliness who always keep their pencils perfectly sharpened and for whom every single object and event in their lives has to have its clearly designated place. "Tidiness is half the battle" is thus the quintessential motto of the obsessive-compulsive, for whom life indeed consists mainly of order and orderliness. Hostile and life-threatening disorder consequently becomes an anti-world, like unto hell itself, which is for the compulsive an extremely messy place full of deterioration and transition. The main reason that hell is hell, in the eyes of the obsessive-compulsive, is not the disorderliness *per se*, but that disorder so quickly demolishes everything. Order means safeguarding life and making it possible in the first place. Because of the deeply felt correctness of the equation *Order = Life*, orderliness is disproportionately important to the compulsive, since, for him, it equals personal survival. The true reason for the focus on tidyness is the fear of transience.

The obsessive-compulsive wants strictly observed rules for all aspects of life. Because of their quasi-religious observance of rules, caretakers, inspectors, and civil servants are over-represented in the ranks of the obsessive-compulsives. Whenever strict rules are lacking, this type all too easily deteriorates into a state of vague disorientation. One should therefore approach compulsives with firmly-anchored rules in place, because they feel elementally threatened by anything anarchic and disordered. Hysterics, for instance, actually thrive on chaos, inexplicably glimpsing order in disorder, able to fish out precisely the desired letter from a huge pile of mail. Messy desks are no disgrace for hysterics, but rather an elixir of life, making them feel free and unencumbered. For obsessive-compulsives, on the other hand, messy desks are unthinkable, since any sign of disorder irritates them at once and, over the long run, makes them quite ill.

For example, an appliance with a missing user's manual will unsettle an obsessive-compulsive. They often wrap users' manuals in foil and store them in a safe place, because they consider them extremely important and indispensable. On the other hand, a missing manual doesn't bother the schizoid at all, since he would rather figure it out for himself. Schizoids are autocrats who prefer to draw up their own

rules, which of course includes instructions and precepts. Obsessive-compulsives have to know, however, how something works, and which rules are to be observed. Until they learn this, they are agonizingly upset and tense. This inquisitiveness does not originate in any genuine thirst for knowledge, but rather the tormented insecurity of being helpless in the face of chaos.

Psychodynamically, obsessive-compulsives have an overly strict superego that manifests itself in extreme skepticism and a very high standard of perfection that monitors them constantly and keeps them in check. They then transfer their monitoring rights to those around them. Because everyone should behave as they do, obsessive-compulsives tend toward despotism. Behind this, however, is the unbending determination to prevent chaotic and unforeseeable situations. Compulsives thus make ideal supervisors, guards, traffic policemen, and teachers. I have already explained the concealed context of love of orderliness as a secret defense of the deep-rooted and primary fears of transience. Because of this fear, compulsives are very keen on collecting, hoarding, and conserving everything under the sun. Something like mummification in ancient Egypt has to have been first thought up by an obsessive-compulsive, ditto for seatbelts, stamp collections, railroad timetables, and 3-ring binders with tabbed dividers.

As with all the character types, obsessive-compulsives come in all possible gradations, and the harmless, normal, seemingly average types can only be recognized as obsessive-compulsives in that they seem somewhat more pedantic and structured than those around them. Not everyone who comes from a very pedantic parental environment or is born into a culture that prizes orderliness is necessarily an obsessive-compulsive, but might just have acquired the love of orderliness with their "mother's milk." One has to take these variations into account in trying to typify people accurately (this of course applies equally to the other character types). In the extreme form, obsessive-compulsives are easy to recognize. They often become know-it-alls and despotic autocrats who have to keep everything under tight control – obsessive control that often exhibits absurd and even paranoid features. In child rearing, for instance, disorderliness may be punished too severely because disorderliness represents, for obsessive-compulsives, a deadly sin.

Obsessive-compulsives are metabolically very phlegmatic, even though it may not be evident at first. Psychodynamically, their phlegmatic nature is partially explained by the fear of loss, behind which lies the fear of unbridled passion, which is imagined to be destructive and therefore greatly feared. In extreme cases, the obsessive-compulsive becomes totally listless and seems lazy and lethargic. A phlegmatic nature manifests itself externally as sociability, complacency, and slowness. "Haste makes waste" is an obsessive-compulsive motto, which expresses their strained efforts to ensure a correct outcome for all processes, as well as their secret enjoyment of lethargic complacency (keyword: *coziness*) and metered-out passion (keyword: *complacency*).

With respect to domestic partners, the obsessive-compulsive finds the easy light-heartedness and jauntiness of the hysteric extremely attractive. Therefore, when an obsessive-compulsive civil servant marries a lively, exuberant hysteric, one can expect a happy marriage for both of them. In such a harmonious environment, the obsessive-compulsive develops decidedly familial, thoughtful, and pleasant characteristic traits with no trace of the despotism or unwarranted strictness that are his characteristic traits. The hysteric character helps the compulsive attain unburdened *joie de vivre* and impulsive spontaneity, which the obsessive-compulsive so urgently needs as a corrective.

The obsessive-compulsive's relationships with depressives are structured quite differently. Depressives' lack of control and excessive emotionality, along with their out-and-out tragic tone, all too often disgusts obsessive-compulsives. After all, obsessive-compulsives already carry around a huge amount of tragedy! So they often cannot stand depressives, and they express this by ridiculing and disparaging them, i.e., calling them "soppy sentimental," "overly melodramatic," and the like. The situation with schizoids is much more promising. The schizoid, a kindred character type, can become the ideal "brave hero" who sidesteps all the petty pedantic stuff and advances with giant strides toward great goals, instead of (like the compulsive) anxiously counting off every single step. Nevertheless, the schizoid's emphasis on overemphasis leads to a neurotic/pathological exaggeration of unfavorable character traits that run contrary to an obsessive-compulsive's true nature. Way down deep, schizoids are anarchists who "don't give a hoot" for values. Everything that is holy and valuable to obsessive-compulsives bores schizoids, and is increasingly devalued by them over the longer term. Therefore, an obsessive-compulsive exhibiting schizoid character traits is a sign of an unfavorable neurotic development.

The 5th Chakra, which relates to communication and keeping emotions under control, is associated with the obsessive-compulsive. Since the Neck Chakra only has two conflict patterns – which seems awfully Spartan – it very clearly reflects the drab and frugal nature of the obsessive-compulsive. The following example contains all important character traits of this type:

Mr. S., 48, businessman, dressed in plain and modest gray, is an exceedingly sedate and gentle, slim man who radiates a great deal of calmness and trustworthiness. In his tidy shop, he explains to each customer, in excruciating detail, how to use the device they bought, and tries to take care of all matters to perfection – but without ever quite finishing with them. Because he is constantly under time pressure and unable to satisfy very many customers in his charming but skimpy manner, it leads to

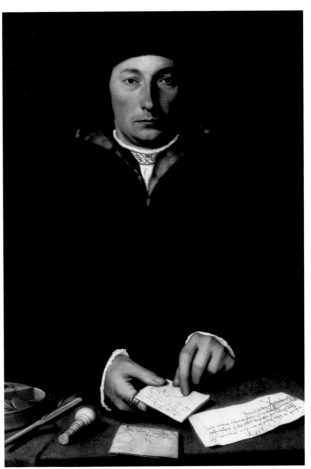

Tidiness, strictness, and level-headedness characterize the basic feeling of the obsessive-compulsive. Simplicity and frugality are cardinal virtues. Many bankers and merchants (as in Holbein's painting) are obsessives, wearing worn-out trousers at home and turning down the heat to save heating costs. Even if they now and then splurge on the heat, it makes them inordinately happy if they have extra cheap fuel to burn so economically. (The Duisburg Merchant, *painting by Hans Holbein, 1533)*

constant dissatisfaction and, on top of that, relatively limited revenues. During a house call, I meet the trained technician's charming wife, who incessantly flutters about the entire time, addressing me without letup while gesticulating enthusiastically and trying to treat and entertain me with a thousand delicacies. His South-American wife is clearly a hysteric matching the classic image of the temperamental smoldering-eyed grande dame *who stages everything with fiery dynamism. She does everything at lightning speed, loves surprises and loud opera music. Her entire life seems to be a multi-media performance, done with enormous dynamism and sparkling vitality.*

Her obsessive-compulsive spouse, meanwhile, sits on the sofa, completely exhausted, complaining about his irritable colon and his frightful restlessness with its tension headaches and sleeplessness. Then there's his brooding, which leads him to rec- ollect, over and over, how comfortable he had been as a techni- cian. He gripes that he gave up his well-paying job to become a businessman. "He's forever crabbing about one thing or anoth- er," his wife interjects. Becoming his own boss, he says, was the biggest mistake of his life. The REBA® Test Device yields read- ings of vital 30% and, for emotional, an extremely low value of only 10%. The disturbed Chakra is Chakra 5, and the con- flict that turns up in the energy test is "Hasty-impulsive, acting before thinking." The patient clearly understands the test result at once – and yet he is not satisfied, because I cannot explain precisely how energy testing works physically. A subtle energy in the body that science has yet to discover – he can't quite go along with that, nor with how one can utilize a method that hasn't been researched and verified down to the last detail.

A few months later, I find out from his wife that the drops did him a world of good and that the headaches have gone away. He is also calmer and more satisfied with himself. She said he's now more casual – which, considering the excessive rigidity of this businessman's character, I take as a great com- pliment.

Evaluation:

The pedant who has to understand everything and explain it down to the tiniest detail is not hard to identify as an obsessive- compulsive character type. Because of his insistence on perfec- tion, the compulsive often carries on an eternally frustrating struggle against time and circumstance – like Don Quixote and the windmills that he mistakenly took to be giants. One sees this in the desperate effort of the above example, where the busi- nessman wastes enormous amounts of time ensuring that the devices he sells are properly operated. In so doing, he loses sight of the practical and profit-oriented aspects of business, which are, to him, quite secondary.

Often, the obsessive-compulsive is concerned from childhood with being especially well-behaved and self-controlled (in which respect he resembles the depressive). He often believes that he has to treat his surroundings exactly the same. This leads to long-lasting educational and correctional efforts aimed at those around him and his environment. Offsetting this are his stolid- ity and hedonism. The obsessive-compulsive is therefore usually only somewhat fanatical, and not very inclined to take on titanic projects for improving his environment. He often drifts off comfortably into idealized worlds, there to indulge in day- dreams that take much less effort than changing the real world. The intolerability of one's own imperfection is not felt nearly as drastically by the compulsive as by the schizoid. Therefore, the compulsive's ability to enjoy life (and to connect with reality) is generally much greater than the schizoid's.

In this case, the obsessive-compulsive's comfort aspect shows up in his tendency to let himself go completely once he's home,

and just dream about possible solutions rather than rolling up his shirtsleeves. He'd rather gripe about reality; lost in wistful daydreams, he tells about a friend who, overnight, won a for- tune in the lottery. That's the kind of luck he needs!

Yet another simple and obvious way to identify one's character type is to compare the listed positive and negative behavioral patterns with one's personality traits. These attributes can be used, point by point, like a questionnaire, to estimate the degree of agreement. The table on the fol- lowing page summarizes typical traits associated with each of the character types:

Typical Traits of the Four Character Types

Character type	Schizoid	Depressive	Obsessive-compulsive	Hysteric
Basic emotional drives & primary personality traits	Strong drive to independence "I am the measure of all things!"	Desire for affection & human closeness "I don't want to be alone!"	Fear of risk and change	Loves change & variety, "I want freedom and risk; traditions and plans constrict me."
Politics	Aristocrat, autocrat	Socialist, liberal	Conservative	Revolutionary
Typical secular occupation	Pilot, spy, researcher, writer, inventor	Nurse, doctor, hostess, social worker, prostitute, group leader	Librarian, civil servant, teacher, scientist	Musician, salesperson, representative, dancer, hedonist, designer
Typical ecclesiastical career choice	Pope, dogmatist	Mother Teresa, nun	Theologian, Church administrator	Missionary, Preacher
Typical brief characteristics of the ideal type	Publicity-shy loner, goes own way unperturbed, often highly intuitive	Only allows self to be happy when everybody else is, pampers others	Underlines main points in instruction manuals, collector, preserver	Gambler, risk-taker, "wine, women, and song," likes to enthuse others and win them over
Emotional fundamental tone	Avoids emotions & human closeness "Don't get too near me!"	Avoids conflicts "I hate arguing!"	Loves detailed planning "Only a clear-cut look ahead can bring satisfaction!"	Loves to be at the center of things "I like to be admired and accepted."
Main character weaknesses	Too factual, cool and objective	Ostrich pose, Victim role	Prejudices, strictness, intolerance	Constant change for change's sake, chaotic
Typical effect on others and basic communicative mechanisms	Aggressive and arrogant, lack of enthusiasm, indifferent to criticism: "Only I know what's right!" Keeps other at arm's length, cynical, impersonal, acts cold and brutal	Selfless and patient: thinks of others first, then self. Childlike/helpless behavior, exerts emotional pressure, provokes guilty conscience, insists on emotional harmony	Perfectionist and consistently correct. Unable to decide, detail-obsessed, nitpicker, gets carried away, bossy, morally strict	Makes promises, doesn't keep them. Erratic train of thought, exhibitionist, puts on airs, prima donna. Confuses everyone, leaves everything unclear, complicates everything, squabbling, coercive, rivaling
Self-esteem and distance	Strong feeling of self-esteem	Little self-esteem, blurts things out, emotionally open and friendly	"No" means "No".	Superficial and easy to influence, emotionally beguiling and inspiring

Schizoid	*Depressive*	*Obsessive-compulsive*	*Hysteric*
Takes clear and uncompromising stands	*Empathetic and cooperative*	*Orderly and diligent*	*Vivacious, spontaneous, charming*
Unsentimental, level-headed and matter-of-fact	*Unostentatious and undemanding*	*Consistent and reliable*	*Only the here and now counts, loves life*
Keen observer, independent, idealist, intellectual	*Little egotism, caring, altruistic, humane*	*Sense of responsibility, self-controlled, fair, conservative (preserving)*	*Lively, pleasure-loving, willing to change, desire for freedom*

These characterological attributions always have a tendentious and negative aftertaste, since each character type is predominantly ascertained on the basis of its shortcomings and failings. One gets the impression that each character type is something bad – but that's a totally one-sided picture, since each character type has strengths – i.e. virtues – as well as weaknesses. These are positive personality traits that give a person personal strength and moral authority. When it comes to virtues, there's no such thing as too many, whereas the vices are a hindrance and a nuisance for ourselves and others. One should therefore develop and advance one's positive traits, while gradually attenuating and overcoming the negative ones – or, as GOETHE put it: "*We should cultivate our qualities, not our peculiarities.*"

At the end of this book, I will address the straightforward option of determining character type by energy testing the associated Central Conflict. In my experience, this simple energy test, which only takes a few minutes, is the most elegant yet reliable way to detect Central Conflicts. In the next chapter, I introduce 28 conflict themes that derive from the four character types, and which represent a kind of emotional proto-language by means of which the various types individually express themselves.

The 28 Conflicts

Our character is created from the ruins of our desperation.
(Ralph Waldo Emerson)

Once we have learned to identify specific character types, we're struck by the great variety of human character within each type. One schizoid bums around as a distrustful and seedy loner while another one is very sociable and energetically manages a big company. Vagabonds and eccentrics are schizoids more often than not. A schizoid's antisocial tendency doesn't necessarily work out to its host's disadvantage: the schizoid company head of our example has achieved great career success despite his characterological predispositions. The schizoid aspect of this person can be seen only in his inclination to make decisions on his own, and his emphatically friendly yet puzzlingly distant attitude toward his employees, including the personal secretary who has worked for him for decades. This multitude of possible internal arrangements of the same character type lets us appreciate the enormous range of variation of the emotional powers: the same character type yields many arrangements and gradations.

Now it is generally thought that the mind is a free, indeed anarchistic territory where everyone can think (do) what they want – after all: "*Thinking is free!*" But reality doesn't work that way. In my energy testing – and long before the discovery of *Psychosomatic Energetics* – I had suspected that there must be a rigorous and universally valid order at work behind the mind's polymorphism. I sensed this because subtle energy reflects the emotions, and the Aura itself exhibits a strict order. Therefore, I reasoned, in all probability the emotional aspect is also subject to a rigorous order.

But after energy testing homeopathic high potentiations[45] on thousands of patients, the issue took a new turn in the form of surprising insights that became the basis of this book. I here have to say up front that we have known for over 200 years (since HAHNEMANN's time, in fact) that homeopathic high potentiations affect the mind. I was able to observe, amazed, as countless patients reacted to the same high potentiations in the energy test. I took a homeopathic preparation and a potentiation, one after the other, brought it into contact with the patient and checked, using energy-medicine test techniques such as Kinesiology (earlier, I had used electroacupuncture), whether the patient exhibited any reaction. A positive test reaction meant that the corresponding homeopathic would have a healing effect on the patient. I would then prescribe these homeopathics for patients and got very good healing results.

The more closely I scrutinized these patients, using the same homeopathic from the energy test, the clearer it became to me that such patients possessed very similar personality traits. Therefore, the common homeopathic reflected an emotional commonality! After years of research, I was ultimately able to collect 28 homeopathic mixtures (compound remedies), each made up of about a half dozen similar homeopathics. It was a mountain of work, but eminently successful in the end. Like a bouquet of flowers, these agents were brought together into a mixture that I called emotional remedy (trade name Emvita®). If there is a positive response in the energy test, the patient virtually always has an associated active conflict with which the emotional remedy has resonated. But the emotional remedies are not just significant diagnostically: they also have a healing effect. Their high potentiations act predominantly on the mind, healing those conflicts with which they resonate.

I was experimenting at the same time with subtle energy centers: the seven Chakras. I was able to relate these energy centers to specific homeopathics, which I gathered into homeopathic complexes and called *Chakra remedies* (trade name *Chavita*®). Using the Chakra remedies, one can quickly determine which of the patient's energy centers is disturbed. Usually, only a single Chakra (along with a specific associated conflict) is disturbed. Since the Chakras are like circuit breakers that can react to overly strong segmental energy stresses, clearly the conflicts are especially nasty troublemakers. In virtually all cases, Chakra disturbances are due to an active emotional conflict.

---

[45] The high homeopathic potentiations above D21 are extreme dilutions that have undergone succussion (i.e., been potentiated) so as to greatly magnify the energetic power of the underlying substance. The healing effect is often the inverse of the initial substance's, e.g., coffee is a stimulant, whereas homeopathic coffee makes one tired. The German physician and pharmacist Samuel HAHNEMANN first discovered homeopathy through the effects of cinchona bark, whose toxic effect resembles that of malaria and that (in the form of quinine) can cure malaria.

The real surprise came from two discoveries I made:

1. *Each Chakra has its own specific emotional conflicts, as if it lived there.* (I now know – as I described in the chapter about the origin of conflicts – that certain conflicts "colonize" specific Chakras due to an energetic affinity, i.e., are stored energetically in the vicinity of the Chakra, such as *Rage* in the Upper-abdomen Chakra.)

2. *Each Chakra can be assigned by depth psychology to a specific character type* (which yields a perfectly-matched cognitive jigsaw puzzle in energy medicine and depth psychology). The 28 Central Conflicts (discussed below) match up perfectly, both content-wise and energetically, to a particular Chakra and a particular character type.

Both subtle-energy and emotional development, along with the related emotional themes (conflicts) are thus subject to a strict logically-structured order. There's absolutely nothing chaotic about the emotional or subtle-energy sphere! On the contrary, it reveals a precise order that, over the course of my researches, led to the third surprising discovery, which was this:

3. *That our subtle/emotional development conforms to a precise organizational pattern that is related to the seven Chakras and energetic/emotional higher development* (which spiritual philosophers such as Teilhard de CHARDIN or religious sages such as Sri AUROBINDO long ago postulated).

I intend to describe all three discoveries in greater detail in the following chapters. The first two discoveries – the breakdown of character types into 28 subgroups and the allocation of character types to Chakras – are closely related contextually. I'll deal with these first two immediately and introduce the third discovery (mental evolution) later on. One thinks of mental evolution initially in terms of DARWIN and the apes from which the human species laboriously developed. In the chapter **The Spiritual Journey and the Civilization Process**, I will elucidate this process (which took millions of years) on the basis of its depth-psychological and subtle-energy logic.

However, one can apply the same evolutionary process to the limited lifespan of individual human beings. The table that follows gives a good overview of this. The principle is that of an upward movement of subtle-emotional energy which gradually ascends the Chakras. As babies, we live in the completely wordless animality of the *Vital Level* (which also has about it something of the divine innocence of the Causal Level); childhood and youth is concerned with the development of the *Emotional Level*. At the zenith of our adult life, we are caught in the wholly rational *Mental Level* (the *logic box*), in order to be able to cope with life in a sensible manner. As we continue to mature, we turn ever more inward and experience the levels of intuition and deeper

meaning and purpose (the *Causal Level*). Spiritually, we arrive at our personal end and our human culmination when we reach the 7th Chakra, where all levels are integrated and a higher understanding of all creation becomes possible, where opposites unite and the cycle of old age and infancy closes in on itself once again.

We can look at our entire life in an overlapping cradle-to-grave panorama as a migration that takes us psychoenergetically through the Chakras and the associated maturation steps (see table on opposite page).

Our emotional constitution clearly obeys a comprehensive maturation and growth plan. During the course of our life, we move through specific Chakras and energy levels that correspond to specific maturation stages and emotional-mental contents. The baby lives in a different Chakra and on other energy levels from the adult or older person. The baby is still struggling for sheer survival – core theme of the 1st Chakra. At higher Chakra stages, the tests get harder and the experiences more profound.

Stressed-out parents, under the burden of their responsibilities, tend to groan: "Tiny children, tiny worries; bigger children, bigger worries." The *Life themes* table row lists the learning tasks to be mastered in each life segment. The learning tasks are more challenging at each new stage – and of course possible failure is more serious. But it seems a lot worse, at first glance, than it really is – because we know, from the soul's viewpoint, that (supposed) failure (reassuringly) doesn't signify catastrophe, but rather simply an even more worthwhile learning task. Therefore, one continues to grow emotionally, regardless of success or failure. **Thus, from the standpoint of the maturing soul, good or bad experiences are, above all, learning tasks that advance us in our spiritual journey.**

The rows underneath depict the energy levels, which integrate seamlessly and logically in the overall picture of the human life stages. To make it easier to understand, I'd like to have the reader picture the following: the first five Chakras are like an orchestra at the start of rehearsal, where the individual instruments (i.e., the energy levels) have yet to be tuned to concert pitch. First, at the baby stage, the Vital Level is tuned up; next, the child stage works on the emotions. The adult then deals with the mind and managing one's life tasks such as career, family, and so on. It is not until maturity that the orchestra – now in the 6th Chakra – gradually starts up (Emotional and Mental Level – i.e., two instruments begin to play), then in the 7th Chakra all the instruments chime in (on all 4 energy levels).

There's one more thing we can learn from this table: the energy levels reflect certain emotional contents that are also found in the character types! Energy levels and character types can thus, in a sense, be viewed as two sides of the same coin. With two exceptions (6th & 7th Chakras) character type and energy level are coterminous, i.e., from the 1st to 5th Chakra; in the 6th Chakra, by way of exception, the emo-

Energy Levels:	Chakra and Active Energy Level						
	Life course →						
Life stages	*Uterus, baby*	*Infant*	*Child*	*Teenager*	*Young adult*	*Mature person*	*Wise person*
Life themes	*Survival and growth*	*First emotional experience*	*Emotional survival, fighting & playing*	*First love, feeling of wholeness*	*Reason, individual life plan*	*Intuition, individual and cosmos*	*Knowledge of God, self-knowledge*
Causal							███
Mental					▓▓▓	▓▓▓	
Emotional		███	███	███		███	███
Vital	▓▓▓						▓▓▓
Chakras:	*Chakra 1*	*Chakra 2*	*Chakra 3*	*Chakra 4*	*Chakra 5*	*Chakra 6*	*Chakra 7*

tional and mental regions mix, leading to the phenomenon of intuition. This is often bound up with a kind of self-enamored dynamism that makes creative livewire types quite an experience for their fellow humans – the reason for which is the all-encompassing positive mood that makes these people so energetic and creative.

Many actors and impresarios belong to this group of exceptional persons, whose enthusiasm and vitality can move and motivate others. However, this group also includes such shady figures as con artists, snake-oil salesmen, and lady-killers – not to mention the famous gurus and spiritual superstars who likewise fall into this category. These hysteric temperaments can transfer their high-frequency psychoenergetic vibrations, like a vaccination, to others – who then say: "He inspired me, and I feel much better now than I used to, I admire him immensely …" These inspiring self-promoters literally make others "fall in love" with them, in which process the furor really does resemble the "high as a kite" feeling of young love. Love is, as they say, blind – and that is the case here as well. In reality, the fascinated ones have been hypnotized by the ecstatic enthusiasm that has been evoked in them. One should therefore be extremely suspicious when you feel overwhelmed like this and, enthusiasm aside, check all statements very critically for their reality content.

There is yet another exception in the 7th Chakra, in that here all four energy levels meld together into a whole. For schizoids, such a powerful dynamism sometimes leads to the (understandable) inclination to consider themselves godlike. Because real gods generally have no need to blow their own horn, schizoids with delusions of grandeur are usually bor-

ing to others, at least as long as they don't bother to present and communicate themselves (since the real adventure takes place, hermetically sealed off, inside their heads). By *megalomania* I don't mean a psychiatric disease, but rather a particular emotional mood in normal-seeming people, usually not even detectable by others.

Many brilliant people belong to the category of highly-gifted persons who inhabit an exclusive private inner emotional world, simply because there is so much exciting and interesting stuff going on inside them. By energy testing people with high levels of 7th Chakra development, one can tell them their secret mood outright – and they will almost always confirm the conjecture. Many writers, inventors, and philosophers are members of this group of gifted schizoids. Of these, I'd like to mention, as a typical example, a writer and former spy who, in conversation with me, said he still misses the many months he spent in solitary confinement during a prison sentence for espionage. The time in solitary was supposed to "soften him up" – but his jailers didn't know that by subjecting him to this gruesome form of punishment (the press was at that time making a big fuss about "arbitrary state-sponsored torture") they were actually doing him a big favor. This person is a schizoid, and in solitary he could finally devote himself unhindered to his rich inner life!

Such examples of extraordinary people once again illustrate the general rule that our energetic mood determines the way we perceive the world. Our inner mood in fact evokes our personality: **"Tell me how you "swing" and I'll tell you who you are!"** Of course, this rule applies without exception to everyone, not just to schizoids. Knowing how we vibrate represents an extraordinarily useful tool for self-knowledge. The descriptions that follow of all the possible character types are intended to help the reader attain this self-knowledge.

With the assignment of character types to energy levels, we find ourselves right in the middle of the topic of the 28 character-type variations. Although there are four character types, there are within these four groups 28 variously structured subtypes. Why this is so will gradually become clear as we proceed. You might think of these subgroups as members of a family who, although they exhibit differing characteristic traits, nevertheless clearly belong to one particular family. I'd like to present these 28 conflict themes in sequence in the pages that follow. My research has shown that there are only 28 Central Conflicts – no more and no less. Evidently, this comprehensively represents all possible Central Conflict themes, somewhat like a language that makes do with a limited number of signs and letter symbols.

Each of the 28 conflict themes is assigned to the Chakra that it best matches up with. Conflicts don't wander aimlessly in our Aura, but rather obey a compelling logic. Everything emotional and subtle-body is subject to a precise logic and a set of laws. For example, the feeling *Rage* will always be situated in the upper abdomen, where it has a particular affinity with the *Earth* element. Temperamentally, the ancient physicians spoke of cholerics. In the choleric's upper abdomen, *Rage* crouches like a devil waiting for its evil and destructive debut. At the beginning, the "Rage Devil" still has the red flush of anger on its face, and people steer clear of such a highly explosive devil.

But a more stable interim state develops over time, as the *Rage* person gets more and more used to the situation, because the *Rage* causes him fewer and fewer overt problems. Finally, one can tell only from the disturbed Upper-abdomen Chakra that an ancient *Rage* must be crouching there. The disturbed Chakra can, for instance, express itself as stomach problems and nausea after eating, which is why cholerics often drink an *aperitif* to stimulate their disturbed digestion. Eventually, the Chakra disturbance disappears, and the conflict then has only a subliminal background significance, acting as an energy drain that reduces the choleric's overall liveliness. Otherwise, the silent conflict generates few overt symptoms, aside from adulterating the emotional sphere with its feeling content – but that's precisely the crucial point! If, for example, it is a particularly big conflict, i.e., the oft-mentioned Central Conflict, then this results in a depressive character.

A depressive character is a person who can become highly enraged astonishingly often, even though he has a "Rage Devil" in his upper abdomen. Why is it that, paradoxically, it is often particularly difficult for rage people to become aware of the especially strong aggressive feelings such as rage? From the outside, the person in question seems quite affectionate and compliant, such that no one would ever suspect that this is a person who is secretly raging inside. The concealment of the deep-rooted rage has to do with the psychological phenomenon of repression, for which there are many explanations: rage is one of the socially unacceptable emotions that tends to destroy a lot of expensive chinaware. Added to this, rage bearers themselves are deathly afraid of letting out their highly explosive rage – afraid of laying waste to everything.

The following description of the 28 conflict themes thus includes both the primary feeling and its repression. When it comes to characterological/emotional shaping, one needs to think along two tracks, always keeping in mind both the original emotion and its repression. This dialectical thinking has its origin in the logic of the Causal Level (divine wisdom). The Chinese sage LAO TSE taught: "*Man uses clay to enclose nothingness with pottery: the nothingness is the point of the pot.*" LAO TSE is saying here that, to fathom the deeper meaning of a pot, you have to understand its hollowness. When it comes to the subconscious, the deeper meaning is particularly well concealed in that it is precisely the contradictory aspect, the totally unsuspected and unknown, that yields the right meaning. Thus, the fact that nonaggressiveness and gentleness are often internally related to suppressed rage is based on a hidden rationale that is revealed only at second glance.[46]

The table on the opposite page summarizes the assignment of character types to the seven Chakras and 28 conflict themes.

From this table one can see that, based on Chakra and conflict, the schizoid is energetically classified with the lower body and head. The hysteric's energy center is the middle lower body and brow region. Energetically, the depressive is at home primarily in the lower abdomen, whereas the obsessive-compulsive dwells in the Neck Chakra. That, oddly enough, leaves out the Heart Chakra. In the case of the Heart Chakra, we have the astonishing phenomenon that we find there, for each character type, at

---

[46] At this point, many people jump to the (logical but wrong) conclusion that meekness is always a cover for repressed rage. By this logic, friendly people are those who have repressed their unfriendliness – just as, according to this simplistic equation, all celibate clergy suffer from strong suppressed sexual desires, all chaste maidens are actually lascivious she-devils, etc. This is of course utter nonsense because, besides faked emotional façades, there are quite obviously genuine feelings as well! External appearances are not always and everywhere Potemkin villages! Especially in analytically-oriented encounter groups, this simplistic assumption (that each and every participant has repressed feelings and fake façades) can easily be wielded as an all-purpose inquisitorial instrument to extort confessions, which can then lead the group down analytic blind alleys and generate emotional confusion. The entire process can be effortlessly successful because psychological conventional wisdom has it that we are all unaware of our subconscious, such that one can well believe the accusation that, behind the façade, one is concealing all kinds of bottomless pits – which of course is very confusing and can make one sick (or even sicker than one was in the first place).

Character type	Schizoid	Depressive	Obsessive-compulsive	Hysteric
Associated Chakra	1st Chakra (pelvis) + 7th Chakra (head)	3rd Chakra (upper abdomen)	5th Chakra (neck)	2nd Chakra (lower abdomen) + 6th Chakra (brow)
Central Conflict (and related conflict themes)	All conflicts from Pelvic and Brow Chakras (1–4 & 25–28)	All conflicts from Upper-abdominal Chakra (8–11)	All conflicts from Neck Chakra (17–18)	All conflicts from Lower-abdominal & Brow Chakras (5–7, 19–24)
Conflict themes of the respective character types in the Heart Chakra	Conflict 13 "Withdrawn, deeply injured"	Conflict 15 "Apprehensive" & Conflict 12 "Mental overexertion"	Conflict 14 "Introverted, compulsive"	Conflict 16 "Panic"

least one and sometimes two conflicts assigned to it. Why does the Heart Chakra occupy such an uncommon special position?

In the Heart Chakra, we are at our most human and most vulnerable. As the emotional center, it represents the gate to our true Self – so it's not hard to understand why the Heart Chakra has a conflict theme and a thematic psychic facet for each character type, in order to be, for all persons, a challenge and a meeting place. The conflicts of the four character types found there are like entryways to a universal language – that of the heart center, where only love and forgiveness reign.

Chakra and Character Type

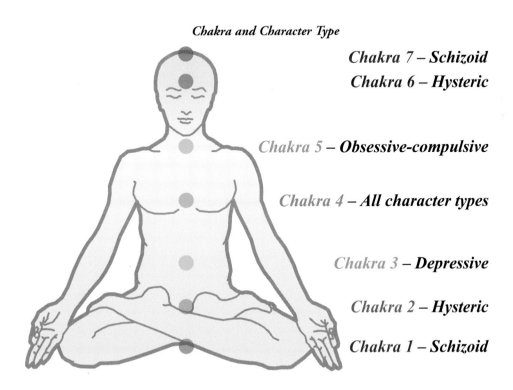

Chakra 7 – Schizoid

Chakra 6 – Hysteric

Chakra 5 – Obsessive-compulsive

Chakra 4 – All character types

Chakra 3 – Depressive

Chakra 2 – Hysteric

Chakra 1 – Schizoid

In closing, I'd like to add some helpful information to the descriptions of the 28 conflicts. Each conflict has its assigned primary theme that, like a headline, summarizes the most important feeling content in a few keywords. One example of this is the emotional theme *Exploding* which, for the suppressed *Rage* conflict, expresses the basic mood of raging destructiveness. However, psychic polymorphism means that the entire issue is not as simple as the "headline" implies. The first problem is **repression**. The person feels deep inside that, despite all the repression (such as meekness), the repressed emotional theme of *Rage* accurately expresses the core of his emotional life. Here, one must simply rely on one's gut feeling in order to see through the repression. For example, those who believe themselves, deep inside, to be on the brink of exploding all the time will immediately recognize the correctness of the *Rage* theme when told about it. They then usually say something like: "I can see myself in that description!"

Another obstacle to understanding is that many feelings represent a summation of various **emotional facets**. Because of its brevity, a conflict theme's name doesn't always reflect all emotional characteristics. One can see this in reading through the conflict descriptions. Another difficulty is that the name of a conflict does not automatically permit one to draw any conclusions regarding the strength of the conflict. Understandably, it makes a great deal of difference whether a towering rage is dominating a person's entire character, or a small rage is only peripherally affecting a person's nature. Therefore, when reading up on a conflict, you need to know whether it is a matter of a small or a large one. Testing with *Psychosomatic Energetics* can be a great help in this regard, in that one can quickly and easily ascertain the size of the conflict.

With respect to the leading symptoms in the following overview, these are short and succinct descriptions of the conflict contents. The reason for the concise telegraphic conflict descriptions has primarily to do with therapeutic intent. Becoming aware of unknown conflicts is known to promote healing processes. However, these are opposed by repression mechanisms that are more likely to make their appearance if one talks too much about the conflict.[47] The more one talks about it, therefore, the more one destroys the healing effect of the words; as the saying has it: "Brevity is the soul of wit."

---

[47] Conflict resistance seems to grow exponentially in direct proportion to rationalization and naming of the conflict contents. And yet it's also counterproductive to leave the contents completely unnamed. The best compromise in this situation seems to be to touch upon it with a few comments. The demonstrable success of quick psychotherapies points in this direction, i.e., that an initial ignition is enough to get the ball rolling and the healing process started.

The Conflicts of the 1st Chakra

In the so-called *Root Chakra* (1st Chakra), we encounter the psychic themes of the schizoid type. The 1st Chakra has to do with themes that schizoids find obsessive and extraordinarily problematic: personal existence and related concepts, such as having enough strength and endurance to survive, possessing an identity, and getting the chance to secure and defend one's survival. According to Indian Yoga, the life force is said to have its headquarters in the 1st Chakra. This is graphically symbolized by the hooped Kundalini snake.

All the important psychoenergetic connections of the 1st Chakra can be found in symbolic contexts. Here, the sexual organs are powerful representatives of the biological survival instinct. Also, the genetic code (DNA), reproduction's material substrate, resembles a rolled-up snake or spiral. The phrase "to stand on your own two feet" has to do with the 1st Chakra, in that, energetically, the legs can not only be conceived as an extension of the pelvis, they're also a symbol of individual centeredness and personal stability. All this relates to the first and most important condition of our individual existence: the 1st Chakra – to borrow from SHAKESPEARE – is all about "*to be or not to be.*"

Basically, the fears of schizoids are relatively easy to penetrate and understand. With schizoids, it is existential threat that becomes the core of their life-fear. In this, the "feeling" is precisely that which mortifies schizoids and threatens their sanity. Schizoids are by no means natural scaredy-cats who are afraid to die: what frightens them much more is the accompanying emotional experience. As the comedian Woody Allen once said: "I don't mind dying, I just don't want to be there when it happens." This perfectly expresses the schizoid's primal fear, which is actually a terrible fear of dying a wretched death and having to suffer horribly in the process. Just imagine courageous schizoid types such as the fictional British secret agent James Bond, in bed exhausted and racked with pain while Ursula Andress washes his behind – anything would be better, in Bond's mind, than to find himself in such a degrading and helpless situation!

The 1st Chakra has four distinct conflict themes:
          1st Conflict: Independence
          2nd Conflict: Lack of concentration
          3rd Conflict: Loss of control / helplessness
          4th Conflict: Extreme self-control

The first theme has to do with personal independence. "Am I good enough to make it on my own?" asks the schizoid in the first conflict. The James Bond character, for example, suffers horribly because of his helplessness in that scene. For schizoids, self-reliance has an obsessive, downright existential significance. Because schizoids are consequently extremely reluctant to imagine themselves in such demeaning situations as a helpless invalid, I have often found that they take no precautions against the eventuality of such situations of helplessness. As schizoids get older, they don't bother, right up to the end, about nursing care or any other health-care resources. They want, always and forever, to remain resolutely autonomous.

In the second conflict, there is a menacing feeling of not being grounded and a lack of concentration, behind which lurk immense fears that lead to a feeling of unreality and being disconnected from the world. The feverish James Bond is forced to watch helplessly as enemy agents take his pistol out of the nightstand drawer. Bond hallucinates and has double vision. The resulting mortifying feeling is the horrific helplessness of knowing that one can no longer rely on one's own powers.

It gets even worse in the next conflict. The third conflict theme is based on total helplessness and the horrible feeling of being at the mercy of foreign powers. Like a puppet, the victim can be completely controlled and manipulated, totally helpless and unable to do a thing about it. James Bond, for instance, lies tied to a carpenter's bench as a huge circular saw blade draws ever nearer. Or a hypnotic command turns him into a villain himself, robotically obeying orders. In these movies, a shout at the last minute usually ensures that the secret agent comes to his senses and shakes off the evil programming.

Finally, in the 4th conflict theme, one does the only sensible thing that can be done in such a hopeless situation, namely play dead and, just to be one the safe side, become totally emotionless. In animals, this is known as "playing possum." Still, this is an emotionally degrading situation, in which one has to throttle down one's liveliness completely in order to stay alive. In a certain sense, it's a kind of internal contradiction that even has something of the perverse about it, i.e., "making oneself lifeless in order to stay alive." Such a situation would give James Bond much to chew on emotionally and for a long time, since it feels so extremely degrading and goes so totally against his nature.

If we want to understand the schizoid's emotional motivation even more profoundly, we need to look behind the curtains of their fears – after all, what is *really* behind this fear of being annihilated and snuffed out? The ultimate and deepest reason is actually the yearning to in fact be obliterated, in order to once again merge into and become one with the cosmic bliss. I remind the reader of the fact that ancient temperament theory says that the schizoid corresponds to the melancholic. Melancholy, as wistful yearning, is somewhat unworldly and virtually suicidal: one desires with all one's might to conjure oneself out of this unloved here-and-now. It pulls one with enormous attraction toward a distant, utopian world. This is why schizoids are, deep down, frequently idealists, all too often devotees of otherworldly utopias.

Behind the schizoid's fear of annihilation there surfaces, unexpectedly, a desire to be dissolved (FREUD's *death wish*!). The problem is, the desire for dissolution is deeply incompatible with life. Anyone wishing to melt back into the cosmic bliss is no longer viable. At this point, the will to survive appears on the scene, since survival is an enormously strong drive – a counter-drive to the desire for dissolution – and it sets up a repression mechanism consisting of naked and monstrous fear designed to protect the schizoid from his self-destructive desires. Psychologists speak of a *double-bind* situation whose true roots are in the schizoid's inner psyche. The more fragile the deep fear becomes, the more susceptible the schizoid is to self-destructive drives. Only after a stable Self and a healthy, mature personality has been put together, can the schizoid afford to eliminate these deep fears.

1st conflict: Independence

Possible problems:[48]

You don't feel good enough for yourself, typically having problems with identity. You lack primary psychic orientation in the form of sufficient self-confidence. The basic trust has been lost or was never present. Melancholy is a frequent tendency. The world is felt to be bad. Children with early-childhood shocks such as divorce, death of a parent, child neglect, unwanted child. Children with an unhappy childhood, for example parents who had hoped for a son (heir) and got a daughter instead. Lack of inner strength to deal with the burdens heaped upon you. Unaware of your strengths. You feel yourself to be smaller than you really are. Tendency to shut other people out and not get attached.

Empirically, frequent pelvic problems. Bladder, prostate, uterus, ovaries, hips, and legs can be affected.

Sought-for solution:
Be cognizant of your strengths and talents. Everyone has a no-strings-attached right to life.

2nd conflict: Lack of concentration

Possible problems:
You are simply not really "here." You don't know your destiny or purpose. This conflict applies even when rebelling against having to be in this world. Your life is lived half-heartedly and with a lack of conviction. You don't trust yourself to show what you are capable of. In stress situations and occasions meant to test your abilities and strengths, you tend to beat a retreat. Tendency to postpone things or do them unwillingly. Inclination to avoid requests or demands. You often give others who meet you an impression of inapproachability or featurelessness. You don't know your own strength. Only a fraction of your potential is ever realized. Deep inside, you obstinately engage in passive resistance. You yearn to be somewhere else very different.

Empirically, frequent pelvic problems. Bladder, prostate, uterus, ovaries, hips and legs can be affected.

Sought-for solution:
Realize that you maintain your own powers and apply them intelligently. Accept being in the world and be thankful for it. Develop and deploy your talents and strong points with genuine enthusiasm.

---

[48] Many thanks to Dr. Ulrike Banis for many valuable tips and experiences. Some of the following descriptions of the 28 emotional conflicts were discussed with her and worked out based on our common experiences in clinical practice. We are also grateful to the many colleagues and seminar attendees who wrote us with many hints and suggestions.

3rd conflict: Loss of control/helplessness

Possible problems:

You feel helpless and in every sense paralyzed. The greater the demands, the less you feel able to find a solution. Life is a never-ending struggle. You never dare fully be yourself, and feel 100% dependent on others. You are never seen as you really are. In a social setting, you feel accepted only if you live up to role expectations. You tend to live for others as a puppet and accomplice. You have learned from experience that giving free rein to your talents, strengths, and needs will be immediately and unrelentingly punished. You therefore dare not do anything at all. You tend to inaction and immobility. You tend to be wishy-washy (undecided, playing for time, keeping things vague, postponing everything until the last second, and so on) or, in the extreme case, to give up entirely. Basically, you do not want to be here.

Empirically, frequent pelvic problems. Bladder, prostate, uterus, ovaries, hips, and legs can be affected. Often helpful also in cases of leg ulcers.

Sought-for solution:

Work on the feeling of being borne by your own powers, don't let others clip your wings any more, and develop more confidence from task to task. Develop steadfastness and rootedness. Stand up resolutely for your convictions.

4th conflict: Extreme self-control

Possible problems:

You don't allow yourself to grow and live your own life. You have put on the brakes completely to your childlike expansionist joy and keep yourself reined in far too much. There are often problems with sexual identity. You try to salvage a ruined family environment by being obedient. You are willing to sacrifice your life to maintain social cohesion. You were too strictly disciplined at too early an age and acted like an adult even as a child. You tend to suppress feelings and spontaneous life-affirming actions. Discipline, rationality, and obedience are top priorities. You expect others to live up to your exacting life standards. You are terribly afraid of giving in to your unruliness and *joie de vivre*, because that exposes you and others to great danger.

Empirically, frequent pelvic problems. Bladder, prostate, uterus, ovaries, hips, and legs can be affected.

Sought-for solution:

Be more loving and accepting with yourself, unconditionally, with no strings attached. Learn to express your wishes and opinions moderately yet vigorously.

The schizoid's four conflict contents revolve around

- Power and powerlessness (slave driver or slave): "Who's in command? Who must obey?"
- Resoluteness and spinelessness (to be or not to be; centeredness or the feeling of losing one's way and getting bogged down)

The schizoid's fundamental feeling vacillates between being weak and being strong. If I'm strong enough, then I've got the upper hand, I can prevail; I'll survive and get whatever I want. But if I'm weak, it'll go badly for me – so badly, in fact, that my situation will become miserable, and the best thing for me to do will be to become completely unfeeling, so as not to notice my misery. Consequently, power and willpower are obsessive states for schizoids, since they represent a bulwark against their biggest fears: helplessness and spinelessness.

Many historical heroic figures were schizoids – the prime example being Alexander the Great, who well illustrates the positive attributes of this character type. As king and a person wielding enormous power, Alexander goes to the limit. He widens ancient man's worldview by extending the territory under his power from Greece all the way to India. The mythological Alexander is said not only to have been a brilliant sovereign, but also to have revealed the secret of longevity. The mythology has it that, at death's door, he ascended into heaven in a basket borne by an eagle. This reflects the tremendous admiration of him by his contemporaries, to whom Alexander the Great must have been – even during his lifetime – an unreal and superhuman Titan.

Their aloofness and independence often endows schizoids with the characteristic traits of the eagle – king of the skies, looking out over everything. Another symbolic animal is the snake which, rolled up as *Kundalini* energy, waits in the 1st Chakra until it rears up like a cobra and shoots up the spinal column (in sexual orgasm and spiritual enlightenment – two profoundly related states). The axe (or hatchet), a symbol of powerful destructive force, and the clock as the symbol of the ability to summon everything together, are further attributes of the 1st Chakra.

"Where there is much, there is also much shadow" is an old folk wisdom, as is "The higher they fly, the harder they fall." Alexander the Great dies miserably of malaria – and his death reveals to us the weak, helplessly vulnerable, and infinitely tragic aspects of this magnificent hero. The dark side of the 1st Chakra has to do with death, failure, and great weakness, even to the extent of being totally at the mercy of foreign powers. The world grows dark and turns into an inferno that, in the extreme case, is represented in *Sodom and Gomorra*. Perversions turn people into demons, and their drives into disorientation in which pain becomes pleasure and the agonies of others enable one's own gratification. The horror of *Sodom and Gomorra* becomes clear in the biblical scene with Lot's wife, whose backward glance at the burning city turns her into a pillar of salt – immortalized as a symbol of "frozen tears."

The Conflicts of the 2nd Chakra

The 2nd Chakra is closely related to the first, in part because the urogenital tract is influenced by both of them. That said, the 2nd Chakra is, by its very nature, totally different from the first. Unlike the 1st Chakra, it is not concerned with sheer existence, but with the kind of life led in this existence. Psychoenergetically, the 2nd Chakra is closely related to the largest human stress organ, the adrenal glands. The most striking attribute of the 2nd Chakra has a dynamic/restless and contentious aspect to it: one never gives up, never yields, and is thus always on the go, so as not (of course) to make any mistakes.

The three conflicts of the 2nd Chakra help clarify important hysteric traits, which are dealt with in the conflicts of the 6th Chakra (also part of the hysteric nature):

> 5th conflict: Hectic
> 6th conflict: Perseverance
> 7th conflict: Show of strength

Having to tie oneself down, to commit oneself, and thus finalize something is the hysteric's biggest fear. Picture a classic hysteric in a situation that is favored and – as critics would have it – actually provoked by his characterological peculiarities. Don Juan has big gambling debts and is being pressured by a number of powerful princes to (at long last) marry their pregnant daughters. Some of the jilted lovers and/or swindled debtors have taken out contracts on Don Juan, and now these hired killers are after him. To prevent their being successful, Don Juan must constantly be on the lookout – which leads to the conflict of the hectic, restlessly anxious, and nervous person. He says to himself: "If I never stop bouncing around inside, then there can be no decision." If he paces back and forth in his room, then it'll be much harder for the rogue at the window across the street to nail him with a crossbow bolt. He can also much more easily put off the tricky decision of who to marry (and who to alienate by rejecting, of course).

In the next phase of indecision, Don Juan attempts to keep a lid on things and banish the emerging fears by simply refusing to acknowledge the feelings. A good friend has "brainwashed" Don Juan and got him to realize that his problems are all in his head. This by no means gets rid of the fear, but instead turns it into an exclusively corporeal matter. Even though, deep inside, Don Juan feels terrible, he acts as if he had the situation well in hand. He struts about with a proud and powerful bearing through the back-streets of the town, even though he has a dreadful headache, because his neck is stiff as a board out of sheer fright. The hired killers could be lurking anywhere, just waiting to stick a knife in his ribs.

The third conflict continues this defiant/snippy mentality that represents the effort to drum up resistance to the misfortunes that have arisen: "They better be ready for major trouble when I hit back horrifically!" is Don Juan's stiff-upper-lip interior monologue, even though he's shaking like a leaf. The entire matter takes on a comic aspect, since his resistance to overwhelming superiority is just a bluff, a show of strength and grandiosity. Many idealists, and even troublemakers, fight like David against Goliath, by (for example) pelting government agencies with a hail of never-ending lawsuits. They delude themselves that they're in the right, without making the least effort to make the means appropriate to the ends, nor allowing common sense to have a say.

The hysteric's anxiety conceals a secret yearning to at long last find the right way to be rewarded by destiny by relieving him of having to make the right decision. The core theme of the psyche becomes: "I can't afford to make any mistakes!" There is no more attractive idea for the hysteric than that of some wise and benevolent providence taking charge of his life and arranging everything for the best. However, the ambivalent and hopeless nature of the situation results from the fact that one can never be completely sure if it really *is* the best solution – maybe there's an even better one? "What if providence goofed and it would be better to wait for an even better opportunity to come along?" the hysteric asks himself over and over again, so that everything remains open and unresolved. This gives rise to fundamental feelings of drivenness, anxious solicitude, and playful flirtatiousness, in order to keep everything up in the air.

5th conflict: Hectic

Possible problems:

Uneasiness and drivenness. Agitation with constant restlessness. High physical stress coupled with the tendency to react to psychic stress with physical symptoms, e.g. tendency to hypertension and deep-seated lower-back pain. Quite often irritable colon symptoms with stomachache, alternating diarrhea and constipation. Tendency to kidney ailments. Above-average work performance, very ambitious and very active. Tendency to perfectionism. You have the feeling of never quite getting going and finishing something. You court recognition and praise from others because you have a very high personal standard. You feel responsible for others' lives. You often talk in a continuous torrent without letting anyone else get a word in edgewise. Incapable of relaxation and rest. Belief that existence is justified only if you force yourself to record accomplishments. You think you have to remain in harness and alert in order to not lose control. You want to be everywhere at once, so as not to miss anything and to extract the maximum from life.

Sought-for solution:

Derive strength from calming down and learn to live life itself instead of the illusion of life, and find peace in each situation. Be contented with yourself and your abilities, even if things turn out less than perfect.

6th conflict: Perseverance

Possible problems:

Tendency to clothe fear in physical ailments. External impression of being completely calm and in control, but very apprehensive deep inside. You are fearful for inner security and your life, but don't want to admit it. You need to act strong and courageous for others and yourself. You are chronically overtaxed. Often irritable colon with diarrhea and stubborn lower-back pain (sacroiliac joint). Feeling of constant overexertion, thereby basically feeling much weaker and constantly exceeding your limits. You are incapable of refusing new requests and are therefore always getting more work piled on. You are unable and too weak to pull out of overtaxing situations and grant yourself the needed respite. You believe that you are only loved and appreciated when doing your duty. You believe that only virile go-getters have a right to live, that betraying weakness and being fainthearted means forfeiting the right to exist.

Sought-for solution:

Develop the ability to recognize and acknowledge your limits, and give in to the need for rest and relaxation. Overcome your inner anxiety and trust that you'll continue to live even in a state of rest and relaxation. Relearn to take notice of your body.

7th conflict: Show of strength

Possible problems:

Actual existence does not agree with self-image. You secretly feel unsure and inferior, but hide it behind a façade of larger-than-life self-confidence. You don't let the outside world look inside. Actual symptoms and problems remain in the dark as you subconsciously baffle and beguile others. You get tangled up in contradictions. Constant alternation between feeling strong and weak, thereby looking unpredictable and unfathomable to others. Another behavioral variant consists of cutting others down to make yourself look better. Large external stresses stand in stark contradiction to actual inner strength.

Sought-for solution:

Honestly see and acknowledge your self-image, with its weakness and helplessness. At the same time, learn to develop and make use of your strong points and talents. "Everyone puts on their pants one leg at a time, too!" Modesty and sincerity are the expression of genuine strength.

> The hysteric's three conflict contents have to do with these antithetical pairs:
> · Fear of failing vs. being infallible
> · Being small and insignificant vs. being big and important

The interior monologue goes as follows: "If I make a decision, I might make a mistake that can ruin me. But it might also turn out to be my lucky break. If I cross the street and a car runs me over, I have made a dreadful decision; on that morning, I would have been better off staying in bed. But if I don't get up, then others will think I'm lazy and useless (e.g., small and insignificant). If I summon up all my courage and cross the street anyway, maybe it'll turn out OK after all! The good fairy rewards my bravery with a kiss and, at the next corner café, as I sit there drinking my morning coffee, I meet a movie producer who picks me on the spot to be the star of his new film and helps me become rich and famous (e.g., big and important) …" In anticipatory pleasure at his fantasy, our hysteric races across the intersection, chest swelled with pride, and takes a seat in the café, where he makes eyes at the waitress with charming affability – they'll all soon realize what a remarkable person he is: "Just wait until the famous director walks through the door and discovers me!"

The hysteric hero-type confronts us in the role of the charming trickster and buffoon who delights everyone (but whom some secretly consider a fool) and is admired by all and sundry for his foolhardiness and gallantry, his elegance and charm. Many movie heroes and seductive historical figures such as Giacomo Casanova can only be properly understood in terms of their hysteric character traits. In their positive expression, wit, charm and courage, coupled with a great drive for freedom, are among the typical attributes of the hysteric. Masks symbolize the ability to play-act and to add variety to expression, which is why they are symbolically closely coupled with the hysteric. We also see the hysteric type in mythology. The Indian god Hanuman typifies the loyalty, devotion, and great strength that is inherent in this character type.

Negative attributes include the tendency to give in – even addictively – to pleasures, debauchery, and temptations. We find these attributes immortalized in the Greek god Dionysus who, along with his cloven-hoofed satyrs, luxuriates in "wine, women, and song" (the modern version is "Sex, Drugs, and Rock & Roll"). No other character type is quite so intensely hedonistic and sensual as the hysteric. The Greek god Pan is also part of this picture (by the way, the word "panic" derives from the name "Pan"). Fear and panic are dominant yet deeply buried hysteric emotions, originating in the finality and inevitability of death. Behind the fear of making a mistake lurks the fear of ultimate extinction – reminiscent of the fear of death of the schizoid, who (unlike the hysteric) sees his peril in the condition of being too weak, raising the spectre of his expiration.

The Conflicts of the 3rd Chakra

The Upper-abdomen Chakra is the psychoenergetic home-land of the depressive. The upper abdomen deals with digestion and processing of external influences, i.e., external substance is transmuted into internal resources. This applies not merely to nutritional intake, it also has a universally valid significance. The foreign is something that depressives need for their inner deficits, like a starving person needs food so as not to keel over and die. Depressives are thus oriented to their surroundings, always on the lookout for something to help them become whole. They are, first and foremost, needy types whose satisfaction and happiness depend on others, and whose lives depend on whether others give them what they unconditionally need: love, recognition, and all other forms of attention and care.

Logically enough, depressives' fundamental fear is the fear of separation and of having to stand on their own. The most awful punishment is thus isolation, which – along with the agonizing loneliness (bad enough in itself) – leads to the loss of other people, who are felt to be indispensable to personal stability. Hence, depressives are prepared to pay almost any price to avoid being alone. Even abasement and total self-sacrifice are possible behavior patterns, understandable because of the enormous fear of rejection. Isolation is the worst: solitary confinement is the worst imaginable punishment for depressives. In solitary, depressives feel cut off from life, becoming completely apathetic and listless, like fish out of water.

This persistent other-directedness has its downside. As with all whose existence feels like slavery, the slave's master-dependency generates an enormous anger and utterly unbelievable rage. This is not a steady rage, but rather an escalating development: because slaves must constantly subordinate their needs to the master's, the rage is built up by the mortifying exploitation and tormenting self-sacrifice, until it turns into murderous hatred. By denying their inner feelings, these "slaves'" self-esteem sinks ever lower, until they wind up hating themselves and – indirectly, of course – those to whom they have subordinated themselves. Yet this is an inescapable trap, since resistance would endanger the "slave's" very existence! Because of the impossibility of rebuffing or (God forbid!) getting angry at other people, the situation culminates in an enormous need to explode.

Thus, in every extreme introversion that can be understood as depression, there exists the possibility of tremendous expansion. In truth, this expansion is only prevented by the underlying fear of a total loss of control ("If I ever flip out, it'll be like ground zero around here!"). Anyone who has experienced a rampaging mob – especially when composed of heretofore suppressed, suddenly unleashed people – can appreciate the monstrous power of pent-up negative emotions. The primary rationalization for authoritarian power structures is based on this. And yet, the fact that an authoritarian regime's repressive acts fuel precisely the explosive rage that it intends to keep in check is a perfect example of circular logic. This is precisely the inner psychic situation of depressives: they do not grasp that, as their own worst enemies, they hurt themselves most of all.

Anyone peeking behind the façade of friendliness and interest that the depressive erects will notice a lurking, ravenous monster. This monster has an insatiable hunger for food, drink, laughter, life's meaning, and a full, rich life. The depressive is therefore a deeply unsatisfied and unhappy person, carrying about an unbelievable emotional hunger. The reason for this inner dissatisfaction lies within the depressive. It is based on the fact that love, the core of true inner contentment, presupposes a balanced mixture of the love of self and of others: *Thou shalt love thy neighbor as thyself.* You have to like yourself in order to be able to love others – yet whoever enslaves herself for others' sake can hardly love herself.

Normally, the first object of love is the mother, who gives the baby a feeling of satisfying comfort, security, and love. The baby keeps a deeply-etched memory of what love really means, namely unconditional give and take between two beings devoted to each other. The depressive lacks this basic feeling, and this spawns an existential greediness. This is greed in the sense of "wanting more." ("If they won't willingly give me what I need, then I'll do whatever it takes to get it!") I'd like to point out that the mother of the depressive should not be viewed as the culprit. Once we realize that depressives are characterologically preformed even before birth, the mother becomes simply an extra, playing her part in a long-ago preordained plan.

Unlike schizoids and hysterics, both of whom are relatively self-sufficient, depressives are fated to become the playthings of their fellow humans. Their excessive emotional dependence on those around them incites exploitative human tendencies. Exploitation and abuse are thus obvious dangers that depressives bring on themselves by signaling to their environment: "Here I am! I'll be nice no matter what!

Do with me what you will!" In a sexual context, this is known as masochism. Depressive character types are all too easily exploited by their fellow humans – sadistically, in the extreme case. This is made quite clear in *Cinderella*, in the scene where she is punished by having to stay behind and count the lentils while the lazy stepsisters (representing the polar-opposite character type, namely the psychic shadow) get to go off to a glitzy soiree.

8th conflict: Isolated

Possible problems:

You live on an island amid strangers. You want to make contact, but are unable to approach the others. You feel like a lonesome outcast Robinson Crusoe, all the more intolerable because there are people all around. You lack the means to communicate satisfactorily with others. The resulting feeling of isolation leads to inner paralysis and lethargy. Therefore, no attempt is made to rebel against the intolerable situation. You become very quiet and lifeless.

Sought-for solution:

You have a right to life in any situation, and the opportunity for happiness and enjoyment.

9th conflict: Pent-up emotions

Possible problems:

You try to win the sympathy and affection of others by being particularly friendly and compliant. You are constantly attuned to the needs of others and try to satisfy them, in the process postponing your own desires, which leads to subliminal rancor and a mountain of unfulfilled wishes. What others think of you is extremely important. An unbearable pressure builds up over time, driven by the contradiction between your seeming lack of desires while constantly being attuned to and fulfilling the wishes of others. This servile attitude magically attracts exploiters and egotists. Moreover, your subconscious seduces other people into egotistical and exploitative behavior. You tend to exceed your limits and overtax yourself constantly. You fantasize someday being grandly rewarded for all this, but the actual reward never measures up to the imagined one. This gives birth to a nagging feeling of dissatisfaction and extreme rage.

Sought-for solution:

Recognize your limits and learn to say no. Above all, learn that saying no does not automatically lead to rejection and destruction, but rather is part of life. "Love thy neighbor as thyself." (But not more than thyself!)

10th conflict: Wanting more

Possible problems:

A persistent feeling of dissatisfaction and the search for happiness makes you want more from life. You are not happy or at ease with yourself way down deep, but rather feel pauperized and extraordinarily needy. You discover that everything in life must be taken by force if you're to obtain satisfaction. However, that which has already been taken is not enough – it is not enough, and therefore you must always take more. Each fulfilled wish generates three more. Good fortune is hoped for at every next turn of the road, making you a driven person. Your self-image tries to hide the drivenness and hunger from yourself and others by projecting an external demeanor of conspicuous calmness and contentment. The hunger for more out of life can find expression in the piling up of knowledge, power, luxury goods, ideas, and countless other objects and energies.

Sought-for solution:

Learn to be thankful and contented for what you have in life, find your center and happiness in your center, without adding (wanting more) other people or objects.

11th conflict: Craving good feelings

Possible problems:

You are deeply discontented. The unhappiness of being frustrated leads easily to a counter-reaction, which consists of the refusal to eat or enjoy life, nor to acknowledge your frustration. This feeling of constant emotional hunger gives rise to unreal fantasies and a nagging driven feeling. Subtle and subconscious tendency to provoke situations in order to experience the frustration time and again, and to over-interpret the rejection. You often fall into a total slave role to garner indirectly a few crumbs from the total satisfaction of the wishes of others. You tend to various kinds of addiction and dependency.

Sought-for solution:

Recognize your needs, learn to nourish yourself emotionally and do the right thing. You should learn to acknowledge that contentment can only come from within, and not wait for others to do the right thing.

The four kinds of conflicts that are situated in the Upper-abdomen Chakra and belong to the depressive character type are oriented around the psychic antithetical pairs:

· "I want everything – but I actually get nothing."
· "I want you so that I can be with myself again – I am not by myself so that I can be with you again."

The depressive is thus stuck in an irresolvable quandary. In game terms, such insoluble situations are known as *checkmate*. Everything that the depressive tries to do to improve the situation ultimately proves fruitless. Nothing seems to lead to a reasonable resolution, so that there are only two options: depression and (covert) aggression. Either stick your head in the sand and be depressed or fight aggressively until total annihilation, exploding with rage and thereby destroying everything that gets in the way.

Depressive character types thus make good soldiers, since they follow orders ideally and are brave fighters; at a battle's crucial moment, they can generate tremendous strength that derives from their concealed aggressiveness. On the other hand, depressives also tend to be pacifists (comparable to schizoids) – I suspect that this is because depressives fear their own highly volatile aggressiveness. Pacifism thus represents a psychic bulwark against their own destructive urges, like carefully placing a live hand grenade inside a thickly padded crate. Basically, depressives have fundamental problems with aggression. Like a beginner learning to ride a powerful motorcycle, at first giving way too much gas, causing the wheels to spin out of control, the depressive tends to go overboard when being aggressive. It's either too much or too little – learning the right dosage is one of the depressive's most important lessons in life.

In order to feel harmonious and centered, depressives are totally dependent on those around them. Depressives are even prepared to neglect themselves to please others. This is again seen in the case of Cinderella – and more than a few depressives clothe themselves "in sackcloth and ashes" in real life. Because of their conformism and their fear of being rejected, the escape route that leads to self-actualization is blocked for them. This is part of the *checkmate* situation – since the more depressives reveal what they really desire in their heart of hearts, the greater their fear of rejection. This generates enormous tension, which is buried in addictive behavior and all kinds of personality "armor" such as a thick layer of fat (obesity), incessant friendliness, or some other masquerade.

The passive and feminine personality element of the depressive character type has much in common with the hysteric: the susceptibility to being seduced by others, a constant dependence on the *vis-à-vis* and a false (because artificially put on) helpfulness. Unlike the depressive, in the hysteric this pose stems from utterly egotistical desires, e.g., to be the center of attention, to gain power over others, and the like. These egotistical motivations are absent in depressives, who are out-and-out altruists.

However, the depressive does possess many positive character traits. These include, first of all, an enormous strength (known in Japanese Zen Buddhism as *Hara*): the gigantic energy of the abdomen. In China, enlightened ones are often depicted as paunchy Buddhas wearing a broad blissful grin. This is not meant to glorify the coarse-material over-weight of these Buddhas, but rather their strength and their exhilarating, enlightening quality. The spiritual-wisdom teacher Graf DÜRCKHEIM has shown *Hara* strength to be a unique opportunity for centering and grounding. Chinese acupuncture views the upper abdomen, along with the region centering on the navel, as the locus of the "Triple Heater" – an energy center of vast dynamic vitality. As early as the embryo and fetus, the umbilical cord constitutes the organism's central supply artery, which is directly related to *Hara*.

In symbology, we find the Bull symbolizing the elemental force situated in the upper abdomen. The Cretan Minotaur cult and the late-antiquity Mithra cult paid homage to the bull's uncontrollable and imposing natural power, which acknowledges the divine in its superhuman strength. The bull is also present at the birth of human civilization, since it was cattle that enabled mankind to settle down and till the soil. The bull is the symbol of naked material survival and hoped-for prosperity. The bull (or ox) has yet another symbolic significance: in Chinese Taoism, the wise man who can ride the ox without having to resort to any auxiliary equipment exemplifies the reconciliation of humanity and nature. Mankind needs to learn to domesticate and subdue its own natural powers in order to live harmoniously. In a figurative sense, the ox is a symbol of the human body along with its drives and feelings – man's "inner nature" whose savagery must be tamed and made subject to the individual will.

If the attempt to tame the unruly inner emotional "bull" is unsuccessful, then the negative character traits of the depressive character type will take center stage. The gargantuan rage is concealed behind a façade of placid conformity. The enormous expenditure of energy necessary to keep the lid on the 3rd Chakra's emotional-energy pressure-cooker generates increasing dissatisfaction and hunger. Just as a cosmic black hole sucks in and engulfs all matter (including passing light rays!) venturing too near it, the depressive becomes an all-devouring giant squid. The Roman Catholic mythology of the "Black Mary" illustrates the all-absorbing gentleness and willing self-sacrifice which also cloaks itself in secrecy and voluntarily stays in the shadows. These spiritual virtues are also part – in morbid and unprocessed form – of the depressive's core theme complex. Unlike Mary, the depressive does not voluntarily enter into the difficult circumstance of self-sacrifice for others, so this gives rise to rancor that threatens to poison the depressive's entire life.

The Conflicts of the 4th Chakra

*The heart is the key
to the world and to life …*

(Novalis)

The Heart Chakra unites the fundamental fears of all four character types. Therefore, the heart is not associated with any one character type, but rather includes conflicts from all the types. Once we realize that the heart holds the psychoenergetic key to an individual's nature, it's much easier to understand why everybody carries emotional baggage regardless of character type. If conflicts are signposts to a person's true nature, then heart conflicts reflect the corresponding basic characterological problem to a very intimate and deeply essential degree.

can be projected onto specific objects and thereby limited in their scope to that object. At the same time, the constant worry and dependence on other people leads the depressive into an additional conflict. The Heart Chakra conflict has to do with the tendency to make enormous psychic exertions, which leads to increasing mental laziness and more and more errors in reasoning. Like a millipede who, if it wonders how it manages the complicated coordinated movement of all those feet, trips and falls over, depressives get all tangled up in their overblown apprehensive solicitude and caring.

Heart Chakra Conflicts and Associated Character Types

Character Type	Schizoid	Depressive	Obsessive-Compulsive	Hysteric
Conflict themes of the respective character type in the Heart Chakra	*Conflict 13 "Withdrawn, deeply injured"*	*Conflict 15 "Apprehensive" and #12 "Mental overexertion"*	*Conflict 14 "Introverted, compulsive"*	*Conflict 16 "Panic"*

We will not be disappointed in this assumption: for each character type, we find in the Heart Chakra a critical and particularly challenging theme which must be worked out and resolved if emotional fulfillment is to be realized. In this obligatory "final exam," each character type is given an especially hard and difficult learning assignment. For the schizoid's fundamental fear of extinction, it is the fear of withdrawing and, deeply wounded, vegetating one's life away. Instead of a redemptive thunderclap that ends the entire horror at one blow, the schizoid is forced to endure an everlastingly long lingering illness. Understandably, the schizoid suffers most of all from the long, drawn-out, constant fear of death.

For the depressive, as for the hysteric, these feeling-states are presented as learning assignments – which represents the most horrifying aspect for these two types, namely being helplessly exposed to an unfathomably enormous fear. The depressive feels abandoned in this fear, like a child that has lost its parents. The depressive then develops phobias about anything and everything imaginable. I believe that the reason for this is that fears become more tolerable when they

In hysterics, simple fear escalates to a terrible fear of death, dwarfing everything else. It rolls over them like a tsunami and literally breaks their heart. Many people with so-called "heart phobia" suffer from such subconscious fears. Amazingly, hidden behind the hysteric's happy, carefree façade is a first-rate emotional drama. The core theme has to do with the heart and the blood that it circulates – a metaphor for life itself. The ancient temperament theory classifies hysterics as sanguine (from *sanguis*, Latin for blood). The sanguine type "cheers hysterically, is deathly sad" – the radical shadowgram of the hysteric's happy-go-lucky demeanor confronts us in this frightening fear of death.

In the obsessive-compulsive, the fundamental fear escalates to the unearthly feeling of being the helpless victim of horrifying compulsions. These are comparable to believing, for instance, that one is locked alive in a casket and is unable to breathe, about to flip out and go completely crazy. Only a superhuman effort can ward off the absolute end – comparable to the schizoid, who has also to survive titanic struggles.

12th conflict: Mental overexertion
Possible problems:

You believe that you can control all feeling through rational thought processes. This need for control is valued more highly than spontaneous expression of emotions. However, since more than 80% of human communication is wordless – i.e., takes place subconsciously – you constantly overtax yourself and cannot keep all your impulses under control. This is of course very tiring, and makes you feel that you can no longer concentrate. You suspect that you have taken on "an impossible task" and have a tendency to take flight internally. This permanent flight tendency makes it impossible to stick to the task at hand. Thoughts of problems and of failure predominate and you cannot trust yourself or others.

Sought-for solution:

Learn that rationality isn't everything. Learn to trust and let life's flow carry you, without always having everything under control. It has to do with letting go of the *idée fixe* that everything has to be preplanned and directed.

13th conflict: Withdrawn
Possible problems:

You feel deeply distressed and believe it impossible to get over such a severe injury. A typical example of such a wounded ego is unrequited love, i.e., the rejection of your amorous overtures by someone who does not reciprocate the emotion. You not only feel injured, but also humiliated and made to look the fool. You withdraw fearfully from human contact because you no longer expect any good to come of it. You are insulted, feel depressed, often can't work up the energy to do anything, become apathetic and dull. You erect walls around your fragile psyche, like a snail withdrawing deep into its shell.

Sought-for solution:

Realize that people are not always "Wicked, nasty, mean, and evil" and that much of it depends on personal context. Thus, certain situations may have negative consequences for you, but another person might get quite a different impression. No everything is a personal attack. Learn to open up emotionally, make your peace with others, re-establish contact.

14th conflict: Introverted
Possible problems:

You have totally shut out the outer world and feel trapped behind walls. Your thoughts go around in circles and you feel worse and worse. This being walled off from others is not felt as being protective; instead, you feel horribly hemmed in, under overpowering compulsion and permanent pressure. Your emotional freedom of movement is extremely limited, such that you become mistrustful and timorous. This anxiety can be felt physically, emotionally, or mentally. The trigger for this emotional retreat is often a severe emotional trauma, which you consider to be insuperable and far too fearsome. You wall yourself into an emotional fortress which, over the long run, doesn't feel protective but rather compulsive.

Sought-for solution:

Recognize who the real builder of your prison is and open up again emotionally.

15th conflict: Apprehensive
Possible problems:

You feel abandoned in a threatening world. You feel anxious and fearful, and would most like to crawl into a hidey-hole somewhere. The threat can be a great heart-wounding sorrow whose consequences now paralyze your initiative. Because of your feebleness, you think your heart might stop beating at any moment. There exists a fundamental fear that can attach itself to real-world objects such a spiders or mice – but it can also remain quite diffuse and generic. Many people develop a "fear of fear itself," which is like an emotional echo chamber.

Sought-for solution:

Fears block energy flows, so you should encourage everything that favors and strengthens psychoenergetic flow.

16th conflict: Panic
Possible problems:

You feel inundated by an overwhelming fear of death, like some gigantic tidal wave. You are unable to put up any resistance to this enormous fear, in fact you feel completely paralyzed. You feel as though the final bell is tolling and everything is irrevocably over, that the catastrophe is inescapable. This fear builds up to huge proportions in your imagination.

Sought-for solution:

Even the worst situations come to an end at some point, and then life goes on as always. Since fears obstruct psychoenergetic flow, you should develop and strengthen your basic trust in the positive and relaxing aspects of life.

It's fairly easy to see that, in the Heart Chakra, the principal theme is the fear of extermination. If we picture the fundamental fear as something that wells up out of our inmost being and is always related to threat, then we see that all fears are dreadful. But are there degrees of dreadfulness? We can endure (tolerably well) the conflicts of the other Chakras for the simple reason that they don't pierce us to the marrow. But with the Heart Chakra, things get serious, and the issue gets to the final decision concerning *"to be or not to be."* Thus, the fear pyramid's ultimate peak is attained in the Heart Chakra!

One may wonder what the deeper meaning might be of such inner psychic terrors. In my experience, the conflict in the Heart Chakra only surfaces after a long developmental period. I'd like to present a typical example of this:

This example involves the masseuse with soft-tissue rheumatism, whose case I presented in the chapter "My Personal Pathway to Energy Medicine." Originally, her rheumatism was based on a conflict with Rage *as the theme. The patient was a depressive character type. Externally, she has an unusually gentle and friendly nature. In the past, many who knew her took shameless advantage of her friendliness, good nature, and cooperativeness. After the repressed subconscious rage was dissolved by administering the emotional remedy* Pent-up emotions, *she became a different person. She dreamed a lot about the repressed rage and became more self-confident. She could finally say "No," which she hadn't been able to before.*

Unfortunately, she had a slight relapse about six months later. A dentist found a focal tooth whose dead root had become inflamed deep in the jaw. Not infrequently, dental foci express repressed emotions, often repressed aggression, which is why they say "It got him in the gums." After the dental focus was eliminated, the soft-tissue rheumatism disappeared as if blown away, but after a while it came back. This time, I found an enormous conflict, Apprehensive, *in the Heart Chakra. This conflict drained off a lot of vital force and emotional energy. After this theme was eliminated, the patient's character was transformed, she became much more open emotionally, and her rheumatism was gone for good.*

If we look at the developmental path of personality, we see that each person goes through a personality development that, at some point, has to deal with working through the Central Conflict before development can go any further. We can see this very well in the case of the woman with *Rage*, where resolving the *Rage* theme enabled her to make enormous developmental leaps. But that's not the end of it! In this case, the soft-tissue rheumatism's resurfacing was a sign that an old conflict had ripened and now needed to be worked on. Yet "ripe" conflicts are not brought to light by illness alone. Often, a necessary emotional/energetic developmental step shows itself in other ways, such as inexplicable problems with other people, or emotional crises.

The final step leads back to the Heart Chakra, where we wind up at the center of the Self. The Crucifixion represents a metaphor in which we must irrevocably give up our false Self before our spiritual journey can continue. From a psychic point of view, we may only go home (find our way back to our true spiritual homeland) after we have given up the false Self and crucified the false personality components. All the symbols of enlightenment, crucifixion, and wholeness point to the process which, through dreadful agonies, frees us from our false identity.

In alchemical mysticism, the search for gold transmutes into the quest for the True Self. The *Philosopher's Stone* and the *Holy Grail* are related images. Androgynous symbols, signs of having overcome the polar opposition of man and woman, surface from the subconscious depths. Angels (androgynous beings) flank our path as our True Self begins to step forward. The beauty of the unfolding lotus blossom becomes the symbol of our rebirth. In Buddhism, we take off the cape of ignorance which consists of the false Self. However, we do not thereby vanish into nothingness: in this context, the concept of *Nirvana* is often misunderstood — because, since nothing is ever lost in the Cosmos, we retain our true personality, which radiates in all its glory. We call it rebirth when we rediscover ourselves in our ultimate indestructible causal body. In Tibetan Buddhism, this is described as the "adamantine truth body," which leads to immortality and heavenly bliss.

The Conflicts of the 5th Chakra

The Neck Chakra is closely related to the obsessive-compulsive character type. Psychoenergetically, the neck has an important function as gate and gatekeeper between thinking and feeling, reason and emotion. The neck constitutes a barrier between head and torso. When we want to suppress feelings such as sobbing or shouting, we tense up the neck region. We can also stifle feelings with the neck, without further ado, like turning off a faucet. When feelings rise up in us, we get a lump in our throat. If we "swallow" feelings such as annoyance or rage and send them back down again, then "the dear soul has its peace," but the resulting extreme condition is emotional emptiness. This open-shut mechanism helps regulate feelings, which can lead in the extreme case to total lovelessness and indifference. "Tit for tat," obsessive-compulsives say to themselves, and they are able to deal with those around them just as coldly as they do with themselves.

Like all control freaks, obsessive-compulsives love regularity and hate change; everything is supposed to stay the way it is for all eternity. We can much better understand the mechanisms of the 5th Chakra if we realize that we are dealing with the mental body itself, which in this context is the center of the entire process. For most people in Western culture, reason forms the core of the Ego, as I pointed out earlier in the discussion of the mental body. The close equation of Ego = reason has a very special emotional significance, since this is how obsessive-compulsives defend something existential, namely reason, as the core of their personality. Behind reason stands the Self's naked existence. Compulsiveness protects the existence of the individual in question, and from this is easily derived the dogmatic rigidity and severity that so often characterizes compulsives.

There are two conflicts in the Neck Chakra:
17th conflict: Emotional emptiness
18th conflict: Rushed

There are two mechanisms with which obsessive-compulsives can get away from upwelling feelings that threaten to throw them off-balance. The first is emotional emptiness: making oneself rigid and lifeless inside, like a cornered animal "playing possum." When we make ourselves emotionless inside, we of course deprive ourselves of the single most important source of *joie de vivre* and sensual depth that we humans possess, namely our emotionality. Emotionally empty people may be free of burdensome feelings, but they have also cheated themselves out of very important and valuable aspects that could have enriched their lives.

Another control mechanism is our mental apparatus, used to think very rapidly and hastily. One cranks up the central processing unit in the head to maximum performance – in order, for example, to drown out the feeling of weakness that is part of feeling at the mercy of emotions, and to use the mastery of reason to become especially powerful and superior. But this isn't so easy to do! Since the sluggish body cannot keep up when the mind goes into overdrive, the entire system begins to get muddled up. For instance, the slower vocal apparatus and its nervous system begins to stutter. Thus, stuttering is often due to inner haste.

Since the obsessive-compulsive is masculine in nature, his character is bound up with the same violent tendencies as the schizoid. Way down deep in his heart, the obsessive-compulsive does not like to admit weakness, since he must always be strong and have the upper hand. Yet I have also noticed the opposite tendency as well, and observed compulsives admitting weaknesses that one would not at all have expected them to. This includes, for instance, a presumably gentle nature or the all-too clearly demonstrated inclination to complain hypochondriacally about all manner of innocuous disorders. This is not what one would expect from a tough guy! And yet, there is a simple explanation for these peculiarities: the obsessive-compulsive finds that these spurious behavior patterns give him an emotional safety-valve through which he can admit weaknesses in order to counteract his emotional impoverishment.

In psychoanalytic jargon, this is known as a compensation mechanism against an overly strong Superego. Just as many workaholics comfort themselves in the evening with sweets and alcohol, the obsessive-compulsive grants himself exceptions to his all-too severe rules, as a way of pampering himself once in a while. I have often noticed that these compensatory actions can include lavish revels and extravagant purchases such as expensive watches and other durable luxury goods. The obsessive-compulsive rationalizes these costly acquisitions on the basis of their durability and permanence, while still keeping an eye out for bargains in the supermarket. The compulsive's predominant stinginess, punctuated by impulsive extravagant spending, is explained by the need to "let off steam" once in a while, so as not to asphyxiate in one's emotional parsimony and severity.

17th conflict: Emotional emptiness

Possible problems:

As the "gateway to feelings," the neck can choke off rising emotions so much that it induces total emotional rigidity. A person acts totally in control, head-guided, as though nothing affects him any more – almost like a robot. Yet the repressed feelings and their expression – crying, sobbing, even screaming – have just been "put on hold" and have not really gone away. Often, these upwelling feelings are associated with psychic shocks and great inner horror, and here the emotional play-dead reflex instinctively insures survival.

People with an emotional "play-dead" reflex have very limited feelings at their disposal, while their rationality continues to operate unhindered. This can can be seen in someone reporting on horrible events very unemotionally, so that listeners get the impression that it means nothing to the reporter, since there is no emotion in the report. Yet such a person is typically in a state of emotional shock, which splits off feeling from thinking, giving rise to the false impression that he or she has no feelings at all.

Sought-for solution:

The aim here is to gradually release repressed feelings from their congealed state, and to re-harmonize heart (body) and mind (reason). These patients need to learn to notice what they are prone to "gulp down" or suppress, and to be aware of and express precisely these emotional contents. This will allow them to be more authentic and straightforward, as they learn to say what they really mean. In this manner, even psychic shocks can eventually be articulated and worked out.

18th conflict: Rushed

Possible problems:

In the neck region (gateway to feelings), so many impulses and drives can rush in, like a flash flood, that the patient panics and feels overwhelmed by it all. Too much gushes forth all at once, and the brain doesn't get a chance to step in and sort it all out. Because so many impulses and contradictory wishes are all active at once, the patient seems rushed and keyed up to others, confused and unclear and, all in all, fairly unstructured.

Such people suffer a great deal from the fact that they cannot express themselves clearly and make themselves understood. They often talk very fast, trying to make listeners understand, but this just confuses people all the more, and in the end no one knows what's going on. Both sides of this attempt at communication are left unsatisfied and feeling like victims of circumstance.

There is often an inner restlessness which is not visible from the outside. Unexpectedly, people with the "Rushed" theme can often seem quite calm and relaxed – but their hastiness is seen in the way their inner stream of thought flows too rapidly.

Sought-for solution:

"Strength lies in calmness" should be the guiding inner theme. Relaxed and calm breathing is often a great aid in restoring inner equilibrium. The patient should be encouraged to do things slowly, yet correctly, and with total conviction.

The obsessive-compulsive's ambivalence consists of:
- Being emotional and vulnerable – being rational and thus invulnerable
- Being calm and having to look at the transgression – being quick and thereby hoping to escape the transgression

Ultimately, the obsessive-compulsive's ambivalent efforts are inadequate and they end up, as they must, in a blind alley. If the compulsive makes an effort to maintain a rational and emotionally neutral stance in order to make himself emotionally invulnerable (a common attitude among intellectuals!), he automatically cuts off his emotional life, thereby ultimately cheating himself out of any joy or depth in life. In Samuel BECKETT's *Waiting for Godot*, one can see what rationality and emotional emptiness has led to for modern rational man: a regular prison, or rather a psychic lunar landscape!

Since we are, historically, living in 5th-Chakra times, in which rationality is king, the obsessive-compulsive problem complex is also the theme of the modern *Zeitgeist*. Modern rational man is interested in cool clarity and rational classification, not in the imponderability and vulnerability of life. In our modern world, reason has attained the status of a sacrosanct, almighty deity. To my mind, modern big-city architecture reflects this collective attitude, which is involved with the vibrational level of the 5th Chakra.

The second insoluble problem is time itself, which for the obsessive-compulsive has the fearful and unalterable property of constantly putting everything into the past. The future is not graspable for the obsessive-compulsive, which makes it seem irrational to him: "The only thing that matters is the here and now!" Thus, for the obsessive-compulsive, there is only the present, in which, like Prometheus (the ancient Greek hero whose name means "forethought"), he struggles against irrevocable transience. This makes the obsessive-compulsive into a symbol of humanity itself. Prometheus outsmarts Zeus, the supreme nature god, at a sacrificial ceremony and brings the gift of fire to man. With this stolen fire begins human civilization and the responsible independence of mankind. Zeus punishes man for this sacrilege with Pandora, a seductive female who brings to mankind a container holding all conceivable ills (Pandora's Box) which

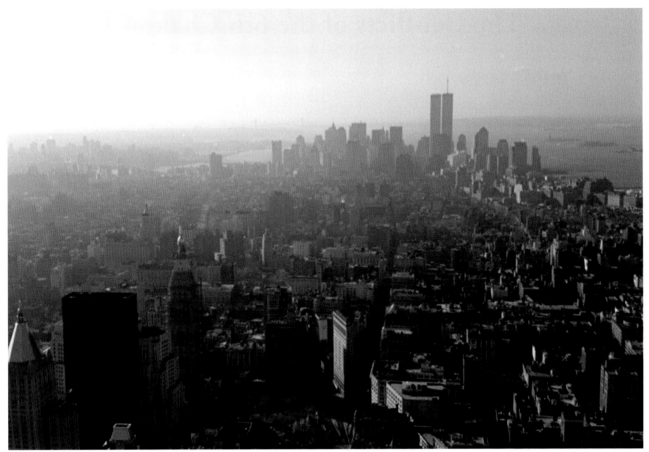

New York, a typical masculine city, embodies many obsessive-com-pulsive characteristic traits – from the rigid rectangular geometry of the canyon-like street grid to the skyscrapers with their aura of lofty perpetuity (divorced from gravity and emotions). The New York skyline viewed from the Empire State Building, looking toward the

World Trade Center, conveys an impression of the grandiosity of human edifices. (I took this picture a few months before the 9/11 attacks in 2001, intending to illustrate the obsessive-compulsive chapter with it. The twin towers no longer exist.)

thereafter bedevil the race of man. These include age, sickness, and insanity.

It's not hard to recognize, in the image of Pandora's Box, the symbolic figure of the false Self with its Central Conflict. The accelerated aging, getting sick, falling out of the psychic center (going insane) is provoked by the conflict. In the ancient antique language, the conflict is called "the Evil." Yet there are still more punishments – for Prometheus is chained to a rock, where an eagle tears out his (regenerating) liver every day for all eternity. The symbolic significance of this gruesome image of torture is that life (here symbolized by the liver) is continually going to be taken away from man and his strength throttled down, just as the conflict steadily diminishes our life force.

Yet another basic problem of the obsessive-compulsive is the sheer impossibility of ever being completely calm and relaxed – because, if the compulsive were truly 100% calm,

the feeling of transitoriness would grow even larger. Amazingly, there are many compulsives who passionately perform meditation exercises, or who engage in calming hobbies such as model building, clock repair, or hunting. All of these activities call for calmness and inner peace. If you consider why compulsives pursue these activities so contrary to their true nature, you come back to the phenomenon of compensation and efforts at self-healing. "Fishing for two hours calms me down completely," says the angler. By engaging in an activity that demands calmness and quiet, he hopes to calm the inner unrest of his obsessive-compulsive nature.

The Conflicts of the 6th Chakra

In the Brow Chakra, we find ourselves once more in the hysteric's emotional world. The 2nd Chakra's emotional themes of the hysteric character type now continue here in the 6th Chakra. The Brow Chakra is associated in mythology with the Third Eye, which symbolizes the paranormal mental abilities of looking within (inner vision). In my experience, people with an energetically strong 6th Chakra are often very intuitive, and they are characterized by a high degree of empathy and creativity. The Brow Chakra contains an enormous creative and intuitive potential which can help leverage people at this vibrational level to surprisingly creative flights of fancy.

But with bright light you also get dark shadows, and so no Chakra has more conflicts than the Brow Chakra. All in all, we find six conflict themes:

19th conflict: Faint-hearted
20th conflict: Self-sufficient
21st conflict: Physical overexertion
22nd conflict: Restless
23rd conflict: Tense
24th conflict: Uneasiness

Like the 2nd Chakra, the Brow Chakra is closely related to stress management. The hypothalamus and the limbic system link internal processes to external environmental factors – for instance, the vegetative nervous system switches to stress mode when our surroundings make special demands on us: heart rate goes up, stress hormones increase blood flow to the muscles, the pupils dilate to improve vision – as they also do when we see someone sexually attractive. In ancient Rome, the sap of the deadly nightshade was used to artificially dilate the pupils and thus simulate sexual interest – which is why this plant's Latin name is *Belladonna* (beautiful lady).

The Brow Chakra synergizes many internal and external interests, as with sexuality, where the individual desire for sexual gratification and emotional warmth combines with the biological interest in gene reproduction, and with the social interest, in optimal pair production of males and females in order to obtain stable germ cells for the society. These varied interests are processed by the Brow Chakra into an overall impression that one can then call "being in love." In reproductive stages of sexual life, the Brow Chakra ensures an orderly course of pregnancy by, for example, secreting the lactiferous hormone *Oxytocin*, and guiding the birth process.

Psychoenergetically, the Brow Chakra follows similar patterns, as in it can arise higher levels of order and new syntheses. It can be counted on to generate new and surprising things, comparable historically to the spirit of the *Renaissance*. The Renaissance revived the heroic spirit of ancient times, and this was bound up with a general enthusiastic feeling of a new beginning. Such buoyancy and reorientation correlate with the Brow Chakra's vibrational level. As in the perceptions of a newborn infant, the world at the Brow Chakra level is marvelously transformed and renewed.

After all these positive "bright" aspects, let us now turn to the Brow Chakra's dark side. People with many facets, such as hysterics, often have an ambiguous nature that is hard to penetrate. This comes out in the polymorphic nature of the conflicts. Hysterics tend to overdramatize convincingly their various problems in manifold ways. You would think that no one else on the planet suffered as much as hysterics; this pose is meant to make anyone in the vicinity rush to their aid. But if you ask the hysteric what the problem is, you often get surprisingly evasive responses.

Hysterics' true emotional theme is their profound aversion to making a firm commitment. In fact, this pertains to the precise description of a disease which, in my experience, often turns out imprecise and hazy. The true fear is of being tied down, being committed, which makes hysterics feel like their freedom is being curtailed. This subliminal fear of loss of freedom leads to constant maneuvering and diplomatic intrigues. This gives rise to the first conflict, which has to do with faint-heartedness. Hysterics think things over a thousand times without ever arriving at a satisfactory solution. Indecisive, ever-vacillating hysterics unnerve those around them. Moreover, their faint-heartedness makes others self-conscious, who then conclude that something might be wrong with themselves – for example, the eager bride-to-be whose boyfriend never gets around to popping the question: it somehow never comes off, to the tune of ever more threadbare excuses, and this can lead her to think that it's somehow her fault, maybe she's not so desirable. Sometimes, a hysteric boyfriend can convince his girlfriend (who would like to be a bride) that the single state is in fact much to be preferred. If so, the vacillating fiancé has elegantly managed to dodge a fateful decision.

The actual cause of procrastination almost always lies with the hysteric, since faint-heartedness results from a profound emotional inability to see things clearly and thus make clear-cut decisions. "What if it turns out to be very different from what I thought?" they ask themselves as they kick the ball down the road. This inner fickleness is a burden to them and is like a debt for which they are made liable. Yet their moral self-accusations don't weigh as heavily as the fear of making wrong irreversible decisions. This applies even to such banal things as buying a suitcase, since even a simple decision can tie a hysteric in knots if different options have differing advantages. If the hysteric buys the wheeled suitcase, that could turn out to be a serious mistake, since wheels can break off, and so on. The string of objections and considerations can be spun out forever. Sometimes the hysteric sidesteps the decision by buying several suitcases. The closets of hysterics often contain an enormous selection of shoes, shirts, socks, and so forth.

Another problem of hysterics is their self-sufficiency. Often, their snobbishness and self-love is camouflaged by a show of modesty and self-effacing behavior. No one would ever suspect a narcissist behind the façade of the always-ready-to-help, ever-smiling waiter, who has some very different hidden sides as well. Only after quitting time does the self-sufficient bloke show his true face, donning the oh-so stylish glittery garb of the star of a local-talent musical and celebrating his triumph onstage. No one suspects the double life he leads – and this is especially titillating for the hysteric, since he's the only one who knows his own true identity. Sometimes, as a special treat for himself, he lets a select few in on his secret. Generally, though, self-sufficient people tend to deal with their problems on their own and keep their secrets to themselves. They also tend to extract the maximum utility and advantage from each situation for themselves – and only themselves.

The next three conflicts deal with the misuse of one's body. Like compulsives, hysterics tend to play power games with their bodies and their essential animal nature. They are forever frittering away energy to get more fun, attention, pleasure, money, dividends, and the like. This results in three conflicts (conflict contents 21–23) whose overlapping themes reflect the exaggerated inner effort that leads to pathological and irresolvable tension and restlessness. In the first conflict, the body becomes a battlefield as these people physically overexert themselves. At one moment, they can look the image of vibrant life itself, only to collapse the next.

The second conflict centers on mental hyperactivity, which involves long-term worries, thoughts crowding in uncontrollably and mental nervousness. Such persons are like washing machines in which thoughts, like laundry, tumble back and forth in an interminable mechanism. This leads to increasing nervousness and fatigue. In the third case, inner tension induces hyperactivity with consequent racing thoughts, being cramped and tense and feeling helpless. These people are like fleeing animals that now and then twitch horribly before relapsing into a helpless spasmodic rigidity.

The Brow Chakra, with its appurtenant diencephalons components of hypothalamus, limbic system, and pituitary, regulates the interplay of cerebrum and body. Imagine an orchestral conductor who watches over what has to happen at the detail level so that we can feel good. If the conductor goes bonkers and starts flailing about wildly, the instruments will play a confused cacaphony, and there arises a great unease, leading to many and varied misperceptions in the audience and, in the extreme case, to lasting pain. The longer this fearsome chaotic state lasts, the more hopeless the spectators become. Finally, the very last spectator is overcome by depression and a feeling of polymorphic bodily misperceptions. This feeling of extreme unease characterizes the 6th conflict theme, which represents a complete disruption of body/mind harmony.

19th conflict: Faint-hearted

Possible problems:

The evasive maneuvering and irresoluteness are rooted in the inability to weigh rationally the relative benefits of different possible courses of action and arrive at a firm decision that won't be regretted later on. The true causes of indecisiveness include the fear of making mistakes and the hope that an even better option might still turn up. Yet every decision involves the possibility of error, and there will always be a better option somewhere, sometime, that can call an earlier decision into question. Therefore, you simply have to summon up the courage to take a stand – but this is enormously difficult for the hysteric to do.

Hysterics want to placate everyone in their immediate vicinity by being friendly and accommodating to them all and scrupulously avoiding confrontation. They try hard to be diplomatic and use delaying tactics, not realizing that they thereby suppress their own wishes and desires. Their disproportionate need for harmony and their drive for freedom in their immediate environment even makes them willing to retreat defensively a great deal. They are interested in many things, but tackle few of them seriously, because any distraction threatens to upset the carefully-cultivated status quo. Such persons appear from the outside to be passive and sluggish, even though they are internally busy keeping things stable and calm. This often makes them emotionally unstable, and they wind up going in circles without making any real progress.

Sought-for solution:

You should work courageously and resolutely to implement your plans, without obsessing about the reactions that others might have to them. Learn to make clear and firm decisions that take the possibility of error into account.

20th conflict: Self-sufficient

Possible problems:

People with this theme often make themselves conspicuous by making abrupt behavioral u-turns. One moment they are extremely shy and reserved, the next they're extroverted and effusive. They can seem very subservient, but also extremely snobbish and arrogant. Like capricious April weather, they have frequent mood swings and sudden behavioral changes. The common denominator underlying these contradictory behavior patterns is that they always and only orbit around themselves, considering those around them to be extras rather than costars or colleagues. Other people are audience or merely part of the scenery; they can be airbrushed away or (u-turn!) wooed passionately, depending on the mood of the moment.

There are frequent rivalries with all manner of people, especially when all are pursuing the same goal and there can only be one winner. Self-sufficient persons nag, are often "badgerers," and have a sadistic tendency to like to see other people in hopeless situations, helpless and at their mercy.

Self-sufficient persons often possess great talents and strengths that enable them to do without the assistance of others.

Such people are hard to get a handle on, and seem unapproachable – precisely because their behavioral pattern can switch so quickly. Deep in their souls, self-sufficient types feel unloved and disliked by everybody. Their egotistical and even autistic behavior tends to unite others against them – which simply reinforces their prejudices.

Sought-for solution:

Most important is learning healthy and positive self-love (not narcissism!) and acquiring social skills.

21st conflict: Physical overexertion

Possible problems:

You feel harried and worn out due to continual overexertion. You are constantly exceeding your limits in order to attain some lofty ideal or other, in the process harming yourself by overdoing it. You are physically driven and tense, often leading to auto-aggressive displacement behavior such as nail-biting, tearing your hair out, gnawing at your lips, and so on. Sometimes, persistent lower-back pain and headaches (and other warning signs) will be indications of a state of permanent overexertion.

You are always on the go, can never let yourself relax – and are therefore constantly irritable and potentially in a bad mood, feeling yourself cheated out of the less stressful side of life.

You suppress your own feelings and work like a maniac, driving yourself to the limit in the absence of any sensible reason for doing so. Behind this are hidden subconscious desires and goals, e.g., wanting to be indispensable and emotionally desirable to others, or being richly rewarded by fortune for having worked your fingers to the bone. Underlying this are a subconscious lust for power and unacknowledged aggressive impulses, as in the "helper syndrome."

Sought-for solution:

You need to learn to recognize and respect your endurance limits.

22nd conflict: Restless

Possible problems:

Internally, it's like being in a strong current, unable to take a break from obsessive thinking. A thousand thoughts whir about in your mind, leading to a state of inner restlessness and compulsion. You would like to do a thousand things at once, and your attention flits from one object to the next like a fidgety bee that can't decide which flower to land on, and so zips about hither and yon among dozens of blooms. Anxiety states are common, of which you might be more or less conscious. For example, there's the fear of missing a one-time chance at something crucial, like the young lady who chases from one potential partner to the next so as not to miss "Mr. Right."

The compulsion is based on a deep-seated feeling of dissatisfaction – or, more precisely: a feeling that anticipates the impossibility of emotional satisfaction even as the longed-for happiness is looked for everywhere, only to be ultimately devalued as undiscoverable and unrealistic. "That won't get me anywhere either! It'll just turn out to be another disappointment!" mutters the restless person, already rushing to the next thought or object.

Much-needed relaxation is made much more difficult – if not indeed impossible – by permanent tension, and this can have physical repercussions such as tension headache, stiff neck, migraine, ringing in the ears (tinnitus), disturbed sleep, and the like. Nervousness, lack of concentration, and irritability are quite common.

From the outside, many internally restless persons seem completely calm, so that nobody has the least inkling what is actually going on inside them.

Sought-for solution:

"Tranquility is strength!" is the "Restlessness Party's" campaign slogan. You need to have the courage to try to get more deeply involved with experiences and feelings, without always anticipating disappointment.

23rd conflict: Tense

Possible problems:

Stressed-out people are always tense and completely unable to relax. This tension is directly manifested as involuntary tics and twitches, writer's cramp, or stiffness, i.e., of the cervical spine – but also in a stiff and stilted manner of speaking, grinding one's teeth, and intestinal cramps. Sometimes, the tension finds its outlet in overdone discipline or exaggerated diligence.

From the outside, people with the conflict *Tense* often seem extra friendly and accommodating. The face is often deeply furrowed and the coloration sometimes ash-gray, a sign of chronic nervous strain which, through hypersecretion of stress hormones, constricts the blood vessels in the skin, causing pale skin and cold hands and feet, as well as prolonged cramping of facial musculature. Yet these people's inner stress is often unnoticeable, and they themselves will only admit that their inability to rest and relax properly is very disturbing and annoying, like a soldier under strict orders to stand at attention during the day, who cannot at home let go of his soldierly rigidity.

The psychic background to tension is grounded in an overly strict Superego. This often relates to a childhood in which an age-inappropriate correctness and self-discipline was demanded.

As with the other similar Brow Chakra conflicts, tension is actually based on a fear of masking mistakes. Basically, one is unforgivingly strict with oneself before any mistake can be made.

Sought-for solution:

Virtually nobody manages to fall asleep by counting sheep, and so, similarly, you should give up trying so hard to relax, and look for an indirect solution, e.g., tiring the body with moderate physical exertion, or taking up a hobby as a distraction.

Emotionally, you should be friendlier and easier on yourself.

24th conflict: Uneasiness

Possible problems:

You no longer feel comfortable in your body, as if wearing a piece of clothing that is the wrong size and shape, so that it pinches and binds everywhere. The body is felt to be a source of discomfort, in the extreme case even of pain and suffering. There can be all sorts of disruptive negative feelings, as if your head or hands were too large, the neck muscles too heavy, or the spinal column twisted. Emotionally, the predominant mood is one of silent and secret hopelessness on up to outright depression. You feel totally out of balance, since everything is unpleasant and most of your body aches.

The predominance of bodily symptoms often causes the underlying depressive basic mood to be overlooked. Nevertheless, the fact remains that the psychic bad mood generates the bodily symptoms.

Underneath the uneasiness is a deeply-rooted feeling of psychic frustration. You are discontented or even hopeless. Deep within, you feel unloved or undeserving of love.

Sought-for solution:

Keep your positive signs and desires in sight, and yield to them – such as the need for rest and relaxation and pampering (i.e., being cared for with nothing expected in return).

The hysteric's six conflict themes are based on the ambivalence of

- Inability to be at ease and satisfied with oneself – but acting on the outside as if everything were in apple-pie order
- Not getting along with reality – thus the flight into busy make-believe fantasy worlds in order to counterfeit proficiency to oneself and others.

In a certain sense, a person in the 6th Chakra lives with the conflicts and problems of a child who is expected to get along in the adult world. This difficult daily world, with all its urgent obligations and unalterable general conditions at first seems to the hysteric like one big game – which, unfortunately, is all too often turned into a huge tragedy by cold, hard reality. Hysterics try to keep up the playful façade, both for themselves and others, for as long as possible. The better one gets to know hysterics, the clearer it becomes that they are by no means innocent victims of external circumstances; rather, they have contributed industriously to the creation of their misfortune. A more dispassionate view reveals that they are the ones tripping themselves up when they fall on their faces.

From the outside, the hysteric is an uncomplicated and cheerful person. However, this façade cunningly conceals a crippling, deep, fundamental self-doubt. In this nagging dissatisfaction, the hysteric resembles the depressive – but is different in possessing a seemingly stable self-confidence. Hysterics are relatively indifferent to what others think of them, as long as they have a good opinion of themselves – or at least that's what they claim (and often believe) – although it actually is not at all true. It is precisely this supposed self-sufficiency that is their big mistake, because the obvious and excellent solution for them might otherwise consist of rediscovering their lost self-love via the affection and sympathy of other people. Hysterics are far more dependent on other people's positive input than depressives, even though it might seem different from the outside – and in fact I would go so far as to say that no other character type is so dependent on the emotional warmth of fellow humans as the hysteric!

Just as children abreact their dissatisfaction through stubbornness, belligerence, and argumentativeness, hysterics tend to have the unfortunate habit of annoying those around them with complaining, even coercive behavior: others, if you please, should be forced to experience some of the discomforts that they constantly have to endure. It is precisely this intolerance with which hysterics tend to enter into disputes that they use to compensate their own dissatisfaction – but also their flightiness and inner strife, as they defend intentionally explicit argumentative positions that verge on the obdurate and paranoid. They often, with coercive effrontery, make go-for-broke plays, even if they have to resort to unfair or dishonest means, such as lying and other immoral behaviors. This shows the predilection for dispute, which for hysterics has aspects of a sporting match; the main thing is getting a chance to win. But if the hoped-for goal is not attained, then the topic of dispute is quickly forgotten, and everything seems to be OK again, as if nothing had happened. Many hysterics conceal their rivalries and intrigues with subtle dodges that, upon closer examination, look like part of a perfidious plan that stems mostly from subconscious drives.

But hysterics also possess surprisingly many excellent and likable character traits that can make one forgive them all their failings on the spot. The positive accomplishments of the 6th Chakra hysteric include increased intuition, delicacy of feeling, and emotional empathy. Whereas the character of the depressive in the preceding 5th Chakra is still enclosed in the snail shell of rationality, the hysteric gets strong creative impulses from the subconscious. While the hysteric on the level of the 2nd Chakra still exhibits wild, libidinal traits (aptly encapsulated in the phrase "wine, women, and song"), the high-level 6th Chakra hysteric develops into a highly civilized hedonist, beguiling others with eloquent intelligence, impeccable manners, and a great deal of charm. Giacomo CASANOVA is a perfect specimen of the 6th Chakra hysteric: he is genteel, charming, creative, playful, and, what's more, clearly enjoys the sensory pleasures of life . The 6th Chakra hysterics also include the hypersensitive and easily-offended *Diva*, as well as the brilliant musician of subtle sensibilities who composes marvelous masterworks – but who, at the same time, can become upset by a fly on the wall.

The increasing inundation of the subconscious makes the person in the 6th Chakra open once more to hitherto buried animalistic and childlike personality components. As we know, when one rediscovers a long-lost object (or ability), it takes a while to learn how to use it again properly. This is exactly what happens to 6th Chakra hysterics, as they find themselves in the well-nigh insoluble dilemma of having to reconcile the inner child (in the subconscious) and the inner animal (in the body) with the adult. This situation is represented symbolically as man-beast: the Centaur (man-horse) or the Sphinx (man-lion). The overwhelming impulses from the animal/sensual body and the creative subconscious at first completely bewilder the hysteric. We say of such people that "He completely lost it" or "She can't get it together." When the 6th Chakra awakes, the undomesticated subconscious drives need to be tamed anew, just like a child has to learn to be civilized and exercise self-control.

The more disciplined and structured that hysterics seem to be, the farther along they are in the maturation process. I have often noticed that mature hysterics seem to belong to a completely different character type. I have not seen this chameleon-like ability to slip into other roles in any other character type to this extent. It corresponds to play-acting ability, which is more pronounced in the hysteric than in any other character type. It's no mystery that the majority of actors are hysterics – although hysterics, unlike actual actors, do not realize that they are acting. Also, on closer examination, it turns out not to be an act after all, but rather genuine feelings that, unlike with other character types, can change quite quickly and abruptly in the hysteric, giving rise to the misleading impression that the person is acting. Thus, the hysteric can, at a given moment, be blubbering like a baby and then, in the very next moment, be as happy as a clam. Or be down in the dumps or even suicidal, then just flip and start making optimistic plans for the future, because someone convinced him that things were looking up and would soon get better.

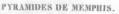

PYRAMIDES DE MEMPHIS.

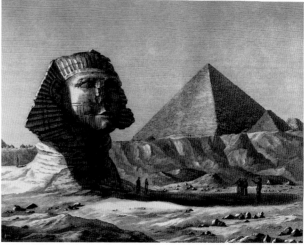

The Sphinx can be viewed as an expression of the awakened Brow Chakra. For the first time in human history, the advanced Egyptians of those times had a clear awareness of their own animal nature. The great puzzle of being simultaneously animal and immortal soul is depicted symbolically in the Sphinx.

The Conflicts of the 7th Chakra

On the material plane, the Crown Chakra corresponds to the cerebrum. Neuroscientists have calculated that the number of possible "wiring" combinations of the cerebral neurons exceeds the number of atoms in the entire universe. This impressive numbers game gives you an idea of the enormous possibilities inherent in the human brain. On the energetic plane, the Crown Chakra reflects the incomprehensibly huge potential contained in human consciousness as an asset to be developed – partly obscured in most people and often only vaguely discernible but (in terms of the sheer possibilities) most certainly infinitely diverse and grandiose. In terms of botanical symbology, the lotus blossom and centaury (a medicinal herb) have been related to the 7th Chakra: the lotus symbolizes the awakening of human consciousness, while centaury is meant to express the enormous potential of the cerebrum.

The Crown Chakra is the pinnacle of human development. We are once again in the world of the schizoid character type that we learned about in conjunction with the 1st Chakra. Looking at the positive attributes of the 7th Chakra, it's as if a bit of paradise has returned. All the ugly, petty fights of the lower Chakras have been left behind, and the world seems once again peaceful and reconciled with itself. The hysteric's inner strife and the monotonous intellectual world of the 5th Chakra have been overcome and seem like far distant trivialities to the person in the 7th Chakra (looking down as if from a mountain peak). Nevertheless, significant parts of the Ego are still present, and important problems remain that address primeval human themes and are extremely difficult to overcome.

The 7th Chakra is home to four different conflicts:

25th conflict: Mistrust
26th conflict: Materialistic
27th conflict: Unwilling to face reality
28th conflict: Wrong thinking

Because 7th Chakra individuals have such above-average farsightedness due to their privileged energetic situation, 7th Chakra schizoids tend to think of themselves as being especially sophisticated and clear-sighted; they see through the egotism and wickedness of their fellow humans and are often very distrustful – without, however, realizing that what they (think they) see is (at least in part) projections of their own dark side. Johann NESTROY once remarked: "*Too much trust is often foolish, but too much mistrust is always foolish.*" The mistrustful person goes to great effort not to have to share anything with or give anything to other people. This definitely includes intellectual property, as in schizoids' use of secret codes to prevent sharing with others. Here, "secret code" can also mean deliberately expressing oneself unclearly or vaguely, so as to make it hard for the listener to understand. People then say "He loves to speak in riddles." Others lock everything up tight.

Because schizoids have a panicky fear of extinction, they will not part with the remnants of their Ego at any price, and fight for it with the ferocity and determination of a bulldog. The "to be or not to be" problem is no longer about material existence (as in the 1st Chakra); the stakes are far higher now, namely: who has the last word, who gets to define reality, and who is a real owner from whom nothing can be taken away. "I've been fighting for so long that I'm not going to surrender a single thing more!" – thus thinks the person in this Chakra. The associated conflict is *Materialistic* (Putting having before being). We're often surprised by the Wise Man that the person at the level of the 7th Chakra would like us to think he is – i.e., by his completely unexpected outbreaks of egotism. We encounter an avarice in which the struggle for personal advantage is fought with a jab in the ribs.

Schizoids want everything for themselves and become extremely miserly, even when it has nothing to do with worldly possessions or power, but rather "just" the immaterial psychic well-being that they have struggled to attain and that they now defend with ideological tricks. Ideological obstinacy and dogmatism, and the power struggles resulting therefrom, are typical negative phenomena of the 7th Chakra. In this view, one <u>has</u> a belief – as opposed to actually living the belief (<u>being</u> a believer). Possessiveness can also manifest itself as attaching greater importance to the packaging than the contents. For example, a person feels his life is more pointless than it seems to be from the outside, but since maintaining the façade is so important, he does nothing to change his unhappy life. The psychoanalyst Erich FROMM, in discussing placing having before being, has noticed a grave character defect in modern civilization, in which genuine human values often count for less than material possessions.

An escalation of self-deception can be seen in two more common psychic conflicts: <u>*Unwilling to face reality*</u> and <u>*Wrong thinking*</u>. If I don't the like the world the way it is, then I have a big problem. Aldous HUXLEY put his finger on the key problem: "*Facts cannot be banished from the world by ignoring them.*" Reality and the claims we make on it sometimes diverge so widely and unfavorably that we can no longer endure it psychologically and go looking for an acceptable solution that can help us out of the "quagmire." Many people build castles in the air, private imaginary worlds in which they cobble together their own new reality. For example, they might twist the facts to cast themselves in a more flattering light. Many people are even trickier: they narrow their field of vision to such a degree that uncomfortable facts are no longer seen at all. Or they don rose-colored glasses to see everything in the most wonderful shades of red. The rose-colored glasses approach includes fleeing into the world of drugs or religious sects in order to escape harsh reality. Even going insane – known medically as *psychosis* – can be a flight from the world.

Another even subtler method uses the perception of the world – a rendition of reality within ourselves – as a lever with which to refashion the world. The idea is: if I think differently, then I am automatically also changing the world. This can take place in manifold ways, though all attempted solutions involve adopting a thoroughly arbitrary viewpoint. As master director of the world, I can invent private philosophies to make puzzling things more explicable, so that the world will seem more consistent to me. I appoint myself director of my own internal **Universal Pictures**, so that I can make what I will of my private world movie. Because if I make myself the center of the universe, I become the fulcrum and pivot around which everything turns, and I can refashion and reinterpret all of history as I see fit. Of course, this all takes place subconsciously, and one does not notice sinking deeper and deeper into the self-made virtual-reality world.

The problem is, however, that the fabricated fantasy world has internal contradictions. If you take these contradictions seriously, then you have to face your own inadequacy and unpleasant character traits, which you would much rather keep out of sight. Self-insight is a painful process which people tend to put off – like going to the dentist. So you develop preconceived opinions and fixed ideas that secure the entire worldview like a fort and, hopefully, cement it in place for all eternity. All these mechanisms are meant to spare one the painful disappointment of true self-knowledge. The resistance to eliminating these ideologies comes from the fear of the *inner bastard* – hence Albert EINSTEIN's resigned remark: "It is harder to smash a preconceived opinion than an atom," which nicely points out the wretchedness of ideological thinking. Experience shows that ideological conflicts are extremely hard to resolve.

25th conflict: Mistrust
Possible problems:
Based on disappointing experiences, you believe that other people have it in for you. You feel surrounded by a hostile world whose sole purpose is to hurt you and steal from you. However, you often overlook your complicity, projecting everything negative outward. A lack of basic trust can often be observed – everything is questioned, critically dissected and broken down into component parts. You refuse to open up emotionally, believing it to be tantamount to surrender. You prefer to lock yourself in, like a snail withdrawing into its shell. You have a fundamental aversion to revealing anything about yourself. You tend to make a wide detour around emotions and situations involving emotional insecurity. You are often very analytical and intellectually oriented, preferring to regard everything from a rational standpoint. People with the *Mistrust* conflict prefer to remain in a distanced spectator role and are reluctant to get drawn into anything that might pull them out of their center.

The real problem with mistrust is strikingly illustrated in the following statement by the billionaire J. Paul GETTY: "*If you can trust a person, a contract is unnecessary; if you can't trust him, a contract is useless.*" Trust is thus to a certain extent an expression of self-love, just as mistrust betrays a lack of self-love – but also a lack of self-confidence: feeling, way down deep inside, bad about oneself. Therefore, trust represents the essential first step toward getting closer to others and in fact being at all viable.

Sought-for solution:
The simplest way to overcome mistrust is to build up trust in yourself.

26th conflict: Materialistic
Possible problems:
There is an obsessive tendency to assign more importance to external circumstances (such as possessions) and to maintaining a façade than to inner values. This can lead to impoverishment notions as well as to greediness, stinginess and a dog-eat-dog mentality. Many people seem from the outside to be very altruistic and friendly and yet, deep inside, they greatly fear large changes: better for everything to stay the way it is, even if it means that life isn't as enjoyable as it might be. Certain ideas are more important than reality – as when you scrimp and save for a future pleasure without, in the process, paying enough attention to your happiness in the present.

It is extraordinarily difficult for such persons to let go of material things and behavioral patterns, or to give away anything. This includes saying goodbye. The same applies to letting go of life itself: the very idea of mortality is denied, and you instead concentrate exclusively on this earthly life.

This wanting-to-have can also apply to certain convictions, such as the belief that you are one of the elite few who "know the score." You can also pile up abstractions such as *knowledge* or *spiritual values* or *good deeds* as possessions – though the distinguishing feature of this emotionally inappropriate attitude is that there remains, deep inside, a nagging frustration that career accolades, fine-looking possessions, or high-quality thoughts and ideas cannot be balanced out.

Sought-for solution:
Learn that life does not work exclusively along the lines of accountant criteria (debit and credit), and rediscover the many modest pleasures, and inner joys, that you have up to now overlooked.

27th conflict: Unwilling to face reality
Possible problems:
Unable to tolerate reality, you banish it from your perception. Airbrushing out reality can include parts of the external world – if, for instance you over- or underestimate the significance of particular people you know. But you might also feel that your entire reality, dark side and all, is so unpleasant that you retreat into fantasy worlds. For most people, taking refuge in their "castles in the air" consists of making changes so extensive that they can no longer remember their childhood; their own life history is foreign to them. Many also block out parts of their inner or outer reality, or they flee into fantasy and proxy worlds. Not infrequently, this reprogramming of reality can be seen externally, i.e., when someone manages to turn a minus into a plus.

In cases of drug addiction or psychosis, the conflict *Unwilling to face reality* is encountered with above-average frequency. Behind all these flight tendencies and repressions lie hidden psychic misery and intolerable frustrations that generate a dark and joyless basic mood in the overall psyche, which you try to escape from for reasons of sheer survival. However, it doesn't change the basic problem, just your viewpoint, by acting as if you lived in a different reality. Good actors with the talent to move people sometimes can transport the audience to a foreign but wonderful world – and forget their own misery in the process. This is similar to what happens to those with the conflict *Unwilling to face reality*, with the difference that they are deceiving themselves.

When you try to escape the pain that is part of being alive, you wind up strangling your own vitality. You need to realize that pain is only a limited part of reality, and that life is much larger than the pain.

Sought-for solution:
Veracity and objectivity are part of attentiveness and living in the present. You should therefore practice being in the here-and-now with full consciousness.

28th conflict: Wrong thinking
Possible problems:
The fundamental problem with Wrong thinking is primarily the refusal to acknowledge reality, so as to be able to derive veridical and rational laws of consciousness. Right thinking leads to a consciousness that is in harmony with both inner and outer reality. But if instead you harbor false ideas that are criticized by the inner voice (the conscience of the True Self), you betray yourself. The same happens if you deny external reality against all reason – i.e., that your opponent in a fight will be a lot stronger than you; you'll pay in that case with a defeat and a broken nose.

In a certain sense, wrong thinking also leads to a type of broken nose, except that the direct visible and perceptible consequences of false consciousness are concealed – namely in the subconscious, as a choking off of vitality. You wind up with a "broken emotional nose" for misjudging reality and indulging bad ideas that have nothing to do with the true state of the world.

You tend to dogmatic thinking. You're unwilling to deviate from your opinion, even if you have to put up with limitations and disadvantages. This includes ancient ideologies and rigid convictions that (in my estimation) could have come from earlier lives. There's not all that much left to be noticed of it in the present life – except that the old ideological rigidity lingers like an undying echo and continues to have an effect in this life. For example, if someone was a member of the privileged nobility in an earlier life, the resulting arrogance can lead to problems if he happens to be a simple farmhand in the present life.

Wrong thinking sometimes comes about because a person, in an earlier incarnation, was forced to pay for her beliefs with her life: e.g., having to die signifies having strong beliefs. You then have a subconscious mental tape loop which says that commitment inevitably leads to dying. Such people are particularly anarchistic and "liberal," in that they never again want to make a commitment: "I'm not getting crucified again for my beliefs!" is the general tenor of their thinking. Refusal to commit then leads to an erratic softness and an exaggerated willingness to conform that stands in sharp contrast to the person's true nature. Actually, the person had been "a tough nut to crack" in the former life, a fact which is now routinely denied in order not to wind up dying for it again.

To this also belong deep-rooted dogmas about oneself. The earlier on in development these doctrines and deep convictions are planted, the harder it will be later on to root them out and give them up. False social structures are often observed in the vicinity of such persons, who in a sense stage wrong thinking as dissonant social structures, i.e., a person paranoically tyrannizes the other family members; or a family member is "disappeared" by never, ever being mentioned, because this (un)person besmirched the family's good name.

Many people engage in wrong thinking by turning overvalued ideas and ideals into standards of behavior – which then constantly collide with reality. For instance, if a woman clings to the belief that "Mr. Right" has to match a very specific laundry list of attributes, then she's going to have problems when her man turns out not to have them all. Therefore, value standards should to some extent harmonize with reality, to give emotional happiness a chance. But if you think wrongly – that is, deliberately "set the bar too high," this will automatically generate a frustrating situation. Right thinking thus means appropriate thinking, i.e., using good common sense when setting the bar height, taking into account both internal and external necessities and facts of the matter – but also allowing for (as yet unknown) future possibilities; in other words, making realistic estimates.

Sought-for solution:
Value yourself and deal attentively with yourself and your needs; this is the most important step toward extricating yourself from the entanglements of *Wrong thinking*.

The common problems of the 4 conflict themes of the 7th Chakra are the deep-rooted convictions that
· No one else has your best interests at heart – you really are your own only true friend
· The world is bad and full of error – you can come up with a better world of your own

Both beliefs, viewed in the cold, hard light of day, are all too justified – for if we look around, the question arises: who really means us well, who would give us the shirt off his back if we needed it? The mistrustful person would answer: the Good Samaritan is kind-hearted only because he believes in a life after death, and he does good deeds to curry favor with God for the afterlife. Those who suddenly lose everything and are cast out by society know how cold and uncaring people can be, and could write a book about their disappointments and letdowns. Understandably, they often become bitter and sarcastic, turning into constant complainers and pessimists.

Because people in the 7th Chakra know a lot about their fellow man and possess a broad vision, they can see through the evil in people all too well – so they scent betrayal and badness everywhere, even when it's not present. In the end, they wind up trusting no one at all, because they suspect furtive betrayal and evil intrigues all around them. "Anyone who gives me the shirt off his back is just trying to lull me into trusting him so that he can bonk me on the noggin when my guard is down!" – thus the mistrustful schizoid upon encountering a Good Samaritan.

The only way to defend yourself against the greedy hordes of humanity is to hoard possessions and defend them doggedly in order to keep them. The problem that arises is, first, that the possessor becomes terribly lonely due to the perpetual defensive posture. But even if you can stand such a horrible situation, there is the additional difficulty that you wind up creating a private universe against the rest of the world – an island of happiness under constant threat from the outside.

Also, walling yourself off from the rest of the world violates the divine principle that all creatures of this world are fundamentally one. The moment you erect a high insurmountable wall around yourself and your possessions, you're halfway to committing a sin – since, presumably, you're prepared to smash in the heads of intruders and thieves if they get too close. *"Those who live by the sword shall die by the sword."* – said Jesus. Thus, in a chain reaction, one wrong decision follows another, i.e., first senselessly walling yourself off, then the resulting isolation and hostility, and finally "wasting" the trespasser (who, in a twisted kind of self-fulfilling prophecy, becomes the *ex post facto* justification that one did the right thing). But killing the intruder is not without consequences, as Jesus' words remind us. Even if no higher justice hurls down lightning bolts from the skies to punish the sinner, you will nevertheless be subconsciously tormented by guilt if you "rub somebody out" because you felt threatened by them, sometimes just for having come too close.

Another widespread schizoid tendency is their predilection for all kinds of mental constructs and (in the most entrenched form) ideologies. By this I mean the tendency for schizoid rationalists to confuse the conceptual world with the real world (or at least to misestimate the degree of correspondence between the two). While the hysteric, for instance, can see absolutely no practical reason to concoct such pipe dreams, and would rather enjoy the pleasures of the senses in the here and now, it's very different for the schizoid, to whom thoughts and ideas are a significant part of reality – the *most* important, in fact! Intellectuals with schizoid character traits thus have a downright erotic rapport with their book collection and with language in general. In fact, rational thinking in the schizoid's reality is the key to any possible changes.

As a result, any change in thinking acts as a kind of anticipatory change in reality. These mechanisms can be seen very well in the schizoid whose ideas have doubtless changed the world the most: Karl MARX. His basic insight (which represents the actual beginning of Marxism) culminates in the thesis: *"Being determines consciousness."* What MARX is saying is that repression in hierarchical societies leads to false mental constructs, after which repression is constantly maintained and solidly cemented into place. For

Brief Overview of the 28 Conflict Themes

Chakra 1
- 1st conflict: Independent
- 2nd conflict: Lack of concentration
- 3rd conflict: Loss of control
- 4th conflict: Extremely self-controlled

Chakra 2
- 5th conflict: Hectic
- 6th conflict: Perseverance
- 7th conflict: Show of strength

Chakra 3
- 8th conflict: Isolated
- 9th conflict: Pent-up emotions
- 10th conflict: Wanting more
- 11th conflict: Craving good feelings

Chakra 4
- 12th conflict: Mental overexertion
- 13th conflict: Withdrawn
- 14th conflict: Introverted
- 15th conflict: Apprehensive
- 16th conflict: Panic

Chakra 5
- 17th conflict: Emotional emptiness
- 18th conflict: Rushed

Chakra 6
- 19th conflict: Faint-hearted
- 20th conflict: Self-sufficient
- 21st conflict: Physical overexertion
- 22nd conflict: Restless
- 23rd conflict: Tense
- 24th conflict: Uneasiness

Chakra 7
- 25th conflict: Mistrust
- 26th conflict: Materialistic
- 27th conflict: Unwilling to face reality
- 28th conflict: Wrong thinking

instance, the worker is too poor to be able to go to school, thus ensuring that the poor will always be dumb and ignorant. Now, if you help poor people attend school, you change their reality (their being), which improves their self-confidence so that they can become proud, successful people, helping society as a whole progress to ever greater riches. That, in a nutshell, is the central message of Communism.

But MARX' famous thesis can also be interpreted in a different way, for it represents (in my estimation) a kind of schizoid self-insight and, in all likelihood, a subconscious self-healing attempt on MARX' part. For schizoids, immediate experience is shaped by the fact that their consciousness is in the foreground of their lives (their *being*). Now, when MARX asserts the opposite, he is thereby standing schizoid feeling on its head. The hysteric – the antipodal type – would be immediately sold on the idea of "being determines consciousness," i.e., when "wine, women, and song," as sensually experienced being, livens up the hysteric's consciousness, or a million dollars won in the lottery improves his living standard. However, such sensations fundamentally fail to characterize the direct experience of schizoids.

How did MARX arrive at this odd and (to his nature) outlandish declaration that being determines consciousness? In my opinion, MARX was attempting in his philosophy to change and repolarize himself completely. His nature would, as it were, become more sensual, grounded, and here-and-now by having his philosophy create a psychic counterweight to his obsessively schizoid rationalistic polarization. Of course, other depth-psychological mechanisms also come into play here, such as self-castigation through self-imposed poverty. MARX was dirt-poor his entire life, constantly having to hit up his rich friend Friedrich ENGELS for money. Was this an attempt to punish himself, because ENGELS belonged to the ruling class? I suspect that this might have been the case, because schizoids, thanks to their obsessively high ideals, tend to castigate themselves when they prove unable to live up to their own overly strict moral standards.

At this point, I could go on forever about the fascinating topic of how the four character types express themselves in the most varied philosophies and historical incidents, but I'd like to wrap it up now because it would take us too far off topic. The descriptions of the 28 conflict themes in these chapters should have made it clear that the four character types can be identified, in characteristic manner and with clear contours, in the 28 themes. Like the letters of an alphabet, the 28 conflicts represent a psychoenergetic language with which the four character types express themselves. As with any foreign language, it takes a while to get oriented and sensitized to the nuances and relevant interconnections.

Because every person is a distinct individual with a unique life history, I have consciously resisted using specific examples and case histories, so as to forestall premature categorization and cookie-cutter oversimplification. Additional useful information on how to identify your character type is included in the next chapter, where I will also recommend the simplest way to implement the entire self-exploratory program in clinical practice. ***Psychosomatic Energetics*** is an invaluable aid here because my experience has shown that the energy test reveals, simply and rapidly, which character a person possesses.

The next few chapters address the question posed earlier, namely: why do there have to be conflicts at all? Speaking generally, conflicts occupy a key position in mankind's evolutionary process. We need conflicts to achieve psychic maturity by having to deal with them. This was touched on earlier when talking about the spiritual journey, at least from the viewpoint of the individual. But the conflict can also be regarded as a superordinate spiritual theme that influences mankind's entire developmental history. Conflicts are then expressions of universal human themes that put their imprint on the spiritual evolutionary process. How that works out in the individual case, and how that changes humans on their energetic vibrational levels, is what I'll be describing in the following chapters. The major theme relates to the fact that the entire cultural and civilizational process coincides with psychoenergetic Chakra levels. "Tell me how you vibrate and I'll tell you how you think, act, and feel."

Some readers may be worrying that I'll discuss these topics in a boring theoretical manner. I'd like to set their minds at rest, because the story of Adam and Eve (starting with which, in the next chapter, the entire theme complex unfolds) – and all the other human developments on up to modern times – touch on core issues which are relevant to every one of us – such as the question of good and evil. These are individual spiritual themes that affect all who are truly interested in self-exploration.

Heaven and Hell –
The Expulsion from Paradise

Paradise tends only to be recognized as such after we have been expelled from it.

(Hermann Hesse)

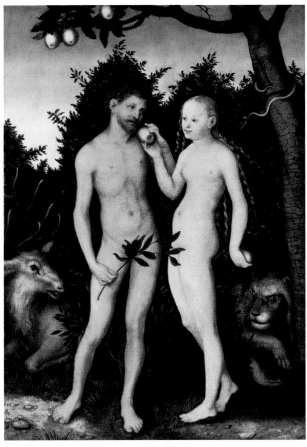

Psychodynamically, Adam and Eve are driven out of paradise by their conflicts (symbolized by the snake). Paradise is a circumlocution for the psychic state in which instincts and actions still coexist harmoniously. The dissociative, discriminating fundamental structure of human consciousness is turned by conflicts into something ugly and evil, leading to the opposite of paradise – namely hell.

After having described the various conflicts in the preceding chapters, I now turn, in the chapters that follow, to their universal effects on the psyche. Unlike much of modern psychoanalytic thinking, I'd like to take an entirely different approach that radically extends the traditional concepts by treating religion and mythology as equivalent partners of depth psychology. That may not at first sound so revolutionary – might indeed smack of superstition and regression to the darkest Middle Ages. Revaluation and integration of spiritual concepts via depth psychology is usually rejected by modern enlightened people with the argument that religion and mythology are just fairy tales and superstitious hocus-pocus – the "opiate of the people," as Karl MARX so scornfully put it – i.e., soothing and anesthetizing tranquilizer pills comparable to telling children bedtime stories meant to lull them to sleep. According to contemporary thinkers, religious and mythological ideas are, in the final analysis, irrational and scientifically unverifiable, hence figments of the imagination.

Meanwhile, more and more people realize that our earthly existence is too constrained and circumscribed by this exclusively rationalistic attitude. Universal human phenomena such as love, nostalgia, the search for meaning in life, and so on are not rationally justifiable either, but they are nonetheless supremely important. Thus, rational scientific thinking can only describe and explain a subset of reality. Human life encompasses much more and even includes the infinite dimensions of the divine! Transpersonal psychology has pressed forward to such revolutionary conceptions. This branch of psychology is an extension of humanistic psychology, which sees an important source of psychological health in man's quest for the divine. From this perspective, religion and science are not antithetical, but rather mutually complementary poles.

C.G. JUNG was the first modern scientist to take the courageous step of acknowledging the value and importance of the psychological content of religion and alchemy for emotional development. JUNG was the first to recognize an extremely important yet normally concealed meaning in spiritual writings, which had to do, in his opinion, with archetypal impressions of the deepest parts of the psyche. JUNG's archetypes are spiritual form and content impressions shaped over millennia, created in the collective unconscious, much like casual everyday habits gradually rigidify into ritualistic rules. Yet archetypes are not only iconic structures; they also have a symbolic and transformative significance: according to JUNG, the soul goes through a maturation process (*individuation*) that is accompanied and guided by the archetypes. JUNG interprets religious and mythological symbols such as the cross of Christianity or the Holy Grail of Arthurian legend as ciphers of inner psychic processes that can only be conveyed to and made directly discernible by consciousness through being formed into archetypes.

At this point, I'd like to adopt a position that goes much farther than this, one that declares archetypes to be actual conditions that by no means exhibit merely significance – like a signpost that tells us which way to go. In fact, I'd like to suggest to the reader that phenomena such as archetypes – as well as abstract religious concepts such as heaven, hell, and the divine – are completely real! In my view, these words describe existing dimensions and qualities of the psychoenergetic world that are as real as the material world, except that – unlike matter – they take place on the invisible and subtle plane. My main consideration here is that the ancient spiritual writings are right when they say that the divine is to be found within. Likewise, of course, heaven and hell, i.e., angels and devils and such, are also within us. These are very old designations, and we can easily be inveigled into not taking them seriously. But I once more point out that, in all likelihood, we are here dealing with authentic psychoenergetic states!

Like the (in principle boundless) universe, our subconscious also enters into a relationship with the divine. In a certain sense, one might say that we are, in fact, God – at least a minuscule part of the divine which is made manifest in us and through us. As "fallen angels" (so to speak), we find ourselves on the way back to the divine, and the conflicts are self-made errors upon which our soul rubs itself raw – but only thereby is able to develop in the first place. Above all, the concepts of heaven and hell play a large inner emotional role. **Briefly put, *heaven* signifies free of sin (i.e., conflicts) and thus being in heaven, whereas *hell* signifies being plagued by conflicts.** Thus, heaven and hell are by no means figments of the imagination, nor are they moral concepts invented to point a patronizing admonitory finger that "puts the fear of God" in us, as many believe. On the contrary, I contend that heaven and hell are very real spiritual worlds!

Heaven and paradise are here very similar concepts: in heaven, as in paradise, we find ourselves in the best of all conceivable worlds. Therefore, I'd like to propose that we consider them to be identical – even though one might object that, according to religious tradition, paradise is where we came from, were expelled from, can never return to. We do, however, have the hope of eventually getting into heaven – i.e., of finding ourselves in psychoenergetic circumstances that will be as beautiful and peaceful as the ear-lier paradise. The expulsion from paradise begins, of course, with *Original Sin*.

Earlier, I compared the Central Conflict with Original Sin. Now, what does the term *Original Sin* mean if one takes it as a symbolic expression of an inner emotional process? First off, modern behavioral biology (ethology) can help us out here, in its view that the separation of instinct from appropriate feelings marks the true beginning of humanity. In wild animals, feelings and instincts are still in harmony, which understandably leads to a paradisiacal feeling of well-being and *joie de vivre*. Nothing stands between the feeling and its experience – neither a critical observer nor any human neuroses. Imagine a cat, stretching luxuriously in the sun: it still exists in this paradisiacal state. In a manner of speaking, this contentedly purring cat is still able to sense

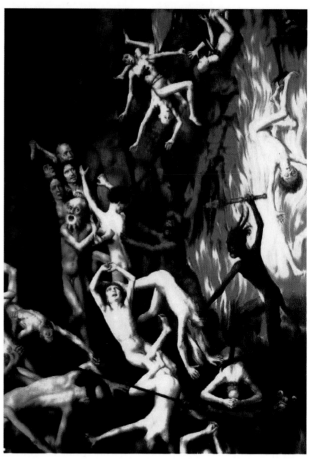

Hell (Hades) represents an inner psychic space that, according to the esoteric traditions of many mystical teachings, comprises a subset of the hereafter. Presumably due to resonance with evil deeds committed in past lives, we are consigned after death to large psychoenergetic worlds that one can designate as hell. There, the evil events recur like an endless litany – except that we have to swap roles (ours was observer and/or perpetrator) with our poor victims.

and enjoy its drives and feelings with all its heart.

Now, I'm not trying to make the absurd assertion that, compared to animals, we humans are to be pitied. No sensible person would want to swap lives with a wild animal, as my experience as a doctor has shown me (even though our more romantic types might occasionally harbor such thoughts). I've asked many people about this, and not a one has wanted even to consider it! We humans appreciate and treasure our free will and our unique human consciousness. When people "lose their minds" – to Alzheimer's, for instance – it represents (at least in the initial stages of the disease) the greatest catastrophe imaginable for the victims. Patients suffer horribly when they can no longer remember and cannot think clearly. They sense, with horror, how their personality slowly begins to dissolve.

The price of our humanity is, as said, the dissonance between drives (desires, instincts) and feelings, by which we lost our edenic innocence. We can of course use all sorts of tricks, but we can never get back to the blissfulness of that state – on top of which, we have also lost the innocence associated with that state. In depth-psychology terms, we feel the expulsion from paradise as being like having to leave the womb at the moment of birth. Our beatitude and our infinite bliss seem forever lost. What happens next, now that we have had to leave paradise? We have become miserable, pitiful creatures, expected to find our way in a hostile world.

We humans stand, naked and freezing, in a complex world that confronts us with enormously difficult tasks and problems. For openers, we're hungry and need a roof over our heads. Animals have the enviable advantage of coming into the world fully equipped with all necessary gear and abilities.[49] More than a few researchers are convinced that it is man's nakedness and homelessness that made man, unlike the animals, have to become cleverer and able to accomplish more. Add to this an uncommonly long childhood, during which the growing child is completely dependent on its fellow humans. We humans simply have to come up with more and better ideas than animals precisely because we have no protective fur coat, no instincts, and no convenient ecosystem.

Of course, these disadvantages also get us our enormously valuable advantages! I already mentioned that nobody would voluntarily trade places with any animal – and, by the way, that also applies to the erroneous assertion that humans could turn back into animals via reincarnation: I hold this to be sheer nonsense in virtually all cases! I'll return to this point later on in the chapter about Karma. For us humans, the greatest treasures are free will and personality. Before I delve more deeply into the advantages of being human, I'd first like to turn in greater detail to the disadvantages. To my mind, one of the biggest downsides of our humanity is the fear that leads to the creation of character types and conflicts, with all the strokes of fate, illnesses, and mental anguish deriving therefrom.

Naturally, animals also experience fear and mental anguish, but it is usually short-term, after which all seems to be OK again. Let's take a look here at a typical scene in a nature film set on an African wildlife preserve. After the male lion kills the lioness' baby (because it had been fathered by a rival male), the lioness has a short period of mourning, after which she lies there placidly, even letting the infanticidal male mount her. In my years of clinical practice, I have yet to see a human mother whose mourning period after the death of her child ever really comes to a close: deep inside, there remains in her forever an inconsolable grief and an enormous ache.[50] Of course, I cannot peer into the inmost recesses of the minds of lionesses, but my empathetic/telepathic abilities, such as they are, were unable to sense any lingering sorrow on the part of the lioness in the film in question.

We humans develop conflicts simply because we live and are thereby forced to deal with all of life's difficulties. One of course wonders what would happen if people were simply left in peace. In the 13th century, the German Hohenstaufen emperor Friedrich II carried out a barbarous experiment on some infants. The wet-nurses were not allowed to talk to the babies; the emperor's instructions were that they were to remain completely mute, but otherwise

---

[49] "Behold the fowls of the air: for they sow not, neither do they reap …" says Jesus to his audience, and he is here certainly not suggesting that we should adopt the carefree lifestyle of our feathered friends as a behavioral model – at least not with respect to our daily work, as many a lazybones might carelessly assume. Jesus was well aware that people must work hard in order to survive. Therefore, Jesus meant something else entirely, namely that animals' lightheartedness and trust in God can be a useful model for people who are constantly worried and apprehensive. The unconcerned and trustful animals reveal to us how we can shed our fundamental fears (i.e., Original Sin). According to Jesus, the way back to paradise is via inner transformation, once again becoming "as a little child" – mentally open, unworried, and with the childlike basic trust that nothing can do us harm and that God will provide.

[50] The persistence of psychic sorrow even seems to affect social groups for generations, if we think of experiences in cases involving HELLINGER's Family Constellations, in which deceased children can continue to have an impact on their descendants for generations. As anyone who has gone through the intense and extremely real experiences of reincarnation sessions knows, a child's death thousands of years ago can still have repercussions in the present for the people concerned. According to spiritual tradition, there is a kind of cosmic memory, such as the Akashic record, in which all experiences (and of course every sorrow) are ineradicably recorded for all time. In my opinion, such experiences are stored in the Central Conflict and are thus part of the psychoenergetic property of the individual who has suffered the particular stroke of fate. The family system merely reflects the spiritual theme complex of that stroke of fate, with the family serving as the sounding-board and theatrical stage for the unprocessed sorrows of the individual member (more on this in a subsequent chapter about the family).

behave normally. Friedrich was curious to see what primeval language a child would begin to speak if it were not exposed to language – presumably the "Adamic language" which Adam and Eve spoke. Regrettably, this question was not able to be answered, since all the children died before the age of ten without having developed a language.

To my mind, this suggests that people get sick even when nothing at all happens. Boredom and its associated "under-challenge" are sick-making stress factors, as is every kind of social isolation (such as silence). Friedrich II's infant experiment seems to have been a case of brute neglect (social deprivation), since the wet-nurses' silence was perforce bound up with an emotional remoteness and coldness that went hand in hand with the emperor's gag order. If someone no longer speaks to us, it amounts to a deeply-felt cruel punishment, regardless of whether the victim is a baby or an adult.[51]

Our everyday experience tells us that we cannot live conflict-free and uninvolved. No matter how much we may try, we'll always make mistakes that inexorably lead to emotional conflicts – and it's probably secondary whether these will be our own or someone else's conflicts: "Broken is broken" we say, and it is of no consequence who the injured party is. Life always involves making mistakes and developing conflicts. The actress Sophia LOREN, as a mature woman took thought-provoking stock of her life as follows: *Mistakes are a part of the debts with which one pays for a rich, full life.* Very generally speaking, we humans push forward, full of curiosity and a zest for action, to gather new experiences.

In order to develop a personality and acquire life experience, we need to make mistakes even in childhood. I must confess that I'm the kind of parent who tends to be overprotective; with well-meant advice, I try to shield my children from harm – but they want to try out everything for themselves and not have it "predigested" for them. My attempts to help are taken as bothersome paternalism. It took a while before I realized that human curiosity is based on natural impulses. My advice was thus actually harmful, in that it impeded the ability to learn from mistakes. We all know about the overprotected child, ejected, abruptly and unprepared, from the crippling condition of overprotection into the adult world, with no transitional period. Being allowed to make mistakes is good for us and is necessary for our development. Psychology calls this (highly efficient) method "learning by trial and error." Bruised young knees

and emotional scars are part of the process.

The first step in the self-exploration of one's subconscious consists of accepting that making mistakes is inevitable ("Nobody's perfect." / "To err is human."). Acknowledging weaknesses leads to being more open and honest with oneself. In this context, many people are under enormous moral pressure to always be perfect, kind-hearted, diligent, and so on. Finally realizing that **everyone** is brimming with error (i.e., conflicts) is, for many persons with too much self-discipline, an enormous psychological relief. In self-help groups, the big therapeutic effect comes from learning that others are struggling with the same (or even greater) problems as you are. "He's even worse off than I am!" you exclaim with relief – from a psychological standpoint an extremely effective consolation.

Let us turn now to the first people in history, who had to pay for their mistakes with their expulsion from paradise. As soon as Adam and Eve have been driven out of paradise, they are first confronted with the difficult task of having to learn to get along with each other as husband and wife. As we all know, that isn't so easy, and leads to this day to prolonged quarrels between the sexes. Yet Adam and Eve have much more serious problems to deal with: they have to cope with all manner of horrors, from famine to fire and other catastrophes. Moreover, Adam and Eve live through terrible wars and much suffering – and they must cope with many strokes of cruel fate in their private lives as well.

At the end of their lives, Adam and Eve will possibly have to endure personal failure, e.g., if life has withheld too many of their lifelong dreams from them. This is known as *midlife crisis* or *senile depression* – and keep in mind that numerous medical statistics show that personal satisfaction has little to do with material well-being. Despite a rising standard of living, the average level of satisfaction in the industrialized world has not risen, when larger population segments are polled. Yet whenever I look out of my taxi window in third-world countries, I am amazed at all the laughter and happy faces that I see, even in the slums.

Material well-being is subconsciously equated with happiness; this presumably originates in prehistoric stone-age experience in which hunger and scarcity signified suffering and death, whereas food and food supplies meant survival. Lately, more and more people realize that true happiness depends primarily on nonmaterial factors such as inner satisfaction and a feeling of gratefulness with respect to life in general, spiritual harmony, and completely nonmaterial childlike states such as the play instinct and *joie de vivre*. Now, all of these states are strongly dependent on inner freedom from conflicts, i.e., people become happier and more contented the fewer emotional conflicts they have. In my experience, wealth has a tendency to promote certain kinds of emotionally destabilizing conflicts (such as envy, fear of material loss, and so on). This would explain why Bombay slum dwellers laugh much more and look happier than

---

[51] In this respect, Frederick II's experiment was hobbled by a fateful "limp" from the very outset, since the nurturing life-essential emotional aspect had been left out of consideration by the Hohenstaufen emperor. This circumstance also betrays – peripherally – something about the nature of the schizoid intellectual that Frederick II had to have been. Such an experiment would not have occurred to a depressive emperor, simply because depressive character types are innately more sympathetic and social.

Zurich pedestrians on *Bahnhofstrasse* or New Yorkers on Fifth Avenue.

Another emotional pain is related to leave-taking and dying. At the end of their lives, Adam and Eve must confront and emotionally deal with their personal finitude. Our subconscious resists facing the inevitability of its personal death; we act as if we were going to live forever. Interestingly, most people feel much younger than their calendar age. When I, as a doctor, ask my older patients how old they feel, most of them reply "Like a twenty-year-old!" – or else "At least ten years younger!" It's very rare that older people feel as old as they really are.

In our secret fantasies, we dream of eternal youth. In this context, an interesting phenomenon: many people, when they fantasize about the Fountain of Youth, nevertheless absolutely want to retain their mature personality! Life experience is immeasurably important to all of us. When, as a doctor, I ask older patients whether they'd want to start their life over again if a good fairy could fulfill this wish (from a medical-psychological standpoint, this kind of question has a cathartic-transformative effect), practically all of them say "Yes, I'd like to start over again – but only if I can keep my life experiences." Older people are aware that experience is an enormously valuable treasure, which they would be very reluctant to part with. To my mind, this makes it extraordinarily clear what our true life values are: not possessions or youth, but rather our life experience with its accompanying mature personality.

Turning once again to Adam and Eve: the Paradise evictees must pay a price for having wanted to stand on their own two feet and not be dependent on God. Man pays a high price for the desire for independence, for individually-lived experiences, and for personal individuation. The Bible says: "*In the sweat of thy brow shalt thou eat bread.*" Life outside Paradise and the Land of Milk and Honey is toilsome: people have to work for a living, surrounded by adversaries, including hunger and thirst. Life, for Adam and Eve, becomes a struggle for survival. Dying of hunger and thirst are part of mankind's primordial experiences, as are freezing to death or being eaten by wild beasts.

But Adam and Eve learn their biggest lessons through contact among themselves and other people. Adam and Eve begin to organize into larger families and groupings. The resulting disputes and fights contain much of the explosive material known in social psychology as *conflict potential*. People learn much more much faster (self-experience) once they have formed into societies. Of necessity, contact with one's fellow humans spans the gamut from heaven to hell. **Hell and evil are thereby – from the point of view of emotional maturity – the most powerful agents for accelerating the learning process.** In what follows, therefore, I'd like to turn to the depth-psychological significance of *evil* – man's dark side, hardest for us to comprehend, and whose deeper implications often leave us doubting both ourselves

and the existence of any kind of higher spiritual order whatsoever.

The naked cynicism of the ancient Roman saying "*Homo homini lupus est*" (Man is a wolf to man) reveals the despairing bitterness that our fellow humans' evil side evokes in us. Like rabid dogs, people torture and slay each other. Pessimists and cultural-values conservatives have drawn the conclusion from this that man is essentially evil and an uninhibited beast that can only be restrained by strict laws, punishments (death penalty), and constant surveillance. The enormous destructive potential of our advanced civilization is best illustrated from recent history during the Vietnam War by the My Lai massacre, in which formerly decent American soldiers turned into monsters who sadistically tortured and slaughtered women and children.

One can't help but wonder how many ordinary people might be latent torturers and murderers, capable of My-Lai-style massacres or concentration-camp cruelties. In a psychological test in America (the notorious Milgram Experiment[52]), walk-in volunteers were instructed to administer ever stronger jolts of electricity to "test subjects" whenever they did not give the desired answer, i.e., whenever they failed to "obey." The volunteers were told that the highest voltage setting might possibly be deadly, but the decision was left up to them. The volunteers couldn't see the subjects; they could only hear their (faked) cries of pain. A vanishingly small number of volunteers refused to take part at all, and virtually all participants tortured the subjects considerably – in fact about 65% of the volunteers went up to the "deadly" setting, upon which, after bloodcurdling screams, the loudspeakers went deathly silent!

Publication of the Milgram Experiment triggered a torrent of public outrage, because it showed all too clearly that passersby – and indeed our very neighbors – were potentially capable of murder if placed in a tempting position of power where they had *carte blanche* to commit violent acts against others. Originally, the experiment had been conceived by Stanley MILGRAM to investigate the psychological root causes of the Holocaust. People wonder how they'd act, whether they would have obeyed as blindly as did the experiment's volunteers. To be sure, most people are quick to convey their loathing of murderers who torture helpless victims to death – yet it was ordinary people, volunteers taken off the sidewalk, by no means sadists or killers, who made up the overwhelming majority of the participants in

---

[52] From the original notes of the social psychologist Stanley MILGRAM (Harvard University, Boston MA): "I observed a mature and initially poised businessman enter the laboratory smiling and confident. Within 20 minutes he was reduced to a twitching, stuttering wreck, who was rapidly approaching nervous collapse. He constantly pulled on his ear lobe, and he pushed his fist into his forehead and muttered 'Oh God, let's stop it.' And yet he continued to respond to every word of the experimenter, and obeyed to the end."

the Milgram experiment. The experiment has since been repeated at other locations, and the results have been much the same.

This is evidently why, in most people's self-image, the scary aspects (that surface in such experiments) are strongly repressed. The only possible sensible explanation for the Milgram experiment's results is that, in the majority of humans, violent and destructive drives lurk just beneath the surface. However, these destructive aggressions are not conscious in most people, which is why very, very few people are aware that they harbor gruesome and murderous impulses. As soon as an authority figure gives permission to be cruel, most people exhibit a frightening disinhibition – as one can see in the experiment with the supposedly recalcitrant learners, who are punished with (simulated) electric shocks of up to "deadly" intensity. It is readily apparent that an authority figure's invocation of violence is enough, by itself, to turn most people into unrestrained aggressors, batterers, and murderers.

I made another horrifying discovery which showed me how close to most people's psychic surface these dreadful anxiety states and appalling horrors lie concealed: time and again I have noticed, in all kinds of encounter groups that use drums, ecstatic dancing, hyperventilation, and suchlike to induce deeper states of consciousness, that most people in such trancelike states quickly begin to shout, whimper, and weep. Afterwards, they tell of horrible childhood memories and well-nigh intolerable emotions, also particularly appalling images and scenes of horrible deeds playing out before their inner eye. Out of sheer curiosity, I tallied the subjects who, at large seminars attended by hundreds of people, had some type of unpleasant to dreadful experience … it turned out to be more than two-thirds of all attendees! By the way, it is obvious that these percentages are much the same as in the Milgram experiment. In my opinion, there are tight correlations between these two groups, which I'd like to clarify in greater detail.

Numerous therapists who treat their patients with hypnosis have confirmed to me the huge extent of terrible emotions and horrible experiences that can be found just under the surface of everyday experience. There, in the subconscious, lurk terrifying fantasy figures in the form of demons and devils who can manifest themselves in spine-chilling ways. In earlier times, it was said that someone was "possessed by the Devil" if he had such experiences and – possibly influenced by subconscious fears – behaved differently than normal.

We moderns see this in another light and speak of nightmares when someone tells of terrifying dreams full of horror figures. If these figures take on a life of their own that negatively influences and affects the person, we speak of delusional ideas. My own take on the phenomenon of subconscious conflicts has already been presented in the earlier chapter on the origin of conflicts. I say that the truth lies somewhere in the middle, in that diabolical conflicts and the like represent real beings, but they only gain power over us if we psychoenergetically vibrate in a similar manner as these beings.

At this point, the interesting question for me is: where on earth does the human evil come from in the Milgram experiment? To me, it's obvious that someone with a subconscious inner horror will "pass on some of the horror" to other people – e.g., as a test subject will in the aforementioned experiment, by torturing and even killing, because the test director okayed it. In this situation, the perpetrator is totally unaware of his deeply concealed psychic pain, while the victim feels the pain that the victimizer himself cannot perceive. The evil projects itself onto the outside world (the victim), even though its origin is in the perpetrator's inner world (subconscious).

Now, one could of course object that the Milgram experiment is an artificial situation, and the evil in our civilization doesn't play nearly such a significant role. I'd like to respond that, in real life, we are constantly in the midst of, and even surrounded by, evil. We encounter evil in the daily war of commuter traffic, in family quarrels, in mobbing at work, in the daily horror of the evening news on TV and in the exploding crime statistics. If we are more self-critical, moreover, we'll notice that, when it comes to evil deeds, we are by no means always unfortunate victims, but rather often enough victimizers as well. We confront our violent shadow as soon as we take a closer look at our daily doings. In the process, we notice our own subconscious, subliminal or overt hostility and propensity for violence.

Since we carry our conflicts around with us, there is practically nobody who can be considered to be "without sin." The later discussion of Karma will make it clear that, in fact, everybody is tangled up in conflict formation. In fact, evil and conflicts are one and the same, as I have emphasized a number of times. Now, this sounds reasonable when applied to other people, but it seems suddenly downright strange and incomprehensible when the crosshairs are on us. Someone reproaches us bitterly and accuses us. We ask ourselves incredulously "How come I'm the bad guy?" The aphorism *"Evil is always other people"* puts it quite nicely. Taking a peek behind our psychic curtain is usually the last thing that would occur to any of us to do. We always look for evil outside of ourselves! The Roman orator Marcus Fabius QUINTILIAN saw the real problem when he said: *"Everyone would rather see others' faults corrected than their own."* Others should change, if you please, but we are unwilling to ourselves.

From a higher observational plane, human faults and conflicts are by no means useless, but rather have a deeper significance that (as already mentioned numerous times) has to do with spiritual maturity. The biblical parable of the Prodigal Son relates symbolically our human destiny to make progress via our errors. Each of us thus represents the prodigal son, with God in the father's role. Eventually, the prodigal son returns from his odyssey, having developed into a mature personality. The prodigal son experienced his true spiritual core, in the sense of "know thyself," only after having lived in a world full of error. Through his own and others' errors, he learned a great deal and grew up to become a mature personality.

In view of human development, the function of evil takes

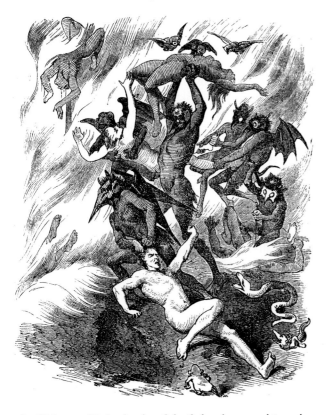

On Walpurgis Night, hordes of devils break out and inundate mankind like a torrent. They torment, torture, and destroy their victims in a nightmarish orgy. What we are actually dealing with here is the conflicts of the subconscious, which are symbolized as devils and which are truly fiendish – also symbolized in the form of the snakes and crocodiles in the lower right.

on another meaning, which can be equated with the meaning of *disease*. Both evil and disease are destructive and hostile states that nevertheless generate life-giving growth and catalytic transformations, just as fire does, which burns up everything and thus allows the new to emerge. This kind of superordinate worldview is, it seems to me, necessary and sensible for arriving at a deeper understanding of medical science (the *healing arts*). "Becoming healthy" (hale or whole) then takes on a spiritual dimension that embraces the whole person.

The Spiritual Journey and the Civilization Process

When the greater sense is lost, it is replaced by morality and duty.

(Laotse)

If we were to open up the morning paper with the idea in our minds that we are embarked on a collective spiritual journey, then we would view the headlines (plane hijackings, child abuse, corrupt politicians) in a completely different light. It's not that such a viewpoint excuses anything, but it is a totally unaccustomed perspective that deviates sharply from the usual way of looking at events. From this viewpoint, the entire global stage looks like a spiritual school in which people – as involved actors – take part in a personal maturation process. The visible outer process would then be that of civilization and culture, the inner one that of spiritual maturation (C.G. JUNG's *individuation*).

While the preceding chapters have dealt with individual spiritual maturation, one can also relate the developmental stages of mankind as a whole to the energy levels and Chakras. Basically, individuals, from infancy to old age, all pass through the same psychoenergetic developmental stages – i.e., they begin at the first Chakra and rise ever higher in their psychoenergetic development; mankind as a whole goes through this selfsame process.

Viewed in this manner, the entire history of civilization becomes an external mirror of internal consciousness developments. Now, at first this association might seem like a lot of "psychobabble" in which a part of human life (the psychological conflict and its appurtenant psychoenergetic developmental stage) is singled out and turned into a cosmic passkey to an all-inclusive explanation of the world. But I hope I can persuade the reader that this radical viewpoint contains significantly more concealed truth than one might at first think. The reason has to do with the tight coupling of Chakra developmental levels and associated mental structures: **"Tell me what Chakra level you vibrate on and I'll tell you how you think"** is the key sentence here that describes the actual meaning context.

When we look at mankind as a collective that must pass through the same maturation stages that individuals do, we learn a great deal about ourselves by studying these maturation stages in human history. I would therefore like to recommend that readers view human development as a mirror of their own personal development. I begin (logically) at the

Psychoenergetic Development of Mankind

	Chakra and associated culture epoch						
	World history						
Chakra	*1st*	*2nd*	*3rd*	*4th*	*5th*	*6th*	*7th*
Culture epoch	Stone age, Indians	First high cultures (Mesopotamia, Egypt)	Antiquity to Middle Ages	Renaissance	Modern (present day)	Future (global village)	???
Age of individual	Womb, baby	Infant	Child	Adolescent	Adult	Mature person	Wise person
Life theme	Survival and growth	First emotional experience	Emotional survival, fighting and playing	First love, feeling of wholeness	Reason, individual, life plan	Intuition, individual and cosmos	Knowledge of God, Self-knowledge
Character type	Schizoid	Hysteric	Depressive	All types	Obsessive-compulsive	Hysteric	Schizoid

beginning with the 1st Chakra, which correlates with the Stone Age and the cultural stage of roaming nomadic tribes. In the 1st Chakra, we find ourselves in mankind's infant phase. This phase is concerned primarily with sheer survival, having to defend against dangers such as starvation, cold, hostile foreign tribes, and predatory beasts.

There are many who look back at these early phases of human development – which seem so outlandish to modern man – with a great deal of nostalgia, idealizing the life of the "noble savage" into something "holy and innocent." Children, like animals, still have a kind of naïveté that we (correctly) designate as *innocence*. Evidently, many people sense a comparable innocence in primitive cultures and become similarly infatuated, just as children enchant us with their natural charm. I have observed a comparable nature in spiritually highly developed persons (about which more later). Saints also have an air of innocence, so that primitives, children, and saints exhibit very similar character traits – at least (regarding children and primitives) as long as they're not spoiled by external influences. Our grownup world, with its sins and failings, gets in the way: people are no longer as naïve as innocent children, nor yet as advanced as pure saints.

The average person lives amid constraints and problems. Simply put, adults have to deal with a potentially threatening and often malevolent world. The Central Conflict plays an important role here, since it represents the actual source of evil, as I have mentioned earlier. Very surprisingly, however, it is quite a different matter (from us adults) when it comes to infants, primitives, and saints. I think there's a simple reason for this, namely that they lack a Central Conflict: primitives do not have it yet; in infants, it is largely still hidden (at least in psychologically healthy, normal children); and saints have gotten rid of their Central Conflict.

Saints are particularly interesting to us, since they have personal development problems behind them that we have to wrestle with every day. With respect to saints, Paradise Lost seems to have been re-found. *Religio*, literally "to bind fast," becomes for the saint an actually experienced, immutable reality. The saint or sage becomes re-aware that man and the world are, at bottom, one – often imparted by a mystical experience of oneness that completely transforms the saint (known in the esoteric tradition as *unio mystica*).

From the time of this **enlightenment** on, the saint once again experiences the world as good and benign; evil no longer holds sway and can no longer maintain the separation illusion. Sometimes, the state of enlightenment takes on altogether unrealistic aspects. States of enlightenment are thus exceptional situations that should not last too long if they are not to seriously jeopardize the saint's life. For instance, the famous Indian saint RAMAKRISHNA is reported to have remained for weeks in a state of divine ecstasy (*Samadhi*), having to be artificially nourished by his disciples. Evidently, people can only linger in paradisiacal

states and "seventh heavens" for a short time.

With the saintly state, we have arrived at the terminus of our spiritual journey. The entire process of civilization unfolds between the primitive and the saint – in the middle of which, presumably, each reader of this book is stuck, since I doubt that all that many saints will be reading it. Still, it makes sense to think about the endpoint of our spiritual journey and to describe such states – because saintliness is by no means an elitist state granted only to a few unrealistic eccentrics. On the contrary, I strongly suspect that our current ideas of saintliness are pretty untrue and illusory! They are based on ancient times, when saints were still something special, because the majority of people had relatively much lower vibrations.

Saints – or, better put: wise and spiritually advanced people – are, I suspect, simply people who inhabit the vibrational level of the 7th Chakra and higher. I have met more and more people in the past few decades who have reached these vibrational levels, yet who are still "just plain folk." I find more and more of these people in my energy testing, so I can safely say that their numbers are on the rise. I will talk about this interesting group of exceptional people in greater detail in a closing chapter. The remark of the French poet SAINT-EXUPÉRY applies to these warm-hearted, friendly beings: "*If you succeed in sitting in judgment on yourself, then you are a truly wise person.*"

We thus find that the best key to spiritual development is self-knowledge: getting to know our dark side and integrating it. We should make an effort to attenuate our errors and recapture our lost emotional aspects in order to reawaken the underlying hidden energy potential. That sounds (and is!) difficult, but the first step, at least, is relatively easy to attain with a simple trick, because we find our most primitive problems reflected in the external world. We therefore need only observe the external world in order to learn a lot about our secret inner life. This applies as well to the much larger world-historical criteria. In this process, every cultural epoch and every stage of our entire civilization deals with differing themes and aspects of the universal human dark side.

In this way of looking at things, we can recognize our own psyche with all its drives, secret wishes, and conflicts in the Stone Age, in ancient India or Egypt, as well as in humanity's other epochs. Just as children play specific games at each age level, we can see the inner emotional processes of the principal participants represented in each respective civilizational level. If we can get a handle on the underlying psychological mechanisms, we can of course learn a great deal about ourselves and our inmost drives. At the same time, an evolutionary rule emerges from the cultural accomplishments of the collective as well as of the individual.

1st Chakra

War as the "father of all things" stands at the beginning of human development. The phenomenon of war is bound up with an extraordinarily powerful and extremely intense fundamental fear that turns on the issue of whether you live or die. Amazingly, this war begins right at conception: so-called "killer sperm" have been found in male ejaculate that can destroy foreign spermatozoa. The killer sperm count rises sharply in men who suspect their wives are two-timing them. We can thus observe the phenomenon of war even in the aggressive behavior of sperm, which view competitors as enemies and try to put them out of the running. So, the very first topic of this world revolves around power and reproduction! A brutal Darwinian struggle for survival of the fittest rages all around us. Will we even survive being born? Are we strong enough to defy hostile climate, aggressive bacteria, human enemies, and evil rivals?

At first, we are still one with the universe, part of the whole – whether as primeval man in the early stages of human development who felt at one with nature, or as fetus and infant living with its mother in paradisiacal harmony. Then, the first serious problems arise, having to do with the fear of dying and being annihilated. Within the psyche, the juxtaposition of the contradictory states of life and death generates a terrible feeling of threat, symbolized by the Hindu goddess *Kali*, who first begets her brood, then slays and devours them. A comparable mythical figure is that of the evil stepmother in fairy tales, in which the nurturing, protective maternal principle is transformed into a deadly danger.

Similarly, the perverted eroticism of sadomasochism intermingles desire and pain, satisfaction and submission, creating new life only to murder it with "painful lust." We also find this admixture of violence and sexual desire in the animal kingdom, all the way up to killing and eating the partner or offspring. Aggression and sexuality are closely-related drives, both serving to maintain life and bound up with desire. It isn't hard to see why such incomprehensible and seemingly contradictory behaviors can arise.

The 1st Chakra is about a free-for-all war of "every man for himself." Everybody wants the biggest slice of the pie – and the sheer survival of the individual takes center stage. The first developmental step is separation and isolation, the first stage of war. This leads to disconnection from the whole and to the first rudimentary aspects of individuation, the contours of which are here already discernible. Thus, a genuine feeling of fear can only arise after a *self*-consciousness has developed.

At this stage of consciousness, mythology refers to the *Great Mother* and the *Great Father*. Since many primitive cultures do not apprehend the connection between sex and birth, the beginning of human development is inevitably mother-oriented: if you don't know "where babies come from," the mother is the dominant figure. In matriarchal societies, the individual merges completely with the group. The social community becomes an external womb, whose protective aspect segues directly to the mother-goddess, who is experienced as sovereign mother and divine nurturer (Mother Nature).

Much later, the Great Father appears as an equivalent or even more powerful mythical figure, and is regarded as the true Creator (*Brahma* in India, *Jehova* in Israel, *Aton* in Egypt). Surprisingly, father and mother are seldom perceived as androgynous creator-parents. This might have to do with the bitter patriarchy/matriarchy enmity. We find this androgynous element of father and mother as creator-parents in the figures of Jesus and Mary.

Turning to the psychoenergetic development of humanity's primeval beginnings, we find many commonalities between the early childhood of the individual and that of humanity as a whole. As long as we are developing our 1st Chakra, we remain energetic and very permeable. Thus, all beings are much more open in this stage to the emotional body and their entire psychic primal ground of being than in later stages. Parapsychological phenomena such as sensing and seeing the Aura were everyday experiences for primitive man. Anyone whose feelings are not this delicate and permeable will likely have a very hard time comprehending this kind of enhanced perception. Modern psychology refers to the view that everything has a soul as *animism*. Infants seem to experience the world in this manner, and can converse with inanimate objects such as wooden toys or dolls.

The actual key to understanding magical thinking is the realization that these phenomena work only if one steadfastly believes in them. In my opinion, therefore, the hunt magic of the stone-age hunter was a real phenomenon and not just wishful thinking, and so cave drawings of prey animals represented a very sensible attraction method. This needs to be qualified: ... sensible as long as one is still in the 1st Chakra. After that, the magic quickly vanishes, leaving behind mere superstition.

From the standpoint of first impressions, all beings whose 1st Chakra is developing come across as downright childlike, open, and friendly. Because of its psychological proximity to the nurturing primal source of the mother-child unity, the young being still experiences much of the original paradise. It still radiates angelically something of the brilliance of the heavens, from whence it recently came. In this first stage of human development, evil is still on the far horizon, perceived at the most as distant thunder, and not yet able to be classified and evaluated as to dangerousness. Amazingly many primitive Indian tribes are strangers to aggressiveness and criminality in the modern sense. Similarly, animals who have not yet been exposed to man as enemy exhibit an edenic trustfulness. One is reminded of the biblical story of the lion lying down peacefully with the lamb. In our journey through the Chakras and mankind's development, we still have one foot in Paradise, in which prehistoric man and the forest Indians dwell.

And yet, despite this, man in the 1st Chakra is already a partial outcast from Paradise. The Self of man in the 1st Chakra is highly sensitive, because it is as yet so little developed. This can lead to serious problems that result in a schizoid character. The schizoid's fundamental problem always has to do with lost basic trust. Schizoids wonder if they have any right to exist at all, or any right to happiness at all.

I'd like briefly to recap the schizoid's four basic conflicts:

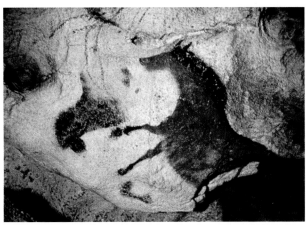

In the Stone Age, prehistoric man's magical hunting drawings were meant to make wild game easier to hunt by showing it already "captured" in the drawing. Horse falling down, from the Cave of Lascaux (Dordogne, France).

Conflict 1: Inferiority complex – Right at birth, the right to exist is put to a hard test: whether one is fit for life and whether one can stand on one's own two feet.

Conflict 2: Lack of concentration – Nostalgically missing the lost paradise in the mother's body, which gave life order and blissful centeredness, and generated a feeling of coherence and groundedness.

Conflict 3: Loss of control – The psychological problems orbit around the feeling of being helpless and totally at the mercy of circumstances beyond one's control, as in the case of a difficult delivery, which for the newborn baby is associated with pain and deadly danger.

Conflict 4: Extremely self-controlled – The unbearable agony of being murdered and of not being loved is completely repressed; one makes oneself totally deaf and emotionless, violently strangling feelings at their first manifesta-

tion, in the extreme case even killing and destroying the objects of one's affection before they can do the same to you.

2nd Chakra

After we're born and the umbilical cord has been cut, the actual struggle for survival begins when we have to stand on our own two feet. The 1st Chakra's basic problems are taken up by the 2nd Chakra in a completely different way. With gruesome enthusiasm, the lion begins to exterminate the lamb lying serenely next to him. A competitive "every man for himself" struggle for survival ensues, in which deviousness and duplicity count for as much as strength and speed. People at the 2nd Chakra developmental level – and this includes those with a corresponding Central Conflict – often surprise those around them with their unusual talents and abilities.

The 2nd Chakra leads to the first clearly recognizable development of individuality. Depth-psychologically, development of the Self begins in earnest at this stage, leading to stable and clearly-discernible individuation. One can see this in contacts with very primitive tribes compared to more highly developed ones: at first, the individual is scarcely recognizable as such but, at ever higher levels of civilizational development, it takes on clearer contour and demarcation.

The 1st Chakra still contains many subconscious and transpersonal themes that transcend the Self. Only in the 2nd Chakra does the infant begin to turn into an individual – and in the process recognize itself as an object of love. It sucks its thumb or sensually fondles its genitals, its own pleasure very egotistically taking center stage. In Greek mythology, Narcissus sets himself apart from the Great Mother, loving himself more than anything else. This is the source of the feeling of being a magnificent champion, largely independent of external love-objects. Other objects are there to be subjugated, pillaged, and exploited, and otherwise have no subjectivity (unlike the 1st Chakra, in which one merged regressively with the love-object).

Everything becomes magnificently violent, exceptionally pretentious and bombastic, dynamic and extraordinarily exhilarating. People at the 2nd Chakra stage tend to boost their relatively weak Self by forming into groups. In the course of this development, the nomadic hunter-gatherer becomes a sedentary farmer, joining forces with like-minded souls into clans and tribes. The first affluent individuals develop in these tribes. The coronation of the first kings and the first territorial battles take place, to defend and expand the first large nations and dynasties.

Early heroic myths reflect this titanic struggle, as in ancient Crete's Palace of Knossos, where the bull (that symbolizes the untamed force of nature) is fought. In this projection of the demonic and libidinal, nature's superiority is transformed into the malevolent dragon that must be slain by the Hero. The dragon myth thus symbolizes the elementary dilemma of the hysteric on the developmental level of the 2nd Chakra.

In the 2nd Chakra, man learns, through cleverness and discipline, how to vanquish what are, in the final analysis, superior forces. This might involve recourse to clandestine dirty tricks, true to the old saying, "no witnesses, no crime." Genghis Khan's warriors and the Vikings are the perfect prototypes of 2nd Chakra man. With splendid headdresses, fearsome horned helmets, and heroic chests swelled with pride, strangers are made vividly aware of these warriors' personal power during the course of riotous carousing celebrations. They feel like proud victors over hostile nature and the vast hordes of enemy combatants.

When things go well, the emotional contents of the 2nd Chakra are a feeling of strength, pride, and power, such as we can marvel at in military parades. Patience and courage, as well as strength, are the positive characteristics of the 2nd Chakra.

2nd Chakra disturbances give rise to emotional disorders that contain polar opposite images of the desirable emotional characteristics of proud warriors. The fragility of the "newborn" Self allows wretched images of failure and defeat to arise.

The hysteric's three basic conflicts are:

Conflict 5: Hectic – The threat of defeat leads to nervousness and irritability which conceal a great fear that is held in check by hectic activity-for-its-own-sake.

Conflict 6: Perseverance – Big fears arise because, basically, despite feeling weakness and inferiority, one wants to be strong and in control. At the same time, Oedipal character problems are developing, which can only be understood through the I-feeling of Narcissism. For Oedipus it's a matter of "me or you" in which the rivalry seems to presuppose equality between the opponents, but which in reality is trying to conceal a stubborn and childish self-centeredness.

Conflict 7: Show of strength – the fundamentally weak warrior cleverly tries to conceal his secret inferiority behind a façade of laid-on-thick arrogance. Irritably and stubbornly, he declares that he is strong enough to emerge victorious. In his heart of hearts, the opponent doesn't bother him in the least, because he always and forever feels himself to be a winner, even if the victory is only a figment of his fevered imagination. In this spirit, that bygone era sees the building of the first huge tombs, which seem to have been erected by Titans, as can be seen in the gigantic stone sculptures of Easter Island or Stonehenge. One can make out, in many ancient cultures, a certain phallicism, from the Hindu Lingam to the modern skyscraper. The Hero needs to prove how fantastic, mighty, and wonderful he is by erecting gigantic edifices.

3rd Chakra

The 3rd Chakra represents an antithesis to the heroic thesis of the 2nd Chakra. These 180-degree "about-faces" can also be seen in the transition from the 1st to the 2nd Chakra. In the 3rd Chakra, it is no longer the lone Hero, but rather the group, that is the focus of attention. All of the 2nd Chakra values having to do with power and rivalry are worthless in the 3rd Chakra.

Systemic processes are initiated because the social group is a surrogate mother. One can easily observe this in the growing child, when it begins to associate with its age peers in order to win sympathy and recognition, and to be able to live contentedly within the protective confines of the group. The effort of conforming to the expectations of others becomes the dominant experience and most important inner emotional *leitmotiv*. In so doing, one senses how much one's own fate directly depends on that of others: "Do **not** do unto others as you would **not** have them do unto you." (in the words of the – lightly modified – Golden Rule)

In the 3rd Chakra phase, people begin to live in their own social sphere, a human world separated from the surrounding natural world by walls and fences. *Out there* it's hostile; *in here*, at home, it's friendly. The cultivated human world and the wild natural world become antipodes to be kept apart.

Nature and its powers are associated with anthropoid mythological figures, whose pantheon becomes a mirror of human desires and weaknesses: we are speaking here of heroes and gods such as Shiva, Zeus, and Odysseus. These anthropomorphized gods fall in love, make embarrassing mistakes, and are subject to all manner of passions and emotions that are, basically, no different from those of mortal humans. However, the humanization of the gods at the 3rd Chakra developmental level by no means signifies that the gods are to be dismantled and dethroned. On the contrary, man in the 3rd Chakra has a strong need for tough and practical reality management, and humanizing the gods is an outgrowth of this need. After all, unworldly gods are of no earthly use to man – and besides, it's not so easy to carry on a conversation with aloof Olympians.

Man's fundamental experience in the 3rd Chakra is beset by frustration and greed. Dionysian orgies and Faustian bargains unleash the enormously strong attraction that arises from the excruciating longing for perfect satisfaction. Even the ascetic who has renounced the sordid material world is driven by the monstrous need created by man's alienation from nature and the divine ground of being. The core theme of the 3rd Chakra concerns power and hunger – and even the ascetic strives to attain a contented state of power and abundant energy through deliberate fasting: spiritual satiation consists of the desire for enlightenment and supernal bliss.

3rd Chakra people populated cities such as ancient Rome, Athens, and Benares; I'd also include most of Medieval

Europe on the psychoenergetic level of the 3rd Chakra. The determinant life-feeling of those times was the ambivalence of hunger/gorging and power/powerlessness – the classic psychic themes of the 3rd Chakra. The fear of starvation and craving enough to eat have crucially to do with the social group, since only within the group can one get enough to eat. Figuratively, nourishment signifies everything that man needs in life, i.e., food, loving care, a meaningful life task, and social contact.

The other dominant theme of the 3rd Chakra deals with power and the lack of it. The subjective energetic weakness and insignificance of the individual is countered by the size and power of the group. On a very elemental and vital level, the group is needed to stabilize the individual Ego and maintain its energy budget. To be sure, the 3rd Chakra still has its heroes, but the group now gives them some stiff competition. In the 3rd Chakra, the heroic loner has turned into a hero by virtue of group recognition: a Caesar without the cheering throngs makes no sense. By contrast, the heroes of the 1st and 2nd Chakra are far less dependent on applause.

The positive character traits of the 3rd Chakra have to do with self-control and group consensus. On the 3rd Chakra level of development, man learns both inner and external moderation. The egomaniacal self-centeredness of the first 2 Chakras has been overcome. Man learns how important the group is, and realizes that *"the whole is greater than the sum of its parts."* Persons at the vibrational level of the 3rd Chakra generally have few problems subordinating themselves; they know that their Ego and its demands have to defer to the group in order to fit in. Since their personal fortune has become identified with that of the group, subordination is not experienced as doing without: they get back far more from the members of the group than they invested at the beginning.

However, the group-centeredness of life in the 3rd Chakra, and the fragile role of the Self, generates numerous conflict themes. Four conflict themes can be distinguished:

Conflict 8: Isolated – The overdependence of the individual on the group can all too easily turn into to its opposite, tipping over into indifferent stupor and lethargy – a depressive emotional state that can arise due to having suffered deep disappointment. In the absence of group support, the individual is oddly cut off and apathetic – in the extreme case like a lazy, secretly despondent, brooding lump. My most intense exposure to this emotional state was, as I recall, on a trip to a remote Indian village in the mountains of Bolivia, in which the entire village seemed, like Sleeping Beauty, to have fallen into a paralyzing slumber of inconsolable apathy. It has been my experience that slaves and slum dwellers easily fall prey to these miserable, vegetating emotional states.

Conflict 9: Pent-up emotions – The image of the sad, pitiful figure can change in an instant if, out of the intense pent-up feelings, a fit of raving madness erupts, in which the emotional discharge is like a cleansing thunderstorm. For instance, mobs are a flare-up of collective outrage, as furious people storm through city streets, pillaging and plundering. Revolutions and popular uprisings are discharges of pent-up rage, always preceded by a long period of oppression which forms the actual "culture medium" of the feeling of "bursting with rage."

Conflict 10: Wanting more – The insatiable craving for material belongings can be seen in the territorial expansion wars of the ancient empires of Rome and Egypt, as well as the subsequent exploitation of the oppressed peoples. The power-hungry despot, autocratically commanding the masses and grabbing everything in sight with aggressive recklessness, is the very image of the dictatorial and uncaring element that is the very essence of avarice. During the Middle Ages, the universal scholar ERASMUS of ROTTERDAM hoarded knowledge like property, just as the MEDICIs and FUGGERs did with worldly goods. Anyone who wants more will have to take things away from others. This is the unlovely and (in the extreme case) antisocial shadow side of the depressive character which, from the outside, so ostentatiously craves community and public spirit.

Conflict 11: Craving good feelings – Inner frustration leads to a lasting feeling of emotional dissatisfaction. One feels bad and unfulfilled inside and tries to fill the nagging, frustrating void with wild parties, drugs, casual sex, and other distractions and diversions. This hunger sometimes turns into its opposite, namely the asceticism of the medieval monks, whose rounded bellies are the last vestige of their earlier appetites.

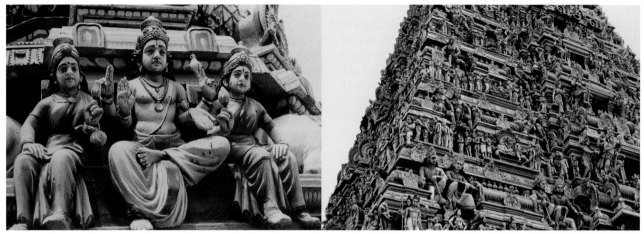

Gods in human form on southern Indian temple, extending on the temple walls seemingly on up to the heavens.

4th Chakra

The Heart Chakra is the midpoint of energetic/psychic development. From its position at the center of the emotional management system, the heart is the mediator of the psychic depths in which we (re)discover out True Self. In mythology, the Hero sets out on a journey to foreign lands in the quest for the Holy Grail. These journeys are self-discovery adventures, since the Grail (or some other treasure) is a metaphor for the True Self, which dwells in the heart. The Hero's journey takes him deep into his heart. The Hero must first undergo many adventures in which he overcomes all the negative dark sides of his psyche and in the end integrates his recovered personality components into a harmonious whole.

We encounter people in the 4th Chakra stage of development in two variations. The first is a preliminary stage in which an early attempt at integration and completion is first attempted. Of necessity, this foolhardy enterprise is doomed to failure because of its enormous difficulty and insufficient inner strength. Nowhere else is mankind's actual mission and purpose clearer than in these heroic struggles, in which the greatest fortune and most abject failure are so very close to each other. Always, at this point, the first attempt at fulfillment will fail, simply because there is yet much to learn and integrate. Odysseus' saga – as likewise that of Prometheus and GOETHE's Faust and other heroic myths – takes place in this first phase, where the attempt to liberate the inner Self fails.

It is not until the second stage that we see, in Jesus' heart, the heart-wrenching symbol of the lost son who returns to heaven – but only after traversing and enduring the thorny path of the Crucifixion in the 7th Chakra; this is equivalent to the renunciation of the Ego. Jesus' words that "*no man cometh unto the Father, but by me*" signifies the necessity of letting go of the Ego, with all its rigidity and self-centeredness, in order to get back to our True Self. First, we must resolve all conflicts and cleanse our spirit of the old pains and entrenched fears stored up there, before we can hope to reach the vibrational level of the 4th Chakra.

The 4th Chakra is a rebirth: the person becomes a newborn lad or maiden, wonderful to behold and equipped with all manner of virtues and talents. In a certain sense, we meet man in his true form for the very first time in the 4th Chakra developmental level. On the earlier levels, we came across the dreamers and innocents, sometimes the downright violent and dangerously wild (1st Chakra), the courageous and sometimes rowdy Hero (2nd Chakra), as well as the vacillating-between-tears-and-laughter insatiable groupman (3rd Chakra) ... all of the characters come across, subtly yet unmistakably, as distorted and phony. One senses their bogus and inauthentic nature. It is only on the developmental level of the 4th Chakra that we can identify with the actors "with all our heart." Only on this level do we finally meet the true person who wins all our sympathy and understanding.

Historically, man in the 4th Chakra belongs to the phase between the chivalrous rituals of early medieval knighthood (courtly love) and the Romantic and Renaissance eras. Artists such as MICHELANGELO and Leonardo DA VINCI convey a good impression of those times, which were characterized by a general mood of change and new beginnings. The enormous range of emotional experiences and the huge stature of those creative geniuses convey an early impression of the dizzying possibilities dormant in us all, which can serve as an expression of our True Self. An ennoblement and refinement of the senses and customs, paired with a fresh and virginal mentality, arouse the beguiling feeling of a completely new beginning. The beautiful lad and the comely, fairylike princess awaken in all people the archetypal dream of the perfect couple that goes from the wedding altar straightway to paradise. For the first time in human history, we see our existence transformed into eternal youth and beauty, and ourselves re-awakened to our True Self, recognized in our actual existence and released from the frightful spell that seems, in hindsight, like a bad dream.

And yet the 4th Chakra has its fears as well, its terrors and dark sides. In the 4th Chakra, we encounter character traits and conflicts from all four character types. There are five different conflicts here:

Conflict 12: Mental overexertion – The 4th Chakra can be conceived of as a locus of integration in which reason and emotion need to be brought into equilibrium with each other. The heart center, however, has a stronger intrinsic affinity for the emotional pole. The first conflict thus has to do with the fact that the tidal wave of erupting emotions tends to drown out rationality. One example is the chaotic state of bureaucracy in emerging third-world democracies: the enthusiasm of a new beginning makes everything "higgledy-piggledy."

Conflict 13: Withdrawn – the large emotional opening in the Heart Chakra gives rise to extraordinarily great vulnerability which leads, in the event of failure, to a feeling of being "shot through the heart" and a retreat into one's shell. The dropout and Robinson-Crusoe fantasies at the beginning of the modern age seem to express these emotional states.

Conflict 14: Introverted – The Heart Chakra can harbor many tragic and extraordinary painful feelings. These include the next three conflicts, all of which have to do with fear and extremely great psychic pain. Imagine the psychological mood of soldiers who are surrounded, trapped in an increasingly hopeless situation, to get an idea of the agonizing feeling of being closed in that makes escape seem impossible. The soldiers dare not even breathe for fear of detection by the enemy.

Conflict 15: Apprehensive – As death draws ever nearer, fear condenses down to a sinister, dreadful emotional state that makes the thought of being left alone seem unbearable. It feels like one's heart is breaking in two.

Conflict 16: Panic – At the point of greatest distress, the constricting feeling turns into out-and-out fear of death, in which the person feels threatened by a monstrous wave that will, any second now, roll over and crush him. This panic feeling surpasses all other anxiety states for sheer frightfulness. Nearly everyone with whom I have spoken, in my capacity as a physician, about states of extreme panic, agrees

that no words can be found to describe these horrific conditions.

I'd like to say a few things about the significance of the Heart Chakra. It is actually erroneous to view the Crown Chakra as the highest Chakra. Spiritual teachers say that the developmental step from Buddhism to Christianity parallels that between the Crown to the Heart Chakra. According to a number of commentators, Buddha had foreseen Christ (he spoke of the *Maitreya* as the future Buddha) and, by the way, had always felt himself to be merely a bridge or guidepost. We find, in the concept of the *Bodhisattva* – an enlightened being in service to its fellow beings – the Buddhist equivalent to the Christian belief in the Redeemer. The Heart Chakra is hardly ever represented in Buddhist illustrations and symbols, which must mean that it is relatively unknown in these cultures.

In Islam and Christianity – as in many other major religions – this is no longer the case. In these, the fully-developed Heart Chakra is regarded as the highest center, bringing together all human potential. We can also view the divine heart as that of Allah, Mary, or whoever else. We are dealing here with coded images that paraphrase a different reality – namely that the highest reality has a good and infinitely loving heart (never-ending love). Once we realize that the **heart is the highest Chakra**, then even an egotistical, monomaniacal quest for enlightenment makes sense. I cannot heartlessly look for something that is the very essence of cordiality (heartiness). From this derives also the Christian concept of *Caritas* (charity), according to which redemption is better served by doing good unto others than by concerning oneself egotistically with one's own well-being.

5th Chakra

In every respect, the 5th Chakra represents the most down-to-earth and unsentimental of all the developmental stages. We find ourselves here in a totally gray and mundane world, where it's all sober rationality and reality-oriented everyday consciousness that accords logic the highest priority. Feelings have only a secondary role as decorative ornaments of no intrinsic value.

This psychic state is like a grand symphony orchestra suddenly going silent: now the cleaning lady goes down the empty rows of seats picking up the litter that the audience discarded. The glamour of the preceding developmental stages has completely dissipated, leaving behind only staid matter-of-factness.

"Dreams are just so much foam! It's all a pack of lies!" the disappointed theatergoer feels like shouting. The only person there, the visitor sits silently in his assigned seat and wonders how the show is to go on. One can imagine the theater owner's responsibility, who has to bankroll the performance. The theater looks very different from his corner: a great number of people must be brought together under one roof in a precisely calculated manner if the production is to succeed. There is a great reluctance to take note of and give free rein to large theatrical emotions – because the wilder and less restrained the feelings lived out, the more unrestrained the theater director's investment in plays that have captivated him, and the dearer the final reckoning. "Experience has made me cleverer, but it has cost me a pretty penny! So let's not get carried away here!" is the motto. Far more important than feelings are tidy rows of seats in sufficient number and a well-stuffed theater safe to pay for it all.

The theater of which I speak is actually a metaphor for modern civilization and its predominant mindset: rationality, purposeful efficiency, profit, and utility totally occupy center stage. Esthetic aspects and grand feelings have become private filigrees decorating the sober routine of rational man, who returns home in the evening after a hard day at the office and goes out to catch a movie or a musical. Emotions no longer have any meaningful function or wider context.

Any feeling of a common bond with nature is derided as sheer wishful thinking; anything unpredictable, visionary, or dramatic is considered dangerous and warded off. The gods have shriveled down to letters in libraries, reminding people of earlier times. The individual withdraws into his shell, whose rigid exterior is constructed of rational thinking. In these snail shells, all are on their own, leading to general egotism and a free-for-all that pits people against each other. Modern man sits, like Diogenes in his barrel, in his casket of reason which is a cross between a prison and fortress. Modern man is accused of being trapped and imprisoned in rationality by rebellious youth – for instance the hippies of the 60's, who denounced and called into question bourgeois double standards. Naturally, rational 5th Chakra man rejects all such accusations, regarding his values as binding on everyone and of the greatest utility. "Anyone who doesn't do exactly as I do is a complete idiot!" is the credo of man in the 5th Chakra.

The characteristic traits of the 5th Chakra also correspond to the overall mental state of the modern scientist, whose marvelous discoveries are taken as cogent proof of what a splendid fellow the scientist is (and, by extension, all of humanity). Privately, even the more grotesque outgrowths of human destructiveness such as the atomic bomb are secret proof of man's gloriousness and near-divinity! The resulting fascination (in the sense of seductive narcissism) is tabooed and kept under wraps from the general public – using the upraised index finger of indignation, for example, against such embarrassing emotions. The thought of being able to blow up the entire world sends a creepily pleasant

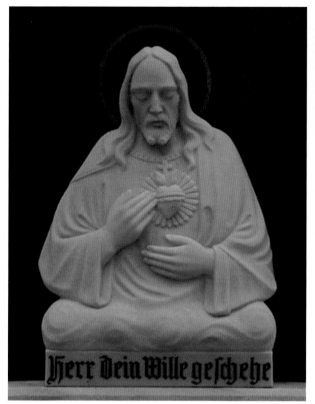

Gravestone in South Tyrol with the two most important Christian elements: Love (represented by Jesus' heart) and Humility (expressed by the words "Thy will be done, O Lord!"). Unlike the other high religions, Christianity is a religion of the 4th Chakra (and not – like Buddhism – of the Crown Chakra).

subconscious sensation running down the spine of *Homo sapiens*. "What a mighty creature am I, to have such abilities," he thinks, feeling so enormously superior. "I'm a member of the powerful species that can pulverize the entire planet!"

Since feelings of omnipotence and deeper intuitions must, before the background of preceding Chakra development, be considered to be enormously anxiety-ridden, there is in the 5th Chakra an extreme inability to grasp the true essence of human nature. Never before has man understood so little about himself and his true essence as man in the 5th Chakra. Sigmund FREUD's revolutionary discovery of the subconscious can be viewed as a *meneteker* directed at a rationalist society whose members are predominantly at the 5th Chakra level, and among whom the rediscovery of the subconscious is a trememdous sensation – felt, moreover, to be a significant act of liberation. But when you think about it, the *really* peculiar thing is 5th Chakra man's astonishment at the rediscovery of the emotional aspect: when something so deeply human as our inner feelings is viewed as a sensational new discovery, it simply points up the monstrous alienation that has screened modern man off (like a gigantic cheese cover) from his own nature and the rest of the world.

Man's alienation from his true nature has its external-world counterpart in our high-tech civilization, which many like to adduce as proof that the modern world represents a great enrichment: even when we have to endure hours of rush-hour traffic, everything is quicker and more comfortable; even if we complain about electromagnetic pollution, we have the Internet and TV as information sources at our disposal; or we have the electric light that lets us stay up late at night.

In the external world, modern man becomes ever more of a homebody, while at the same time becoming ever less familiar with his inner world. Modern man has set up house in the world to such a degree that it's as if the intent were to subjugate every last blade of grass. Following in the footsteps of Christopher COLUMBUS' voyages of discovery, people travel to ever more distant corners of the outer macro-world – just as they (with the aid of the microscope and the physical sciences) explore the depths of the micro-world. Paradoxically, the more that man explores the outer world and sets up shop there, the more alienated he becomes from his true nature, in a manner that is incomprehensible and was previously totally unknown.

The positive character traits of the 5th Chakra include virtues such as dependability, practicality, and fairness. Since the 5th Chakra, as the communications center, is much concerned with exchange, a new and previously unknown type of advanced civilization has developed that has immense communication and distribution capabilities. Both human rights and the DIN standardization of electric wall plugs can be counted among the accomplishments of people who psychoenergetically vibrate on the 5th Chakra level. Classic 5th Chakra roles include the dutiful, routine-ridden white-collar worker, and blue-collar workers whose untiring diligence and modesty have created a secure world filled with material riches.

For the first time in human history, we have a reliable, clean, and decent world, in which we can all live like kings, drive our cars everywhere, and be enormously wealthy. Modern remote controls and washing machines replace the king's slaves, and all of modern man's accomplishments, such as television and jet travel, represent a mind-boggling affluence that would have seemed incomprehensible and grandiose to earlier generations. When civilized man books a vacation to a tropical jungle, he realizes the enormous difference that has been set up between the wilderness and our advanced civilization. Now, I have nothing against adventure vacations that project us back (in well-dosed moderation) to the Stone Age and such – but most survival training participants, when they return from the wilderness, feel an intoxicating rush at being able to toggle a light switch and know that it will work every time. Even such banalities as the indoor flush toilet and clean drinking water from the tap are some of modern man's marvelous accomplishments.

Yet where there is much light, there is also much shadow. When you start dealing with the negative characteristics of the Neck Chakra, you first have to understand its psychoenergetic function as an emotional sluice-gate which attunes emotions and thoughts to each other. It's like animal training: man's animal nature – symbolized in mythology as Centaur or Sphinx – is tamed and trained. Training the inner animal and suppressing feelings in man leads, on the level of the Heart Chakra, to a great feeling of relief which is bound up with, for the first time in human history, a feeling of dependability and security quite unknown to earlier evolutionary stages.

The Neck Chakra's Spartan nature is also seen in the fact that the associated conflicts consist solely of two differing variants.

Conflict 17: Emotional emptiness – the inglorious dark side of the 5th Chakra includes fending off all emotions, so that a cold indifference is disseminated. The coldness conceals extraordinarily painful emotions, which are thereby fended off. This lack of emotions and feelings is completely incomprehensible and inexplicable from the outside. Worst-case developments include a couldn't-care-less indifference and lovelessness that can even carry over into how people take care of their own body. The total lack of empathy opens the door to barbarism and giving free rein to negative emotions, inconceivable in earlier periods of human history.

Puritanism represents a pure form of this intellectual and emotional state. It's easy to see why the North American Indians, still on the 1st and 2nd Chakra levels of development, would find the Puritan colonists completely outlandish and downright mechanical. I'd like to add that each psychoenergetic developmental level represents an independent world in which other worlds are incomprehensible. The farther apart Chakras are from each other, the less they can understand one another. We can thus understand the psychic shock and the destructive conflict potential when two psychoenergetically very disparate cultures converge.

Conflict 18: Rushed – 5th Chakra man's second basic problem is the tendency to always "step on the gas" of the rational mind and force it to hurry more and more. Over-wound reason then pushes the entire organism too hard, so that motor functions and emotions can't keep up with the hectic pace of the rational mind. Hectic activity often conceals power-hunger and greed, which we learned about in a less adulterated form in the 3rd Chakra. Such people simply want more out of life, and, in their insatiable ravenousness, they whip themselves up to ever greater effort.

Another basis for this bustling activity is modern man's altered time-sense. The leisurely pace of native cultures that tourists encounter can get them terribly upset, since it seems to them to be laziness, bad attitude, and the like. Mutually incompatible psychoenergetic developmental stages contain an enormous conflict potential. "These poky native waiters are gonna drive me bananas!" complains the annoyed tourist, thereby precisely expressing the conflict's key problem – except that the tourist doesn't realize that his pedal-to-the-metal pace is making him sick. (He'll find that out after his heart attack, after which he'll be forced to "take it easy.")

The speeded-up time-sense led, in the Christian West, to the building of church towers, from which the clocks' precise rhythms carved the day up into uniform segments. Using one's time to do something sensible with one's life was one of the paradigms of Calvinism and the dawning industrial age. Making good use of one's time was equated with virtues such as rationality, suitability, and modesty. Behind these lurk unpleasant emotions which these are meant to compensate: above all such negative emotions as feelings of inferiority, weakness, and fear – e.g., the capitalist's fear of impoverishment if one doesn't work hard enough.

6th Chakra

The 5th Chakra represents an apparent high point in personality development, yet development actually goes much farther. Whereas man at the developmental level of the 5th Chakra exhibits compulsive and clearly understandable characteristic traits (most distinctly in Puritans and bureaucrats), the Brow Chakra effects a creative explosion, thanks to the revitalizing effect of the 6th Chakra's intuitive nature. The 6th Chakra develops inspiration, creativity, and sensitivity, making possible peak artistic and scientific performance. The awakening of the 6th Chakra can thus be compared to a rebirth (Renaissance), such as we observed in the transition from the 3rd to the 4th Chakra.

The Brow Chakra has been associated with supernatural powers for ages. In the ancient Egyptian and Tibetan cultures, the Third Eye symbolized clairvoyance and inner contemplation (Eye of Horus, Ajna Chakra). In my experience, many people in our Western culture develop more socially acceptable abilities via the 6th Chakra – in science or art, for example. As we know, clairvoyants get little recognition or respect in our enlightened society. Yet the talents of the 6th Chakra also emerge in other ways, although not under the designation *clairvoyant*: many inventors and scientists speak of "inspiration," "intuition," and a "sixth sense." These scientists thus use the awakened 6th Chakra's abilities to attain very mundane, rational results – although, in the cold light of day, what they're doing looks just like clairvoyance.

There's the well-known discovery of the structure of the benzene ring by the chemist KEKULÉ, who, in a dream, saw a snake loop around and bite its own tail (it's not hard to recognize the *Ouroboros* motif here): the researcher realized at once that benzene had to be a ring, just like the snake! The annals of parapsychology (which deal with the fringe areas of psychology, including all paranormal phenomena) are full to overflowing with reports, experiments, and eyewitness accounts that confirm beyond a doubt the existence of extraordinary human powers and abilities that go beyond those of our five senses and our common sense. In my opinion, all of these abilities are related to the 6th Chakra.

The elevated energetic vibration in the 6th Chakra leads to a revitalization of previously unknown potentials, which increases not only creativity and intuition, but also energy as well. People with an active 6th Chakra make do with uncommonly little sleep and can draw on unsuspected reserves of strength.

Looking along the time axis of human evolution, the first signs of an awakening of the 6th Chakra can be found in ancient Egypt: the most advanced initiates – of which the famed Greek philosopher PLATO (from *Bal-Aton*, "disciple of *Aton*," the first Egyptian monotheistic god) is said to have been one – had an active 6th Chakra which connected them to deep spiritual wisdom. The next wave of 6th-Chakra awakening is found at the end of the Middle Ages, above all among the artists of MEDICI Florence. Art history terms this period of rediscovery of buried abilities the *Renaissance*. Long-lost possibilities were developed (present in nascent form as early as the 4th Chakra). Nearly every genius and great artist had the awakening of the 6th Chakra to thank for his creative works. Without this potential, MICHELANGELO or RAPHAEL would have been inconceivable.

However, the new possibilities of the 6th Chakra endow not just the genius, but practically every person on this vibrational level, with an energetically fresh and cheery disposition. Intellectual ability is also enormously stimulated, making possible an inventive type of thinking in which complex interrelationships are intuitively and holistically grasped. Geniuses such as PARACELSUS, GOETHE, and DANTE have primarily the awakened 6th Chakra to thank for their capabilities.

Historically, we are still at the 5th Chakra vibrational level – but we can even now detect the early phases of our future world, which corresponds to the vibrational level of the 6th Chakra. Esoteric groups look forward eagerly to a so-called Age of Aquarius in which the new intuitive capabilities of the 6th Chakra will (hopefully) lead to a better world. All of these newly-awakened abilities will presumably make people more ecologically and socially aware and more peaceable –

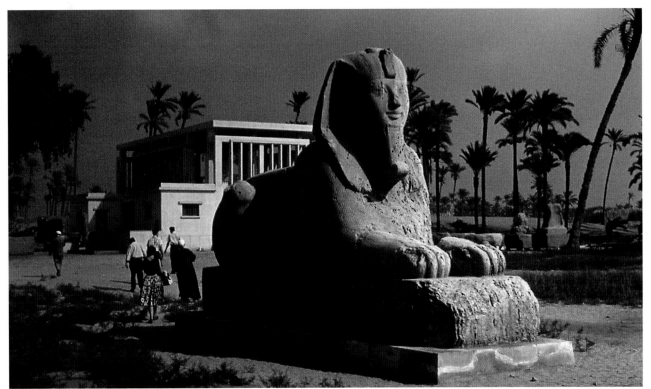

The Sphinx, a beast with human head, expresses the deeply sensual experience of the awakened 6th Chakra, where, for the first time, a strong, magically-experienced consciousness of being both man and beast comes into being.

The Sphinx of Memphis, 1600 BCE.

in short: people should become better persons once their 6th Chakra is awakened.

In the more than ten years that I have been investigating the psychoenergetic vibrational level of people from diverse social groups and nationalities, I have come across a fair number of people with an awakened 6th Chakra, and I can confirm the positive descriptions – yet my sobering experiences with these people can only partly justify some of the utopian expectations and idealistic transfigurations: people do not necessarily become better when they vibrate at a higher level. The so-called "new human being" with activated 6th Chakra has, besides the virtues, many negative characteristic traits that may be termed unappealing and antisocial. "Much light means much shadow."

I already mentioned that hysterics can be quite self-involved. For such egomaniacs, their mental body and the indwelling individual Ego becomes the central world axis from whose hub all activities and sensations radiate. Hysterics and people with an awakened 6th Chakra often resemble each other in their important character traits so that, character type aside, one can observe many similar characteristics. Many people are infatuated by the awakened 6th Chakra's innate multifaceted and fascinating potentiali-

ties, seducing many into explicit self-love that elevates them to the level of a personal Sun King: *"L'etat c'est moi!"* This god/king affectation is clearly visible in famous fashion designers, who absolutely must be the center of attention at all important social events, and who make embarrassingly certain that everyone knows who they are.[53]

This egotism occasionally goes to extremes, taking on a despotic aspect due to the 6th Chakra's hysteric nature. Although I have not personally examined certain indisputably brilliant but morally controversial autocrats, in my experience all the indications are that (for example) HITLER must have had an awakened 6th Chakra. In all

---

[53] I heard the following revealing anecdote from the head stewardess of a major airline. A world-famous passenger in first class was complaining about some petty annoyance. When a young stewardess tried to mollify him by pointing out politely that they'd be landing very soon, which would automatically solve his "problem," he barked at her "Young lady, don't you know who I am?" Unfortunately she didn't, whereupon the world-famous celebrity, livid with rage, told her his name. He was going to complain to the management, he said, that their inexperienced personnel was not even familiar with the most basic principles of high society, and so forth and so on. For him, it was a personal affront not to have been recognized at once and been treated accordingly. It only remains to be added that this celebrity must be a hysteric character type.

likelihood, HITLER was a schizoid character type with strong hysteric traits, lending a strongly paranoid cast to his overall personality. HITLER believed in parapsychology, was a strict vegetarian (like many highly sensitive individuals with an awakened 6th Chakra), and was, beyond the shadow of a doubt, the century's leading talent in the art of demagoguery.

People at the developmental level of the Brow Chakra tend to commandeer their surroundings and fellow humans as theater and extras to the service of their power hunger and personal showmanship. Other people often don't really interest 6th-Chakra persons, so they all too readily use them as "cannon fodder." However, the despot's highly sensitive and energetically open nature makes him need more coarse-minded underlings to do his murderous dirty work for him. The French revolutionary ROBESPIERRE reportedly became quite ill the first time he personally attended a guillotine execution, despite having signed hundreds of death sentences with no conscience pangs.

Many charismatic leaders have shocked their faithful followers when something goes wrong at a staged spectacle and it takes on questionable aspects: from one instant to the next, their beloved leader becomes a quite ordinary person whose negative character traits suddenly burst forth.

Because of their lack of self-insight, 6th-Chakra persons tend not to rue the wrong they have done unto others; instead, they project everything negative outward onto some bogeyman figure that then has to be ruthlessly exterminated – or else they turn into weepy weaklings, injecting pathos into even the most minor complaints.

And with that, I'd like to wrap up this enumeration of the positive and negative character traits of Brow Chakra people. I'd like to make clear that the piling up of negative character traits in my description should not mislead the reader into coming to the erroneous conclusion that the negative aspects predominate in the 6th Chakra. This is by no means the case! I merely wish to dial down expectations of a dawning *Age of Aquarius* to a more sensible level. Of course, once you've seen through the Brow Chakra's pitfalls and trap-doors, you're much less likely to fall for the hypnotic tricks and seductive ideologies of the 6th Chakra.

Historically, the Brow Chakra largely relates to the future, so it's understandable that I won't be able to produce any historical references to the individual conflicts. However, in the interest of completeness, I'd like briefly to recap the important conflict themes and identify by name the beginning phases of their modern manifestation. No other Chakra presents as broad a palette of psychic conflicts and emotions as the 6th Chakra.

There are, in all, six conflicts:

Conflict 19: Faint-hearted – Due to the enormous abundance of possibilities available to 6th-Chakra persons, they are often indecisive: if they commit themselves prematurely,

they might pass up a better opportunity. Since they don't want to alienate anybody, they seem faint-hearted and they dither diplomatically, evading clear-cut decisions. The Internet, symbol of our modern information glut, intimidates many people into hesitant behavior. Marketing research has shown that over-choice has a paralyzing effect. American Internet investigators have shown that (possibly for this reason) more and more Internet users always use the same entry portals.

Conflict 20: Self-sufficient – Basically, self-sufficient types proceed from the assumption that nobody really loves them and they had best therefore look out for themselves. This egocentricity sometimes leads to a narcissistic snootiness whose smug vanity is often camouflaged behind a façade of modesty and servility. Self-sufficient people thus often seem, from the outside, to be particularly pleasant and conciliatory.

Modern urbanites exhibit all the symptoms of self-centered modesty associated with this conflict. There's hardly another emotional theme that involves so much Ego concealing an enormous need to be loved. For this reason, modern humans are easily manipulated, since their lack of roots and self-involvement lead to inadequate groundedness and weak self-determination.

Conflict 21: Physical overexertion – Because of the great energy load that corresponds to the thrust of a jet engine, 6th-Chakra people tend to be physically restive and constantly tense.

Conflicts 21–23 are typical emotional themes of modern civilized man, who is becoming ever more tense, restless and nervous. The hectic life of the big city is more and more becoming a significant source of disease, because the needed counterpoise – relaxation, rest, and grounding – gets short shrift.

Conflict 22: Restless – Mental overmodulation leads to permanent worries for Brow Chakra people, who never get a moment's peace.

Conflict 23: Tense – Overmodulation can become extreme, leading to involuntary actions (tics) and cramps that give rise to a spiral of long-term helplessness and tension.

Conflict 24: Uneasiness – Many people with the *Uneasiness* conflict prefer permanent physical pain to unbearable psychic pain, because it's easier to cope with and endure.

As a physician, I've observed that chronic pain has been on the rise for some time, and I take it as a sign of the times. Physical pain takes on a manifold safety-valve function because modern life more and more blocks off other pressure-relief options – e.g., vigorous wood-chopping when one is boiling over with rage, or being able to have a really good cry in the presence of one's family when feeling totally feeble and miserable.

7th Chakra

The Crown Chakra is viewed as the pinnacle of spiritual development and as the symbol of enlightenment. The halo symbolizes the great radiative power of the fully-energized 7th Chakra. Unlike the 6th, 7th-Chakra people have the painful transformation of a mini-crucifixion behind them: they had to transform and shed the overly narcissistic self-centered Ego of the Brow Chakra in order to continue growing emotionally. As with any transition from one Chakra to the next, this involves crises and emotional upheavals that often seem like the end of the world. You rub your eyes in amazement afterward, finding yourself in a similar and yet unmistakably transformed world.

The childlike innocence and peace of the 1st Chakra is rediscovered, but at a higher level of integration. 7th-Chakra man simultaneously radiates the dignity of the sage and the innocent friendliness of the child.

The smile playing around the corners of Mona Lisa's lips echoes the seductive charm and the majestic, downright divine beauty of the Crown Chakra. Most of Leonardo da VINCI's paintings – not just the Mona Lisa – have this enchantment about them, presumably because Leonardo himself was at the 7th Chakra vibrational level. Based on my investigations, the music of Johann Sebastian BACH, with its understated magnificence and mathematical elegance, belongs to the 7th Chakra. In the current era, I'd like to name two outstanding representatives of the Crown Chakra: the violinist Yehudi MENUHIN and the DALAI LAMA. Both stand out through a number of character traits that identify them as inhabiting the 7th Chakra vibrational level: they are extraordinarily humane and very modest; their demeanor in public is almost ostentatiously unostentatious, unusually friendly, humorous and warm-hearted, psychologically poised; on top of all that, they are passionately dedicated to their true mission in life.

The beauty of nature manifests itself to the Crown Chakra person as a "golden section," and the wisdom and laws of the cosmos can be experienced, quite literally, sensually. Animals, flowers, and children become friends by nature, through whom the Crown Chakra person rediscovers much more than from the countless fellow humans whose emotional sclerosis and ego games seem ever more incomprehensible and alien. At some point, he had played all these games and knows them by heart; on the other hand, he has grown increasingly weary and bored with them.

The high degree of openness with respect to the subconscious stimulates creativity, thereby increasing the creative urge and the bandwidth of creative possibilities, compared to the Brow Chakra, even more. This is easily seen in the tremendously multi-faceted opus of Johann Sebastian BACH, as well as in the restless exploratory spirit of

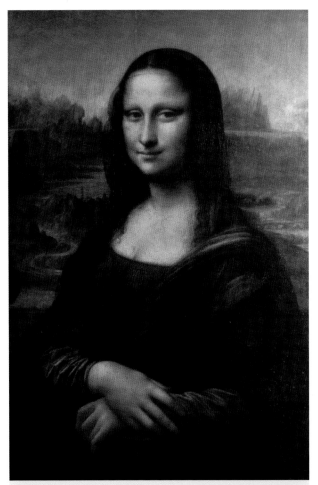

Mona Lisa, with her enigmatic smile and her natural beauty, conveys to us an impression of the loveliness and grace of the Crown Chakra.

Leonardo DA VINCI. In my experience, 7th-Chakra people are terrifically enthusiastic hobbyists who love to design and implement their own sophisticated devices. Work itself, like being creative, is tremendously enjoyable to the Crown Chakra person, who is constantly researching and discovering new things. We can also see, in Leonardo DA VINCI, that the go-getter and the playful aspects can rise to such dynamic heights that most works of art are simply not taken to completion, simply because the Crown Chakra person instinctively senses that "the journey is the reward" – and anyway, nothing is permanent: why then agonize about putting the finishing touches on works of art?

By the way, I have observed similar behavior in many highly-talented children: at school, they are relegated to the "Fidgety Frank" category, nobody suspecting that their high level of development makes them bored very quickly.[54] One occasionally finds such "Albert Einsteins" stuck in special schools for the learning impaired, because their constant inattentiveness misleads people into thinking they're simply stupid. They're also sometimes adjudged to have behavioral disorders because they're difficult to integrate into social groups. In the US, they are known as "indigo children" because clairvoyants describe their Aura as having a violet coloration. One may indeed regard the vibrational level of the 7th Chakra as a summation of all vibrations, as when colors are mixed together. Evidently, this summation appears as violet to clairvoyants (or, alternatively, as "white"). In a later chapter on "emotional growth and conflict healing," I'll discuss these people in greater detail, whose high level of psychological development makes integration into normal life very difficult.

Readers might ask how in the world I can know on what level a person is vibrating. I don't intend to withhold the answer for long, plus I'll reveal technical details in a later chapter on the Psychosomatic Energetics testing method. Basically, after hundreds of measurements, I've found out that one can measure a person's overall vibration with the right testing equipment. Now, for years I never encountered a person at the 7th-Chakra vibrational level among my patients. I did come across many unusually inspired, creative, and fascinating people at the Brow Chakra developmental level, yet not a single one at the Crown Chakra level.

Surprisingly, this situation has changed in the last five years, and I am now running across (especially among young children) more and more "superior souls." These spiritually advanced children often have enormous problems trying to lead a normal life. Their troubles put me in mind of a race-car driver trying to manage his high-powered vehicle in normal traffic. Another more ancient image is that of the heroic breakdown of the highly-talented artist who just can't make it in a disdainful, unappreciative world. The reputed close affinity between genius and insanity was a popular theme at the end of the 19th century, which was often dismissed as a delusion. Yet I believe that this idea was and is valid; one can find many geniuses and spiritually advanced persons in psychiatric institutions, although they have only two problems: they have overly high psychoenergetic vibration and, on top of that, usually an active Central Conflict that pulls them completely off-center and off-balance.

Historically, less can be said concerning the 7th Chakra than about the preceding Brow Chakra. The Crown Chakra will be a formative influence in a future phase of human development – but not for at least a hundred (or maybe even a thousand) years. Still, one now and then notices subtle precursors of this upcoming phase, such as the spiritually advanced indigo children. The future Crown Chakra world will, in my estimation, externally be significantly simpler and more modest than today's world. On the other hand, the people will have a substantially richer inner life, and they will much more appreciate the beauty of unspoiled nature. Thus, in terms of harbingers of this future Crown Chakra epoch: protection of the environment; the hunger of many people for spiritual sustenance; simpler esthetics in their immediate environment (architecture, domestic interior design, Zen gardens, and so on); the increasing desire for the so-called "simple joys of life" (a hike in the spring, living on a farm, and so on) – all these are signs of an emerging Crown Chakra consciousness. I will return to further indications of spiritually advanced consciousness.

The four conflicts of the Crown Chakra have some common features that can already be observed in contemporary society – even though the Crown Chakra represents an as yet relatively distant future stage of human development:

Conflict 25: Mistrust – Crown Chakra persons tends to regard most other people as bothersome nuisances with evil intent, who want only to take advantage of them. This makes them secretive and embittered. Deep inside, it's clear to them that they cannot trust anybody. The fact that the deep subconscious conceals a great lack of ability to love, and a hunger for love, is covered over and repressed. Mistrust is an omnipresent feature of our modern advanced civilization. Locks and keys, cryptography, and espionage are expressions of this basic mental attitude. Moreover, more and more wealthy people live behind the prison-high walls of gated communities that require passwords for entry: these people, too, are afflicted with mistrust and the fear of being robbed or otherwise harmed.

Conflict 26: Materialistic (putting having before being) – Schizoids tend to look ahead too much, which makes them pile up possessions so as not someday to be plundered and become impoverished, then die in poverty. Often, this materialism is expressed in other ways, such as paying more attention to the outer façade of one's life than to the inner content. As in the previous conflict (*Mistrust*), the material-

---

[54] I'd like to make it clear that not all bored Fidgety Franks are unsung geniuses, as so many parents are all too prepared to believe. Many such kids are quite average, some are even subpar. In my experience, however, Fidgety Franks (ADHD children) are almost always burdened with emotional conflicts and/or geopathic stress and/or electrosmog, which lowers energy levels, causing their attention to suffer. Add to this too much watching TV, computer games, and the consumption of way too much chemically-saturated candy.

istic element and the emphasis on crassly superficial appearance is omnipresent in modern society.

Conflict 27: Unwilling to face reality – In Crown Chakra persons, the surging subconscious leads to all manner of possible conceits and hallucinations that they wander about in like an enchanted forest. Withdrawing into their dream world seems better than confronting harsh reality which, in any event, looks rather squalid to them. This flight from the world and avoidance of reality is manifested through drug addiction and the retreat into contrived dream worlds – both typical elements of modern culture.

Conflict 28: Wrong thinking – The hubris of those who go around telling others "what's what" is based on the subtle self-deception of making oneself the measure of all things. This conflict also includes dogmas and overly rigid abstract standards. Sometimes, the conflict is expressed by making one's Ego the center of the universe. Putting ideology ahead of human lives is a classic expression of *Wrong thinking*, as is deliberately overlooking looming environmental problems and other inconvenient facts – all character traits of the wrong and short-sighted politics of our advanced civilization.

This is precisely what happens with each of us in our evolutionary development. Besides external pressure, there is an inner one that can express itself in the form of disorders, diseases, or a certain longing: more and more people strongly need a truly fulfilling search for meaning, for religious orientation and a totally fulfilled life. The inner pressure thus compels us to embark on a difficult inner quest. Like hiking in the mountains, when the path steepens and narrows, one has to keep discarding baggage in order to be able to grow spiritually. The resolution of conflicts serves the same purpose as letting go of heavy and nonessential gear in order to progress more quickly.

The end result is that these efforts help us rediscover our concealed spiritual heart. According to the spiritual masters, our spiritual center – the *True Self* – is said, at the moment of **redemption**, to rise in the Heart Chakra as a brilliant and sympathetic spiritual sun. We then find ourselves in a spiritual space in which personal belief and religiosity have their deepest roots. Without the faith that Creation, at its deepest essential core, consists of love, the True Self would be inconceivable. The heart of Jesus, as well as the sympathetic heart of the Buddha *Amithaba*, feels every creature's pain. Love is the supreme principle that must apply to every being, and so only the redemption of all beings can bring the process to a felicitous conclusion. Jesus will wait until The End Of Days for us and our liberation. In Buddhism as well, the sympathetic and merciful *Bodhisattva* forgoes his own redemption until the very last being in the Cosmos has attained it.

This closes the cycle, ending where it began with child-like innocence – but with the momentous difference that the soul, during its developmental journey through life's painful and agitating experiences, has ripened into a personality, like the biblical parable of the Prodigal Son who returns, after a prolonged odyssey, to his father's house. Finally home once again, his father showers him with gifts and honors him by allowing him to become his successor and heir. Just so do we hope to return, after an eternally long absence, to the home of our True Self. We re-enter the paradise lost in which we had previously been totally happy and at one with ourselves and the world. But, according to religious tradition, we don't just get back our lost paradise (for then the entire spiritual journey would have been nothing more than an incredibly arduous yet totally pointless detour): we also receive immeasurable riches as the reward for our efforts, which we would never have received were it not for the painful path of personality maturation. These riches are our imperishable, individual, and matured soul,

Upward Spiral of the Chakras

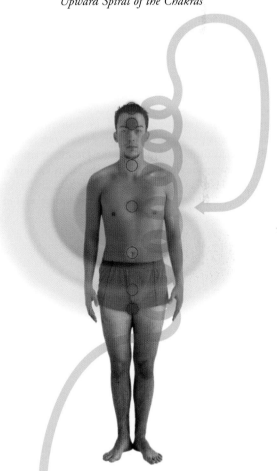

261

which has become immortal during its evolutionary development.

The entire process of spiritual maturation can be represented graphically as an upward spiral (see previous page). The human development process begins with the 1st and ends with the 7th Chakra: keep in mind the innocent child of the 1st Chakra and the enlightened sage of the 7th Chakra. The 2nd and 6th Chakras create a shell-like (or onion-layered) structure. We approach closer and closer to the core of becoming human, since the hysteric character type already possesses significantly more primordial human characteristic traits than the schizoid. We get even closer to the actual core of being human via the 3rd Chakra, which builds on the preceding and which belongs to the depressive disposition. In the 3rd Chakra, we develop our emotional life most completely, and the totally material-sensuous "being in the here and now." The 5th Chakra frames the entire picture from above. The 5th Chakra and its obsessive-compulsive structure develops the rational aspect, which is of inestimable value for the development of the individual.

The Heart Chakra can be considered the most important energy center, forming the center point of the entire spiritual development. The Heart Chakra funnels together all the developmental paths like a whirlpool and unites them in itself. This gives rise to the image of a Mandala-shaped human representation that we admire in many medieval illustrations. The esoteric interpretation of the Mandala-shaped circles is: "As the inner, so the outer," making man a representation of divine order and the cosmos. The microcosm of man's personality and energy structures reflects the entire macrocosm. According to the Gnostic writings, the closer we approach the true center – the Heart Chakra at the center of the Mandala – and our True Self, the more we become the *All* and can reunite with the cosmic soul of the world.

Interpersonal Conflicts

Whoever is dissatisfied with himself is always itching for revenge.

(Nietzsche)

Up to now, it's been pretty clear how the Central Conflict impinges on the individual and on entire cultural epochs. I have so far deliberately excluded human interaction so as to more clearly emphasize the dynamics of the process. I'd like to assume that the divine plan is interested in neither our little family problems nor our workplace mini-feuds. By "divine plan" I mean the great evolutionary idea that is behind the aforementioned spiritual journey – but I also include the individual soul which, according to depth psychology, is of interest only to a few select individuals: parents, partners, and children.

Still, social behavior is supremely important to our psychic health – for if you look into what most upsets individuals, it turns out to be problems and quarrels with other people. Strife and conflicts are part of everyday life even for the most peaceful people: you might, for example, take a seat in a restaurant that happens to be the regular seat of someone who has sat there at lunchtime for years. If this person shows up, he'll either aggressively tell you to get lost or – if he's too timid to do that – grumpily let it be known that he's unhappy with you, although you don't have a clue as to why. "I simply had no idea!" we say by way of justification – although here too, as so often in life, ignorance is no excuse.

Despite the surface calm of modern society, strife is an omnipresent background phenomenon. I've already mentioned the latent violence that psychological investigations such as the Milgram experiment have revealed. Beneath a veneer of normalcy, an enormous aggressive potential smolders in most people. Whenever the mask of rules, commandments, and moral decency slips, unsuspected aggression is released: in rush-hour traffic, in the family, and at work. The high number of civil lawsuits dealing with arguments that got physical, quarrels with neighbors, spousal abuse, and the like makes this all too clear.

The more we turn our attention to it, the more aware we become of the overt and covert violence that dominates everyday life. Locks on doors, traffic signs that tell you what you must (and may not) do, moral pre- and proscriptions – all are an expression of violence: for instance, we speak of the "power of the state," which holds an exclusive monopoly on the use of (deadly) force in civilized societies. The state exercises this power when it punishes us for running a red light. Force is thus one of the omnipresent phenomena that shape social life. A look at history shows that one war follows the next *ad infinitum*. Now, the obvious question is: what significance does strife have for psychic development? We already know that fighting is always a bad idea from which neither side will derive any benefit, over the short or long term. So why do we fight anyway? Why do we have to fight at all, what drives us and what's the underlying hidden motive? What psychoenergetic consequences does strife have?

I'll try to answer all these questions in the following pages. Bringing the psychoenergetic mechanisms of disputes into the foreground leads to surprising new insights. We usually adopt a moral pose, either repudiating fighting wholesale or else pigeonholing the parties to the conflict into "good guys" and "bad guys." In so doing, we overlook the background psychoenergetic processes. I'd like to start by saying that a dispute can be conceived as an unsuccessful energy transfer: **psychoenergetically, disputes are nothing more than blocked energy exchange processes!**

In what follows, we turn to the oldest dispute in human history. The Bible reports that Cain and Abel quarreled – yet the cause of this dispute is of absolutely no interest to our analysis, since knowing the reason automatically means adopting a moral viewpoint, and that's what we want to detach ourselves from, the better to be able to see through to the psychoenergetic processes. One of the two estranged brothers started it because he wanted something that the other one didn't want to give him. If we want to study the energetic processes of the dispute between Cain and Abel, we come up with basically four possible energy-transfer outcomes:

Cain wins
Abel wins
Cain and Abel both lose
Cain and Abel both win

I contend that the winner of a dispute will wind up with more energy than before! Normally, we attribute this to the triumphant feeling that (consciously or subconsciously) promotes well-being – but this isn't just an emotional matter. To all appearances, the winner has actually received more subtle energy as well. The fact that one feels better after winning a dispute is thus primarily an energetic phenomenon and less dependent on emotional circumstances. That might sound unusual to modern ears, but it seems in fact to be the case.

The American clairvoyant Lea SANDERS describes the scene of a dispute from the viewpoint of her clairvoyant perception, in which the winner sucks up, like a vacuum cleaner, the shards of the loser's Aura that have fallen to the ground. My investigations in Psychosomatic Energetics have confirmed very similar phenomena – namely that the winner of a dispute will consistently have higher Vital and Emotional Levels than the loser! In my experience, the increase in energy rests on the simple fact that the winner has stolen it from the loser. The loser, in turn, loses emotional energy, which can lead (in the worst case) to extremely low Vital and Emotional Levels. From the outside, this kind of energy emptiness will look like complete emotional rigidity or depression.

In short, I claim that the trauma suffered by the battered wife or mistreated child is followed by an energetic weakness that should by no means be viewed as a purely emotional problem – as so-called "reactive depression," say. It is mainly an energetic phenomenon, which can be improved, and even eliminated, much more quickly and lastingly by supplying subtle energy and breaking up energy blocks than by treating the victim purely on an emotional basis with comfort and consolation. My experiences in daily practice have taught me that here, out of sheer ignorance, an enormous amount of humane support vanishes into thin air – wasted, and treatment success is jeopardized, simply because nobody has grasped the significance of psychoenergetic energy theft. The stolen energy must be replaced in order to improve the victim's overall condition quickly and lastingly!

The story of Dracula (and other vampire figures) is really about the theft of energy – not blood, which is ostensibly what is taken from the victim. **Vampirism** fascinates us because it archetypically depicts the phenomenon of energy theft. The stolen blood symbolically stands for stolen life energy. If we think about the topic of conflict that we are here dealing with, the vampire in these narratives is always the winner: he steals the victim's blood, and thus his or her life force. The vampire thus typifies, on the psychoenergetic level, the winner who steals his victim's energy discreetly and silently. The vampire is the furtive winner, operating under the cover of darkness, whose crimes are expiated by his being one of the *living dead*, or a *zombie*. I'll return later to this important circumstance.

Against all expectation, vampirism seems to be a common phenomenon. Once we become aware of it, we can find energy vampires all around us. After contact with them, we tend to feel leached out, while the vampire looks visibly rosier and more vital. "Talking with Ms. X has really worn me out," the poor victim groans. The vampiric Ms. X, on the other hand, looks rosy, even as her victim turns pale and is drained of energy. According to the British sensitive David TANSLEY, energy thieves connect up to people by bewildering, beguiling, and distracting them with gushing praise

and other distraction techniques, thereby exploiting a tiny moment of weakness in their victims. This moment of *not being centered* seems to be necessary in order to penetrate the victim's mental defensive armor.

Amazingly, many artists are addicted to vampirism, living off the adulation of their fans and draining away their energy. The energy theft generates a "pseudo-kick" that additionally fascinates their admirers. Young people in particular, because of their abundant energy reserves and their inexperience, are relatively insensitive to energy piracy. The

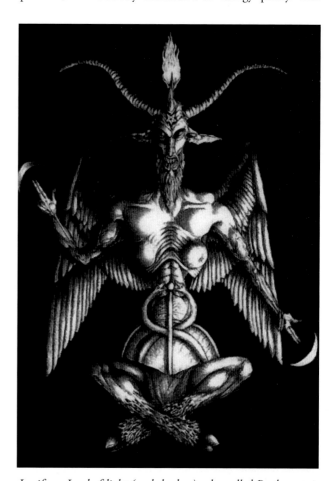

Lucifer – Lord of light (and shadow), also called Baphomet, is worshipped by Satanists as the supreme demon, and is also regarded as the highest "black" god. The female breasts on the male god are clearly recognizable: his hermaphroditic nature transcends gender differences. Actually, Satanism is a nature religion on the level of the 3rd Chakra, i.e., a low level of development; Lucifer's Kundalini snake ends there. Satanism derives its energy from black-magic sexual practices and is based energetically on the phenomenon of vampirism, as mankind's greatest adversary – the Devil – can kindle strong sensual energies. With the aid of magic, a strong, transforming energy can be recovered from life force – a first experience of the divine at a low psychoenergetic level.

young fans just feel energetically different, which somehow feels stimulating and exciting. In both parties, the entire interaction demands repetition, since it creates addiction mechanisms. This is known in Kinesiology as the *pseudo-kick* phenomenon, in which the addictive pseudo-kick generates a demonic, stimulating suction effect that a person can eventually no longer do without. I consider phenomena such as body piercing to also be part of these quasi-addictive, energetically often extremely disruptive fads, based on the fascination with the *pseudo-kick*.

The American Kinesiologist DIAMOND describes such auto-destructive mechanisms above all in heavy metal rock music. This violent music genre seems to have a particularly negative effect on psychoenergetic harmony. Revealingly, adherents like to use black-magic symbols such as swastikas and death-heads, which makes explicit the union of both black-magic practices. Experiments on dairy farms have shown that playing heavy metal recordings drastically reduces the milk output of dairy cows, whereas classical music markedly increases it. On the basis of the failure to crystallize of water exposed to heavy metal music, the Japanese energy researcher Masuru EMOTO demonstrated what is evidently a valid underlying rule: such music vibrationally represents pure destruction and negative-polarity aggression. The crazy part of the whole thing is that the fans of this kind of music, and other energetically harmful practices, become thoroughly addicted to them.

Evil influences induce, on a deep psychoenergetic level, the flow of great quantities of life energy that was previously blocked! Satanism and other black-magic practices are based, I think, on the pseudo-kick effect. Everybody is familiar with the phenomenon of obsessively looking over and over at a gruesome picture with unpleasant content, even though it makes one nauseous. Sensationalist tourism and the crowds that gather to gawk at an accident are based on such emotional attractions, which excite the destroyed and mangled in us. Ancient Rome's gladiatorial combat also exploited these base impulses. In some people, this process seems to switch over to its opposite, in which the unpleasant conditions are compensated by an increase in life force. These people look at the gruesome, nauseating picture and feel better. This seems to be the case with many perverts, whose videos and horrifying photographs can turn the stomach of even the toughest vice cops.

Another aspect of the psychoenergetic effects of evil can be explained through vampirism, because when we injure another living being, allow it to suffer or torture it, we first steal its energy. We thereby acquire foreign energy that we're really not entitled to, and for which the law of Karma will someday call us to account. This seems to be a matter of total indifference to people who commit evil deeds – as when a pervert horribly tortures a child to death. Just as "every pleasure longs for eternity" (Nietzsche), so also does evil look only to itself and its absolutist demands. Moral objections are thus completely beside the point, since they go right past the core problem.[55]

Black-magic practices exploit these regularities in a very comparable manner. Trying to cast a magic spell on someone is condemned in all cultures. In the first place, everyone is afraid that spells might someday be used on themselves. But the main reason for our aversion to black magic is that we instinctively sense that, through it, evil could become independent and slip out of control.[56] I am convinced that significantly more of the world's insoluble problems can be traced back to black-magic practices than our enlightened minds can possibly conceive. The enormous damage caused by such practices in the third world, where belief in the efficacy of black magic is widespread, needs much greater awareness and scrutiny. To me, black magic is basically the same as a felonious criminal act, except that it takes place out of sight. The best protection is learning the harmfulness of such practices, and the dissolution of subconscious conflicts (in victimizer and victim!) – since these magic practices can make contact only at the victim's subconscious conflicts.

The question as to whether man is basically good or bad leads, in my estimation, to an insoluble dilemma, for as long as people, in the process of maturing between the 1st and 7th Chakras, continue to make mistakes, they will have evil within themselves. It is only in those who become enlightened saints that evil's chances are vanishingly slim – but even then, the game is not entirely over. I like to call patients who suffer from an overly strict Superego "Jesus," because, according to the New Testament, he was also tempted by the Devil. If even Christ, God incarnate in human form, exhibited such human traits that the Devil could try to lead him into temptation, then we can probably go a little easier on our own fallible selves.

Of course, the issue of man's essential nature has some very practical consequences, which influence political convictions, the legal system, and group norms. If one believes that all people are evil – which of course includes the believer – then we need strict laws and conservative-value politics to tame the beast in man. If we hold the opposite view, we become liberals who see personal freedom as the guarantee that the good in man can develop and flourish. I personally

---

[55] Instead of totally ineffective moral preaching, life sentences, or castration (of sexual criminals), what is needed is to raise perverted perpetrators' energy levels, resolve their huge psychic conflicts and alter their badly-programmed automatic mechanisms (the wrong kick) with behavioral therapy in such a manner that healthy and normal reactions once again become possible.

[56] Of course, the Law of Karma also worries us: that our bad deeds will someday catch up with us. Obviously, black-magic practices do great harm simply from a self-interest standpoint. Some might get away with it over the short term, but over the long term, they'll be forced to believe in it, and be punished quite severely. In my opinion, many inborn handicaps should be viewed in this context. In the chapter on Karma, I deal in great detail with the subconscious background of these karmic laws.

believe that the lower the vibration of Chakra development of a population (as in many third-world countries), the stricter and more conservative the group norms have to be. When individualization progresses and vibrations go up, a liberal stance makes more sense (as in modern democracies).[57]

Now, if the good is already potentially present in the bad, then we can view evil as the error of those who, in Jesus' words, "*know not what they do*." If bad people could know what idiots they really are, what the karmic repercussions of their badness are, and that – from a depth-psychological/ spiritual standpoint – they mostly hurt themselves, they would at once cease to be bad. As the DALAI LAMA said in his book on the nature of love, correct logic must coexist with love. Evil is always illogical, short-sighted, and dumb. The more that people discover their deep Self, the more they come to regard their negative character traits as superfluous armor to be discarded. They rediscover their original life impulses, and thus their basic attitude turns from unhappy and frustrated to happy and satisfied.

Getting away from evil, I'd like now to delve more deeply into the strife between Cain and Abel – because the possibilities have not yet been played out, i.e., when one of the two wins, or both lose, or both win. First off, strife is always a struggle for energy and power! Strife mechanisms of course also apply when the bone of contention is "materialized" energy such as money and property. The foreground fight is about material things, while behind the scenes the contenders skirmish over subtle energy. "I want to feel better! Give me the energy!" is what the squabblers seem to be yelling at each other – utterly subconsciously, of course. **No one seems to have the slightest inkling that the struggle is really about a sense of well-being and energetic satisfaction!** Underlying this is the background motivation that no one wants to admit: how bad things are going for them, and that – psychoenergetically – they are forced, like a starving beggar, to grab at other people's food. Nobody likes to be cast as the miserable loser, as some pitiful kind of energy-starved "petty thief" – especially not in the presence of rivals.

[57] An important qualification is needed here. Just as more light often creates more shadow, the aggression potential at first grows ever greater with increasing civilization and higher cultural development. Stone-age cultures didn't have concentration camps, genocide and atom bombs – simply because the aggression potential was not yet so great. Fascism, an extreme form of aggression, is a product of modern advanced civilization. Because it is exceedingly seductive to try to recapture lost life energy by stamping out other human beings perceived to be hostile (and by means of other vitalizing mechanisms such as mass marches and parades, etc.), we humans must, in a sense, protect ourselves from ourselves. Since, moreover, a society always consists of a mixture of the most varied individuals, we have to presume that it will always include some especially violent and criminal elements. Therefore, excessive liberalism would make the majority of people victims of a violent few – just as a rigid "law-and-order" mentality would limit the spiritual developmental possibilities of many highly developed persons. The truth lies somewhere in the middle.

The slightest scruples over a conflict will later on haunt the victors, since to them it's OK that they won the conflict. The energy transfer that has taken place has satisfied them in the truest sense of the word, and so, in retrospect, the strife that (for them) turned out so well also gives them something good. They seem to be saying to themselves: "If I'm better off afterward, then there can't have been anything wrong with the conflict. Somehow, the struggle did indeed benefit me (and maybe my rival, too)." This is why experience shows that winners are supremely uninterested in the mechanisms of the game. Whether it's the Old Testament Cain, wife-beating husbands, or someone else – winners always have a clear conscience. The reader will understand that I am speaking here of the secret corners of the subconscious where victors stash their true motivations! Publicly, winners often affect contrition, pretending to be penitent sinners, while totally different things are going on behind the scenes. Abusive husbands tend to continue beating their wives even while putting on a big public show of repentance. Their justification is often that women need a good beating now and then, sometimes even accusing their victims of giving as good as they get.

At this point, it's worth taking a closer look at the energy-transfer processes between perpetrator and victim – for if we do, we'll see that the real reason is based solely on the energy deficiency of the contending parties. A sated lion is a peaceful lion – and the same principle applies on the energetic plane. But satiety is not a permanent condition, and the lion will eventually get hungry again. Trying to communicate with a hungry lion is difficult, and it will snap at us ever more aggressively until it eventually bites us. Once it has ripped off half our arm, we'll have to concede that a hungry lion in a state of inner frustration is not very friendly. We realize – transferring this to our strife topic – that **conflict readiness depends quite crucially on the energy situation of the parties involved.**

At this point, the Central Conflict now comes back onstage, since it is the psychoenergetic phenomena triggered by the Central Conflict that make the strife truly comprehensible in the first place. Our energy situation is decisively impaired by the Central Conflict, which of necessity raises our conflict readiness. Like a ravenous lion, the Central Conflict makes us energetically hungry. Due to the great **dissatisfaction and energy vacuum** that the Central Conflict engenders, our vitality and sense of satisfaction is throttled, leading to a constant agonizing energy deficit. The obvious solution is to take energy away from other people, so that we'll have more of it. The underlying psychic hunger and the constant feeling of dissatisfaction are thus the actual triggers of conflict readiness.

In my considered opinion, gnawing inner emotional frustration is the crucial motivating force driving us to commit and suffer evil in the form of disputes with our fellow humans. By *evil*, I mean all factors that even children identify as harmful and painful factors, that are not sympathetic to us. Frustrated inside, we begin to hate and become aggressive; we envy other people for what they have or are. The philosopher NIETZSCHE recognized the real roots of human envy: "*Whoever is dissatisfied with himself is always itching for revenge.*" Deep inside, we are totally unsatisfied and much angrier than we'd like to admit, plus emotionally injured and secretly dreadfully unhappy.

Earlier, I mentioned the enormous emotional pain that surfaces in psychological encounter groups. One might of course wonder why it is that so little of this psychic pain is noticed in everyday life. The fact is that we use our *persona* mask to repress our inner emotional unhappiness and hide it from ourselves; we hide it from others by putting on a false identity, acting completely normal and well-adjusted. Experience shows that this doesn't work over the long run, though, and patching up the external façade becomes harder as time goes on. The more impossible our repair attempts, the more angry, violent and destructive we become. Eventually, the inner frustration and hate erupts violently, and many take refuge in some pseudo-solution or other to try to preserve their psychic equilibrium. This might take the form of drugs, or obsessive industriousness (workaholism), or some other surrogate solution in an attempt to ease the compulsion and make the emotional frustrations tolerable.

Now – with this background of the very deep emotional frustration – what subconscious dynamic underlies the phenomenon of strife? It's true that strife can occasionally relieve frustration (like when you want to "let off some steam"), but generally strife just amplifies internal frustration. What to do with the adversary who makes you totally crazy with rage and anger? You slay him without further ado, as Cain did to his brother Abel in the Bible. At this point, I'd like to put forward two daring theses that will, very likely, shock many readers. I contend, first, that murder is generally accepted in our society as a surrogate solution for emotional frustration (at least in veiled form) – in crime novels and movies! By their 14th birthdays, German children will have witnessed, on average, 25,000 murders on television. (It is not my intent here to bemoan the passing of some presumed "good old days" that most likely never were. Children have always been exposed to murder and manslaughter, in the gruesome horror stories known as *fairy tales*, just for openers.)

Which brings me to my second thesis, long known to depth-psychologists: murder is a very interesting phenomenon because (according to depth psychology, no matter how unbelievable and bonkers it may sound) in reality it represents a proof of love! If we take hate and destruction to be a response to spurned love, then annihilation of the object of hatred leads to a subconscious reunification with its essence. In psychological terminology, this is known as a "regressive fusion" with the slain object. Like a predator devouring its prey, the slain enemy in a sense becomes the exclusive property of the slayer.

One can observe similar processes in the practice of cannibalism. Ritualistic anthropophagy is based on the magical idea of appropriating the powers of the slain victim. The cannibal – unlike the murderer – thus performs a conscious and deliberate act of unification with his victim. The expression "I love you so much I could just eat you up!" captures a fading echo of this subconscious dynamic – because, in our culture, cannibalism has become taboo, and is considered abhorrent. It is only practiced by perverts such as the homosexual serial killer Fritz HAARMANN, who murdered 24 male prostitutes in the 1930s, and sold some of their flesh as sausage: he "hospitably" (if that's the phrase in this gruesome context) wanted others to share in his cannibalism, even though those who ate the sausages were unaware of the source of the sausage contents.

For modern man, the idea of devouring the slain enemy is intolerable. To my mind, this is basically due to the fact that, since the Stone Age, our capacity for hatred has expanded considerably! The cannibal still feels a certain degree of pride and sympathy for his victim – and, for the slain warrior, to be devoured counted as a kind of tribute, since this honor was only accorded to a particularly strong and courageous warrior. A cowardly, "wimpy" soldier would not be eaten but rather, at most, buried as an act of mercy, so that the wild beasts would not eat him. In today's wars, the dead are often simply left lying around on the battlefield once the carnage is over.

In modern society, murder and cannibalism are considered marginal phenomena, so that aggression has to be worked off (abreacted) in some other manner. Modern society has become increasingly stressful emotionally, especially in the lower socioeconomic strata (due to unemployment and homelessness), which increases the predisposition to violence: The crime rate in the USA went from 60 violent crimes per 100,000 in 1957 to 440 by the mid-nineties. The military psychologist David GROSSMANN attributes this above all to – besides increased inner emotional stress and other factors – the role-model function of television. While the biologically-based inhibition against killing members of one's species is lowered in the military via brutalization and systematic deconditioning, the same thing is done in children, according to GROSSMANN, predominantly by television. When children are exposed to a great many TV murders, their inhibition against killing is more and more diminished.

My own experience with infantile violence has taught me that large conflicts play an especially significant role in triggering violence. The bigger the conflicts a child has, the more the child tends to antisocial behavior and violence. Whether such conflicts are activated by depictions of violence on television – as the violence expert GROSSMANN believes – needs to be looked into more closely. I think that

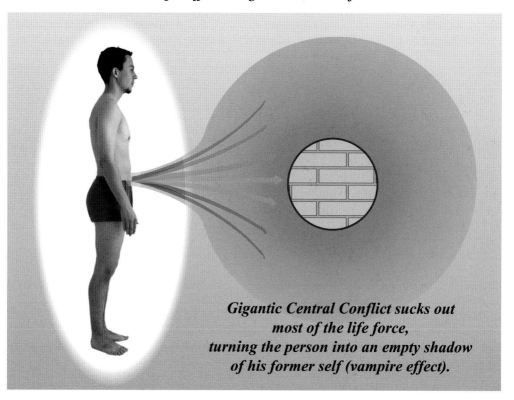

Gigantic Central Conflict sucks out most of the life force, turning the person into an empty shadow of his former self (vampire effect).

conflicts are (at least latently) already present before a child sees its first TV murder scene. From a prophylactic standpoint, we should be treating children's conflicts so that they'll be happier and more authentic, while at the same time becoming socially better adapted and friendlier. They would then be able to watch TV murder scenes with a different consciousness.

I'd like to illustrate this with a typical example taken from my daily practice:

Patrik is a nine-year-old boy with a life history of upbringing problems and severe behavioral disorders. Teachers complained about his antisocial behavior even in kindergarten. Patrik is extremely self-conscious around other children; once he starts to play with them, he systematically torments them until they run away in tears. Patrik has no interest in learning, he doesn't obey, and he often plays monotonous games for hours in his room. Testing Patrik with Psychosomatic Energetics revealed very low readings (20% each) in the Vital and Emotional regions, plus enormous conflicts with the themes Uneasiness and Mistrust. After two months of therapy, the conflicts have been considerably reduced. The mother, overjoyed, reports that Patrik is a completely different child: he now uncomplainingly does whatever his parents or teachers ask him to; he's much more contented and stable; lately, he has begun to play enthusiastically with another child from the neighborhood without trying to pick a fight.

Patrik's example, which I present as representative of hundreds of other children, illustrates very well the effects of large conflicts. Patrik is energetically "hungry" because the conflicts drain off a good deal of his life energy. This makes Patrik a frustrated, dreadfully unhappy boy who doesn't feel loved. It is understandable that, under the circumstances, he is not a loving son, obedient student, or a pleasant playmate; quite the contrary, he turns himself into an out-and-out little devil who alienates everyone around him. Only energetically dissolving the conflicts breaks the wicked spell, allowing Patrik once again to become the pleasant and friendly fellow that he had been as an infant.

In children, one seldom notes another problem that increases conflict readiness, particularly in adults. It has to do with distortion and narrowing of perception, in which the Central Conflict makes a big shift in the direction of **subjectivity**. In a certain sense, we become "dis-placed," because we acquire a far too subjective and egotistical point of view. We then see the world as we believe it should be rather than how it really is.

So if you have a Central Conflict with the theme *Rage*, you'll perceive the world as a dangerous bomb that might go off at any moment. The Central Conflict gives people with latent *Rage* a skewed worldview that can get harder and harder to correct for. For them, other people are perceived as furtively violent monsters, to be feared and constantly

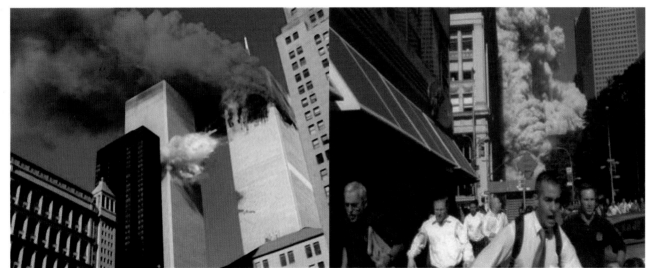

In terrorism, the hate-driven annihilation of the enemy becomes the primary motivation, behind which lie hidden psychological conflicts, provoked by an emotionally hungry and a latently violent and malevolent mental state. The terrorist hopes to find peace through destruction; actually, he projects his unhappiness onto the outside world. Basically, he hopes that destroying the enemy will rid him of his psychic conflicts. This is, of course, a completely erroneous supposition.

appeased. People with the *Rage* theme are therefore extraordinarily nice and obliging, since their imagination leads them to believe that only constant exaggerated accommodation and friendliness can prevent the rage-bomb from exploding. They act like hostages who have been kidnapped by extremely violent psychopaths ("Just don't say anything to upset them! Don't be rebellious! Always act friendly and never stop smiling!").

Depending on the specific fundamental fear, we perceive the world filtered through the "spectacles" of our conflict theme. "You're way too nice and obliging, you let sneaky and self-centered people take advantage of you!" we say to people with the *Rage* theme. "Can't you see that you're just imagining their rage?" Yet people with the *Rage* theme often don't grasp right away what it is we're trying to tell them – because, tragically, their conflict themes get mixed up with prevalent conceptions of the nature of contemporary society. This makes it much harder to detect the conflict theme and its off-kilter worldview, especially when it's bolstered and substantiated by rational-sounding arguments.

For instance, conflict hosts with the *Rage* theme will dislike other people in the society based on certain societal preconceptions; they'll be mad at asylum-seekers, politicians, pit-bull owners or some other group. In people with the *Rage* theme, I very often notice that they develop particularly peaceable convictions, i.e., to appease a "wild world" with their pacifism. They are totally unaware that their lofty ideals and noble political concerns conceal great dynamite-like loads of subconscious feelings. Even skilled outside observers have a lot of trouble noticing the skewed worldview, since the repressed emotions have been so expertly camouflaged. No one suspects a gentle and friendly pacifist of concealing a *Rage* theme.

Among the Central Conflict's dangerous and even diabolical traits is that of imputing wicked, ignoble and negative motives to other people. Seeing in others our own vices and shortcomings is what psychologists call **projection**. We fail to notice that our perception is pure imagination. Our nonsensical and ridiculous fantasies threaten to conjure up precisely that which we fear the most – namely, that the other person, thanks to our (over)reaction, will become truly nasty and mean. We project onto others our veiled and repressed negative, undesirable attributes. Afterwards, we are surprised to get back as an echo that which we have shouted out – but since we fail to notice what we had shouted, the reaction of others simply reinforces our original opinion.

So what happens when people don't have a Central Conflict? We can expect that social groups with few Central Conflicts will be extraordinary peaceable. Based on what I've seen, this seems in fact to be the case. For example, among the Australian aborigines, competitive games with winners and losers are totally unknown. In fact, they cannot comprehend how anybody could like games with winners and losers. They especially don't understand the covert sadism behind the disappointment, frustration and humiliation of the loser. The Aborigines much prefer to play games in which everybody wins (their motto is: "If no one loses, then nothing can go wrong."). As far as I can tell, Aborigines don't yet have any Central Conflicts – or at least didn't yet, in those paradisiacal times before the white man's arrival in Australia.

Eventually, however, everyone gets kicked out of paradise. This includes the knowledge that it is impossible to live in this world innocently and aggression-free. A closer look reveals that even the act of eating food involves the destruction of life. There is a nice little story from ancient India which illustrates the impossibility of living an innocent life:

A wise man refused to help carry the royal sedan chair, contending that, if he did, he might inadvertently step on insects, since he then wouldn't be able to look down at the ground, and that stepping on an insect would be bad for his Karma. Whereupon the king had the wise man beheaded.[58]

The wise man was executed for refusing to bear the royal sedan chair, which refusal caused the spiral of aggression to take yet another turn (which the wise man, in his stubbornness, failed to anticipate!). We also live with the paradox of perennial guilt: we'll be guilty no matter which way we decide. This applies particularly to our involvement in arguments and quarrels. Clever teachers are fond of the notorious solution (attributed to Solomon): "It doesn't matter who started it, I'm going to punish you both!" Now this is of course sheer nonsense, since it draws the punishing teacher into the spiral of guilt for unnecessarily – unjustly – punishing an innocent person. One can conclude from these two examples (wise man and teacher) that Indian sages and teachers are often subject to similar thought processes: in trying to be particularly clever and wise, they often bring about the exact opposite!

Because of the impossibility of emerging unscathed from a strife situation, important learning processes are set in motion in both parties. The king is guilty of having had the wise man beheaded; the wise man loses his obstinate head – with some justification, of course: one can argue that the wise man's attitude led him into a type of suicide, which leads in turn to further guilt. After all, the wise man could have given in, which would have saved his life, but evidently the insects (and his principles) were more important to him than his very head – a foolish stubbornness whose logic and erroneous fundamental assumption is based on equating one's bliss with the inflexible observance of certain behavioral codes. *Dogmatism* is a good way to characterize these pig-headed ideologies.

Since interpersonal relationships lead to energy theft and the exercise of power, this saddles both parties to the conflict with insoluble role assignments and standpoints. This can be seen particularly clearly in any well-established power hierarchy, such as master/slave or guard/inmate. Because certain fixed roles have been pre-assigned, both parties become immovably fixed in their social roles. They are forced to act in a manner that, as in a game of chess, inevitably leads to conflicts. This leads to psychic learning tasks having to do with guilt and expiation.

As civilization advances, aggressive pressure and compounded frustration rise ever higher. Instead of satisfactory solutions and harmonious outcomes, the cauldron of aggressive emotions bubbles all the more vigorously. Laws and moral codes – invisible walls – are erected to protect individuals from each other, giving rise to ideologies and dogmas[59] that try to reclaim paradise by force – whether Marxist Communism or religious fundamentalism. It's easy to see that the final goal of ideology is subconsciously equated with one's personal redemption. The Marxist thinks: "When Communism finally triumphs, I'll be rid of my tormenting inner frustration!" Understandably, this kind of attitude triggers very drastic actions, since one is fighting for one's most profound bliss! Ideologues and demagogues are perfectly humorless and intellectually rigid, since they have gotten themselves tangled up in an insane concept of salvation.

In our advanced civilization, we no longer go at each other with clubs, like our stone-age progenitors; instead, we press a button to launch a missile. To that extent, the destructive potential has risen steadily with the rise of civilization. Missiles do not slumber in their silos forever: at some point, they will be used. A warhead's detonation kills many more people than a blow from a stone-age club. Thus, the number of war dead rises ever higher in our modern civilization, as the instruments of war get ever more refined; the atom bombs dropped on Hiroshima and Nagasaki are tragic examples of this.

Yet even in peacetime, the frequency of aggressive acts and energy theft in our modern civilization continues to grow. As in the example of the hungry lion, energy-restricting Central Conflicts emerge that keep on raising the level of aggression. People become bellicose and try to establish who is the strongest within the context of hierarchical power structures. This will of course be whoever can lay claim to the most energy, kicking off a Social-Darwinist struggle of "every man for himself." As far back as ancient Rome, man had come to the unsettling conclusion that man is his own

---

[58] In modern India, these ideas are still current. Jains, for example, wear a cloth over their mouths to prevent from inhaling (and possibly killing) flying insects. Logically enough, orthodox Jains may not drive cars either, since flying insects can be killed by the windshield. But since, on my trip to India, I met orthodox Jains on trains, I assume that these things are not interpreted as dogmatically these days, since the locomotive of course kills insects constantly.

[59] I refer here to the phenomenologically interesting **similarity between dogmatism and psychosis,** with respect to the intolerance, rigidity and totalitarian attitude in defending one's worldview. To a certain approximation, our Ego structure – even that of "normal" contemporaries – exhibits dogmatic and psychotic aspects. The [quantitative] difference with pathology is ultimately gradual, but qualitatively totally different: totalitarian types always have an appetite for destruction and negativity. And yet experience has shown that psychotics – other than at the peak of the their psychotic episodes – are peaceable people, and they destroy more passively than actively, particularly their Ego and their social connections. In a certain sense, the dogmatic fundamentalist is also a psychotic – although a much more dangerous one: the dangerousness of dogmatism is based on its projection outward, in which the bomb (the materialization of the fundamentalist psychosis) explodes outside of his head!

worst enemy ("*Homo homini lupus est*" = Man is a wolf to [his fellow] man).

In war and strife, one can no longer withdraw from the predefined options for action, because the warlike other party has forced its own view of reality on the opponent:"Give up or I'll bash your head in!" In the militant hordes and clans, there now initiate various psychic processes based on insoluble paradoxes. These paradoxes – dialectical exchange processes – are the starting point for learning and maturation opportunities, because they contain enormous conflict potential. One may speak in terms of the "explosive material" concealed in social pecking orders, castes, and power relationships.

The best example in social psychology is the dialectical relationship of **master and slave**: on a subtle level of interpretation, the presumably powerful party becomes the powerless one. We know it has to be that way because the master is and remains master only because the slave exists as counterpart. It doesn't take long for the slave to realize this dependency – and this realization threatens to upset the power-relationship applecart. Similarly, the prison guard becomes the victim of his strategy of locking up the prisoner, since he must then constantly watch the prisoner in order to foil any escape attempts.

But wars do not take place only outside the four walls of the family home. In many families, dramas are staged in which children are cast as tiny tyrants tormenting their parents. In my experience, energetic disturbances due to conflicts play a crucial role. Because of conflicts, people have deep-seated frustration which they try to discharge in some way or another. Children do that, for instance, with power plays that serve, first, to prop up their own fragile egos and, secondly, to discharge inner frustration. As Patrik's example made clear, healing the conflict terminates these family dramas.

Increasing cultural development and the awakening of the higher Chakras (above the diaphragm) leads to a counter-movement. People begin to suspect that, when it comes to strife and energy theft, there are no winners or losers as such, **since it ultimately doesn't matter whether Cain or Abel wins – in actuality, there are always only two possible outcomes: either there are two winners or two losers!** I think that we can only understand this simple yet irrefutable fact by dealing with psychoenergy and the phenomenon of karmic compensation. **Karma,** as the consequence of guilt and error, ensues the moment we harm another person. In plain language, this means that we'll all have to pay our karmic debt some day, and need to come up with a peacemaking compensation.

Both parties lose in a dispute, as they accuse each other and get entangled in mistakes. When we begin to be aware that there is such a thing as Karma, we learn that eventually, guilt forces a karmic compensation. Jesus pointed out the stupidity of ostensible victors when he said "… *for they know not what they do.*" Since we perceive neither the subconscious part of our psyche nor the invisible workings of Karma, we erroneously think that one is the winner and the other the loser – but in reality every destructive dispute that harms someone results in two losers. Energy theft will thus eventually work out unfavorably for both parties: the loser pays his dues immediately (as it were) by having painfully lost, whereas the winner will have to make good his karmic debt later.

Anyone uncomfortable with the concept of *Karma* is free to speak and think in terms of *higher order* or *sense of community*. The fact is that the egotistical, short-sighted, and unilateral behavior of winners can and should be rejected for entirely rational reasons, since their victory is entirely at the loser's expense. So-called "Manchester capitalism" is an excellent example of this: underpaid workers work their fingers to the bone to create surplus value for the capitalist bosses. When the goods are sold, the energy-robbing play continues, as each businessman tries to get the better of the other. Later, the fight is continued at the consumer level, as exorbitant and exploitative profits are made. By now, we're all aware that this kind of "predator capitalism" has enormously detrimental consequences for all involved – and it becomes even clearer from a global ecological perspective. The old saying "We're all in the same boat" aptly expresses the state of affairs.

The idea that you can get away with stealing another person's energy and quickly running away ("Player A wins, player B loses") is based on a dim-witted and short-sighted viewpoint. People at the developmental level of the 4th (only feelings count) or 5th (only reason counts) Chakra do not yet empirically understand that there is an imperceptible bond uniting all living beings; these intuitive and authentic insights don't emerge until the 6th Chakra (and even more strongly in the 7th Chakra). It is thus possible to see laws and moral precepts as (to some extent) anticipated wisdom for those who are not yet advanced enough to intuit it on their own.

With all the violent images that beset us, one can't help wondering if what we have here might not be a patently sick world. Many readers will no doubt accuse me of painting an overly dismal and apocalyptic picture of our world. They will remind me (correctly) that, all over the world, most people lead quite normal (often even cheerful and happy) lives – while I, on the other hand, like a scandal-sheet reporter, portray an exclusively negative, outrageous, and totally distorted picture of real life. After all this negativity about strife, I'd like to wind up this exposition with a "happy ending" – because, in contrast to the unfavorable possibilities mentioned above (where there's either a winner and a loser or two losers), there is a far better one that we can conceive, namely that **both parties can profit from a conflict!** This kind of outcome is not just conceivable, it is highly desirable, since we end up with two winners who benefit and profit from each other. I'd like to define "two winners" as the advantageous situation, worth striving for, in which two people affectionately help and enrich each other, instead of injuring each other and taking something away energetically.

The DALAI LAMA speaks, in this context, of the "logic of love." We may define **love** as a form of communication that generates maximum benefit for both parties, and thus emphasizes the "we" aspect of the relationship. Jesus commands us to "... *love thy neighbor as thyself*' – meaning the egalitarian *Philia* [Greek: brotherly love, affection] in which one pays precisely as much attention to the other's well-being and happiness as to one's own. One thinks and acts in terms of mutual benefit, which leads psychoenergetically to more life force and greater spiritual development. Nature shows us, via the example of sexual love, how this works even on the coarse-materials level of two bodies coupling. Parenthood transforms sexual partners into winners – i.e., father and mother, who have begotten a child.

A closer examination of our world (whether human society or the physical environment) reveals that *Love* and the so-called *Good* clearly have the upper hand. Inasmuch as nature's powers cause food to grow and ripen, the sun to shine, and to bring many situations to a favorable conclusion, we plainly live in a predominantly beautiful and good world. But there is not only a good world that sees to the birth of healthy babies, grows food, and creates a good and friendly place (for the most part) – there is also an everyday world. The banal uniformity of that which we call "everyday" and "normal" has great significance for psychic development. This *everyday-ness*, along with our emotional center, forms something like a layer of humus in which our personality can grow and develop.

If we didn't have this loving goodness within us, then traits such as conscience, trust in others, or the ability to love would be inconceivable. Without normalcy and trust in the world, our psychic stability – and thus our personal growth – would be seriously jeopardized. Despite this, I'd like to stick by my portrayal of evil and the world as a kind of *battlefield*. Only a dreamer and visionary could fail to take into account (at least partially) the world's badness – e.g., by leaving his car, with valuables in it, unlocked, or carelessly falling for a con-man's blandishments. We call it paranoia when a person's worldview is completely dark, and evil is imagined to be all around. A paranoid attitude is not the point here, but rather the fact that we need to take the undeniable factual existence of evil into account, just as we do the dark side of our psyche. The point is to have a realistic picture of the human environment that spans the gamut of our human existence.

The Soul Within the Family

All bad traits develop in the family.
It begins with murder and proceeds via treachery and alcoholism on to smoking.

(Alfred Hitchcock)

The preceding chapter dealt with interpersonal conflicts and the phenomenon of evil. To a certain extent, this is a great game in which our psyche learns, as it matures, to harmonize its own wishes and needs with those of other people in such a manner as to generate the maximum possible benefit. I'd like to designate this benefit as an expression of "love" (in a completely non-romantic sense), because both parties derive maximum profit from it. Now, for moralistic reasons, we tend to think of love and profitable dealings as being mutually exclusive, so many readers will no doubt be shocked at my choice of words. Yet **I can't discover any essential difference between dealings that turn out profitable for both parties and the phenomenon of love**. The end result is, psychoenergetically, a "more" in both cases. Afterwards, all persons involved are happier and more energy-laden than before – and that's the point.

I'd like in this section to address the depth-psychological interrelationships within the family. The principle of family dynamics seems quite simple to me, since we learn much more easily and quickly in groups. The family is the oldest, most proven and stable group that there is. Since it is tremendously hard to grapple alone with one's fundamental fears and overcome them, we form social groups with other people in order to advance in our spiritual journey. Inside the protective walls of the family, we can develop the foreign and rejected personality traits that we need for emotional stability. This can take the form of missing personality components being mirrored within the family by other members, so that we learn from them how to "bring out the best in others."

When we empathize with the spiritual journey (mentioned often already), in the last few decades more and more therapists have come to the view, based on their experiences with depth-psychology in daily practice, that the individual psyche must come into the world multiple times – otherwise, many psychoenergetic connections (and reports from persons under deep hypnosis) simply cannot be explained. In the chapters that follow, I'd like to apply the subtopics covered so far in this book – the origin of conflicts, character types, the spiritual journey – to the topic of the family and the inextricably related issue of *Karma*. In so doing, I'd like to sketch out an overall view of the psychoenergetic processes of personal death, birth, choice of family, and on through dying again.

I'd like to say up front that the perfect intermeshing of depth-psychological and spiritual views speaks for the correctness of my conception. My core theses match up perfectly with the views of "The Perennial Philosophy," as Aldous HUXLEY called the remarkable commonalities between all of the world's religions and Gnostic philosophies. Also, the knowledge and experiences of traditional shamans, humoral medicine, and modern energy medicine corroborate the theses I am presenting here. Admittedly, from the viewpoint of diehard skeptics, all this might seem conjectural. Nevertheless, I'd like to be so bold as to assert that the following account can claim a degree of truth that agrees with the experiences of skilled depth psychologists.

The triadic family of father, mother, child is of course one of the great mysteries of the deeper layers of the psyche. The image of the Christ child in the manger illustrates the mystery of our earthly existence. Looking into the manger, we see the newborn child, psychoenergetically open and with the heartwarming innocence that all babies radiate. Most manger scenes reinforce the impression of the child's openness by depicting its diminutive arms outstretched. Many people have been deeply moved by the image of the Godchild in the manger, because deep inside they feel that the manger scene is actually about themselves: every human comes into the world as a defenseless baby, just as the Christ child in the manger did.

The miracle begins when opposites (in this case man and woman) unite to create new life. From this perspective, one can view all living beings as torchbearers of an enormously long chain of begetting and birthing, in which the flame of life is passed on from one generation to the next. At the deepest spiritual level – that of the causal body – a great love unites us with father and mother, which has about it the air of a divine gift, or sacrament. The holier and more transpersonal we become, the more we are united by a deep love of creation, which we also re-encounter in our relationship with our parents.

We leave the realm of the sacred and enter that of the profane, where we have to deal with changing diapers, skinned knees and the chaos of pubertal self-discovery – for the child inexorably grows bigger and older, eventually becoming an adult. Only now does psychic development begin in its individual and personal uniqueness. For the first time, the young person begins to speak about herself in the first person, and at some point insists on being addressed more formally. The child, by contrast, still speaks in terms of "we" because it does not yet have a firmly-established consciousness of itself. As the Self develops, the number of role models increases. Inside the family and other social groupings, we adopt a fixed position that conforms to our character type. At the same time, our social life begins, and we have to deal with other people at school, work, and elsewhere.

Then there's the core issue for each of us: which people do we get along well with and which not? Experience has shown that human happiness depends crucially on whether, during the course of one's life, one finds enough other people who are on the same wavelength. This includes good friends and marriage partners. The scope of the problem becomes evident when we think about which people we get along well with, without reservation. Even with many friends and acquaintances, we meet very few really close friends. For similar reasons, partner-search agencies have a lot of trouble making good matches, even with many, many potential partners in their databases: the great number of variables entered into the computer in the search for statistical compatibility only turn up a small number of "hits" even with thousands of candidates. With respect to this core issue of social well-being and flourishing human cooperation, the DALAI LAMA once remarked that it had always puzzled him that the world was not more violent, since, after all, only one person in a thousand suits us even a little.

An even more exciting question emerges from thinking about how people inside a family get along – because we seem, at first glance, to be completely uninvolved in the composition of our family – choice of marriage partner aside, and the choice to have children or not. But what kind of people these children will be, or which relatives we wind up with when we choose a marriage partner – all this is beyond our control. We're subject to all kinds of imponderables and surprises – and yet this seems not to be the case, when people under deep hypnosis or ecstatic states such as those induced by hyperventilation[60] are asked about the deeper reasons why their family has the particular members it does, and not others. Amazingly, virtually all people in such trance states report **having had a prenatal hand in the choice of their family members!**

It's precisely at this crucial point that things get extremely interesting! An amazing perspective opens up that uncovers new and unusual insights, if we assume a prenatal choice in putting together our family. The theory of reincarnation

has long maintained that we choose our parents before birth; this includes all other general conditions. The fact that so many people in deep trance talk about having chosen their parents seems to me an important indication of the correctness of this thesis. What's more, in my energy testing of spiritually advanced persons, I was often told that they considered such an option to be an immutable part of reality. Since, in most areas (i.e., having premonitions of illnesses), these highly-advanced people have such a good "nose" for such things, I respect their judgment.

To me, having this choice with respect to family seems utterly logical, since the entire sense of the spiritual journey implies that such laws and regularities must exist. The alternative – e.g., that it's purely random chance – makes much less sense, since only a freely-choosing soul can have karmically sensible and valuable experiences. Of course, I cannot allay the skepticism of readers who reject the whole thing, or are suspicious of it. I admit that I too, as a scientifically educated academician, used to think it was all sheer nonsense. My own experiences, and the detailed observations of the thousands of people I have encountered during the course of my medical career (including many families), have caused me to rethink my position a step at a time, to the point where I am now firmly convinced of the existence of (preincarnational) parent selection.[61]

This concept of parent selection (so foreign to mainstream psychology) also raises the question: What made us choose precisely these parents in the first place? Why on earth do we do it – especially when we wind up in a difficult family with bickering (or already divorced) parents? Or why do we accept having stupid, annoying siblings who get on our nerves; or coming into the world as a lonely only child even though we secretly wish we had brothers and sisters; or being born in a country where we don't at all feel at home?

In view of the prenatal options, one has to ask oneself why some voluntarily choose a bad fate. Better to reincarnate in the bosom of a super-friendly multimillionaire family, where one can lead a carefree happy life, feeling completely at home and secure. Why do so many choose a

---

[60] A very simple, free, and highly effective deep entry can be effected via hyperventilation. From a relaxed position, breathe more deeply and rapidly than normal. After a while, you'll usually enter a trance state. The initially distracting tingling in the extremities and mouth quickly fades. To terminate the state, simply resume your slower normal breathing rate. This method is generally safe and free of risk for emotionally stable and physically healthy people. It is a good idea not to undertake your first attempts alone, but rather find someone else who is experienced in these matters (this method is practiced by many reincarnation therapists).

[61] Shortly before his death, the current DALAI LAMA's predecessor mentioned some precise details of his reincarnation: a farmstead in a specific remote region of Tibet, the color of a flag fluttering in the wind in front of the house, family details, and more. Some years after the DALAI LAMA's death, an expedition found, after months of searching, a child in a situation where all the details were exactly as described. As a secret test, personal possessions of the former DALAI LAMA were placed underneath appealing toys; a normal child would not be interested in these objects and would instead choose the interesting-looking toys on top – yet the child unerringly chose these personal possessions. Moreover, certain physical details (such as striking pigmentation marks) bore out the correctness of the supposition that the child had to be the reincarnated DALAI LAMA. As the child got older, close friends of the former DALAI LAMA recognized many of his character traits in the new DALAI LAMA.

difficult destiny? My deliberations here are oriented toward answering this interesting question – for the answers confront us with the mysterious interaction of Karma, family, and character type.

If we want to understand the mechanisms of family formation from the karmic standpoint, we have to put ourselves in the position of the unborn soul. There are mystical writings on this topic. In the *Tibetan Book of the Dead* (*Bardo Thödol*), the soul normally chooses a parent as a desirable partner who will later become the opposite-sex parent. A female child thus chooses the father, whereas a boy chooses the mother as a sex partner. Identification with the copulating parents then leads to rebirth, as we – like a honeybee drawn to the flower – are attracted by our parents' mating act. Psychoanalysts will point out (correctly) that we are then in an oedipal situation even before having been born. Evidently, our spiritual journey begins with a voyeuristic, very erotically-tinged crucial experience.

When we put ourselves in the place of the soul of an unborn child, we are by no means dealing with a blank slate. The young soul is not inexperienced in matters erotic; indeed, it experiences sexual lust and desire – as we can read in the *Tibetan Book of the Dead*. According to Buddhism and Hinduism, carnal desire keeps us chained to the well-known "Wheel of Life" (as the karmic reincarnation sequence is known in Eastern religions). We must consequently keep on reincarnating, simply because we feel so much sensual lust for life. Moreover, the soul is a personality that has grown and firmed up over the course of many reincarnations, and cannot be regarded as inexperienced. The soul brings with it the associated Central Conflict, as well as all previous karmic experiences that comprise the individual's spiritual history.

We now come to the decisive point at which the parents are chosen. Modern psychology and psychoanalysis says that a large part of our personality is shaped by our parents and our childhood. On the other hand, if we have selected our parents before birth, then we have, in a certain sense, prefigured the whole thing – and very likely even foreseen and therefore knowingly accepted it! According to everything we know from reincarnation experiences, parent selection seems to conform to certain intents and preferences. This applies as well to the choice of the future society, with its nationality and geography. We thus don't reincarnate just anywhere, randomly as in a lottery: according to spiritual masters, we invisibly circle the loving couple that are to become our parents for months before the act of procreation. In this process, we seek out suitable parents based on specific ideas.

Parent selection can be compared to phenomena that have been observed on long ocean cruises: groups of like-minded people wind up getting together due to a number of guidance and control systems. Distinguished travelers in 1st class, for example, pay a higher ticket price, which lowers the likelihood of their coming into contact with uncouth members of the lower class. The lower classes, for their part, find the upper-class persons to be unfriendly (arrogant, affected, and so on). Through mutual understanding and the recognition of accustomed behavioral patterns, people of like speech, race, and social standing gravitate toward each other. All voyagers are interested in making things as pleasant as possible for themselves, and to this end they seek out the "right" people. Similarly, we seek some prenatal options in order, like the passengers, to further our particular interests. In this endeavor, we seek out both the journey and our traveling companions.

Our traveling companions will be those with similar previous experiences, who preferably already know each other and who are united by common preferences and interests. We thus don't choose our parents, in the pre-birth situation, arbitrarily and thoughtlessly, but rather from a mixture of conscious and subconscious motives, as happens in setting out on a normal journey. We make our choice based on certain conceptions and intentions predetermined by our personality and history. Basically, we seem to prefer traveling companions whom we know, since we think we then know what to expect from them in the future. Of course, it can turn out later that one's choice was completely erroneous.

Some people may not care where and to whom they are reincarnated – as long as they have a roof over their heads and life goes on somehow or other. This might indeed be the case with the huge number of dirt-poor people in the third world. However, I am of the opinion that any impulse toward pity is out of place here. For one thing, I already mentioned that amazingly many destitute persons seem to be relatively happy – compared, that is, to bitterly miserable materially-rich Westerners. On top of which, the soul might have much better maturation opportunities if it is reincarnated in a third-world slum than in a safe and secure Western family home. Therefore, the soul's selection should be respected and regarded as the best one possible.

When they are under deep hypnosis or in a trance state, one will get a wide variety of answers from patients to the query as to why they chose this reincarnation and not another. As we know, daily life is about higher stakes than merely taking it easy. Our souls are guided by various motives and desires that play a role in parent selection. I'd like to shine a spotlight on these different subconscious motivations. Over time, certain indicatory cardinal motivations emerge in most persons that point to why they chose to reincarnate in the specific body they did. It often takes a relatively long time before, in a deep trance state, the answer to such questions is found in a person's subconscious.

One reason for the choice of a certain reincarnation might be, for instance, wanting vengeance for a suffered injustice. You've waited a long time for payback, and now the right time seems to have arrived. Another desire might be to get together again with especially beloved persons. The desire to reunite with a loved one seems to lead extraordinarily often to reincarnation. Often, the interest is directed at a group of people, a particular countryside, or the opportunity to develop a particular talent once again. Thus originate regular dynasties of artistic families, in which the special talent of the individual leads to like-minded people finding each other and combining into a group.

The individual reasons for reincarnation can vary quite widely. This means that we can't subsume all reasons under a single rubric. We'll probably have to lower our sights somewhat on our wish list, because the saying "You can't have everything" applies to (p)reincarnation selection as well. So, those who absolutely want to reincarnate in their beloved homeland might not find the ideal parent candidates there, and be forced to make do with less. Or if you want to see a beloved person again, you might not be 100% thrilled with the family or the region in which you wind up.

Our families represent, first of all, a choice we made and that, generally speaking, we wanted to be the way they are. All by itself, this is a fascinating idea. The most informative aspect seems to be who the persons are that we specifically selected, and which ones we had to accept as part of a "package deal" – for instance, when intense yearning has driven us to choose an especially beloved family member, we might also acquire unknown, less congenial – or even hostile – persons in the bargain.

In my experience, therefore, previous especially happy incarnations can lead to big problems because, after such a magnificent life, we tend to measure future lives against that one! Such a comparison is bound to lead to emotional disappointment, since "the better is the enemy of the good" and it is unlikely to be as good again as it was in the "good old days." So, my feeling is that not only horrible incarnations are hard to cope with: so are the terrific ones. Of course, this applies particularly to people that we associate with this good fortune. We then can scarcely tear ourselves away from these beloved persons, and we willingly make great sacrifices – including entering into foolish constellations – to be reunited with them.

I'd next like to turn to the problem of the "unhappy childhood." As we know, many traditional psychologists and psychoanalysts tend strongly to blame parents for people's mental problems. "My mother withheld affection!" – so goes the accusation. The mother is a popular villain for depressive character types who overeat, presumably because they didn't get enough motherly love and are now trying to compensate by stuffing their faces. "My father was too hardhearted and strict!" – thus the shy person who can't make a go of it in life, presumably for lack of a father figure with whom to identify, wherefore the father (so it is thought) must be the chief culprit.

Now, over my many years as general practitioner, I have come to know hundreds of families from whom I acquired my own experiences in this respect. Besides obese depressives, I also treated their parents, so I could see for myself whether the depressives' claims to have horrible parents were warranted. I had shy loser types in therapy whose parents were also patients of mine. Because of this, I was able to make some amazing discoveries that deviate sharply from conventional psychoanalytical wisdom.

Even Sigmund FREUD treated individual patients without – in virtually all cases – knowing anything much about family members. Psychoanalysis is thus based on the viewpoint of the individual who has been artificially crystallized out of the familial clan. And even family-oriented therapists are at times presented with a false front, i.e., in order to make a good impression, or the better to "put down" another family member. But GPs – thanks to years of treating these patients – get a much better picture of the actual situation. In particular, I have learned a lot from the kind of gossip that neither psychoanalysts nor other specialists would ever hear.

It's really astounding how subtle are the acts that people relate – about themselves and others. I would hear details from the hairdresser or some gossipy neighbor that I would otherwise never have found out about. Yet the most important aspect of my family research wasn't the gossip; it was meticulous observation of the people themselves. I have observed hundreds and hundreds of parents and their children, in order to check out the "unhappy childhood" theory. However, I won't deny that this widespread theory does indeed apply in numerous cases. There is hardly a criminal or antisocial person who has not had a cheerless childhood characterized by lovelessness and/or abuse.

Let's take a look at the fate of a person who grows up with "extreme parents" – by which I mean unusually unpleasant. At this point, critical readers will accuse me of overlooking that the evaluation of "pleasant" and "unpleasant" is highly subjective – to which my (equally vehement) response is: are these two concepts *really* a matter of entirely subjective gradations? Psychological experiments have emphatically shown that, when larger groups are questioned, there is amazing consistency as to who is considered particularly pleasant or unpleasant. To the statement "Nick has nice parents," most people who know Nick's parents will nod in agreement. Most of those who know them well will also agree that "Sibyl has a loathsome father, and her mother is a pain in the neck."

In the following section, I'd like to designate pleasant parents like Nick's as "dream parents," and Sibyl's unflatteringly described ones as "nightmare parents." Now, what happens to Nick and Sibyl, having to grow up with these dream or nightmare parents? Any sane person would congratulate Nick on his luck of the parental draw and predict a bright future for him, whereas for Sibyl, they'd expect her future to hold obesity, alcoholism, multiple divorces, or at the least serious mental problems once she moves out of her parents' home and has to make it on her own. Nick, on the other hand, will make rapid progress as a successful businessman, have a charming family, and become as nice a father as his own father had been. These are, at any rate, the predictions that independent observers will make if asked to speculate about Nick and Sibyl's respective futures.

Against all expectation, experience shows that children of dream parents are likely as not to become "gray mice" or have disagreeable character traits – not in every case, but relatively often all the same. For instance, as a doctor I met the parents of a shy, neurotic failure – and they turn out to be extraordinarily pleasant and emotionally level-headed dream parents. Their closest friends also confirm that no one understands how it is that such a loser of a son could have come from such nice parents. The parents gave him all their love and understanding, but it didn't help.

At first, I filed these away as outliers (i.e., exceptions) and paid no attention to such remarkably inconsistent details. Evidently, the conventional wisdom regarding unhappy childhoods is sometimes wrong, I thought to myself, surprised at first. Yet these outliers continued to pile up as time went by – and I encountered the opposite extreme more frequently, in which nightmare parents, unexpectedly, occasionally raise charming and friendly children (although admittedly less often than the opposite variant). In the case of Nick and Sibyl, it's Sibyl who becomes the successful businesswoman with a charming family, while Nick surprisingly turns into a depressive failure, muddling through one low-level job after another, overweight and alcoholic, and even, at one point, attempting suicide.

Patients would often warn me about their parents when I made house calls, predicting that I would think them horrible – yet time and again, confusingly, the purportedly atrocious parents turned out to be extraordinarily nice dream parents whose only flaw was a noticeable (but by all means likable) quirkiness. Clearly, the children's description of their supposedly dreadful parents was based on a distorted mental picture.

I'd like to make clear that I am (of course) not the only one to have noticed these striking breaches in the conventional views of developmental psychology. These phenomena – when noticed at all, which is seldom – are usually blamed on the genes. I will discuss the significance of genetics in the next chapter, where the topic is the profounder interrelationships of Karma, but I'd like to remark here that the karmic context has nothing to do with the basic issue under discussion, since, from the viewpoint of the prenatal soul, one obviously also selects the genes with which one wishes to be reincarnated; this is clearly an option, and one will instinctively choose the appropriate genetic equipment.

Looking at dream and nightmare parents from the viewpoint of the prenatal soul, it is clear that the soul knows, before reincarnation, which parent type it will get. The soul thus makes a decision that will lead to either pleasant or unpleasant results regarding the parents-to-be.

There are three prenatal options:

1. *The hard (problematic) way:* **choose parents with whom the outcome in life will be indeterminate.** You can learn a great deal from hard experience, and if the soul chooses this option, it guarantees itself an eventful and instructive life journey.

Or the exact opposite:

2. *The easy way:* **choose friendly parents who will go easy on you.** The reason for this choice might be a harrowing and as yet inadequately processed previous incarnation, so that you want to "take a [long overdue] break" in the next life.

Or in between:

3. *The middle way:* Most choose a totally average **way full of compromise and mediocrity,** as far as their prenatal selection is concerned. Strictly speaking, they don't choose at all well, but they feel drawn to the most comfortable and middling solution, predominantly subject to random chance and with relatively few underlying selection criteria. This middle way is different from the easy way, but not nearly as instructive as the hard way.

I estimate that about 50% choose the middle way, while the other half opt for one of the extremes representing either minimum or maximum challenge. Those who select dream parents intend to take it particularly easy. In deep trance, you find out from their subconscious that they need some R&R and want to be very comfortable – say, because the parents are quite well off.

In the safety and security of the psychic hammock one has crawled into by growing up with dream parents, all incentive to personal growth atrophies. Personal initiative is extinguished in these pampered children, quite a few of whom become lazy and deviate from the family norm. I've mentioned the surprisingly large number of drab children who have unusually pleasant parents. These constellations likewise give rise to the typical children of filthy-rich parents, who fill the headlines of the tabloids with their escapades. Evidently, people who are too comfortable all too easily develop disagreeable character traits. So the supposedly gentle solution of choosing a comfortable reincarnation soon turns out to be a dead end as far as spiritual growth is concerned.

On the other hand we have the ambitious souls who have chosen nightmare parents. These want to learn a lot in this next incarnation, and so choose the hard way that leads through darkness and difficulty to the bright light of day (*Per aspera ad astra* – To the stars through hardships – to use the felicitous Latin phrase that is the official state motto of Kansas). Yet the nightmare parents are often only so difficult in the eyes of their children because they belong to the polar opposite character type, which makes the parents' strangeness seem unpleasant to them. It's not hard to recognize parents about whose unpleasant character traits my patients have preventively warned me, which I was not able to confirm during my house calls, since the alleged nightmare parents were really very pleasant. The discrepancy arises from the fact that the child cannot stand his or her parents because their character types are so opposite.

Next, I'd like to describe the important role the different **character types** have within the family. Let's take a closer look at the already "nonblank slate" of the infant that brings with it certain experiences from earlier incarnations. As a father of three, I can bear witness to that which all experienced parents know, namely that babies by no means come into the world as mentally amorphous beings. On the contrary, one can very early on see the beginnings of character traits that will become ever more pronounced as they grow older.

We look at the personality, already preformed through many reincarnations, that has declared itself in the young infant to be made flesh once again. How will the baby get along with the parents and siblings it chose before birth? Clearly, a great deal depends on how the different character types impinge on each other – since, in the relationship of the four character types to each other, we can make out opposing and attracting character traits. The interplay is like a bunch of magnets whose poles attract or repel each other – except that the character types give us four poles to take into consideration, which determine sympathy or antipathy.

The four character types yield four combinatorial relationship possibilities:
1. Essentially identical (+/+)
2. Dissimilar attracting (+/–)
3. Similar ambivalent (–/+)
4. Dissimilar repelling (–/–)

If we put ourselves in the unborn child's situation, we see that, surprisingly, it can't choose its parents from four character types! Since the parents have already chosen each other as partners long before the child was conceived, the child no longer has the choice of four different character types of a single person, but rather only two character types of two people: that of the father and that of the mother. Let's look at the entire process as a math puzzle: the parents' relationship has already been fixed when they became a couple, which means that the unborn child's options are fewer.

The child no longer chooses from among four character types, but rather from 4 x 4 = 16 constellations. When the child's type is added to the mix, making up the triad of father-mother-child and its added component, this then yields 16 x 4 = 64 possible combinations, e.g., hysteric-hysteric-depressive, and so on. The number 64, by the way, corresponds exactly to the number of possible hexagrams in the Chinese oracle, the ***I Ching*** (book of changes), which begins with *Yin* and *Yang* as the primal polarity. I consider this to

be no accident, so it's no surprise that, in the view of the ancient Chinese, the *I Ching's* so-called "yarrow-stalk oracle" is thought to emulate perfectly the possibilities of the material world. Numerous authors have pointed out the surprising correlations between the genetic code and the oracle book's 64 hexagram signs.

In the discussion that follows, it should be kept in mind that the newborn child brings its predetermined character type into the world. Even the first contact with its parents yields many combinatorial possibilities which can be assigned to good, fair, or poor constellations. The situation gets complicated for all concerned if the child subconsciously rejects one of the parents because it belongs to the polar opposite type. You can then truly speak in terms of the child having selected a difficult karmic path in its prenatal decision. For the child itself, there is the unfortunate addition of the wish to be loved – a child needs love – by the unsympathetic parent, which that parent of course cannot do: you can't jump over your own shadow, so that way lies neurosis.[62]

As we get older, our true character type emerges more and more. Nevertheless, it can happen that the true character type can be hard to recognize in its repressed and displaced form. The many reasons for this – repression, conforming to family and social environment – have already been mentioned, so the interested reader is referred to those earlier chapters. Yet despite all the hide-and-seek, there is an unmistakable indicator of your own character type which I consider to be extraordinarily useful in practical everyday use: **whomever you like right off the bat and whomever you absolutely can't stand best reveals your own character type!** As a rule, you'll tend to like most those people who belong to your own character type, whereas you'll feel the dissimilar repelling type to be strange to unpleasant. Based on character type, there are four possibilities we can realize in our relationships with others, which derive from their attitude to our own character type:

---

[62] One will now, for the rest of one's life, subconsciously grumble at the longed-for parent for having chosen the rejected partner – even though, as a child, one would never have chosen the person if one had been asked at the time. One feels one has been bypassed as a child, and this gets one into a completely insoluble stalemate situation. To my mind, the greater part of a presumably erotically-tinged Oedipal problem complex can be traced back to these character-typical incompatibilities – and the erotic context is of strictly secondary importance!

Similar and Dissimilar Character Types

Character Type	Schizoid	Depressive	Obsessive-compulsive	Hysteric
Identical relationship = best friend (+/+)	Schizoid	Depressive	Obsessive-compulsive	Hysteric
Similar character trait with ambivalence (attracting/repelling) = repression level (–/+)	Obsessive-compulsive	Hysteric	Schizoid	Depressive
Dissimilar (attracting) = ideal partner (+/–)	Depressive	Schizoid	Hysteric	Obsessive-compulsive
Dissimilar (repelling) = high conflict potential (–/–)	Hysteric	Obsessive-compulsive	Depressive	Schizoid

We can virtually predict certain constellations of a relationship if we know the character type involved:

1. In the case of the (in character or nature) *identical relationship* (+/+), for people with the same character type as ours, we "click" immediately and directly on a deep emotional level. We understand these identical people with very little effort, at the so-called "gut level." Our best friend should be of the identical character type, since that gives the friendship an effortless and spontaneous note. For all the mutual sympathy, one misses the tingly tension of the differentness that is felt in relationships involving the other character types.

2. For every character type there exists a particularly favorable polar opposite power, commonly known as the "missing half of the soul." We should definitely marry the *favorable opposite type* (+/–) and declare it to be our "better half," since there is enough of an energetic difference to evoke erotic tension. Yet another advantage is that the characterological compensation process makes us feel much better than we did before. The polar opposite type sees to it that – despite the psychic imbalance that our character type involves – we once again feel complete and centered. In the ideal case, we get back a piece of "heaven on earth" and experience something of the joy of wholeness that our soul lost way back at the beginning when it was consigned (and confined) to a single character type.

3. With respect to the type with *similar character traits* (–/+), experience shows that you get the initial impression of having met up with a highly attractive kindred soul – but it's almost always a case of a treacherous trap into which you've fallen. As time passes, you'll notice that the relationship to this character gets increasingly difficult. You have "two souls in one breast" as far as the relationship to the similar character is concerned, such that conflicts trigger sharply ambivalent feelings that (in the extreme case) can vacillate between love and hate. This tends to lead to an unending succession of quarrels that can't be brought to a satisfactory conclusion. Basically, we can take the similar character trait to be the negative reinforcement and accentuation of our own character type. In a certain sense, it's a parody – which is, however, only amusing for a limited time since, ultimately, our relationship with a similar character type becomes basically neurotic.

4. The last of the four combinatorial possibilities is that character type that stands in *complete polarity* (–/–) and antithesis to our own. These people seem totally inscrutable to us, as if they came from another planet. Their behavior seems odd and illogical to us. At the beginning of a relationship, there might be a great attraction, but the crackling tension often leads tragically to sheer incomprehension. Estranged parties, I have noticed, almost always consist of antipodal character types. One can justifiably say that the antipodal character type represents the biggest stumbling block in the path of personality maturation. A worthier adversary – in the sense of a perfect psychic shadow – cannot be found.

On the basis of the combinations of the four character types, we can accurately predict what will happen with people within marriages and partnerships.

I'd like to summarize and recap the most important points with respect to reincarnation:

- • Each person keeps the same character type over many reincarnations, which type correlates with the person's deepest fundamental fear and is the starting point for personality maturation;
- • Each person prenatally selects the parents (along with extended family, country and society) he wants to reincarnate with;
- • Each soul, at reincarnation, chooses the family (and its general conditions) that gives it the best chances to grow, to make mistakes, to produce friction, and to develop before the background of the search for love.

I'll deal with these points in sequence, because this best brings out their deeper significance. The **_first point_** explains why people develop such a robust character type that can remain intact and stable over the course of many reincarnations. The reason for this stability has to do with the Central Conflict, whose psychoenergetic solidity is sustained over many reincarnations. If we had no Central Conflict, we would in all likelihood wander around aimlessly like amorphous spirits and would be totally incapable of developing. A house needs a solid foundation – and so, it would seem, does our soul.[63] To be sure, our "spiritual house" may be furnished differently in each successive incarnation, but its basic floor plan remains essentially the same.

The **_second point_** regarding prenatal selection of one's parents has also been thoroughly discussed here. At reincarnation time, everybody has a choice as to which parents, family members and other relatives – and, furthermore, in which country – with whom they wish to come into the world. I've already mentioned that it is a subconscious process. I sometimes get the impression that certain people were unable to come to a decision before birth, and now suffer from the problem of being psychically stuck in their indecision.

We tend to assume that parental lack of feeling is the cause of later miseries and emotional illnesses ("It's all your fault for having been so cold and unloving to me!"). From the reincarnation viewpoint – under hypnosis and in deep trance – we consciously chose these parents in order to have certain experiences. The reincarnation therapist and JUNG disciple Roger WOOLGER has thought long and hard about the amazing and unusual-sounding inferences that follow from accepting reincarnation as a real phenomenon: "_In looking for the causes of psychic trauma in former lives, we stand all of Freudianism and traditional child psychology on its head. If one traces the problems that children have back to events in earlier lives, then these difficulties can no longer be ascribed exclusively to parental misdemeanor._ (cit.n. WOOLGER)"

Therefore, if we complain about our parents, we are simply retrospectively bemoaning our own erroneous decision: "How nice if I could have been the son of a popular millionaire Hollywood star!" Or if we meet some particularly kind and warm-hearted people that make us wish they could have been our parents instead: "Oh, if only I had had these good-hearted parents!" For some reason, we did _not_ choose these good-hearted folk. The same thematic complex applies as well to our choice of society (capitalist or fascist, rich or poor, and so on), so that we are forced to the unsettling conclusion that we are completely responsible for our fate.

To my mind, the feeling (during a hypnotic trance) of having consciously chosen to reincarnate in this current life is (in reality and nevertheless) an after-the-fact interpretation. We most likely deceive ourselves because too much passivity in the selection process would be uncomfortable. Evidently, as unborn souls we choose our new life from deep in our psyche, quite subconsciously, such that our Central Conflict plays a decisive role in the process. Crucial to our later considerations is the belief that we didn't make a stupid choice, but rather would like to give our soul, in this new incarnation, the best chances for growth and maturation.

When it comes to selecting parents, we choose the type with whom we are most familiar. Our soul's inner wisdom plays an important role in the final decision, since we choose the family with the best growth opportunities. As with a strong magnet, we are drawn to a family whose character-type makeup and emotional problems best match up with our own themes (**_third point_**). It's like a jigsaw puzzle whose individual pieces interlock perfectly.

Most families I have examined show a mixture of character types subject to certain rules and regularities. And since we can best develop when we're exposed to as wide a variety of character types as possible, we tend to choose a "variegated bouquet." I'd next like to present a family structure that is very widespread in today's society with its high divorce rate: families characterized by much strife and disharmony, and split into two warring camps.

[63] Symbolically, the house or home has always been equated with the people themselves. We say that someone comes "from a good house" or grew up "in a broken home." In depth psychology, the home is equated with the psyche – and that which, in dreams, takes place hidden within the walls of a house is occurring figuratively in the psyche.

Here is an example of a dysfunctional family:

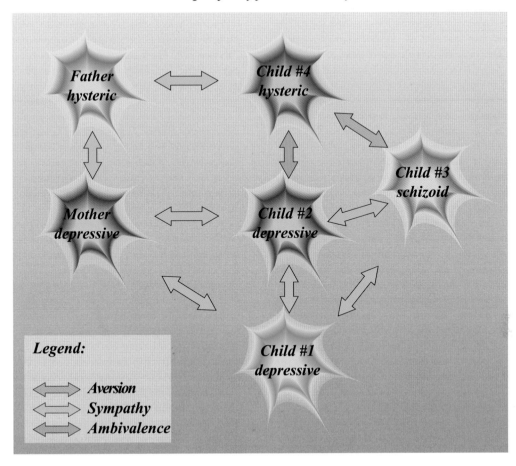

The couple married quite young and, over the years, it became increasingly clear to both parties that they didn't understand each other at all. The wife said that they had been too inexperienced, at the time they got married, to notice this ("... almost children still ..."). This couple's actual marriage problem is rooted in their character-type differences, which constitute an opposite/ambivalent relationship (hysteric and depressive). Empirically, such couples have a sharply divided emotional relationship in which rejection and affection alternate constantly – which is of course no basis for a reliable relationship of mutual trust. People in this situation are forever talking at cross purposes because each basically doesn't understand the other, being of essentially different natures.

This frequently leads to vicious power struggles ("Who wears the pants in this family?!"). In these kinds of relationships, the man often becomes a tyrannical dictator who exploits the woman as a slave and accomplice. Behind the scenes, the tyrant turns into an emotional wimp who preserves his authority by beating his wife, afterwards often tending to self-pity, while his wife comes to despise him, becoming emotionally embittered

and sinking into mute resignation.

In one specific case, the man tends to play down the marriage's problems ("We're doing basically OK, really ...") and to erect a façade of familial contentment and a seemingly intact marriage. In the American town that the couple lives in, "keeping up appearances" is extremely important, thanks to the gossip and rumors that pervade such communities. The father, moreover, tends as a hysteric to return quickly to the order of the day after their brief but vicious arguments, thus seeing to it that the world around him is once again in working order ("beer, broads, and baseball" are his core concerns). Drinking so much beer has made him severely overweight, and his high blood pressure puts him at high risk of a heart attack.

The depressive mother throws herself into raising the children and running the family. She only complains if you ask her pointed questions, otherwise trying to be as inconspicuous as possible. As a depressive, the weekly "hen parties" with her girlfriends and her volunteer community work are more important than anything to her. The mother is a short chubby type who likes to scurry about the house in a dressing gown until noon, and whose daily schedule is filled with trips to the supermarket, to the kids' various schools, and to girlfriends' houses.

Of the four children, the youngest – whose nature is most like the father's and who also has the hysteric character type – became the father's declared favorite rather quickly. This child can "read" the father better than the others can, and dares criticize him fairly strongly without fear of retribution. The oldest child shares the mother's character type, trying to get along with all family members and, in particular, to referee parental arguments and be a conciliatory influence. The second depressive child tags along in the slipstream of the older sibling.

The middle child (schizoid character type) is the outsider ("Cuckoo"), quickly having mutated into the Black Sheep of the Family, and with whom the others have developed a kind of love/hate relationship. It was reported to me unanimously that each family member has a bone to pick with the "Cuckoo Kid." In fact, the reason for the medical consultation has to do with the problems the family is having with the "Cuckoo Kid" – who, on top of everything else, has a physical disability. He lives during the week in a home for the handicapped, coming home for the weekends. Evidently they all expected me to do a miraculous makeover on the "Cuckoo Kid," turning him into a healthy and fully integrated family member. During the family's visits, I also examined the rest of the family, so that I became familiar with all their various little aches and pains, plus the psychoenergetic readings for each person. I also tested out the Central Conflicts of each family member, which became the basis for the family description presented here.

When I (somewhat shocked) asked the mother whether the "Cuckoo Kid" had a good relationship with <u>any</u> family member, she replied: his grandfather. Only between these two does there seem to exist a noticeably cordial and close relationship – as if they had known each other forever. Based on my experience in similar cases, I suspect that the "Cuckoo Kid's" reincarnation into this family was due exclusively to this very beloved person – who, by the way, had also always been considered an outsider in the family fold. The "Cuckoo Kid" had simply (resignedly) accepted the other family members when making his prenatal selection. This is easier to understand if you keep in mind that schizoids (such as the "Cuckoo Kid") don't care all that much for the company of most people anyhow, which surely made the prenatal decision easier in this case.

Evaluation and discussion:
In this example of a dysfunctional family, we find many regularities that illustrate the dynamic processes within the family – processes which bear the germ of numerous conflicts and psychosomatic disorders. To begin with the youngest members, the siblings, in early youth still exhibit very few sources of friction or conflict material. Despite character type differences, children often get along amazingly well. It's usually with the onset of puberty that the crisis-laden disputes begin, with the family members whose character types are antipodal and hostile.

Our initial question – i.e., why some people create difficult situations for themselves by choosing inappropriate or discordant parents – applies of course to all four children, where the oldest and second-oldest have a discordant character type relationship with the father and the youngest with the mother. The "Cuckoo Kid" has it especially bad; he doesn't feel at ease with any of them. The children (as likewise the parents) are separated by a "character type ditch" – so it's no surprise that shouting and arguing has been a constant in this family.

In closing, I'd like to reveal what the final outcome was in this case: the Central Conflict of each family member was treated, after which they all felt much more relaxed, better and more energy-laden – which is what most patients report once they're rid of their major conflicts. Family harmony has been increased greatly, and all of them counted it a great success that the "Cuckoo Kid" was now much friendlier and more accessible and (for instance) no longer made a mess of the sisters' bedroom, nor broke things, which had earlier often led to quarrels. Also, the physical handicap (epileptic seizures = schizoid character type = Central Conflict in Crown Chakra!) was much improved, with milder seizures occurring less often.

This dysfunctional family example reveals a number of regularities and patterns. All parties were strong, distinctive characters, each having his/her own will and clearly delineated personality. Evidently, these people didn't make it easy for themselves, but chose each other as representing particularly demanding challenges. One reason is their strength of character: in my experience, strong personalities tend to grow up in difficult families. Critics will object that I am confusing cause and effect, but I stick by my assertion and repeat that I'm firmly convinced of the reality of fixed character types and prenatal parent selection. It seems to me that the most striking proof is the fact that children come into the world with a fixed character type; experienced parents can confirm this. Moreover, you can psychoenergetically detect Central Conflicts even in newborn babies – yet another strong argument in favor of my thesis.

Now begins the whole drama of the "quarrel marriage" of the parents who, in their youthful inexperience, made a characterologically unfortunate partner choice and then compounded the mistake by getting married. How the choice of partner comes about in terms of individual steps, and which psychoenergetic mechanisms (such as sympathy and antipathy) result therefrom, which can be derived from the various character type combinations – will be covered in greater detail in the upcoming chapter. At this point, all that interests us with respect to family formation is the finished "nest" that the candidate parents place at the disposal of potential children for their reincarnation by consummating their pair formation through copulation. The child then has only the choice between various "nests," but at the time of its conception has no influence on the parents' choice of partners, since it is far too late for that!

Family members can learn a great deal from each other

precisely *because* of the huge character differences between them. Particularly piquant dramas emerge in those cases in which one, as a child, becomes the misfit (cuckoo) of the family. Whereas most people choose at least one parent with similar vibrations (of the same character type), there are some particularly brave souls who (as in the case of the dysfunctional family here described) for reincarnation seek out totally foreign parents, and must then eke out their lives as lonely "cuckoos." In my experience, the opposite-sex parent will then often belong to the opposed/attractive character type, so that there is usually a particularly strong Oedipal complication as well – which, as it were, puts the capper on the whole affair. Such persons seem to want to make it particularly hard on themselves – and this dovetails perfectly with the physical disability that the "Cuckoo Kid" in our example also chose prenatally: clearly, the "Cuckoo Kid" wanted to leave no instructive stone unturned and therefore opted for every conceivable adversity. From the viewpoint of the eager-to-learn soul, it thereby made the best possible choice, no matter how bizarre it might seem.

Choice of Partner

Frankly, I am not a fan of long engagements: they give couples time to discover each other's character before the wedding – which is, I believe, never advisable.

(Oscar Wilde)

When doing psychoenergetic testing on married couples, I often noticed that happiness and stability of the partnership depended crucially on the relationship between the character types. One reason is the subtle-body processes that are analogous to the polarity of magnets. The well-known geopathic radiation researcher Ernst HARTMANN recognized that people are either *Yin* or *Yang* polarity, and that same-polarity couples often were childless. Opposite polarity thus seems to be very important to fertility. There has to be a gradient, so that sufficient life force can flow for impregnation.[64]

The reason for different polarities is the different character types, each of which brings about a particular orientation of our energetic force field: either positive or negative, Yang or Yin (This has been mentioned in earlier chapters.). We perceive functioning polarity as an essential coherence and physically as a good, correctly sensed feeling. With proper polarity, we experience the unmistakable sensation of having arrived at our true center; only then do we begin to feel really good. We speak in terms of other concepts such as our "essential nature," by which we mean specific preferences and (in part) even quirky peculiarities. We excuse ourselves to others by saying "Well, that's just the way I am!" We don't mean anything biological by this, just our character type, expressed via physical sensation. "Character" is therefore not only an attribute of our psyche, but also (and above all) of our body!

The other factor crucially affecting the ultimate destiny of a relationship is not energetic/physical but rather psychic attributes of the respective character type. Obviously, the better people understand each other, the better they can live together. Now, another person's psyche – for some initially obscure reason – seems to get more veiled the more the sexual element mixes into the relationship. We know all too well that many lovers fall prey, in the beginning, to a dire delusion that can always be traced back to a strongly-felt erotic and emotional attraction. "Love is blind" as the saying goes – and there's no denying that, without the befud-

dling and befogging effect of Eros, it would be quite a different world (much less populated, at the least). Thanks to sexual attraction, Mother Nature has seen to it that humanity does not die out, and that people are drawn together to form couples. During the continued course of a relationship, however, one spends more and more time in the everyday world and correspondingly less of it in the snug coziness of the connubial bed. Sex recedes into the background, until one eventually realizes that the partner is (or, better put: should be) becoming ever more important as an emotional support, friend, and conversational partner.

Over time, all intimate relationships work their way into the subconscious, there to impinge on ever deeper layers. The partners bare themselves emotionally to each other as they get to know each other better, and become aware of mannerisms that they had not noticed earlier on. The French philosopher VOLTAIRE once commented ironically on this: "*The first month of marriage is honey and the second is absinthe.*" It helps to know that absinthe is a major ingredient in vermouth, considered to be an excellent pick-me-up (i.e., if you're "down"). My own grandmother was fond of saying: "*Whoever has problems also has liquor!*"

However, many couples are not prepared to go so far with each other that it might lead to mutual "dis-illusionment." One can see that many couples "fake" harmony, in the firm conviction that they won't (or at least shouldn't) hurt each other because that's simply not done. Often, external problems will then be the stumbling block that rocks the boat of pretend harmony – overdue bills, say, or an extramarital affair. A state of pretend harmony is characterized by the fact that, in these relationships, "the sun always shines," only until the first serious problems crop up and the façade begins to crumble. Pretend harmony can also consist of the refusal to develop further. People can drift apart as soon as they develop more clearly-outlined personalities – and so, in order to avoid this tragic turn of events, the relationship is allowed to stagnate at a low level by not allowing either person any freedom of movement for development.

Going against the conventional wisdom of many marriage and relationship counselors, I'd like to say that the concept of a "relationship ability" is often just a fairy tale! Couples quarrel, shout at each other, and, after a while, get

---

[64] Because couples exposed to strong geopathic radiation are often childless – which likewise leads to energetic blocks – subtle energy seems to be a major factor in fertility. The ancient fertility cults such as the Cult of Dionysus took such factors into account, but all knowledge of the energetic component of fertility has been forgotten today.

divorced – simply because they are incompatible types. Or couples notice after a while that they have nothing more to say to each other (which amounts to the same thing). Or they develop in different directions and then notice that they can no longer live together. It usually has nothing to do with the inability to enter into a relationship per se – and a counselor who tinkers around with "relationship ability" (as so often happens) doesn't improve matters. In my experience, many couples' unhappy marriages have nothing to do with any fundamental incompatibility between men and women – as many a smart-aleck would have us believe – but simply with hasty and unconsidered unions of differing character types.

I'd next like to present the different constellations resulting from the combination of the four character types. Each of us, with our respective character type, is constantly faced with the choice of whom we want to live with and whom not. Even in the remotest regions of India, where bride and groom are assigned to each other by the parents, the roll-of-the-dice outcome among the possible constellations will be the same: drawing from a large uniformly-distributed population of marriageable candidates, there is a 25% chance of hitting the jackpot and winding up with the ideal partner. By this I mean the dissimilar attracting type, i.e., for schizoid, depressives; for obsessive-compulsives, hysterics. In my experience, these marriages are usually happy and harmonious. Later in this chapter, I'll get into why this is so.

The second-best alternative is also a 25% possibility, namely the essentially identical type, i.e., when a hysteric marries another hysteric. Both partners having the same character type, this constellation also has good chances of resulting in a satisfactory and harmonious marriage. The remaining 50% is evenly distributed between the two worst alternatives: the similar character type (e.g., schizoid/obsessive-compulsive) or the dissimilar repelling type (e.g., schizoid/hysteric). Based on what I've observed in hundreds of couples, these last two variants are always problematic over the long run, often leading to divorce, because the parties are unwilling to compromise or feel increasingly unhappy. In these unfortunate marriages, an affair is often the alleged grounds for divorce, even though the real reason is the mutual incompatibility of character types.

I've noticed that the pairings observable in daily life are evenly distributed among the four variants. I can only speculate why that might be – but I suspect that the remote rural Indian practice (parents choosing marriage partners for their children) would not deviate significantly from the randomness with which modern people seek out marriage partners. One can thus also understand why it is that, statistically, roughly half of all couples have chosen the "wrong" partner. You have about a 50/50 chance of falling in love with the right (or wrong) partner, and it speaks for the correctness of my supposition that the divorce rate in

Austria and Switzerland, for example, is approximately 40% – with a rising trend toward 50%.

I'd now like to describe the pairing variants, starting with the best and ending with the worst:

In my experience, only the **_dissimilar attracting type_** is a long-term ideal partner, because only this type ideally complements our essential nature with what we are missing for emotional wholeness. Most happy partnerships are composed of dissimilar attracting types. This means, specifically, that a schizoid prefers a depressive partner, and a hysteric an obsessive-compulsive. Why is this? The first reason is the antipodal energetic orientation: schizoids, like obsessive-compulsives, have Yang polarity, while hysterics and depressives are Yin-polarized. This leads to antipodal types being good for each other: you simply feel better with your "better half" by your side. Another benefit is that counter-polarity markedly elevates fertility.

Dissimilar attracting types are also the best choice from the standpoint of complementary character traits: obsessive-compulsives learn to "take it easy" from hysterics, while hysterics learn the importance of clear-cut structures from obsessives. For schizoids, depressives – with their strong emphasis on emotions and sociability – counterbalance their intellectuality and solitariness, whereas depressives learn from schizoids to draw personal boundaries and trust their intellect. The beneficial partnership of dissimilar attracting types is like the story of the blind and the lame: they combine their (dis)abilities to their mutual benefit.

The second-best pairings are the _identical_ or harmonious character types: you simply choose your own kind. This is logical, since no one understands you better. To others, such married couples often come across like brother and sister (like Hansel and Gretel, say), seemingly made for each other and having an ideal marriage. However, the downside is mounting boredom and stagnation, since the tension-generating antipodal element is missing. Consequently, there is not only diminishing sexual interest, but in many cases even infertility – and even when they succeed in these respects, harmonious couples often have apathetic children who are usually the same character type as the parents. From the outside, such families look like perfect, model families, and I don't deny that this harmony arises from genuine feelings and real circumstances – yet these families not infrequently disintegrate when the boredom simply gets unbearable.

The next-worst alternative involves what I reckon as the problematic relationships, made up of _similar_ types: a schizoid marries an obsessive-compulsive, or a depressive a hysteric. Like the harmonious identical types, these couples lack energetic dissimilarity, since both are Yang (schizoid/obsessive-compulsive) or Yin (depressive/hysteric) polarity. Such couples are often childless and, with time, sexually disinterested. Yet the real problem with these pairs is the neuroticism: the partner's character type is a caricature or a pathological exaggeration of one's own traits. Thus, for

Own Character Type	Schizoid	Depressive	Obsessive-compulsive	Hysteric
Dissimilar (attracting) = ideal partnership (+/–)	Depressive	Schizoid	Hysteric	Obsessive-compulsive
Identical relationship = friendly, but often non-erotic (+/+)	Schizoid	Depressive	Obsessive-compulsive	Hysteric
Similar character trait (neurotic) (–/+)	Obsessive-compulsive	Hysteric	Schizoid	Depressive
Dissimilar (repelling) = often unhappy marriage (–/–)	Hysteric	Obsessive-compulsive	Depressive	Schizoid

schizoids, obsessive-compulsive partners induce neurotic amplification of undesirable character traits, making them more pig-headed, cranky, and morally authoritarian (a "head case"). For depressives, hysteric partners lead to emotional distortions, as the depressive's tragic but genuine nature thereby suddenly turns flirtatious, manneristic, and deformed ("too shrill"). Similar rules also apply, in reverse, to the other two character types. Obsessive-compulsives should actually develop compensatory playful traits, but are inveigled into even greater intellectual strictness by schizoid partners. Hysterics should really structure themselves better, but instead get more emotionally charged up by depressive partners, magnifying their lability.

The worst option is the dissimilar repelling type. There is often a great deal of erotic sexual tension in the stormy initial phase of such an antipodal relationship, occasionally with addictive overtones (similar to the pseudo-kick discussed earlier on). Film fans will recall the German classic *Der blaue Engel* [*The Blue Angel*] with Marlene Dietrich playing the hysteric showgirl and Emil Jannings as the schizoid Professor Unrat [Dr. Garbage] who falls head over heels for the vaudeville hoofer and tragically winds up in the gutter. The tragedy of these pairings is based, on one hand, on an erotic attraction which can lead to sexual bondage,[65] and on the other hand on profound essential differences: those involved characterize such extreme differences as "fire and water." The extremely antipodal partner not only has a completely unfamiliar nature, but also (in conflict situations) an argumentative style that wears down and quickly exhausts the other person. So far, I have found very, very few long-lasting happy marriages composed of antipodal couples. They dominate the divorce-rate statistics.

Like flipping a coin, we have a 50/50 chance of a happy future when we enter into a relationship. The big hurdle in selecting a partner is that the ideal partner cannot be found immediately. The big question, it seems to me, is how, from the outset, we can improve the odds of a happy partnership. To do this, we have to know in advance where we stand with the other person. But how do we tell whether the other is the "Mr. (or Mrs.) Right" who will be good for us over the long run? Only experience, and taking a long, hard look at what our partner's psychic core consists of and what his or her external shell (*persona* mask) is made up of.

For instance, a person with a tough emotional core, such as is found in schizoids and obsessive-compulsives, often has a soft shell ("soft on the outside, hard on the inside"). The opposite is true of the depressive and hysteric types ("hard on the outside, soft on the inside"). The dissimilar attracting type will always have precisely the opposite kind of emotional core than we have – i.e., a hard one if ours is soft (and vice-versa). The tricky thing is that we often mistake the shell for the core, and are thus quite easily deceived. Any woman with life experience has known plenty of men who

---

[65] Owing to the soul's great vulnerability, I am against free polygamous love for fundamental reasons. In my experience and that of many patients, nothing good comes out of **polygamy**, although there are, to be sure, phases in life – e.g., puberty and early adolescence – in which polygamy, as an inexperienced, groping quest, represents a transitional solution. There may also be societies having other social groupings such as polygamy, but these societies have nothing to do with us. In our culture, monogamy is the best solution for all concerned. It's precisely because of the harmful emotional consequences of extramarital affairs that the choice of partner seems to me to be of paramount importance for our whole happiness in life; two-timing is in all likelihood the result of unfortunate relationships.

act tough at first, only to be unmasked, later on in the cold light of day as "wimps." Conversely, many a man has found out, to his amazement, that a tender, cuddly woman can, in crisis situations, reveal an unexpectedly tough emotional core – and is then daunted and paralyzed by such a "mannish" woman.

The trouble with finding the right dissimilar attracting type is that, in the initial stages of a relationship, we can so easily delude ourselves into mistaking the shell for the core. For example, if we personally are soft inside, then we need to look for a partner with a firm core to give us much-needed stability. On the other hand, a "hard-core" person will be on the lookout for the gentility and peaceableness of a "soft-core" type in order to strike a balance. That's exactly what would happen with a dissimilar attracting type, if we could find one right off the bat! However, because we often camouflage our actual character traits and put on an antipodal mask, the potential partner is often deceived – at least half the time, in fact – which leads to a predictably difficult and unfortunate relationship.

In the light of all this, one naturally asks what practical advice should young people get who are actively seeking partners. The simplest solution would be for all potential partners to wear badges (like branded cattle) that would make singling out the right partner a lot easier. In a sense, these "badges" do exist, even if they're not visible, and making use of these identifying features is better than relying on random chance. Those who familiarize themselves with the personality traits of the respective types as I have carefully described them in earlier chapters will have fairly little trouble finding a suitable partner, because I have identified enough traits to aid in distinguishing between the different character types.

My second suggestion is to practice being honest with yourself with respect to your type because, in order to find the right partner, you must first know what type you are. Here too, I hope I have given enough useful tips. An important source of self-knowledge can also be found in character descriptions of yourself by close family members, since they know very well where your weak points are and what your sometimes concealed nature actually amounts to. And the third (very useful) tip is the spontaneous feeling of antipathy when you meet an unsuitable partner ("internal alarm bells").

Now I'm sure that many readers will be rubbing their eyes in bewilderment, wondering what on earth I mean by such a strange-sounding sentence – since it seems like a really bad idea to choose a spontaneously unappealing partner. In fact, my own experiences and my detailed questioning of numerous good friends and many patients have brought to light the astounding realization that most people sense right away, in their first impression, that something or other isn't quite right about partner X – be it an instinctive feeling of antipathy, fear, anxiety, or other feelings that signal danger.

But, shortly thereafter, the seductive siren songs of eroticism becloud the mind, and we quickly forget that initial uneasy feeling. However, we should take this initial feeling quite seriously! And, assuming that we're not yet aware of such feelings, we should stay on the alert until we notice these inner warning signals – which are, after all, trying to save us from impending calamity. We would do well to trust our inner voice and give these unsuitable partners a wide berth.

In closing, I'd like to add that it's entirely possible for couples to be perfectly happy even though their character type pairing indicates otherwise. Now, I myself have yet to meet such a couple, but I suppose that such strokes of luck are possible in the individual case. In this context, it seems to me that the most important prerequisite for happiness is mental maturity and a minimum of large active conflicts in the partner. To simplify somewhat, what is needed for contented partnerships to develop – independently of the respective character types – is especially loveable, emotionally mature, and spiritually advanced people.

Karma

*Many people lead lives of such stupefying routine
that it's hard to believe they were ever alive.*

(Stanislaw Jerzy Lec)

I had already mentioned in earlier chapters that depth psychology tends to confirm that something like Karma and rebirth must exist, since otherwise many incidents and events – and many aspects of our energy-medicine measurements – make no sense. Karma is the essential missing piece of the puzzle that makes the phenomena of the spiritual journey and psychoenergetic upward development comprehensible. For example, it is only through rebirth that one understands why newborn children come into the world with gigantic conflicts and spiritually highly developed souls (which they could not have picked up and developed in the womb). Basically, this can only have come from former lives, just as MOZART's highly developed talent must have, because such abilities are inconceivable without a certain amount of training and education, which these geniuses bring with them from past lives.

Now these are not the only arguments that substantiate the presence of multiple earthly lives. Researchers such as STEVENSON have collected persuasive evidence that children can remember earlier lives in surprising detail that corresponds precisely to historical fact. A careful study of the available data should persuade even skeptics that there might be something to the phenomenon of rebirth – keeping in mind that nobody can prove beyond the shadow of a doubt that it really does take place. I'd like to repeat that there is a very high correlation between being spiritually highly developed and believing in the possibility of reincarnation. This should compel an opinion shift in favor of reincarnation, since more and more people are becoming ever more spiritually highly developed.

The doctrine of Karma and rebirth is by no means a recent discovery, since it is the ancient empirical knowledge of many spiritual systems.

Great thinkers such as PLATO, GOETHE, and NIETZSCHE were convinced of the reality of rebirth. As we know, the doctrine of Karma is an essential element of Eastern religions such as Hinduism and Buddhism. According to experts, there are strong indications that early Christianity included a belief in the repeated return of souls to earth. Jesus is said to have more than once referred to reincarnation as fact – which is not surprising, inasmuch as Judaism maintained that the newborn child incorporates the soul of an ancestor. The Talmud (the Bible of Judaism, so to speak) says that Adam was reborn as David. Since Jesus interpreted the Jewish scriptures with the scholars in the temple, he would have also accepted reincarnation as fact, because any unheard-of departure from tradition would have surely been remarked upon by his disciples.

The well-known church father ORIGEN was convinced that souls return to earth repeatedly, and in their choice of return are likely motivated by earlier victories and defeats – an idea that I can fully confirm from my own experiences! The Council of Constantinople in 533 A.D. banned the doctrine of rebirth from Christian orthodoxy, evidently because reincarnation's imponderability called the church's authority into question. After the ecclesiastical ban, the knowledge of rebirth went underground and became a secretly held belief of mystic sects such as the Rosicrucians and other secret orders, which has not necessarily promoted its broad acceptance in the general population. The Romantic Era saw a revival of belief in reincarnation that continues to this day, being particularly widespread in intellectually open minded and spiritually oriented circles.

I mentioned that research into the deep subconscious has yielded strong indications of the validity of Karma and rebirth. Modern investigations of people who, in trance and lucid dreams, reported on earlier lives, have yielded contradictory results. In some cases, the experiences of supposed former lives could be traced back to newspaper articles or novels that the subjects had read as a children or teenagers and then forgotten, only later on to mistake these stories for their own earlier earthly lives. One should therefore not blindly believe such karmic narratives, but rather exercise skeptical common sense.

Still, the most important argument in favor of rebirth lies in the logic of the soul itself, in which an overall picture coalesces that, without rebirth, would simply make no sense whatsoever. Skeptics will object that this hardly constitutes proof, but I'd like to counter by pointing out that modern science has always made use of hypotheses that have only later turned out to be correct. Certain basic assumptions of EINSTEIN's theory of relativity have been confirmed only recently by cutting-edge technology. Most physicists were nevertheless long ago convinced that EINSTEIN's hypotheses must be correct. I am confident that future research will confirm the existence of Karma and reincarnation.

In my experience, belief in rebirth seems increasingly to become certainty the higher a person's causal body readings are in the energy test.[66] This should come as no surprise since, in the view of all great spiritual leaders, our remembrance of karmic experiences begins the moment our personality has become strong enough to face its own karmic past – i.e., the point at which the soul, through its own strength, can withstand these extremely repressed and emotionally agitating experiences. This is the case when the causal reading has become larger. I further suspect that false rebirth narratives (such as the woman mentioned earlier, who reported as belonging to a former life excerpts of novels she had read as a child) are much more frequent among those with low causal readings. A high causal reading thus seems to be an important guarantee that a person has reliable memories of earlier lives.

The researcher Ian STEVENSON has queried children about their earlier lives and then sought out the locations and the people of these presumed earlier lives. Children seem to recall former lives more easily, which I think is due to their open causal body (which closes up more in late adolescence with the emergence of conflicts). STEVENSON was able to confirm fascinating narrations of former lives in great detail, in which the children could not possibly have had – in any way, shape, or form in this life – any knowledge of the persons named or events described. Other researchers have come up with similar results, such that the majority of those doing research in this area now consider the phenomenon of reincarnation to be highly likely.

Because the first two Chakras are still quite active in the first few years of life, and thus enable direct access to deep subconscious levels, we can as children much more easily recall past earthly lives. Later on, memories get deposited so deeply in the subconscious that we can no longer recollect them. To my mind, this is definitely a sensible protective mechanism that forces us to look toward the future. As in the biblical story of Lot's wife, who was turned into a pillar of salt for looking back, we would all most probably suffer great harm if we could remember our earlier Karma. Many experiences would be too painful to endure without losing our emotional equilibrium.

In fact, some psychic ailments and distresses affect us so strongly because the sensible "backward-look barrier" to earlier lives has become perforated. The former life then acquires a magnetic/hypnotic attraction, such that the people involved seem to be "wistfully" chained to their long-ago destiny and can no longer get free of it. Such cases usually involve extremely large conflicts that hold the victims cap-

tive in their spell. To break the spell you have to dissolve the underlying large conflict. Thus, any resuscitation of huge ancient karmic themes carries the risk of psychotic derailment – particularly if such painful topics are activated prematurely. I have seen more than a few patients whose severe psychological problems began when overly stimulating psycho-techniques were employed that reactivated ancient karmic themes.

When I was in medical school, I was one of the skeptics who thought that rebirth was sheer speculation. In this book's introduction, I mentioned an earlier phase in my life during which I had some strong spiritual experiences that led to considerable opening up of my causal body. Since then, I have become increasingly convinced of the reality of rebirth, and I have been discovering countries and landscapes – that I am magically attracted to – which are ever more clearly sites from former lives. The same applies to certain hobbies, passions, and preferences, which also seem to be strongly shaped by former existences. It seems almost redundant to mention that, among the people close to you, you'll recognize many who were part of your former life.

Certain trends in therapy, such as "Rebirthing" from the USA, specifically work with trance/hypnotic states, which are supposed to help people remember earlier lives. I have come to believe that this can just confuse people, and it doesn't much help them to be looking for solutions to current problems in their past lives. When reincarnation memories arise of their own accord, that's certainly a normal process in the context of self-discovery – but this kind of recollection should not be forced. I therefore don't think it's a good idea to think too much about past lives and drag up old animosities: "In an earlier life, my wicked boss burned me at the stake … ," and similar nonsense that I get from some of my patients.

Ultimately, these supposed experiences serve as "collateral" to confirm hostile patterns in this life through earlier karmic misdeeds and thus reinforce one's righteous indignation ("My boss is an even bigger bastard than I thought!"). Also, I very much question whether such recollections have any basis in fact, or are just figments of a fevered imagination.[67] In fact, my own experience has revealed to me a very divergent background, in that many clairvoyants or reincarnation therapists can subconsciously give free rein to their own hostile impulses by leading their clients astray into unfavorable situations.

Psychoanalytic research tell us that patients' subconscious subject matter tends to adapt to what their therapists expect/want to hear, e.g., patients talk Freudian to classical-

---

[66] The depth psychologist and Jungian Roger WOOLGER has arrived at some fascinating observations based on reincarnation sessions. He comes up with the same evolutionary interpretation that I put forth in this book, as he writes: "A universe without good and evil is as inconceivable as one without highs and lows – for about this axis turns all of spiritual and phenomenal reality. They generate the dynamic tension of opposites without which created reality could not become aware of itself."

---

[67] Even supposed child abuse (so often reported) very often has its source in subconscious fantasies! Often, Oedipal entanglements and ancient previous karmic experiences are projected onto the accused parent, relative, or teacher, even though they're figments of the subconscious imagination. This leads to situations that are very hard to straighten out.

ly trained analysts but Jungian to depth-psychologists from the Jungian school, and so on. In my experience, patients with bad reincarnation experiences often seem not to be experiencing actual material from their own subconscious, but rather products of their imagination having to do with "shadow impulses" – or the reincarnation therapist's own subconscious. If therapists are harboring any subconscious hostility – which is frequently the case, in my experience – they can wind up subconsciously transferring these feelings to their patients.

And even when therapists and clairvoyants only wish the best for their patients, they wind up harming them anyway by making them sicker with such depictions and experiences. Moreover, the resurfacing of old karmic matter always carries the risk that "You'll never be able to banish the spirits you've conjured up!" (GOETHE's *The Sorcerer's Apprentice*). Subtly, new and fresh energy is infused into the old conflict pattern in the form of attention, emotional turmoil, and vital life force, whereby the conflict is charged up and unnecessarily invigorated. It's much better to dissolve energetically the underlying conflicts in order to deprive them of the "culture medium" for further sick-making activities.

One can see that (in the case of the aforementioned secretary with the evil boss – as soon as her own conflicts have been healed, that is) her supposedly evil boss is just an unhappy person who can easily be coaxed out of his frustration with a few kind words, instead of constantly holding up to him, as the secretary in our example did, "What a bastard he really is." Thoughts are vibrations that are subconsciously transmitted to other people, which makes it easy to interchange cause and effect. When you are centered – by having had your conflicts dissolved – you have much friendlier thoughts, which quickly and lastingly improves the workplace climate (as in the example of the secretary who was mobbed).

Next, I'd like to define the term **Karma** a bit more precisely. Hinduism and Buddhism see Karma as the law of cause and effect – often misunderstood as a purely moral venue of divine power that (sooner or later) punishes evil deeds. But the significance of Karma far surpasses any purely moral venue and, because of its importance, I'd like to describe this in greater detail. The Karma doctrine is indissolubly bound up with the idea of rebirth. The gist of Karma is that past deeds must be viewed as the actual cause of present and future events – as in the old saying "You can't get something from nothing." The ancient Indian view is that it is a law which permits no exceptions and cannot be circumvented. This means that one can't do something bad and then run away. If the consequences don't catch up with you in the present life, the expiatory Karma-extinguishing effect will happen in a later one. Karma is thus equated with guilt that must at some point be expiated.

Good deeds also generate Karma, so that it doesn't automatically mean being guilty of having done something bad. Obviously, good deeds also have consequences, and they must also be "repaid." In this case, we wind up with a positive balance in a kind of karmic savings account, in which Karma "owes" us. To use another analogy, there is a differential that needs to be compensated. Since compensating good Karma means a reward of some kind, we tend to think of it as being much better than bad Karma – and yet, there are indications from spiritual masters that bad Karma (as in the form of poor behavior patterns) enables us to mature and grow significantly faster. This should not, of course, be taken as *carte blanche* to commit evil deeds.

To the modern Western way of thinking, it seems utterly absurd and irrational to think in terms of spiritual connections that depend on the beliefs of the individual, as is the case with Karma. Unlike "enlightened" Westerners, people who believe in rebirth and Karma consider behavior to be realistic and rational when it takes higher realities such as Karma into account. For now, I prefer not to go into who's right, since there can never be ironclad proof that Karma exists, just indications (but, as I'd like to stress once more: strong indications!).

But whether or not we believe in Karma seems to me not so much a question of right or wrong as of morality, as far as the mass of humanity is concerned. Since "to err is human," even people who believe in Karma will do wrong, and then regret it. It's just that, unlike the Karma deniers, they know that they'll eventually have to make reparations for their misdeeds. You might ask at this point what difference it makes if a person believes in a punishment to come or not. Criminology has long known that even draconian measures such as the death sentence don't lower the murder rate. Still, after everything I've observed, I'm convinced that belief in Karma has a far greater downward effect on the crime statistics than earthly retribution. People who believe in Karma inhabit a different kind of consciousness that gives rise to more careful, friendly, and gentle behavior – as one can clearly observe in the Asian cultures. Reviving belief in Karma would be very beneficial in raising the overall level of morality.

The question is this: what does one imagine *Karma* to be? Since the widespread image of rebirth is from ancient India, I'd like to start off by elucidating Karma in more modern terms. The easiest way to understand what Karma is about is by visualizing everyday occurrences. When I do something, I have to reckon with the consequences of that act. Being conscious of this is considered to be realistic and rational. So, I drill a hole in the wall with my electric drill and carelessly hit a water pipe. As water spurts in my face, it becomes clear to me that I'm going to have immediate unpleasant consequences. With my electric drill, I have kicked off a chain reaction of cause and effect. In this tense situation, many people innocently try to symbolically "undo" the event – say by very quickly putting down the drill, acting as if they hadn't drilled into the water pipe after all. Unfortunately, this doesn't work – nor can the law of Karma be "fooled" like this.

Yet another secret (and often well-hidden) impediment to self-awareness is the phenomenon of synchronicity. The vernacular term for the concept first coined by C.G. JUNG is "blind chance." Those who learn to keep an eye out for instances of synchronicity will be astonished beyond belief.[68] As the old saying has it: "There's no such thing as coincidence!" Diehard rationalists speak of self-fulfilling prophecies whereby, without being aware of it, one does exactly that which leads to realization of the prophecy. But C.G. JUNG and other keen observers recognized that there must be more to it than that. Evidently, some part of us has made itself independent and – "somewhere up there" – runs something like a karmic lottery. People and events are brought together such that – based on a person's fundamental psychic melody, character type, certain fixed impulses, and "wishful thinking" – a harmonious consonance results.

The actual meaning of Karma is nothing other than *repetition*. This is my personal interpretation of Karma, and in my considered opinion it goes much deeper and gets closer to the real root of the universal law that underlies karmic phenomena. Usually, Karma is understood to be a moral law of cause and effect. Yet when we take a closer look at the nature of Karma, it turns out to be a type of habit pattern that strives for repetition. Therefore, at bottom, every repetition is an instance of Karma, and consequently the most dissimilar things, from laws of nature to human customs, are laden with Karma. Different "habits" are more or less firmly rooted. We know that a person can give up a nasty habit such as smoking, while the law of gravity represents a constant that is (to put it mildly) harder to change. Thus Karma exists in differing characteristics, just as habits have different characteristics. **The more distinctive the characteristics, the harder it is to alter the respective Karma.**

---

68 There are of course countless calendar mottoes, books about Positive Thinking and Bible stories on this topic – basically, sin and its negative consequences, as well as the forgiveness of sins and its positive consequences. Scientifically trained positivists, with their belief in so-called "random chance" and the nonexistence of God, categorically declare this kind of thinking to be sheer nonsense. They then (at first) turn out, in their own minds, to be right – if only because such a mental attitude prevalidates the very idea one had in the first place, as Max PLANCK was forced to realize in his investigations of quantum phenomena. Over the longer term, these "realists" will, I think, die out, because energetic and spiritual development will also increase public acceptance of synchronicity and other spiritual phenomena. Numerous authors are of the opinion that the probability of "dumb coincidences" (i.e., synchronicities) goes up the more we accept such phenomena and the more emotional life force we carry about – i.e., the more psychically/energetically open we become.

Karma, in the sense of an explanation of how laws of nature come about, has relatively little significance in our daily lives, since the underlying laws proceed unusually sluggishly and arduously. This applies generally to all physically graspable processes, such that the law of repetition has little (and unpredictably random) significance in daily life. Let's take as an example the antitheses of good and bad luck: to be sure, we know from experience that luckiness and unluckiness tend to repeat for an individual, as they randomly accumulate, but the significance in daily life is limited. If you break a cup while washing dishes, that doesn't mean that the rest of the day is doomed – but the odds of it have increased. Many people observe the exact opposite and assert that "broken crockery brings you luck." Still, bad luck tends to be self-reinforcing, and one tends to get clumsier from then on – an instance of a very common psychological mechanism, simply because one has gotten clumsy.

But now something different comes along, as higher powers see to it that we mysteriously attract more bad luck once we have had one unfortunate thing happen, even though we by no means desire it and can't do anything at all about it. Our everyday experience shows that misfortune has the regrettable tendency to develop into a chain of events we call an "unlucky streak." For instance, my experience has been that, if you're driving and in a hurry, you're hindered much more by traffic jams and red lights than if you have a lot of time, at which point all the lights turn green, even though you'd welcome some red lights to dawdle away the excess time. We call these concatenations of favorable or unfavorable circumstances the "perversity of inanimate objects." Depth psychology speaks of synchronicity, as objects of similar content seem to want to flock together.

Karma comes in different degrees of severity, giving rise to different amounts of karmic debt calling out for indemnification. If I double-park and don't get ticketed, this is an example of lightweight Karma; if, on the other hand, I cause a serious car accident, I have created weighty Karma. Now, let's assume that the "fickle finger of fate" lets me get away without being identified as the cause of the accident. Possibly I wasn't even aware of the accident I caused, or possibly I justify my hit-and-run act based on my being the breadwinner for my litter of little children, who would starve if I were brought up on charges and found guilty – i.e., I rationalize my fleeing the scene of the accident by bringing up my parental obligations. Am I then, from a moral viewpoint, free of Karma because I have a good excuse? All spiritual teachers agree that Karma admits no exceptions or extenuating circumstances, and that excuses are meaningless.

What really makes the law of Karma interesting is that it is a spiritual law. Even if I think I'm innocent, I still have to pay because, on the spiritual level, the sin remains and must be atoned for someday. This is why Karma is more than the law of cause and effect. Karma has three components: first, a universal spiritual memory function that most likely has to do with storage in the causal body; secondly, a moral dimension coupled to compensatory justice. The third factor is indemnification (redress, reparations), which is inextricably bound up with the concept of rebirth, because punishment in the present life might not be possible. At some point, the law of indemnification goes into effect (even in a future life, if needs be), and one will have to pay for something which one, in all likelihood, no longer remembers.

It is the opinion of most sages and esoteric teachings that the primary cause of the creation of Karma lies in our conscience. When we die, our life is said to "flash before our eyes" like a fast-forwarded movie. In this manner, a personal balance of the past life is struck. We become our own judge, deciding on a fitting punishment and seeing to its execution. We recognize the *True Self* (covered in great detail earlier on) in the participating conscience. Basically, the True Self knows what the false self (our current sinful personality) has done wrong. The only way to regain emotional peace and expiate the guilt is through Karma. Evidently, the choice of specific parents, societies, and countries – and, later on, meeting people known in former lives – leads to such karmic stagings in which guilt is expiated. According to many spiritual teachers, diseases as well as accidents are related to the affected person's Karma.

As we delve deeper into the riddle of Karma, the opinion of most esoteric teachers is that Karma works, first of all, because there is a causal body.

In the causal body – an eternal, all-embracing form of energy not coupled to the individual – are stored all memories of former lives. Indian mysticism speaks of the *Akasha Chronicle*, in which all our good and bad deeds, experiences and everything that has ever happened is recorded in a kind of huge cosmic ledger-book. In my chosen terminology, it is the causal body. C.G. JUNG spoke in the same context of the collective unconscious, in which archetypes and symbols are stored – meaning the causal body. The way that JUNG discovered the causal body is basically a banal story: at some point he noticed that his patients dreamt about ancient myths and alchemical secrets that they couldn't possibly have known about. It was these unexplainable dreams that raised the concept of the collective unconscious to a necessity in JUNG's depth psychology. JUNG realized that only a universal collective unconscious could produce such archetypes.

We can picture the causal body as a huge memory bank in which nothing ever gets lost. In addition, the rules and regulations having to do with Karma are stored there. The fundamental rules of the major world religions – the Christian Ten Commandments, the Buddhist Eightfold Way – teach us to not stray from the "path of righteousness" and to avoid bad Karma: "*Without staff or sword, conscientiously and compassionately, he (the believer) is concerned about*

the well-being of all fellow creatures" (Gautama Buddha). Or the same meaning with greater emphasis: "*Whosoever shall smite thee on thy right cheek, turn to him the other also*" (Jesus Christ). The rules for avoiding Karma can be reduced to the primary insight of avoiding conflict and always heading toward a good outcome. According to the teachings of the religion founders Buddha and Jesus, the well-being of our fellow creatures should be our highest and noblest goal.

It has long been clear that we humans are mostly not saints, if only because we're dragging around with us way too many conflicts that we first have to process and resolve. As imperfect sinners, we will continue to do wrong despite our good intentions, provoke conflicts with neighbors and inevitably create new Karma, whether we want to or not. Although we can try to live up to the commandments of the world religions, we'll mostly not succeed. And even if the commandments mean nothing to us, "*ignorance is no defense before the law*" – because we know very well, way down deep, when we have done wrong: our conscience (True Self) tells us in its quiet clear voice. The errors committed generate a moral debt we must repay. The divine law of compensation, in the form of Karma, will see to it that we don't get away unpunished. According to the esoteric teachers, many (if not indeed all) diseases and mental suffering are said to be karmic in origin.[69]

If this point of view is correct – and there are many indications that it is – we therapists very much need to be addressing these issues. I don't think this means we have to turn off critical rationality. We can do ourselves and our patients a very practical and realistic service by simply leaving out all the religious trappings and looking at the matter with a thoughtful and pragmatic eye. From this thoughtful point of view, **Karma functions as a law of compensation just like a law of nature – it keeps on reconstructing the conflict-laden situation in similar form until the matter comes to a "happy end" and is thereby resolved**. Surprisingly – and quite contrary to the popular view that yesterday's victims are today's victimizers – in my experience, Karma functions predominantly as a repetition machine in which ultimately everything stays the way it was! Perpetrators thus remain perpetrators and victims stay victims, even if that seems quite unfair to us.

Karma is thus just a rerun of a movie that has a disturbing scene in it. The disturbing scene (a murder, for instance) is recapitulated in a new life. Now, in this "rerun," the mur-

---

[69] The habit many therapists have of asking new patients (before beginning therapy) whether they may treat them from a karmic viewpoint, or let events take their course (by means of energetic test procedures such as pendulums, kinesiology, etc.) I take to be a false and deplorable approach. To my mind, this is an impermissible arrogation on the therapist's part of the role of umpire. If some higher providence has led a patient to my practice, it is my mission to therapize that patient with appropriate humility. Whether the patient becomes well is not in my hands anyway, but rather is based on the healing powers of "mother nature."

derer is often not, in the name of justice, murdered "to personally experience how terrible it feels," but instead (amazingly) often becomes once again a murderer – or at least someone who still has murderous tendencies. All the actors keep the same roles, which horrifies and repels us. As with a particular shot in a movie, the scene is rehearsed and repeated until the director declares "It's a wrap!" to the perspiring and disheveled actors: he's satisfied with the "take." As a rule, directors try to cast individual actors in the same roles. But, lacking suitable actors, an "as if" situation is often good enough, in which one acts as if the story is once again the same old scene, so that the murderer from a former life can only be recognized as such by his murderous emotions, even if no actual murder is committed – even if only due to lack of opportunity.

In order to study what goes on in the karmic process, I have lurked like a hunter stalking an easily-frightened prey – and the more I watched, the more certain I became that Karma amounts to nothing more than a chance-event generator that, working behind the scenes, brings forth karmic arrangements of the most exquisite perfection. This perfection involves a subtle camouflage that ensures that the entire story seems accidental and unplanned. Unlike a movie and its director, in real life we're not puppets with no will of our own, having our strings pulled by an unseen director. Like their eventuation, this camouflaging of karmic events is not staged by some higher power: it's based on the noiselessly functioning precision clockwork mechanism that we know as Karma. Since there are no superordinate beings involved in this game we are simultaneously director and actor, at once victim and perpetrator.

In my experience, many serious mistakes are made in the interpretation of individual Karma, and these often result in much unnecessary suffering, since nobody can say with certainty how Karma will proceed in the individual case, and whether the inauspicious incidents are based on earlier guilt. Therefore, hasty judgments can generate a chain of further karmic entanglements, the repercussions of which the individual will be unable to assess. Thus, telling a person whom a serious car accident has confined to a wheelchair that his quadriplegic state is a just penance for past sins can be total nonsense that needlessly causes the wheelchair-bound victim additional grief. No one can say with total certainty that this assertion is correct, that the accident could not have been due to blind chance and karmic causes thus played no part whatsoever in the event. Therefore, I'd like to approach the concept of Karma a little differently – in a way that is fairer to our accident victim in the wheelchair. Maybe the poor man is completely innocent, and an accusation of guilt will simply inflict needless emotional distress. As we know, the Bible cautions against judging others![70] The thing is, their limited mental horizon makes humans exceptionally obtuse and singularly poor at reading the hand of providence with the requisite accuracy. We should thus sit in judgment only over ourselves, and ask whether there is something of which we are guilty.

I'd like to show in an example how such analyses can be done. For instance, inner self-exploration can lead to someone recovering, in the inner image, the situation just before the accident – as the hypnotherapist Werner MEINHOLD once told me concerning one of his patients. Under hypnosis, the accident victim re-experiences the enormous sorrow that had befallen him on the day of the accident, and he realized his secret desire to ram the car into the bridge abutment – shortly after a woman he adored had so painfully rejected him. But the man had not before been aware of his subconscious suicidal intent. Now let's try to imagine being this man who in actuality wanted to commit suicide. Holding up to him that he only has himself to blame for now being in a wheelchair because, as a spurned lover, he had had his feelings hurt, would only be an unnecessary added burden – as long as the man remained unaware of this himself. This example shows why it's so important to learn to bring to light the causes of our difficulties on our own, instead of having them forced on us by others.

From a medical and depth psychology viewpoint, belief in Karma and rebirth induces a dramatic shift in our customary thinking about causality. The entire conventional worldview collapses and has to be replaced by a new one, which is why many people shy away from the far-reaching implications of the concept of Karma. If, that is, our parents are not responsible for our miserable earthly destiny – as conventional psychology maintains – but rather a prenatal decision of the soul has insisted on being (re)born to certain parents, then the entire affair gets very thorny and difficult. All of the psychology textbooks would have to be rewritten, and familiar worldviews replaced by new ones. And the conventional worldview goes completely haywire when we consider the role of Karma as compensatory justice, because our unhappy life would then be the consequence of bad Karma, which we at some point evoked and deserved ("It's not

---

[70] To exploit karmic entanglements to wash one's hands of guilt and comfortably shove it all onto Karma is responsible for a great deal of the resulting social misery – as reflected in India to the present day, with its caste system and offhand attitude to the day-to-day problems of existence. I think that the right attitude consists in, first, recognizing the intertwined nature of personal responsibility and karmic entanglement, in which the existence of Karma helps clarify and mitigate our guilt without automatically exonerating us. Basically, we need to understand that Karma kicks in at some point – but we cannot know when that is. There is thus the important point of the innocent beginning behind which lies our personal freedom. The biggest moral/intellectual error of Karma theory is to ascribe a karmic cause/effect relationship to all events. In the case of the innocent beginning, however, there would be no predecessor drama, so that an overly rigid cause/effect argument goes off in the wrong direction – and, moreover, leaves personal will out of the picture altogether. Because we never know exactly what is really going on in the karmic rule system, my feeling is that postulating karmic guilt is extremely error-prone – and in many cases leads, absurdly enough, directly into karmic guilt!

enough that we've made a mess of things, we then also have to live with the mess …").

I'd next like to try to introduce the reader to a worldview that integrates the concepts of Karma and rebirth into our Western worldview. It's important to me that this view be as realistic as possible, one that doesn't conflict with rational thinking, but also isn't so rigidly and small-mindedly structured that it rules out psychological and spiritual factors. I hope to produce proof that our modern scientifically oriented worldview by no means has to exclude phenomena such as Karma and reincarnation.

First, I'd like to describe the most important **forms of expression of Karma**. After we have decided on reincarnation and settled on a particular couple as future parents, the Wheel of Rebirth begins to turn and the Game of Life can begin. In Indian mythology, the dance of the God Shiva symbolizes the interconnectedness of cause and effect which makes life a cyclic process. To us humans, life seems to proceed linearly because we are yoked to the continuum of birth and death. From the soul's point of view, it is a circular process centered on the True Self – like a hurricane, in whose central "eye" reigns total stillness.

Basically, we have to familiarize ourselves with the unlikely-sounding idea that our soul seeks out its future Karma like an actor chooses a role and a costume in which he "struts and frets his hour upon the stage." An actor will of course try to make the best choice, especially when one considers that it's in fact not a stage play, but rather the actor's future life. But the actor has already made the decision to choose a particular type of theater at a yet earlier stage, when he decided on a particular character type.

Depending on character type, he will have decided on a particular type of theater, one which can be more …
- Comedic-sad (depressive),
- Theatrical-playful (hysteric),
- Tragic-thoughtful (schizoid) or
- Objective-controlled (obsessive-compulsive)

The soul's choice depends crucially on its prior experiences and its character type. "Prior experience" summarizes that which is commonly referred to as *Karma*, while the character type is critically shaped by the individual Central Conflict. How a choice is arrived at in the particular case is a very controversial issue even among the experts, because (of course) one is forced to rely on speculation when it comes to the mysterious murkiness of prebirth existence. Still, larger-scale studies on children, such as STEVENSON's, indicate that reincarnations are preferred in which one can encounter known persons and deal with familiar regions and cultural groups. I'd like to pass over such relatively broad selection criteria at this point, simply because they're hard to get a grip on – and because, in my opinion, they reveal little of our inmost secrets (or at least not with the requisite clarity and vigor for extended analysis). There are better distinguishing features of Karma – lying right on the surface, so to speak – that can yield deep insights into the riddle of Karma.

I'd like to single out two options that the unborn soul has in choosing its future Karma, which to me seem particularly important. There is first, the body we choose and, second, the parents who determine our future family. No other factors influence future Karma as strongly and irreversibly as these two: obviously, one cannot *ex post facto* change either one's body or one's parents, however much one might want to. Whoever is born into an ugly body and a poor family will simply have to learn to live with it. I won't go into the significance of the family in any more detail here because I've already covered that thoroughly elsewhere.

I'd also like to mention two more karmic forms of expression in which we can discern individual problems and large emotional conflicts particularly clearly. The birthing process brings into clear focus everything that determined our prior existence, as well as that which will characterize our future life. Secondly, we can see what kind of Karma we have in our strokes of fate and severe chronic ailments. In fact, many people regard Karma exclusively from this strokes-of-fate aspect – which is of course an overly narrow perspective. Since many chronic ailments (like many strokes of fate) are genetically based, we once again confront the role of the genome to which I made reference earlier on. In this chapter, I'd like to explicate the karmic significance of our genetic makeup, and then delve into the meaning of strokes of fate and diseases in the following chapter.

Briefly, the way I see it, Karma can manifest and express itself in four ways, namely via:

1. **the genotype (genes) and resulting phenotype (body);**
2. **the family and early childhood situation;**
3. **birth and its individual order of events;**
4. **strokes of fate and diseases.**

If we want to understand what our mind is really about, we first have to look at our body. This raises a number of questions, of which I'd like to single out the most important: Why did we prenatally select this particular body? What feelings and longings do we associate with our body? What unwanted feelings and experiences do we suppress with our body by numbing and deadening ourselves in certain areas? Which bodily traits and attributes express deeper psychic attributes, and which are in fact relatively insignificant? Why do so many people select such unfavorable bodies, while others get the most beautiful body imaginable?

The **genome** constitutes the most unalterable element shaping our personality. Our body, along with its metabolism, accurately reveals our character type. Because, from the standpoint of the theory of the elements, every body can be associated with one of four elements, this results in a strict exclusive assignment to one of the four character types. The vernacular says – quite rightly – by way of explanation when someone's thoughts and actions are inflexibly set: "After all, a leopard can't change its spots." This expresses the fact that the body has a specific emphasis or attitude (i.e., preference) that is preset by the corresponding metabolic element-theory element. People can only act and feel within the limits imposed by their own bodies. By the way, we have thus solved the biggest riddle of psychosomatics – which I had mentioned before – because, namely, the soul prenatally seeks out the appropriate body.

In element theory, each element is precisely associated with a specific character type. This yields a strict psychosomatic allocation, in that the body senses exactly as the mind does. As a rule, then, body and mind are consonant so that, for instance, a choleric will generally be a good-natured and often somewhat overweight person who, due to a lack of energy in the 3rd Chakra (upper abdomen), enjoys eating a lot, but who flares up tremendously when annoyed, and can become frightfully enraged, which is likewise pre-programmed by the predominant element (bile). Thus, the choleric's choice of body also selects a psyche with a depressive character type and its corresponding metabolism. This applies to all the other character types, such that, in most cases, our body and its metabolism is the perfect expression of our basic characterological structure.

As we all know, to every rule there is an exception. Therefore, I'd like to call attention to the largely unfamiliar viewpoint that many people seem to find themselves in a body that does not match their psyche. When questioned closely, some people have told me that they feel very odd and unwell in their own body. There are psychological ailments for which this feeling is adjudged to be an expression of the disease: many depressions, schizophrenia, or mental illnesses that include a tendency to self-mutilation.[76] There are, however, mentally normal people who also have these strange feelings – because, it turns out, they prenatally chose the wrong body. If, on top of this, one selects the wrong biological sex, this will have serious repercussions (as I explained in detail in the earlier chapter on sexual polarity).

Many people seem to try prenatally to escape from their intolerable Karma by not identifying with their body. This gives rise to the phenomenon of **pupation** (as I call it), which can take on all manner of variations, the far-reaching consequences of which go mainly unrecognized by outsiders. Psychoenergetically, it has to do with a soul that apparently has only half-heartedly incarnated, such that part of it remains stuck "somewhere out there." In such cases, these people can feel totally strange in their bodies, and sometimes the only visible symptoms are a tendency toward bizarre and inexplicable behavioral disorders, and escapist tendencies such as addiction or other self-destructive behavioral patterns. In the extreme case, pupation can lead to inborn mental retardation, simply because a large part of the psychic personality remains unincarnated. In such cases, our goal as therapists should be to melt away the underlying intolerable Central Conflict and to make life in this world more attractive for the "pupated" personality. It is of course no longer possible to "undo" the regrettable prenatal choice, but one can at least try to alleviate the consequences in the present life.

That the genetic contribution does not constitute 100% of the total personality can be seen particularly clearly in the mentally handicapped. In these cases, a large part of the personality is often "stuck somewhere out there" asleep, as it were, in a holding pattern. My observations suggest that, with a great deal of care and training, the mentally handicapped can actually be persuaded to reincarnate a little bit more – which can mean the difference between "special" education and a normal public school diploma. In my estimation, inborn mental handicaps virtually always have a strong karmic significance. For example, the concealed agenda might be the seductive possibility, for the psyche, that the handicapped person can

---

[71] In contrast to transitory states of alienation in psychiatric cases, "pupated persons" are constantly confronted with the feeling of foreignness in their own bodies. I'd also like to point out that this alienation can of course be extended to one's family, one's society, or even the country into which one is born into this life.

remain in a lifelong infantile role, thereby forcing other people to "love me this time around."

Of course, one can ask why a soul has done something so foolish as to select an inappropriate body, or not to reincarnate fully.[72] One of the reasons might be the need for stronger spiritual growth. More than likely, such unfamiliar-feeling bodies (i.e., genes) become spiritual "pebbles in the shoe" by means of which a pupated soul acquires additional maturation opportunities. Characteristic traits and behavior patterns, when viewed from the outside, seem strange and inappropriate, so that they keep on causing various and sundry difficulties for the pupated person and his relatives. We see this most clearly in cases of physical handicaps. In Alfred ADLER's Individual Psychology, physical weaknesses become the initial challenging opportunities for individuals to surpass themselves. Amazingly many politicians (the most famous being NAPOLEON) have been strikingly short people. They evidently compensate for their feeling of inferiority by exercising their power. Intrinsic bodily strangeness and isolated "dropped stitches" in the form of handicaps are extraordinarily widespread, and they must help many people to surpass themselves.

Pupation as the refusal fully to expose oneself as a personality leads to various disorders. This can be seen in cases of Minimal Brain Dysfunction (MBD), legasthenia, and many severe infantile behavioral and learning disorders. I suspect that virtually all especially difficult and petulant children want to prevent revealing their true personality. The reason might be fear of once more (as in former lives) being punished or hurt. They are trying to prevent the earlier karmic situations from recurring, in which their personality was not accepted, by retreating like a snail into its shell. Other possible reasons include obstinacy and the desire to punish in this incarnation, to "punch the hated world in the nose." In individual cases, the motives can be extraordinarily many and varied.

But the options of the soul desiring reincarnation to express itself can also manifest in a very contrary manner, in which the parents' genes are not a hindrance, but rather lead to new expressive possibilities. The child forces, with its Karma, a new arrangement of the genetic material. The child's personality thereby expresses its character traits especially energetically and clearly, instead of (as in pupation

and mental retardation) hiding them. The well-known (and hard to explicate) biological-psychology phenomenon of ***Emergenesis*** corresponds precisely to this process of partial re-creation of genetic material. I interpret Emergenesis as a particularly clear-cut indication of the existence of Karma – and it gives us, moreover, indications of a personality that remains stable over the course of multiple incarnations.

In Emergenesis, the parents' genes are reshuffled so that traits emerge that cannot (or can only with difficulty) be traced back to the parents. This gives rise to traits that are not present in the parents in this form, e.g., two unattractive parents of average intelligence giving birth to an especially good-looking and clever child. In my estimation, these emergent characteristics accentuate particularly striking aspects of personality which are karmically preformed. We can view them as characteristics that are particularly important to the individuals in question, such that they "by all means want to get them back in this reincarnation" – for instance, a particularly handsome and clever child had these traits in a former life and doesn't want to do without them in this one.

Well-known emergent characteristics include:
- EEG Alpha preferential frequency (consciousness mood)
- Habituation (i.e., growing weaker due to familiarization), psychophysiological variables (such as learning ability)
- Occupational and intellectual interests and talents
- Creativity (ingenuity, for good or evil)
- Strength of one's influence on others ("social impact")
- Extroversion (optimistic, socially open-minded, feeling of personal control, low susceptibility to stress)
- A "good" physical appearance

(from: Birbaumer/Schmidt: Biologische Psychologie [Biological Psychology], Springer: Berlin, New York 1999)

We can detect – particularly clearly in the above-named emergent characteristics – which karmic components belong to us. For example, if we were especially beautiful and creative in earlier incarnations, we'll be reluctant, in the present one, to do without these aspects that we've grown so fond of. Even if we reincarnate with unattractive and uncreative parents, we'll push through our brought-along characteristics, simply because we never want to do without them. Talents and occupational and intellectual interests are also part of the indispensable personality components that we would sorely miss. They will therefore be reflected, opposition notwithstanding, in the new genetic material, just as are our predominant emotional moods and social interests.

I'd next like to turn to birth, through which karmic themes are likewise expressed – very intensely, in fact. The ***birth setting*** (re)presents particularly large fundamental

---

[72] Reincarnation as an animal or plant I consider to be a horror story meant to scare people out of their wits. Based on my observations, the closest thing would be semi-reincarnation as a mentally handicapped person. In these cases, part of the personality simply refuses to take part in the reincarnation – often in connection with extremely traumatic experiences in an earlier incarnation that have not yet been fully assimilated. The soul then says: "This time the show goes on without me." Faced with the dilemma of having to choose a reincarnation in order, as a new personality, to get charged up with life energy in order to be able to go on living – or else die forever – it opts for a half-hearted solution in which the greater part of the mental body remains outside, sending in only the vital and emotional bodies along with a minimal fraction of the mental body.

fears and important core themes of earlier existence. At birth, particularly traumatic situations of earlier karmic terrors often resurface symbolically, reflecting themselves right at the beginning in the circumstances of the birthing process. Thus, a child born with the umbilical cord wrapped around its neck, almost strangled by it during birth, will later on, under hypnosis, recall having been hanged (or a comparable theme) in a former life. Being hanged has its self-destructive aspects – but a strangled baby can also be the death of its mother. Thus, there often exists a difficult relationship with the mother as well, who not infrequently represents a person known from a former life with whom one "has a bone to pick," a "score to settle."

Surprisingly, birth almost always perfectly illustrates the themes of the Central Conflict that the child being born brings with it. This, it seems to me, is the reason why transpersonal psychologists such as Stanislav GROF view the birth process as the key to the nature of the personality. GROF found, in deep LSD-induced trance states (and later drug-free ecstatic states brought on by ecstatic music and hyperventilation), that many people relived their birth as an extremely agitating emotional experience. GROF then came to the obvious conclusion that the kind of birth has a formative influence on the future personality – which is, in a certain sense, completely correct; one just needs to keep in mind that birth represents just one part of the total karmic possibilities.

For instance, if during a difficult birth the baby resists being born, then it will, as an adult, remarkably often exhibit similar characteristic traits, such as being shy and introverted. Schizoid or pupated people often have strikingly difficult births, and those whose birth went smoothly will later on often turn out to be uncomplicated and easy-to-please creatures. One is reminded of the saying that "first impressions are crucial": in our very first entrance onto the world stage, basic structures of being become clearly visible, as if we wanted to make it clear to the world exactly who it is that they'll be having to deal with in the future.

However, I have to mention some limitations regarding birth and its informational value. Since modern birthing methods such as Caesarean sections limit many karmic expressional possibilities, it's important not to over-interpret the birth circumstances. I'd also like to point out the many misinterpretations made possible by some strongly subjectively-toned elements of the birthing process. For example, an apparently complication-free birth might be experienced by the infant's soul (or the mother's sensations) as having been much more dramatic. Evaluation thus has a strong subjective element, such that one needs to take into account all the factors involved.

In the next chapter, I'd like to talk about so-called chance (or coincidence), about which the poet Marie von EBNER-ESCHENBACH once wrote: *"Chance is veiled necessity."* From the outside, we don't recognize the karmic rules that seem to us like mysterious destiny, although (from a higher perspective) they proceed according to a logical plan. In what follows, I'll be correcting a lot of mystical and superstitious ideas having to do with the concept of fate by showing that the Central Conflict (i.e., our largest subconscious psychic wound) plays a pivotal role in Karma formation. If we clean up our psychic chaos and re-attain psychoenergetic harmony, we are freed from the clutches of our previous Karma and once again become the true masters of our fate.

Fate and Chance

Accidents are Destiny's way of implementing its most important plans for us.
(Charles Tschopp)

From time immemorial, people have believed in a predetermined destiny, and have paid astrologists and fortunetellers to predict their future. As a scientifically trained physician, I had long held fortunetelling to be total nonsense – until a personal crisis drove me, in my desperation, to seek out a fortuneteller. This woman was an actual gypsy whose forebears had died in a concentration camp, and whose mother and grandmother had also been clairvoyant. Evidently, the gift is passed on to the descendants: the fortuneteller's 3-year-old granddaughter once said to a departing blonde client of her grandmother's, passing her by chance in the hallway: "Your husband's hair is black." This was in fact true, as the blonde lady admitted, who had come from far away and who had never previously visited the gypsy woman.

My first encounter with this clairvoyant took a dramatic turn: in the session, she related precise details from my past, off the top of her head, which she couldn't possibly have known about – such as how many siblings I have, what their occupations are, what certain people think of me and suchlike. After the session, I was at first completely convinced and understandably very enthused, because I had absolutely no doubt as to her abilities. Later on, I realized that clairvoyants' statements are limited both in content and temporally. After my initial enthusiasm, I delved very deeply into the phenomena of chance and fortune, read many books, queried experts about clairvoyance, sought out other serious fortunetellers and spoke to patients of mine who had visited clairvoyants. I now think I have developed a fairly comprehensive picture of the possibilities and limits of clairvoyance, which I'd like to summarize here.

The basic question is whether our fate is predetermined and, if so, in what way. In this context, I'd like to present two very informative anecdotes relating to fortunetelling:

1. The *Huna* instructor Max Freedom LONG tells about a Hawaiian friend of his who was told by a clairvoyant woman that he would have a serious car accident in the immediate future. As a precaution, he had a friend (for whom the woman predicted no accident) drive his delivery van. A few days later, a big semi-trailer bore down on the two at high speed, and they would have had a bad accident had it not been for his friend's alertness in steering the van out of the path of the oncoming semi.

2. One of my patients refused to sign a million-dollar contract with a major building contractor because the clairvoyant woman had advised against it. A few days later, he got the news from his bank that, although his signature would have kept the bankrupt contractor in business for a little while longer, it would have eventually dragged him down into financial ruin as well, because the contractor's debts were simply too huge. He was so relieved and excited that he forgot another of the clairvoyant's prophecies, remembering it only after it was already too late: a tire blowout on the Autobahn crashed him at 125 MPH into the center divider. The car was totaled, but he walked away unharmed. The urgency of the financial transaction had made him forget the serious accident that the clairvoyant had predicted would occur in the next few days.

After hearing these two examples, one would assume that fortunetelling really does work and can boast reliable results. It is not my intent here to do a commercial for fortunetellers, but rather to clarify the underlying mechanisms of chance and destiny that are revealed by fortunetelling. Basically, fortunetelling is only possible for a limited time-span. In fact, good fortunetellers seem to be able to predict the future for a few days in advance. Numerous parapsychological investigations have confirmed that short-term predictions by gifted mediums are definitely possible, and their accuracy is far greater than would be possible due to sheer coincidence.

If one is wise enough to take timely precautions (as in the example with LONG's friend), then it is possible to deflect one's predicted fate. But after a few days, a clairvoyant's predictions get less and less accurate, becoming totally unreliable over longer time-spans. An example of this is the incredibly high error rate of famous clairvoyants who on New Year's Day predict important events for the upcoming year – and mostly wind up having missed the mark entirely when, a year later, their predictions are compared with actual events.

Many prophecy fans from the true-believer fortunetelling faction point to the prophecies of NOSTRADAMUS as proof that long-term prognoses are possible. I, on the other hand, consider all long-term predictions to be sheer superstition. Every time that fateful events such as Cold War crises, the collapse of the Soviet Union or the 9/11 attacks get people all frightened and upset, along come the professional doomsayers and predict The End Of The World, often citing NOSTRADAMUS as proof. NOSTRADAMUS was a famous astrologer during the Middle Ages who, according to his followers, predicted the entire future course of mankind's history – but his writings, upon closer examination, turn out to be mythic, ambiguous, and essentially undecipherable descriptions of murky nightmare worlds. The tenor of the text resembles that of the Revelations of St. John in the New Testament – which can also be viewed as a depth psychological description of emotional infernos (rather than of actual future events). A good imagination can read just about anything into such texts.

Some people also refer to the Indian palm-leaf manuscripts in which, thousands of years ago, clairvoyant seers supposedly wrote down the detailed destinies of all the people who, thousands of years later, would visit these libraries. To anyone thinking this obscure and unbelievable, I can assure them that a number of trustworthy people, independently of each other, have insisted that they have read, in one of these palm-leaf manuscripts, similarly amazing details from their past, as happened to me with the aforementioned clairvoyant woman. Particularly with respect to the more respected palm-leaf manuscripts, the reports of past events and life circumstances seem to be unusually unerring.

Parapsychological researchers now know that clairvoyants use mind-reading to amaze their clients with details from their past, simply by doing a "readout" of the person's memory. After that, the client blindly trusts the clairvoyant, and no longer doubts the clairvoyant's ability to foresee the future, especially if the predicted events should happen to extend far into the future. I suspect that clairvoyants use the palm-leaf manuscripts much as seers use a glass ball to go into a trance.[73]

Of course, clairvoyance is by no means restricted to the near future; the diviner also sees future possibilities that will come to pass if everything remains as it is. Just as one can predict the trajectory of a soccer ball once it has been kicked, this seems also to be the case with future events. Unlike the soccer ball, however, which cannot alter its trajectory once it has been kicked, we humans have free will. **We can change our mind, thereby also changing our future.** As a confirmation of this, I point out that soothsayers have repeatedly predicted future events in my life which would certainly have occurred based on earlier ideas and plans, if I had not in the meantime changed my mind.

The next question that comes up is: by what is our future predetermined? Experts agree that our future has something to do with our thoughts, hopes, and fears. In particular, the subconscious and emotions seems to influence our future much more than our thoughts. We all know that just thinking "I want to be rich!" is not going to win the lottery, nor conjure up a bagful of money with a million dollars in it to trip over while taking a walk. In order to become a millionaire, most people will have to work like a dog for a lifetime ("The first million is the hardest!"). Some few "get rich quick" with a bright idea, others through trickery or even criminal endeavors such as embezzlement.

Basically, consciously expressed wishes must be followed by actions if the wish is to come true. You can't just dream, you have to do your part if the consciously expressed wishes are to be fulfilled. It seems to be different with subconscious programs, which are realized much more easily, especially when it comes to negative emotions. Psychological investigations have shown that some people are just jinxed, and have far more than their share of accidents. I have been flabbergasted time and again at certain people who seem to be misfortune magnets. We speak colloquially of jinxes and bad-luck streaks, and the insurance companies know from their actuarial data that some people are more accident-prone than others.

For example, I know a feminist university professor in Germany with a guest professorship at an American university who, during her frequent travels, has been sexually assaulted or threatened any number of times. After each one of these disturbing incidents, she would take even more precautions against such attacks, only to have them happen again and again. I found it particularly ghastly that a feminist should so often be a rape victim, as if the rapists were trying to prove to her, in the most extreme manner possible, that all men were indeed "pigs" – a prejudice that she is now fully convinced of thanks to her traumatic experiences.

We all know a jinx or two among our friends and acquaintances, those who magically attract accidents and bad luck. As the saying goes: "The Devil likes to sh** on a big pile." Although Sigmund FREUD was, fundamentally, a very rational and skeptical person, he noted the vagaries of fate as well. In his words, if one were to throw a banana peel onto the sidewalk in front of an apartment house every day for many consecutive days, the same person would slip on it every time. FREUD was familiar with the subconscious mechanisms that play such an important role here, in that

---

[73] There's an additional aspect, based on the fact that symbolically-charged objects and concepts such as Tarot cards, I Ching yarrow stalks, the bowels of butchered animals, certain astrological symbols, and some numbers, etc. tend to depict subconscious processes. One can think in terms of a magical quasi-materialization in which certain random arrangements occur significantly more often if sufficient magical concentration is in play. Experts speak of morphic resonance, with reference to the discoveries of the English biologist Rupert SHELDRAKE, who interpreted all real-world phenomena, including the laws of nature, as customs in the sense of ingrained courses of action which repeat all the more often the more they have been psychoenergetically rehearsed and ingrained. There are still other mechanisms that resemble the well-known inkblot (Rohrschach) test. Like the clairvoyant's crystal ball, the seer's interpreting subconscious sees patterns and contents of the past and future that reveal themselves in certain random-seeming arrangements, analogous to the way a Polaroid snapshot gradually comes into view.

jinxes seem to carry around in their subconscious something that attracts bad luck. For instance, if you carry around certain fears, you tend somehow to attract incidents involving these very fears.

Even if our more distant future, beyond the next few days, is (thanks to free will) undetermined and more or less shapeable, our subconscious emotions nevertheless shape our future, even though we consciously don't desire that at all. **It is because of our subconscious conflicts that we are not free to shape and determine our future!** In this, the Central Conflict (the largest subconscious conflict) plays the leading role. For instance, if you have a *Rage* Central Conflict, this exerts a strong direct influence on your destiny – which I'd like to elucidate with the example of a woman who had this conflict:

Ms. S. comes in for energy testing because she always feels tired, listless and tense. Her painful lumbar spinal region and stiff neck are particularly big problems because nothing she's tried has alleviated these bothersome ailments. By nature, Ms. S. is a friendly and sympathetic person who, for some reason, keeps falling into fairly long-term emotional lows. She has a people-oriented job and is happily married, so there seems to be no social or family component to her problems.

I measure in her an enormous Central Conflict with Rage *as the theme – which, experience has shown, often accompanies tension and depression. When asked whether this made any sense to her, she said that in fact she had been getting into enraging situations all her life, but without suspecting that it could have something to do with her. As a child, she had been beaten by her father, for no reason, on a number of occasions. In school, her classmates were only too happy to copy from her – because she was an above-average student – but her cooperativeness was not rewarded with friendship because they all thought she was weird, so they avoided her. Even as a young lady, she had numerous liaisons with married men who strung her along for years with empty promises, taking advantage of her longing for love. Later on, her first marriage was to a man who turned out to be a brutal wife-beater and rapist, and whom she was able to divorce only after great effort and torment. She is now happy in her second marriage, but still suffers from the emotional wounds inflicted on her in her earlier relationships.*

Even in nonsexual relationships, people exploit her, simply because she's so ready to lend a helping hand and can't say no. Even her best friend tends to use her as a shoulder to cry on, pestering her with hour-long late-night phone calls in which she is forced to listen to every last detail of her friend's problems, even though she can barely keep her eyes open. She just can't work up the courage to tell her friend what she really thinks, that she shouldn't call so late at night, and that she's sick and tired of listening to her complaints in such excruciating detail.

In this description of the life of a person with the *Rage* theme, one can easily see how manipulative, sadistic and egotistical people keep turning up in her life, whose common denominator is that they provoke a furious rage in her. In her revenge fantasies, she likes to imagine squashing her abusive first husband like a bug and strangling her pain-in-the-neck girlfriend with the telephone cord. The problem is, however, that she's not even capable of modest and innocuous forms of resistance; it's only in her imagination that she can hatch huge revenge plots in which she shows the entire world, once and for all, what's been going on inside her the whole time.

Empirically, people with the *Rage* theme are unusually aggression-inhibited (to use the psychological term): they cannot say "No." Understandably, depressives are quite popular, and they themselves like to play the role of "everybody's darling." If you think back to the character types, you'll recall that the *Rage* Central Conflict is assigned to the depressive character type. Depressives have in common the characteristic of excessive longing for love, plus deep-seated feelings of frustration – and a conspicuous friendliness in their dealings with others that is frequently taken advantage of. Depressives are socially very accommodating and self-sacrificing persons who'll do anything to make sure that things go well for the other person – but in the process they neglect their own needs and desires.

That's just how it was with the woman of our example, who is in fact a depressive character type. She has always attracted sadists and egotists into her life. Evidently, exploiters instinctively sense that "I can have my way with her" – and then pretend to love the depressive and act as if they were seriously interested in them, although the primary motivation of such exploiters consists entirely of satisfying their egotistical drives. Finally, I'd like to round out this case by reporting that she cut off all contact with the exploiters in her life once her *Rage* Central Conflict had been cured. After that, she was finally able to say no, and to distance herself from other people's excessive demands.

If you know a person's Central Conflict and put their past under a microscope, you'll be surprised to note, time and again, that everything dovetails perfectly. You just have to take care not to make overly superficial equations, e.g., of the sort: *Helper Syndrome = Depressive character type* – because, for example, schizoids with the *Helpless* theme likewise tend to let themselves be exploited and thereby wind up in a helpless emotional situation. After having analyzed many hundreds of patients, I can say that no other factor so strongly influences a person's individual destiny as the Central Conflict. Chance events and strokes of fate nevertheless do reflect (with some qualifications) – *not always*, but surprisingly often – precisely that emotional theme which corresponds to the person's Central Conflict.

There are exceptions, of course: our external reality is *not completely* influenced by our secret negative impulses, but rather just to a greater or lesser degree. We are by no means robots, nor are we puppets dangling will-lessly from the puppeteer's strings and able to be manipulated at will; we do in fact have free will. What's more, our fate is interwoven with that of countless others, so that the interconnections inside social groupings sometimes outweigh personal destiny (as in the case of racial persecution). Therefore, that which befalls us does not have to lead, straight as an arrow, directly to our subconscious conflicts. In many cases, our fate is just as likely to have its source in completely unrelated factors that we cannot see through to in their entirety. We should thus guard against hasty conclusions that shove everything into the subconscious, because other factors could always be involved.

Let us return to the banana peel and the subconscious conflict. I'm using the cliché banana peel as a general symbol for bad luck and karmic entanglements. The conflict stores up our secret subconscious negative ideas that, through their desire to be realized, at some point land us in unpleasant situations. Conflict contents strive to re-attain reality – which is ultimately nothing other than Karma. Karma thus represents the increased probability of the repetition of subconscious conflict contents. One's subconscious assembles personal failure scenarios, thereby reinforcing the conflict contents' significance. At this stage of the proceedings, the famous banana peel now makes its entry.

For example, if someone has a subconscious fear of helplessness or is subconsciously enraged, then the banana peel is the perfect vehicle for shaping that person's individual fate. It helps the subconscious act out its hidden feelings. The subconscious directs a person's footsteps straight to the banana peel so that the subconscious feelings of rage or helplessness can be expressed and reinforced. The poor victim slips on the banana peel and is then terribly enraged or else feels helpless, like the world's biggest fool. The banana-peel victim then thinks: "This unfair world, so full of accidents waiting to happen, simply makes me furious!" – or: "Well, I'm really useless, since I can't even stay on my own two feet, slipping on every dumb banana peel that comes along!" We recognize that the conflict has here attained its goal of once again setting this person into subconscious emotional vibration, thereby recapitulating the conflict and psychoenergetically reinforcing its intrinsic dynamics.

And even though I have warned against simplistic thinking, because it generates a lot of guilt feelings and unnecessary suffering, we can't avoid the fact that we subconsciously direct our own fate to some extent – as a Sad Sack, say – by being likely to slip on banana peels. The following deals with our personal contribution to this process. We treat first of all the "famous coincidence" that leads us into all manner of possible fates and catastrophes. Later on, we'll derive a universal logic: namely that the Central Conflict fundamentally represents a karmic problem.

In our life with other people, projection, synchronicity and Karma play such a great and destiny-determining role that, when we look more closely, we're tempted to believe in something like Providence. Of course, terms such as Providence and Destiny are reassuring excuses intended to shift our responsibility onto Higher Powers. But the difficult process of acquiring self-knowledge includes recognizing our own role in our personal destiny. Based on my observations, this gets easier the higher we vibrate energetically and the more emotionally open we are. As our Chakra development increases – particularly from the 5th (rational) to the 6th (intuitive) Chakra – "the scales fall [more and more] from our eyes" and we realize that we are the true masters of our fate. For a long time and over many incarnations, we entangle ourselves in a web of guilt and error, until we gradually come to know the truth.

Only after we have rid ourselves of conflict will we be able freely to shape our future. I mentioned earlier that the conflict has a tendency to repeat which makes its occurrence (against the laws of chance) more likely. At this point, it's easy to see that Karma and conflicts have something to do with each other. Therefore, we can clearly derive from the conflict's repetitious tendency how the laws of Karma unfold.

The common denominator of all conflicts and karmic events consists of the fact that an incident

1. is experienced with a great deal of emotional and psychic excitement, and
2. does not come to a good end.

The great excitement at the origin of the conflict leads to Karma in the first place, while the effort involved in "wanting to bring the affair to a good end" makes the later-on application of Karma necessary.

I'd first like to address point 1 above. In the chapter on the origin of conflicts, I mentioned the shocks that are bound up with the great agitation and intolerability of emotions. At the time of the origin of the conflict, the psyche says to itself, as it were: "I can't take this anymore!" – and constructs a conflict so that life can go on and the intolerable tension associated with the shock is moderated. The organism attempts to shift the intolerable emotional contents out into the Aura ("Just get it outta here!") and psychoenergetically constructs a conflict. The shock (the great agitation in conflict formation) thus automatically activates causal-body energy, which flows into the conflict and which, ultimately, is to be viewed as the true reason for the origin of Karma, since the whole thing is cemented in place and equipped with long-term memory by causal-body energy.

On the material plane, causal-body energy represents the brainwaves associated with great stress and heightened attention (beta waves). The teacher raps our knuckles with a yardstick and shouts: "Now don't you forget it!" The activated stress brainwaves lead to the teacher's words being stored in the deep subconscious of the causal body, in which are stored all the important primeval programs essential for survival. The commands and programs of the Causal Level are "burned" into us, like a cow branded by the cowboy. The worse the shock and agitation, the deeper the program is pushed down, to become part of our "flesh and blood." In fact, the Central Conflict, with its immense fundamental fear, becomes a permanent part of us.

In the causal body, the conflict is reshaped into **deep-seated convictions** (paradigms) that are known in psychology as **conditioning**, and whose contents are stamped deeper into the subconscious the larger and older the conflict is. Of course, the largest and most important conflict is the Central Conflict, about which much has already been said in great detail. The Central Conflict leads to deep-seated convictions that predetermine our character, our overall mood and our worldview. To some extent, the effect of the Central Conflict can be compared to *dressage* (training a horse to be ridden), as it predetermines our nature and our actions in fixed and predictable ways.

The basic principle of this kind of *dressage* is based on psychoenergetically imprinting (conditioning) the causal body. The Russian researcher PAVLOV discovered the phenomenon of conditioning near the end of the 19th century. PAVLOV got his laboratory dogs to salivate at the sound of a bell by creating a reflex association between the bell sound and being fed. At the beginning of the dressage, the bell was sounded just before the food was presented. Finally, the bell sound alone would trigger reflexive salivation, thus proving that behavior can be channeled and fixed through habituation. When these research results were first published, it caused a first-class scientific sensation that kicked off the triumphal march of Behaviorism, that school of psychology that reduces virtually everything to behavioral conditioning.

Of course dressage is effective not just on dogs, but on humans as well. For example: "Whenever I see a yardstick, I can't help remembering the teacher's words!" says the former student, now (50 years later) an old man for whom the fixed connection between yardstick and teacher is still stuck in his memory. The effects of conditioning are amazingly long-lived. In humans, conditioning acts above all on the subconscious, thereby lastingly changing behavior. When interpreting such conditioning, it needs to be made clear that, due to the extended time perception that dominates in the causal body, contents of the causal body tend strongly to be perceived in eternal categories.

This kind of perpetually active dogma might go something like this: "I'll never again be healthy!" or "Really, there's no point to it all!" or "I'll never again put all my trust in another person as long as I live!"

Many people are understandably shocked when confronted for the first time with such paradigms (of which they had hitherto been completely unaware) as they are brought into their awareness by means of trance and hypnosis. "I would never have believed that I could have such negative feelings!" is what most people say spontaneously. And yet, on the outside they seem to embrace life and to be happy – while, down deep, the conflict harbors an entirely different, anti-life, and deathly miserable worldview. "*Two souls, alas, reside within my breast!*" is how GOETHE's *Faust* expresses it.

The nature of the conflict not only enables us to grasp the abysses of our psyche, with its deeply-rooted preconceptions and fears, but also allows us to understand the psyche's desire for everything to turn out well in the end. The origin of a conflict is thus automatically bound up with the wish for a Happy Ending. It's not just the moviegoer who wants one; so does the conflict host, being eaten away by constant frustration. I just compared the conflict to a movie, which contains scenes that take a bad turn, these being repeated by the director until they lead to the Happy Hollywood Ending. And in fact the conflict really is like a movie that's gotten stuck in the middle, relentlessly pushing the spectator to a Happy Ending. Our psyche, with the aid of Karma and chance, sees to it that the movie ends on a happy note.

In a certain sense, Karma and conflict are two sides of the same coin. Spiritual teachers tell us that Karma comes to an end because everything earthly is subject to transience. Karma abrades over time, but it can take an unbearably long time. However, using the appropriate naturopathic aids, it's possible to break up the conflict completely and permanently in a relatively short time – which means that the associated Karma is brought to a good end. For I believe that, without conflict, there is no Karma, and then the psyche is no longer remote controlled by its deep subconscious dark side.

In my experience, illness often represents a subconscious attempt to work off Karma via painful experiences, and get rid of it. This will be dealt with in the next chapter, but I'd like to anticipate it a little, and say that dissolving conflicts works off Karma in illness form much quicker and less painfully; in this manner, many diseases can be causally and permanently cured. By going to the real cause of many diseases and ill-fated event sequences, you attack the problem at its root. This way, the psyche can more rapidly and less painfully find its way back to its true center, and the body's energy once again flows full strength and the overall metabolism recuperates.

Disease as the Search
for the True Self

From the viewpoint of psychoenergetic medicine, most diseases arise for reasons other than the ones normally considered to be responsible. I've already named the most important reason, but I'll repeat it here because it is so important: **the most frequent cause of disease is psychic conflicts that lead to psychoenergetic blocks!**[74] In an earlier chapter, I described in detail the circumstances of conflict genesis. Most people don't notice their psychoenergetic block, and often cannot recall when the illness that gave rise to the block began. The only detectable part for most people is the disease and its symptoms, i.e., that they are plagued with headaches, feel nervous, have skin eruptions or some such symptom.

In addition, there are further energetic disease causes such as geopathic stress zones, electrosmog and such (see the earlier chapter on geopathic stress zones), or metabolic disorders conditioned by harmful bacteria and fungi (bad intestinal flora) as well as by inflammation foci (such as root-dead teeth). These situations lead to hyperacidity and displacement of the mineral balance, plus blood-vessel (capillary) spasms. At a rough estimate, about a third of the population is ailing due to geopathic stress, with an additional third due to disease foci such as harmful intestinal bacteria, dental foci, and chronic sinus inflammations – but which, nevertheless, in 99% of all mankind is due to emotional conflicts! Emotional conflict therefore represents the largest and most important hidden cause of disease.

There are of course other causes of disease besides these, all just as real and logical – for instance, someone might be "sickly" due to an emotional conflict, but the present ailment can be ascribed to other causes. One example would be a car accident involving broken bones, caused by the driver being overly nervous and thus accident-prone. The broken bones must be treated before one can address the underlying emotional conflict. Another example: obesity coupled with diabetes; in this case, the blood sugar must be brought down before any other measures are taken, such as eliminating the emotional frustration that is the root cause of the excessive appetite. All possible causes of disease can thus be graded according to current relevance and importance – always, of course, treating the current disease first when necessary for practical reasons, before addressing the deeper causes. The following tragic case from my practice shows that even this simple rule of thumb is often not heeded:

Ms. X. is a friendly, attractive middle-aged woman who has come in for energy testing due to a number of vague symptoms. I detect geopathic stress as well as poor intestinal flora. Her extremely bad metabolic readings worry me, so I recommend a thorough gynecological examination. Six months later, I see this patient again. This time, it's because she found a small nodule in her breast that the palpation indicates has the typical stiffness and non-relocatability of an incipient cancer nodule. I strongly advise her to undergo a thorough breast examination. A little over a year later, the patient shows up again, and, to my horror, the nodule is now the size of a tangerine. When I ask, appalled, why she hadn't taken my advice, she tells me about a renowned therapist who had promised her that his method would completely cure her. He turns out to be a notorious charlatan who had been convicted and sent to prison a number of times for violations of medical ethics laws, and who ascribed cancer to emotional dreams that allegedly caused lasting damage to brain tissue. According to this therapist, our patient's breast cancer was traceable to a partner conflict. Right after he told her that, the patient recalled a key incident in which her (now ex-)husband had teased her about her small breasts, which had hurt her feelings.

The therapist had thereupon assured her that her recollection of this emotional trauma would lead automatically to the cancer's disappearance. I was unable to convince her that she was laboring under a delusion, and I found out to my horror that this therapist's ideas had, from the beginning, kept her from getting a cancer diagnosis, so that my words had just bounced uselessly off of her, even back when the tumor was still tiny and the healing prognosis would have been unusually good. She hadn't told me that at first, because she'd been afraid that I would take it as a professional insult if she consulted someone else. Six

---

[74] The Swiss psychologist Jakob Bösch is one of the few doctors who has had the courage to collaborate with a faith healer. He describes the typical case of an internist with vague and incurable symptoms resembling those of a stroke. Bösch calls in the faith healer, and she sees, in a trance, that a shocklike drowning episode from about ten years ago is the actual cause, and thereupon completely cures the man's ailments by eliminating this shock. Bösch mentions that this healer sees shocklike emotional experiences as the true disease cause in the majority of cases, in which (in her words) a piece of the psyche is lost. All of the shamans and faith healers that Bösch knows share this view, he says. It's not hard to see that the healer recognizes psychoenergetic conflict formation as the true cause of disease, and that her viewpoint is completely congruent with the one I set forth in this book.

months later, her breast was a reeking open wound, and she only survived a few months more before succumbing to the cancer.

Looking back on it, I of course blamed myself for not having insisted more forcefully on a sensible course of cancer diagnosis and therapy. More than likely, though, subconscious self-destructive motivations proved to be too strong in this case.

One can see clearly from this case that an incipient cancer nodule should be operated on at once. All the statistics from thousands of cases, as well as clinical experience with individual patients, confirms that this is the best way to go. In fact, it's considered a professional error to deviate from this course of action. It goes without saying that concomitant causal factors (such as emotional conflicts and geopathic stress) should not be ignored. Many patients rightly complain that their conservative therapists fail to take into account their more deep-seated causes adequately, and some have begun to "vote with their feet" – for instance in the USA, where the amount spent on complementary medicine (Chirotherapy, vitamins, Ayurveda, and such) is now greater than that for conventional methods. People simply want to be treated causally and profoundly.

Quite often, laypersons confuse the urgency with which a particular causal factor of disease needs to be addressed therapeutically with the importance of the cause itself. There is much that is urgent yet relatively unimportant, simply because it makes the person acutely sick. After all, you almost always first put out the fire before looking into what may have caused it. Therefore, it is of foremost importance to proceed pragmatically and logically, and many patients instinctively choose a two-track process by, for example, entrusting the basic diagnostics and the operation to conventional medicine but the post-operative (follow-up) treatment to natural healers who work with energy medicine. In my experience, they are taking the best course of action under the circumstances, especially when it comes to diseases such as cancer.

The detection and treatment of the true causes of a disease often takes on a confusing multi-layered aspect, depending on which level you consider the matter. This befuddles many people and makes them doubt their own and their therapist's judgment. And yet, the answer can be found in most cases, even if it often takes a great deal of effort, i.e., visiting specialists and submitting to various exams. To illustrate this, I'd like to describe a commonplace case from daily practice. An elderly woman, after physical exertion, feels so leached out for months that she can't recover her strength and is plagued by terrible lower-back pain (lumbago). Understandably, she looks despondent and perplexed, she has prolonged sleep disorders and deep rings under her eyes. The therapist would like to be able to help her, and casts about for the best solution to her problems.

The patient and her therapist can interpret the lumbago and the prolonged tiredness on very different levels, which leads to specific therapies and strategies:

1. ***In the here-and-now and derived directly from external injurious factors:*** "I've been working in the garden, often bent over, and wasn't wearing enough clothing, so that the cold crept into my back. I should have dressed more warmly. The lower-back pain has tired me out. Warmth and rest will help."

2. ***In the here-and-now and directly explained by social relationships:*** "I've been fed up for quite a while with the miserable social climate at the office, where I'm always held up as the departmental dummy, and so I've brought this ailment on myself in order to get some rest and have time to think things over. My mind refuses to kowtow any more. I should at long last simply bang on the table and quit …"

3. ***In the here-and-now and viewed from the orthopedic point of view:*** "My orthopedist explained to me that a slipped disc is the cause of my lumbago and that my bending over wrong is why the disc 'slipped.' In the worst case, I'll need an operation, and I need rest and painkillers."

4. ***In the here-and-now and with a pain-therapy/psychiatric explanation:*** "I am subconsciously depressed and my lower back represents my emotional resonance organ, as my psychiatrist explained to me in an extended conversation – and, to make things worse, the pain ratcheted up and got stronger and stronger. I was told that the most important thing is to treat the depression with psychotropic agents and the pain with analgesics. After that, I should see to my psyche; I need dialogues and relaxation exercises …"

5. ***In childhood and from the psychoanalytic point of view:*** "Behind the lumbago lies my depressiveness, which stems from an unhappy childhood. An additional aggravating factor is the fact that my partner ruthlessly exploits my emotional weakness."

6. ***In the here-and-now and from an energetic point of view:*** "My acupuncturist has found some weakness in certain meridians that has allowed a cold wind energy to slink in. He plans to heal me with needles and moxibustion …"

7. ***Grounded in family history:*** "I cannot emotionally bow down before my father because I've always thought of him as a sissy."

8. ***Explained by reincarnation memories:*** "In some long-ago battle, I suffered a terrible blow to the lower back before I died. I need to learn to forgive my one-time murderer …"

You can get a good idea, from the variety of different answers, how hard it can be in the individual case to recognize the true cause of an illness and to do precisely the right thing. In and of itself, each answer seems right and logical. But the instant we leave one explanatory model and turn to the next, our doubts begin, as we ask ourselves: how can the psychoanalyst and the orthopedist both be right? And even if they are both right, there's still the question of what actually is primarily responsible: the shattered disc or the shattered childhood? Does the big bad boss at the office or the cold wind energy (in the sense of Traditional Chinese Medicine) hold the key to the puzzle? You can see that the best answer is often very hard to find.

The surprising solution to the puzzle is that the patient's psyche foreshadows the true reason for its illness. This applies above all to the psychoenergetic background factors, but sometimes to traditional medical diagnoses as well. For example, one study checked whether patients suspected the cause of their disease in advance. Before gynecological check-ups, women at a university clinic filled out a questionnaire, and more than 80% of the time they checked off precisely the illness that was then later on diagnosed, such as benign or malignant breast tumor. They guessed fairly accurately what the disease was that led them to come see the doctor. I should add, by way of qualification, that patients of a university clinic represent a select clientele, coming in as they do for a prophylactic gynecological check-up that could be done by any gynecologist on any street. This study thus deals with a select subgroup that is not representative of the population as a whole.

Therefore I'd like to say from personal experience that highly intuitive, well-informed patients do the medically right thing amazingly often, even though they are, medically speaking, laypersons. When such people trust their instincts and think logically, they often, on their own, head in the right direction as far as the diagnosis of their illness and its best-possible treatment is concerned. Many specialists don't like hearing this, since they hold the conventional view that patients are by nature ignorant and need authoritarian leadership, as an underage child is told what to do by older and wiser grownups. Lately, many specialists have been rethinking and realizing that patients and their instincts are often right and that they should be paid attention to. This applies especially to the psychoenergetic background of diseases: it's here that I experience, to my never-ending surprise, how many people of the most varied educational and age levels unerringly sense what kinds of energy blocks they have, even if they can't identify the subconscious contents. I'd like to make it clear that most people don't directly sense their energy blocks, but rather sense intuitively that there's a foreboding something lurking behind their symptoms. It's these feelings that lead them to energy medicine – which means, from my point of view, that they've made the right decision.

Let us return again to the woman with depression and lumbago. My experience has shown that patients often take the right steps on their own, representing the best thing to do in their case. Thus a typical answer from a lumbago patient might be: "I have the feeling that the disc has slipped out." She would thus do well to go to an orthopedist to be thoroughly checked over. But I've also noticed that patients are unsure of themselves, and are prone to misjudgments. As an experienced General Practitioner, I of course have a better overview than most patients, and in critical cases I also make use of energy-medicine tests. There's a spectacular case from my practice that aptly illustrates this:

Ms. M. is a corpulent 65-year-old lady who has for years been plagued with lower-back pain (lumbago). She's tried everything medically possible. I first treat her depression with St. John's Wort and recommend that she move her bed location (geopathic stress zone). Also, a root-dead tooth needs to be treated, which leads to an appreciable alleviation of the lower-back pain, which the patient describes as "being stabbed with knives." Finally, in the acupuncture test, the only disturbed organ to respond is the spinal cord. Given that, up to now, all neurological examinations had come back NAD, I recommend NMR tomography as a last resort, which is best at imaging soft tissue. Three months later, I am sitting across from a freshly-operated on and cured patient. The NMR had revealed a rare protrusion (myelocyst) that was triggering the pain by pressure on the nerves.

Patient histories such as this show that, in individual cases, both orthodox physicians and their unfortunate patients can be equally at a loss when it comes to the cause of a disease. However, I don't want to give the impression that I think I always know best what's really going on. In more than a few cases, I have been grateful to the lab technicians, other experts, and specialist departments whose findings have provided the crucial clues for solving a case. I too find myself groping about in the dark, dependent on the help of colleagues. So I'd like to make it clear that I am basically calling for more and better collaboration between scientifically-based orthodox medicine and naturopathic energy medicine. The above case of the lumbago patient is a striking demonstration that this approach usually leads to the best healing results.

Now, there are always cases in which the disease onset goes totally unnoticed. Time and again, people get cancer out of the blue or helplessly suffer the agonies of a stroke or contract some other horrible disease, even after having led healthy lives for decades.[75] To all external appearances, they enjoyed emotional harmony and were bursting with health before the disease so unexpectedly broke out. My advice (as a fellow sufferer), to trust your inner voice when you've become sick, breaks down if the onset of the disease has gone unnoticed. And although, as a physician, I can be as thorough as I like in a prophylactic examination for disease, it's impossible for me to peer into every last nook and cranny of the body, simply because the human organism is too large and complex – just consider the number of cells in a body, each of which can, in its own way, degenerate and, over years of unnoticed growth, cause cancer.

The question arises as to what the individual can do in order to stay healthy and take note of incipient ailments in time. It seems to me that the most important thing is psychoenergetic harmony and a subtle sensibility. As long as we are in psychoenergetic harmony and feel good about ourselves, we are most likely to remain healthy and to notice emerging discrepancies in our body. Depending on character type, certain methods can be helpful and supportive, which I'll go into in greater detail in the next chapter. While one person might prefer meditation to achieve psychoenergetic harmony, another might turn to quite different means having nothing to do with meditation.

A new situation begins when people get sick – this is especially true of serious diseases such as heart attack or cancer. Most people who have fallen seriously ill want to know what the deeper cause of their disease is: "Why me of all people? What did I do wrong? What's the point of this illness?" – these are the questions running through their heads. I'd like to present some hints that can help answer these questions better. In previous chapters, I introduced a model that places our lives and our psyches in a larger context that builds on ancient spiritual knowledge, according to which all people, in their individual lives, are on a kind of spiritual journey in which they inexorably develop spiritually.

From this viewpoint, disease represents the soul's attempt to rediscover its true homeland. In a realistic view, disease is a special case of general human destiny, in which we find ourselves embarked on a great journey that

leads, via personal maturation and psychoenergetic growth, to our soul's true core. In this process, disease often represents a big growth opportunity – which one can see in the increasingly higher readings of energy testing. For instance, during the course of the disease, causal readings keep rising, which is an expression of psychoenergetic higher vibrations that are directly and primarily bound up with spiritual maturation. I'd like to present a typical example of this:

I have known Mr. G. as a patient for many years, but he hadn't been in my clinic for three years since there was nothing wrong with him. I know him as a quiet, friendly, and sedate 70-year-old with refined manners. Before his retirement, he had been a department clerk in a specialty store, and he always keeps his documents in perfect order. The Energy Check reveals an enormous Central Conflict in the Neck Chakra with the theme Rushed. *He confirms that, although he might seem calm on the outside, inside him everything is happening very rapidly, and that he thinks a lot faster than he acts. Evidently, Mr. G. is an obsessive-compulsive character type.*

In obsessive-compulsive types, it's often the 5th Chakra (and the associated 3rd Upper-Abdomen Chakra) that's disturbed – and so it is in Mr. G.'s case, who had often suffered from colds and neck ailments. Now he's come in because of a tragic development: he has, surprisingly, contracted liver cancer. An experienced physician can read the diagnosis in him at once, since he is strikingly emaciated and his skin has a sickly yellowish tinge to it. I measure very low emotional readings and a causal reading of 60%, i.e., a rather high reading that later on rises to 80%. At the same time, during the intensive treatment of his Central Conflict with the appropriate homeopathics, Mr. G. becomes emotionally more relaxed, he loses his depressive sadness and in general "gets a new lease on life." He feels much more balanced and stable and is able to make peace with his life circumstances. As had been expected, he dies after six months, because the disease was already far too advanced when the cancer was discovered – but he remains largely pain-free right up to the end, and is able to bear the increasing jaundice-induced itching relatively well. Yet the most important thing, it seems to me, is that, at the end of his life, Mr. G. experiences an enormous spiritual development that enables his soul to mature greatly. I hope that, thanks to this maturation, he will experience a better fate in the future than the unhappy end that took him so quickly away from this life.

Severe chronic diseases take us to our personal limits and force us to grow beyond ourselves. In the case of the above patient with advanced liver cancer, this spiritual maturing did thankfully take place. But we also have to be realistic and admit that spiritual maturation and transformation does not always succeed, since not all people emerge from a serious illness spiritually sublimated, wiser, and more mature. Many miss the goal, and their ill fortune makes them angry, bitter, and withdrawn, because they have suf-

---

[75] These seemingly incomprehensible diseases that come out of seemingly nowhere and seem to occur for no reason also affect quite admirable persons leading exemplary, very healthy and emotionally well-balanced lives. To the amazement of many disciples, many saintly and respected spiritual leaders die quite unexpectedly and very mundanely. To be sure, the response to that is often that the holy one took on, with the disease, another person's bad Karma in order to expiate it. Far be it from me to deny this, yet it does seem a bit odd that so many wonderfully drawn up rules now and then fail to function after all. To that extent, such incidents should teach us to be humble, and to realize that true healing must always involve an extra bit of extrinsic and (to us) inaccessible Grace.

fered too much for too long. Such people even seem to become spiritually uglier and more deformed, instead of bursting their characterological bonds and emerging sublimated from the disease.

Somewhat taken aback, you ask yourself why many sick people exhibit such joyless emotional changes. In my experience, in these cases the Central Conflict is too strong and the awakening personality as yet too weak to survive the disease's "crucifixion" unscathed. Sometimes relatives will then say, very disappointed and with a sarcastic edge in their voice, that the true nature of the person is now emerging – which is of course not so, from this limited viewpoint, because a person's true nature never includes wickedness and bitterness: the ugly character aspects belong to the false self that underlies the Central Conflict and its associated smaller conflicts.

It is thus necessary to resolve the psychoenergetic conflicts in these emotional embittered patients, in order to free them from their heavy psychic burden so that they can again be hopeful and friendly – as can be seen so well in Mr. G.'s case, who, despite his grave illness did not lose heart. We basically get, with each disease, an opportunity for reinvigorated psychic growth – but with no guarantee that we'll actually mature. By eliminating the conflicts, one can help patients seize their psychic growth opportunity and make the best of it (but the patients have to do the growing on their own!).

If we once again consider what illnesses hold within them in terms of opportunities for insight, we see that it has to do with key existential questions that – because of the disease – all of a sudden urgently have to be answered. The illness confronts the soul with the elemental life questions about its true needs, feelings, and intentions:

—What do I really want? What really motivates my actions?

—what do I really truly feel? What are the real feelings hiding behind my surface feelings?

—What do I really believe, really think?

—Who am I, really?

If therapists truly want to help their patients as much as possible, they should point out the way back to their True Self and help them recover themselves and their true needs, longings, and attributes. It's normally very hard for us to recognize our dark side, which detaches us from our True Self, so we are often dependent on others for help in this quest. Disease disrupts the dependence on other people by abruptly and brutally throwing us back on our own resources, like a thunderclap that, with its frightful implacable strength, challenges us to face the truth.

A thousand questions race through the head of the despairing patient who has, for the first time, been confronted with the diagnosis of an incurable disease: "Why has this happened to me of all people? If only I had done the right thing and quit smoking sooner! How the hell do I get out of this mess? Am I going to come out of this agonizing experience in one piece?" Oddly enough, the attitude of most seriously ill patients changes with time, because the disease guides them to a kind of quiet humility that to my mind has to do with the fact that the patient's psyche knows the real reason for the illness. Deep inside, the seriously ill person senses the hopeful promise of a spiritual renewal that is bound up with the disease. Friends and relatives, on the other hand, tend out of ignorance to curse the patient's fate as an injustice and a burden, since they don't grasp the deeper psychic background.

The true cause of many serious diseases is apparently a difference of opinion between the True Self and the false self that needs to be resolved. As long as we act in harmony with our True Self, we'll be sick much less often. This can be seen quite well in that our psychic sense of well-being is directly related to a stable and familiar social milieu. Disease is much more common among the socially uprooted and marginalized. The same holds for separation and divorce, which are two of the greatest stressors and the most important disease causes. Our health is thus a product of external and internal factors. Therefore, only those who attain inner peace and psycho-energetic harmony will be able to stay healthy over the long run.

307

Paths to Psychoenergetic Harmony

The greatest and longest-lasting revolution that we know of took place when man discovered his soul and learned that each soul has individual value for itself alone.

(John Steinbeck)

In the next few chapters, I'd like to present some proven and practice-related ways with which a person can become psychoenergetically more harmonized and healthier. This also elevates one's general feeling of well-being and optimally prevents disease. Many existing diseases can be ameliorated through psychoenergetic harmonization – or even permanently eliminated. One feels more full of energy and more creative, has more *joie de vivre*, is emotionally centered and can live a freer, more self-determined life. When one personally changes for the better, it often leads to positive changes in the social sphere as well. Therefore, personal psychoenergetic harmonization changes one's entire social environment and life circumstances.

People have tried since time immemorial to raise their general sense of well-being and obtain more pleasurable sensations. Traditionally, drugs, sexuality, and trance-inducing situations such as ecstatic dancing have been used, all of which have the shortcoming of not lasting very long, or being associated with unfavorable conditions such as unwanted pregnancies or sexually-transmitted diseases (STDs). The question is how one can feel better, sexier, and more centered – permanently and with no drawbacks.

Basically, there are two routes to greater well-being:
1. The first way is to increase and harmonize one's energy. Typical examples include meditation, fasting, and sports, as well as certain meditative physical exercises, all of which can harmonize energy and increase its circulation.
2. The second way works on the blocks that prevent the body's energy from flowing freely and in harmony. Typical examples are psychotherapy and shamanistic and energy-medicine healing techniques for ferreting out and healing psychoenergetic blocks.

Comparing these two approaches to a garden hose, the first one (meditation, sports, and so on) figuratively opens up the faucet more, while the second eliminates knots and kinks in the hose (i.e., tries to eliminate energy blocks). If you then ask which is better, the answer can be derived from the garden-hose image: you need to get rid of the kinks before opening up the faucet more. And so – transferring the garden-hose image to our own problems – we need to first dissolve the energy blocks before raising the overall energy level.

Because everyone has energy blocks (which are of course active in some people, hidden and compensated in others), everyone benefits from the dissolution of these blocks – those with active blocks more than those with well-compensated blocks who feel healthy. Therefore, dissolving energy blocks can give healthy persons much more life energy and vitality by making them even healthier and energy-charged.

In what follows, I'd first like to list and evaluate the significance of the most important ways to dissolve psychoenergetic blocks, and then present my own method, in which I make use of philosopher Ken WILBER's hierarchical model of the subconscious (see illustration on p. 309)

I'd like to start with the superficial layer of consciousness associated with mental concepts and motivations. These are the surface personality components that I earlier identified as the **persona**. This is that aspect of personality that primarily deals with social communication and thus most directly with career success. The *persona* corresponds to our outward self-image and what others (ostensibly) think of us. Because much of the *persona* is learned and acquired, the *persona* comes across as masked and phony. Even so, it's very important for "first impressions" and for our self-image. The *persona* can be massively manipulated by thoughts and attitudes – which many already consider to be a type of therapy (but which of course comes up way too short in the subconscious).

I'd like to sketch out in broad strokes the therapy of the persona, simply because, in our modern world, it is often (erroneously) taken to be genuine therapy – but this isn't possible, due to the narrowness of the persona level. The history of persona therapy shows why. In ancient Greece, many educated people considered the dissolution of energy blocks to be a philosophical matter. Interestingly this is, to this very day, the view of many intellectuals: they think they can pull themselves up out of the swamp by their own bootstraps and won't let go of the notion that their own and the world's key problems are purely philosophical.

We see a vestigial minimalist version of this basic approach in the doctrine of positive thinking, which took the world by storm in the fifties. The origins of the positive thinking concept are found in the animated sermons of

Spectrum of Consciousness and Associated Psychotherapeutic Therapies
(in part modeled after Michael LEVIN & Ken WILBER's book *Meditation: Path to Deepest Self*)

Consciousness Levels	Personal Trait	Split-off Trait	Type of Therapy	Significance	Chakra / Energy level / Conflicts
Persona	Persona	Shadow	Basic counseling, chat, basic role-playing, positive thinking, Transactional Analysis (limited behavior therapy)	Impoverished self-image with denial of negative character components (character mask)	Upper emotional level, current conflicts
Self	Self	Body	Psychoanalysis, psychodrama	More profound self-image that includes the shadow (personality)	Medial emotional level, small conflicts
Organism as a whole	Centaur (organism as a whole)	Environment	Humanistic psychology, Bioenergetics (limited behavior therapy)	Dawning awareness of being a conscious animal (deep personal levels of the soul)	Deep emotional level, Central Conflict
Awareness of wholeness	Transpersonal	Universe	Transpersonal therapy, hypnosis, religion	Merging feeling of being one with the cosmos (transpersonal)	Causal Level, Central Conflict

temperamental evangelical preachers in America who, in the late 19th century, drummed into the heads of settlers the promising idea that the individual could move mountains with no more than his own strength and faith in God. In the middle of the 20th century, people such as Dale CARNEGIE and Joseph MURPHY were two of the most important protagonists of positive thinking. "You can do anything if you just think you can!" – these and similar optimistic mantras were presumably able to mobilize reserves and effortlessly, automatically disintegrate negative mental concepts.

The feeling thus triggered of embarking on a new and exciting journey often leads to mere pseudo-solutions, and in my clinical practice I have many times actually observed an increase in psychological disorders when mentally unstable persons subject themselves, via positive thinking programs, to even more internal pressure to succeed. For their failure – which manifests itself in the form of joblessness, an unhappy marriage, or depressions – is often not eliminated by positive thinking and, for them, the world remains a "vale of tears." To make matters worse, they then think it's they who have failed and can only see one solution: to try even harder and motivate themselves even more.

Another criticism is that the goals of positive thinking often have no authentic content that is of any use to the personality and its well-being. For instance, it makes little sense to desire to be rich and so, as a salesman, use every immoral and unethical trick in the book to "sell refrigerators to Eskimos." High sales volumes and healthy bank balances are not the truly rewarding goals, but rather just partial aspects of good business. The main emphasis should be placed on people and their needs! And even those who earn a lot of money honorably should clearly understand that wealth has no intrinsic value as a worthwhile goal that gives meaning to one's life – as the positive-thinking apostles so tirelessly proclaim. One should thus concentrate on truly meaningful goals, such as living more contentedly and sensibly (authentically).

Of course, we shouldn't dismiss positive thinking out of hand, but rather acknowledge its good points. Basically, our thoughts very likely do create part of our future (along with many other imponderables), so that positive thinking can indeed help pave the way for a better future. Also self-evident, however, is that it takes more than just positive thoughts and good intentions; you have to take concrete steps in the real world if your dreams are to come true. A big obstacle to reaching the longed-for future is subconscious negative thoughts and conflicts. In my experience, these psychoenergetic blocks in the area of the superficial subconscious cannot be resolved by positive thinking alone; you have to first confront and deal with your *shadow*. This is the psychological term for the suppressed feelings of envy, wrath, inferiority, and such that prevent us from reaching our goals and leading a self-determined and contented life.

What can one do to get to know one's dark side and work on it? Therapeutically speaking, the therapist enters into a conversation with the patient, to bring about a change of mind. There's the example of the conservative Turkish man whose consent is required for his daughter to marry: "Why don't you want your daughter to marry this man? He's not a bad fellow and you don't have the right to run her life like that, just because the prospective son-in-law is not a Moslem." Or take the opposite tack and pretend that something bad simply doesn't exist: "Think positive! Act like the good-hearted father that, deep in your heart of hearts, you really are, who can't deny his daughter her slightest wish!" The conflicts of that level are felt quite directly and immediately, as the father in my example gets stabbing pains in his chest because of his heartache at the thought of his daughter marrying the unwanted son-in-law-to-be.

The organ language reveals what is happening in such almost-conscious conflicts in terms of psychosomatic relationships, and how the (emotional) feeling gets directly translated into a (physical) sensation: "A lump in the throat from grief, or anger eating a hole in the stomach, and so on." So, you don't have to make any great effort to sense your true feelings, because you experience them directly. Equally simple and obvious are the suggestions we give people to help them solve their problems: do this, don't do that, look at it this way – and so forth and so on. Naturally, most such advice dispensers are not professional advisors, but rather spouses, good friends, and immediate family members, who want to help when they hand out their simple and yet valuable advice.

Simple role-playing, as done in Transactional Analysis, is likewise a good way to get at the *persona* level. This way, one learns to change one's role expectations and develop new social concepts. The most important ground rule for the fairest and best possible communication is: "I'm OK, you're OK." To my mind, the real art here is not to deny one's own and the other person's dark side, but also not to obsess on it so that the feeling for good and right things is preserved: "Of course I have my faults and you have your quirks, but still we're both pretty much OK the way we are, and we can work it out." With this kind of humane attitude, serious interpersonal problems can much better be resolved. No one

is forced to be the loser (or, worse, a "bastard"); instead, face is saved all around, and the resulting peaceful coexistence between the conflicting parties is clearly the best solution.

A folksy way, found all over the world, to confront your shadow is the Carnival [such as New Orleans' *Mardi Gras*]. In it, you learn not to take yourself so seriously, and you reestablish contact with deeper psychic components that have been covered over by the *persona* mask. Those who can laugh at themselves have already gotten past the hardest part of accepting their own shadow. In my experience, the real core of neurotic disorders seems to be an irate humorlessness when it comes to one's own self-image. Consequently those who feel compelled to quarrel with others about the merits of their personal traits usually need to do so because their fragile self-image cannot tolerate any doubt nor the slightest criticism.

After a certain age, children are amazingly good-humored when someone makes fun of their shadow side, i.e., laziness or sloppiness. Very young children still have too fragile an Ego to be able to take rebukes, but that changes later on. On the other hand, children are the most keen-eyed critics of the hypocritical adult world. "But the emperor has no clothes on!" the child exclaims in the fairy tale "The Emperor's New Clothes" (which only exist in the imagination), where the adults, before the child's exclamation, had been completely blind to the emperor's state of undress. Children thus see through psychological façades with astonishing insightfulness. If you want to know the truth about yourself, just ask any moderately perceptive ten-year-old.

The next deeper subconscious level is known as the *Ego level*. It is here that we find the true roots of the feeling of selfhood which, according to developmental psychology, can be traced back to experiences in early childhood. The subconscious contents at this level are of a preverbal nature, so we can't refer to it with words, but instead must resort to emotions and images. As soon as someone can consciously remember something without being in trance state, that which is recalled usually touches on subconscious material at the Ego level. This also highlights the foremost problem of all conversation therapies: that which can be grasped and remembered in words is usually of limited importance, whereas the truly significant parts of our memories remain wordless and intangible. Because of this, I've noticed that most conversation therapies tend to go in circles, getting nowhere.

Vivid and emotionally-charged therapies (psychodrama, gestalt therapy, bioenergetics) can then take it further, as can creative therapies (painting therapy) and contact with animals (horseback riding, swimming with dolphins). Clearly, the great number of therapies and possibilities for re-establishing contact with one's emotional child makes it impossible to get one's bearings very well, and dispense sensible advice – which is no doubt best in the individual case. I imagine that dissolving psychoenergetic conflicts is the simplest route to establishing contact with one's inner child. In addition, one can then choose a therapy with which one is most comfortable.

In the modern notion of what's important in the life of the individual, the idea of the "inner child" occupies a prominent position. In our society, the predominant attitude is that a life of physical pleasures is the only kind worth living; one thus speaks quite properly of a consumption- and pleasure-oriented society. Spinning out this basic attitude, there are widespread ideas as to what right and true living consists of, all related to maximizing fun and pleasure. In order as adults to revive our inner child, the general consensus is that we should do anything that our inner child enjoys, and what an actual child would do when we adults are not around to prevent it. According to this widespread belief, one only needs to develop a sense for what the inner child likes and wants. At first glance, this sounds very simple and quite logical – but in my opinion the entire approach is fundamentally wrong!

Turning the inner child loose without first working on its conflicts and resolving them leads, in the extreme case, to a society of ill-bred, egotistical "Peter Pans" who childishly indulge their own self-interest to the exclusion of all else. The increasing obsession with youthfulness of a society composed entirely of self-centered individuals leads to the dismal end result of an atomized collection of solitary seekers. Only in old age do people tend to notice that their superficial and egotistical attitude has led them to ignore and neglect the deeper meaning of their own life. The reason for this is, quite simply, that the inner child cannot possibly be an end in itself, just as fun or autonomy cannot be intrinsic values. Clearly, its opposite – a cheerless anti-pleasure attitude – is every bit as bad, and no one is pining for a return to the ascetic severity and bleakness of earlier eras. As is so often the case, the truth lies in the middle between the extremes – and of course adults must not forget their inner child, but they also should not lead a 100% childish and superficial life.

Meanwhile, we live in a modern society that is starting to suffer more and more from the wrong-headed concept of the inner child that supposedly needs to be set free. For many people, self-actualization means throwing overboard their entire life so far and starting a radically new one, never realizing that you can't run away from your inner problems. The liberation of the inner child is thus, I firmly believe, not the final goal, but rather a single step in the direction of a more authentic life. The sexual liberation of the seventies was an important collective step in this direction – but exclusively egotistical self-actualization eventually leads down a blind alley. The happiest and most emotionally balanced people I've ever met were those who never gave a thought to their own self-actualization. They were either very spiritual people (deeply religious) or were too poor or uninformed to be able to afford any luxuries, as one can see in the poor people of India, so many of whom have radiantly happy expressions.

The inner child relates to the middle level of the subconscious, the region where childish needs are located – but also animalistic drives. Therefore, when we adults strive to liberate the inner child by re-establishing contact with our deeper emotional layers, it's not just the three-year-old who enjoys eternal affection, uninhibited dancing, monkeyshines, and sweet chocolate who pops up: at this middle level, we also automatically come into contact with our sexual and power drives. We thus find ourselves in the area of the so-called "sexual roundelay" and of hierarchical power struggles. Earlier on, I mentioned that erotic love and social acceptance are among the most important subconscious drives of our existence.

Psychoanalysis is concerned with seeing through enslaving and negative games which lead to our perceiving and acting (from early childhood on) against our true nature. Subconscious blocks prevent us from claiming and enjoying our due share of power and love. There is no denying that psychoanalysis (and its derivative disciplines) is a valuable way to establish contact with oneself and one's inner child – but it is by no means the only way. An awareness of the limitations of traditional psychoanalysis is growing even among psychotherapists themselves.

I'd like briefly to address some problems and limits of psychoanalysis. It seems to me that one of psychoanalysis' core problems is the inauspicious power position that the analyst ends up in as omnipotent master of the therapeutic situation; this position imparts a tilt that's hard to straighten out. In this context, some of the key concepts include: therapist encroachments on their patients in the form of sexual abuse; hindering patient autonomy because the therapist always has the last word. There are other problems common to all speech-oriented therapies. Time and again I have noticed, especially for very intelligent and eloquent people, that psychoanalysis doesn't help them at all – and in fact simply winds up supplying ammunition for the defense of their neurotic disorders. Intelligent people quickly figure out what the analyst wants to hear and integrate this into the therapeutic process.

It seems a good idea at this point to take a critical look at the psychoanalytic concept of "resistance." This is understood as the patient's attempts to prevent painful subconscious contents from being made conscious. This resistance manifests itself in all kinds of boycotts, strikes, and the patient's general refusal to cooperate in the analysis. To this day, it seems to have occurred to virtually no psychoanalysts that maybe patients rebel against the therapeutic strategy because they simply don't see the point in just talking about their problems. Just as many homeopaths attempt to reassure wavering patients by assuring them that each undesired effect of treatment is just a so-called "initial worsening," ostensible "resistance" is often a lie that therapists try to maintain to themselves and their patients to avoid having to admit their own ineptitude.

My encounters with hundreds of patients who had undergone years of psychoanalysis, and who spoke very frankly about their experiences, have reinforced my view on this – which, to any psychoanalyst, will of course sound offensive and even unsound. One could accuse me of simply parroting what people say, and of jeopardizing sound medical opinion, but I firmly believe that the "resistance" concept, and many other psychoanalytic notions, are largely figments of the imagination. "If everyone is saying the same thing, then it's most likely true" is the unstated slogan here. I am aware, despite all my criticism, that there is indeed such a thing as subconscious resistance on the part of patients defending their psychological problems – it's just that this resistance is often confused with rebellion against a talking therapy that seems pointless to them.

Besides the agonizingly long psychotherapeutic learning curve, another problem psychoanalysis has is its inadequate healing possibilities. Sniffing out subconscious problems is not the same thing as curing them – not by a long shot! For a long time, it was believed that simply bringing the suppressed feelings up to the conscious level and activating them would jumpstart the conflict healing process. This erroneous assumption is the seductive mirage which constitutes the actual foundation of psychoanalysis – and its feet of clay. In this context, I'd like to point out that psychoanalytic inquiries have revealed that FREUD had feigned therapeutic progress with his own patients in an effort to make psychoanalysis respectable; detailed review of the treatment protocols (such as "Wolfsmann") showed that there had been no actual observable improvement in symptomatology or personality traits.

As a doctor, I have occasionally even noted in my patients an intensification of symptoms and psychoenergetic blocks that, based on my experience, had been provoked by various different psychological and psychoanalytic therapies. Instead of becoming psychologically healthier and energetically more harmonized, these poor people were made even sicker by such therapies! This is because emotionally provocative procedures supply conflicts with extra energy and thus make them stronger. Therefore, the foremost therapeutic guideline is to bring about a happy and harmonious resolution to all churned-up negative emotions. Unfortunately, this banal basic rule is ignored by amazingly many therapists, so it's no wonder that stirring up emotional blocks and pains only makes things worse.[76]

Despite the criticism, psychoanalysis is, in many cases, indisputably a worthwhile healing method. An obligatory precondition seems to me to be that the patient's positive character traits be fortified and positive emotional solutions found. Then, psychoanalysis can definitely foster personality development and growth that otherwise wouldn't have

taken place (at least in that manner) without therapeutic assistance. It is by no means my intention to engage in a wholesale condemnation of psychoanalysis and psychotherapy, but rather simply to "trim" their territory back to a sensible size. For people with average to mild emotional disorders (which I reckon to be about 70–80% of the population) psychotherapy is usually unnecessary – and even harmful if done wrong.

This still leaves plenty of emotionally suffering people (for which the number of practicing psychotherapists is not nearly enough) who would most likely benefit from psychotherapy. Personal growth and the development of positive emotional qualities seems to me the true domain of psychotherapy. But one must absolutely resolve psychoenergetic conflicts, after which psychotherapy can much better get to the point, can progress much more quickly and effectively and can concentrate on restoring the personality (its true domain!). Emotional blocks heal much more quickly when they're energetically dissolved. In the next chapter I describe how to accomplish that most easily and simply, as I explain the strategy of Psychosomatic Energetics.

The next lower subconscious level deals with body awareness. We tend (wrongly) to believe that we are aware of our bodies – yet we normally only consciously perceive a small fraction of the sensations constantly being generated in it. Babies and very young children still have very strong unfiltered sensations in some parts of their body such as the mouth and tongue, but even babies perceive much less of the body as a whole than is generally assumed. Research has shown that their perception of skin temperature is still little developed, whereas the mouth excites exceptionally strong sensations. Therefore, we as adults need to develop gradually an overall body awareness, during which process we will dredge up extremely strong emotions and ancient memories concealed in stressed and unresponsive body regions.

Many ancient meditation and healing systems work with body awareness, with breathing and posture playing key roles. Breathing and posture directly influence our psychoenergetic well-being. People who take quick shallow breaths and stand hunched over are much more likely to feel nervous and unsure of themselves than those who breathe slowly and calmly and stand up straight. You can quickly make good progress through simple self-observation and attentiveness, but expert assistance is required to address more profound processes. Which kinds of therapy and pro-

---

[76] When therapy succeeds anyway, it's actually due to the strengthening of the feeling of self-worth. As for a flood tide, the "dikes" are therapeutically raised, but the real cause is not eliminated. Although such people are still emotionally every bit as disturbed as before therapy, from the outside they seem more self-confident. Also, disagreeable and egotistical character traits are not toned down; on the contrary, they're unpleasantly amplified – it's just that the analyst has encouraged the patient not to worry about it any more. This entire unfortunate development reminds me of the behavior of ill-mannered children who (on top of their bad manners) have also become impertinent and conceited.

cedures are right for whom – this I can't generalize on, and so intuition plus trial and error yield the best results. But in the next chapter, I include some tips as to which procedures are best for which character types.

Descending to the next level, we arrive at the deepest regions of the subconscious, which are beyond the reach of traditional speech therapies. We here come into contact with those parts of the subconscious that relate to our true spiritual core and transpersonal cosmic consciousness. We are moving away from the interpersonal power struggles of the intermediate emotional regions toward individual spiritual themes located in the deep emotional and causal regions. Down at this level, we are really not interested in what other people think of us, nor what our place is in the pecking order. In this most intimate region of our psyche, we feel like the little child that drags about its extraordinarily painful emotional wounds and is animated by a single overpowering longing to be once again hale and whole, to feel again completely at home emotionally and totally centered spiritually.

This has absolutely nothing to do with what is known in psychological terminology as regression, but rather with a great spiritual longing that is the true root of all genuine religiosity. "What is a man profited, if he shall gain the whole world, and lose his own soul?" [Matthew xiii:26] is an expression of this awareness. At this depth of our psyche, we are moving about in a totally existential region that challenges our entire being. Here is where the psyche is most vulnerable and needs to be handled with the utmost care. Here, it seems to me that the best (and most effective) way is the psychoenergetic dissolution of the Central Conflict. In the next chapter, I'll describe my experiences in treating the Central Conflict of countless patients – and show how best to get in touch with one's deepest spiritual center.

Healing the Center of the Soul

Compassion is an effective antidote to fear.
(Seneca)

We all have, deep in our heart, a longing for our true center, where genuine happiness is to be found, and wholeness with our Self lies hidden (the mythological equivalent of the Garden of Eden). Only at our emotional center can we find our way back to ourselves and be truly happy in our heart of hearts – even more so than in the happiest days of our childhood. People who have found the way back to their emotional center, when they talk about it, all agree that it is an abidingly blissful emotional state.

How does one achieve this on one's own? On this point, all doctrines of salvation and belief systems claim that the only possible solution is to adhere to their doctrine and none other. I'd just like to mention decades-long meditation paths and time-consuming religious practices that are among the oldest traditional paths to salvation. Most of

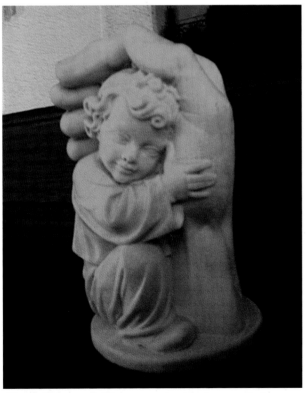

The child is guarded by a protecting hand – a symbolic representation of the inner child that corresponds to the emotional center and the True Self.

them demand of their initiates that they totally renounce their present lives and (for instance) join a monastic order. As a practicing physician tasked with alleviating human suffering and (when possible) healing, I am not interested in such difficult and time-consuming healing processes. I'd therefore like to report on other ways that seem to me more realistic and simpler, and which lead more quickly to lasting positive changes.

In my experience, there are basically three ways to establish contact with one's deep emotional center (the True Self):

1. The first option, namely elaborate **spiritual practices**, I have already mentioned – and rejected as being too arduous and time-consuming. Nowadays, we need quick and effective ways to mature emotionally and eliminate emotional conflicts. Above all, we need non-elitist methods that benefit as many people as possible. Many of the world's urgent problems can be traced back to subconscious conflicts that need to be resolved as quickly and lastingly as possible – or else the world will continue to sink into ever more war and chaos. To counter this trend, we desperately need quick and effective methods that are also affordable and easily accessible.

2. The simplest option that fulfills the above-mentioned criteria is the **melting down of the Central Conflict** (which I'll be covering in next two chapters). When the Central Conflict becomes smaller, the repression and defense mechanisms of the false self disappear automatically, and the True Self can emerge. There are two ways to shrink the Central Conflict: first, reinforcing positive character traits and reducing negative ones (the topic of this chapter) and, second, energetically melting down the conflict itself (the topic of the next chapter, in which Psychosomatic Energetics is described).

3. The third (and most frequent) way to contact the deep subconscious is via existential crises and the extreme psychic stress associated with life-threatening situations and shattering emotional suffering. These are sometimes referred to as **borderline experiences**, and they represent the most spontaneous and unpredictable way to discover one's subconscious. With borderline experiences, you never know exactly what might happen and

what the consequences could be – which makes them extraordinarily hard to control for therapeutic purposes. I therefore advise against all drastic therapies associated with borderline experiences. Still, in isolated cases they can be very efficacious – as can be seen in the magnificent success that LSD psychotherapy has had with some alcoholics. Heroin addicts and violent criminals seem also to benefit from borderline situations as they, in certain kinds of therapy, are forced to suffer through extreme emotional agony. This is, understandably, a matter for highly-trained and experienced therapists only.

Borderline experiences don't have to involve a horrible accident or some other catastrophe; they can also have pleasant and sensual contents. A transforming borderline experience can be an enormously stimulating amusement such as riding the rollercoaster or going through the haunted house at an amusement park. Children and animals, with their unsophisticated instincts, fear for their lives and scream piteously for help. For modern man, on the other hand, the nervous tension instinctively associated with deadly danger has an unexpectedly enlivening and emotionally expansive effect. So it's no wonder that so many people have become addicted to thrills and chills – such as jumping headfirst off high bridges with bungee cords tied to their ankles.

When mountain climbers and extreme-sports athletes are asked what motivates them, they often say that they want to experience themselves and the world more intensely. Actually, these ecstatic experiences and peak emotional excitements seem to be about the search for the True Self. Also, all forms of ecstasy and trance (such as dervish dancing or wild, abandoned sex) can lead to eruptions of deep subconscious psychic contents. Therapies involving hallucinogenics or trance states use the borderline-experience phenomenon to open up the subconscious, as do all methods that work with sensory deprivation (Lilly tanks, for example).

Sometimes the beginning of self-perception is bound up with rather painful agitation – which are definitely not voluntarily sought out, but rather must be painfully endured. Such emotional shocks include the death of a beloved relative or a painful divorce. At the beginning of the book, I described the agonies I underwent in my own divorce. These negative borderline experiences tend to punch the external persona mask full of holes. One thing that extreme-sports athletes and mountain climbers have in common is the intensification of sensory perceptions. I well recall that I lived much more consciously and intensely during the time of my divorce, notwithstanding the associated grief and sorrow. Therefore, it seems to me that both positive and negative borderline experiences seem to be coupled with stronger sensory perception. But borderline experiences can

just as well tip over to the opposite extreme in which one no longer feels anything at all physically. For example, a friend of mine once made fun of his co-workers' horrified faces – until he realized that the reason for their horror was his own torn-off thumb, which had, just seconds before, been caught in the mechanical press he operated. It took a while for the pain (and the realization that he was permanently maimed) to sink in.

Borderline experiences sometimes open up the subconscious, so that vivid dreams, flashes of insight, and the like can take place. Mountain climbers have told, when they fell, how their whole life flashed before their eyes or, trapped in a snowstorm, they encountered mythical creatures whose form and radiance were of extraterrestrial loveliness – and that these creatures told them what was happening at that moment to relatives thousands of miles away, the details of which later turned out to be completely accurate. Many people with paranormal abilities have told me that shock-like and moving experiences triggered their psychic transformation. Starting from the time of some accident or emotional shock, their subconscious opened up, and this opening-up brought with it unsuspected paranormal abilities such as clairvoyance, which then stayed with them for a long time as an adjunct of their transformation.

Many people also experience feelings of inner hopelessness that intensify intolerably, in the absence of any discernible dramatic external influence. From the outside, one hasn't the slightest inkling that these people are suffering horribly. Like the mountain climber who fell off a cliff face, these cases are also genuine inner emotional "crashes." Here certain patterns come into play, e.g., at times of biological transformation such as the oft-cited midlife crisis. These transformational phases are capable of calling into question a person's entire life-plan. Thus, menopausal patients often tell me "… but that can't be all there is, all that I've lived for!" – thus expressing the enormous emotional disappointment associated with the summing-up of the dismally dreary life that many people have led up to a certain point. There's yet another disappointment that accompanies these phases of life: the feeling that one has grown old without having realized any meaningful goal; this (understandably) intensifies the hopeless feeling even more. I often also notice a third sore point that leads to a crisis in middle age: many people have magnificent secret dreams that they carry about their entire lives, that eventually everything will turn out for the better – but then, someday, they stand before the shattered remains of a gigantic disappointment.

I'd like to describe the typical case of a female patient with depression and lower-back pain, whose case is representative of so many who, in middle age, are confronted with a dramatic emotional crisis stemming from decades of disappointment:

Ms. S. lives alone, works as a secretary and lives a normal but rather lonely overtime-dominated life as a single person –

when, at age 43, she's struck with severe lower back pain. She undergoes intervertebral disk surgery and visits numerous health spas, all to no avail. The pain and the forced inactivity of the illness trigger ever more severe feelings of emptiness and hopelessness. She also complains of a constant bloated feeling and of constipation. When I first meet Ms. S., she looks much older than her age (48), is very overweight (she was full-figured before the illness but still relatively well-proportioned), and seems extraordinarily tired and listless – a stark contrast to her basically friendly and empathetic nature.

In the energy testing, I measure extremely low vital and emotional values, as well as a huge conflict with the theme Wanting more *in the Upper-abdomen Chakra. My conversation with her reveals that she has felt extraordinarily dissatisfied for many years. Neither her desire for a husband and children nor any of her other secret wishes (beautiful vacation journeys, a career as an independent business woman) have been fulfilled. She is therefore very deeply dissatisfied. The* Wanting more *theme matches up with her enormous inner frustration, which she anesthetizes with food orgies and reading stacks of novels.*

Only after her Central Conflict is healed does Ms. S. become aware of the full extent of her grief and despair, and she wrestles with herself for a long time over whether to "throw it all away" and move to Australia, where a good friend of hers lives. But then she realizes that running away is not the answer. She takes numerous trips with a women's group, in which she can pour out her heart to kindred souls. She gradually comes to accept her fate and, in time, loses both her depression and her lower back pain. The irksome upper abdominal symptoms and the constipation go away as well. She opens up her own shop and tells me, bursting with pride, that she's managed, despite everything, to realize a part of her dreams. A family is probably out of the question because of her age, she says, but her own business and the companionship of her women friends is enough to give her life some meaningful content.

In Ms. S.'s case it's easy to see that her real life and her inner demands kept moving farther and farther apart, and that this was a crucial factor in the outbreak of her lumbago and depression. The inner emotional pressure got so unbearable that it triggered lower back pain, which can be viewed, psychosomatically, as a form of somatized depression. Later, the emotional depression also began; this, along with the lumbago, can be understood as the screams of her frustrated psyche that her life needs to change from the ground up. "I can't take it any more! I get older every day and none of my wishes is ever going to come true, so I just can't go on!" This is, more or less, the sound of the messages from the deep layers of the psyche that are bound up with Ms. S.'s becoming ill. One can interpret her lower back pain as the physical expression of her emotional inability to go on, because she has been "broken" inside.

This example focuses on a Central Conflict in the upper abdomen having to do with deep-seated and intolerably strong frustrations. It's typical of feelings that are part of the depressive character type that there is a displacement reaction in the form of excessive consumption. Such persons either eat too much and devour anything and everything (like Ms. S.'s stacks of novels), or they put up a façade of ascetic frugality that keeps their Central Conflict hidden from the outside world. They'll even strive to compensate the emotional contents of their Central Conflict with an exterior that looks like the exact opposite, presumably because their emotional shadow is too embarrassing. Yet deep in their soul they're probably harboring an overpowering feeling of hunger, full of frustrations, even though on the outside they seem to have no needs at all. By the way, I find the Central Conflict *Wanting more* fairly frequently among therapists and teachers. Such people often sacrifice themselves selflessly for others – the technical term for which is "helper syndrome." Emotionally, these overeager helpers have, unsuspected by anyone, a shadow side of great emotional hunger (or psychological problems involving similar themes). Helping others is an attempt to generate gratitude with which to feed their emotional hunger.

In appraising Ms. S.'s overall problem complex, once you realize that the Central Conflict had been present long before her condition peaked and became an unendurable crisis, the focus of the situation shifts dramatically – because people who carry around a *Wanting more* conflict are constantly (yet subconsciously) manipulating their own actions. This means that Ms. S. is not really a victim, but rather the secret shaper of her own misfortune! Ms. S. is frustrated and unhappy because that's the way she wants it, subconsciously. In a moment, I'll address the background dynamics driving the process …

… but first I'd like to emphasize that Ms. S. hardly represents a unique case; she's a fairly typical member of a subgroup that gets bigger every day. Day after day, as a doctor I see a growing number of patients with these and similar complaints whose basis is, ultimately, an emotional/energetic block. This is what is known as an active Central Conflict because, when they're tested, one always find a huge conflict that corresponds to the patient's life theme. People with an active Central Conflict find themselves in an extremely difficult spot, because orthodox physicians and psychologists don't usually succeed in finding the real reason why they feel so bad and what the actual problems are.

Typical symptoms of people with active Central Conflicts include:
- Therapy-resistant and chronic ailments of all kinds
- Mental and/or physical complaints of all kinds after severe shock states (such as post-traumatic stress disorder)
- Conspicuous behavioral disorders and severe character dysgenesis

- A strong feeling of being pulled away from one's emotional/energetic center most of the time, and of no longer being able to get back to it under one's own steam
- Persistent "spiritual crises"
- Moderate to severe psychosomatic and psychiatric disorders such as depression, anxiety attacks, psychoses

My book thus addresses, first, the ever-growing group of people with active Central Conflicts who cannot be healed by conventional methods. I can make this assertion because I have seen scads of patients with active Central Conflicts who, before they came to me, had tried every conceivable therapy – to no avail. Only Psychosomatic Energetics gives these patients the crucial healing impetus for finding their way back to their psychic center. Like a piano that has been out of tune, after their Central Conflict is resolved, they once again vibrate in harmony, which then permanently dissolves most of their remaining ailments and disorders. Plus, they get crucial information about which character type they belong to (which corresponds to their Central Conflict), which of course enormously eases both my therapist's advisory role and the patient's path to self-knowledge – since, if you know what your character type is, you know the most important thing there is to know about yourself. A therapist can make much better solution proposals, and patients have a far easier job of self-discovery, once they know what their emotional center consists of and what it is that they really, truly, deeply desire.

This brings me to the crucial point behind the entire disease dynamics when a Central Conflict gets activated. In Ms. S.'s case one can clearly see her psyche subconsciously precipitating an ill-fated life situation that corresponds to the Central Conflict's dark side. For instance, a latently furious person will time and again get into emotionally intolerable tense situations that enrage him, but in which he dare not give vent to his rage. In Ms. S.'s case, the *Wanting more* conflict is an intolerable condition of deep frustration that she herself subconsciously brought about, and which winds up leading her into a blind alley.

Thus, many people subconsciously assemble a tense life situation in which they're actualizing their emotional dark side instead of living in the real world! There are some key questions that can aid the self-discovery process, having to do with the gap between inner and outer reality, and culminating in the key question as to why this discrepancy exists: "Why do I act, in some situations, against my own wishes?" Another question: "Why do I live a life other than the one I really want to live?" Yet another is aimed at fear as the primary source of psychic disorders: "Why do some things scare me so much they actually paralyze me?" Or one can ask oneself: "What kind of power is it that makes me think and feel other than the way I'd actually like to?"

In earlier chapters, I spoke in detail about the significance of the Central Conflict, that largest of conflicts that shapes our thoughts and actions. The Central Conflict, as the False Self, forces thought and behavior patterns on us that, deep in our heart of hearts, are foreign to us and make us slaves of a foreign power. All good (i.e., truly healing) methods, and honest introspection, reinforce our authentic personality components and gradually unmask our False Self and thus make the façade less and less necessary. I'll get into how, specifically, this takes place by means of the different procedures for the four character types. Each character type calls for a different procedure in order to reinforce its positive parts and weaken the negative ones.

The first step is knowing about one's own character. For this, I recommend reading the earlier chapters that describe the character types – or ask close friends and relatives which character type they think you are. You can also visit an energy tester, who will test out the Central Conflict with the aid of Psychosomatic Energetics. Once you know your character type, the simplest path to mental harmony, and the best personal maturation possibility, consists of reinforcing the dissimilar attracting personality components – i.e., those of the schizoid for a depressive, or of the obsessive-compulsive for a hysteric (and vice-versa).

We need the missing half of the psyche in order to take the biggest and most important step toward personal wholeness. Like a one-legged person, we need the second leg "to stand on" to reach our psychic center. In an ideal partnership (and marriage) we choose a complementary partner for this, one who becomes "our better half." Now of course the ultimate goal is striving for character wholeness as a "quaternity" by at some point actualizing the positive traits of all four character types. But the leap over to dissimilar polar characteristics is too hard for most people – i.e., the schizoid over to hysteric, or the obsessive-compulsive to depressive – which is why we (wisely) first try it out with our compensating character psychic half.

C.G. JUNG speaks of the necessity of developing our feminine (*Anima*) and masculine (*Animus*) psychic sides. I'd like to remind the reader that each character type has either predominantly masculine or predominantly feminine traits. Thus the depressive and hysteric types are feminine, while the obsessive-compulsive and schizoid types have masculine polarity. Each character type needs, for balance, a gender-appropriate counter-polarity. There's some confusion as to the true meaning of **Anima** and **Animus**, insofar as a sexuality is being simulated that is not at all intended. Ultimately, it has to do with inner psychological qualities that are completely unrelated to biological gender – for, way down deep, it doesn't matter whether a person is a man or a woman. So *Animus* and *Anima* are not about sexual orientation, but about expansion of the psyche into traits that have a more masculine (or feminine) character.

Ultimately, it has to do with very simple recommendations, e.g., that the stand-offish schizoid needs to acquire social skills and warm-heartedness in order to become a whole person who is more lovable and can better express love in return. Or the depressive must learn to stop wanting to be everyone's darling, and practice setting limits so as not to overcommit and be constantly exploited by others. At that same time, one can recommend to each of the four character types that they dismantle their most obnoxious negative character traits in order to moderate their personality and rein in their egotism. Ultimately, we are dealing with "outmoded" concepts such as virtues (which have to be acquired) and vices (which should be shed).

One can assess the psychic health of the respective character type by how much individuals develop Anima and/or Animus characteristics, and how much they've toned down their negative character traits. A "harmonic character" is one who has struck the right balance among the various polar opposites. Of course, you need to be careful here not to con-fuse psychic harmony with artificially-imposed indoctrination, exemplified in such phrases as "a good upbringing" or "well-mannered." This process is not about a mere display of external traits, but rather about "nobility of the heart" which comes sincerely from within.

I'd like to run through the most important positive and negative character development aspects of each character type.

Schizoids exhibit more positive character development the less their egocentric withdrawal tendencies and their unapproachable nature come to the fore, in favor of socially friendly and emotionally open character traits that confront the external world in a positive manner. These are the depressive's Animus/Anima components that schizoids very much need for balance, and that do them an enormous amount of good once they develop them. Neurotic schizoids get very compulsive, tending to perfectionism and overly rigid control. The psychotic disorders of schizoids exhibit hysteric characteristic traits. This includes the ostentatious

Character Type and the Positive and Negative Character Traits to be Developed and Eliminated, Respectively

Character Type	Negative Character Traits to be Eliminated	Positive and Harmonizing Anima/Animus Character Traits
Schizoid	*Egocentric behavior, insensitivity and excessive callousness, walling oneself off from the outside world, cynicism, rigidity and brutality*	*Pay attention to one's feelings, feel oneself to be a social being, look out for others and their feelings, be gentle and yielding, be able to say yes*
Depressive	*Always docile behavior, helplessly at the mercy of feelings, too soft and conformist, self-deception, emotional terrorization of others, exerting pedagogical dressage*	*Trust one's intellect, learn to listen only to oneself and one's inner voice, be able to exhibit outward toughness, be able to say no*
Obsessive-compulsive	*Emotional rigidity and immobility, wanting to control and hold fast to everything, know-it-all, despotic autocrat, nitpicker and petty*	*Learn to be relaxed and playful, live life carefree and informally, accept the transitoriness of the world and one's own existence, relinquish control*
Hysteric	*Living with the façade, outsmarting oneself and others, being dishonest and egotistical, avoiding decisions, living in the present, coercing others, confusing one's fellow humans, getting violent*	*Learn to be structured and disciplined, adopt firm positions and make clear decisions, consciously set limits for oneself and voluntarily forgo alternatives*

paranoid (Trickster), who works off sadistic impulses by making fun of God and the world, refusing to take anything seriously. In this psychotic situation, everything is mere façade that turns into a two-dimensional robot world in which only theatrical posturing can impart a trace of defiance and liveliness.

Depressives exhibit greater psychic health the more honestly and courageously they promote their own interests with respect to others, while the overly emotional and socially conformist side is scaled back. As neurotics, depressives tend to superficial exaggeration as they eccentrically try to please those around them and view everything as one big game. They then develop the less attractive traits of the hysteric, which are of course latently present in the depressive character type and emerge in neuroses. This leads to psychotic disorders if compulsive control mechanisms and apprehensive pedantry set in. A washing compulsion, in the sense of an isolated psychosis, can thus represent a psychotic personality deformation.

Hysterics who develop properly structured character traits that correspond to the positive compulsive character traits participate in a good harmonic development. Moreover, the weaker their negative character traits – for instance, paying more attention to substance than style – the healthier and more harmonic they'll be. On the other hand, the traits of the other character types (depressive and schizoid) have an unhealthy effect. Hysterics who go neurotic (and thus depressive) will fall tearfully into a regression of addictions and emotion-laden passions, with no ability to set boundaries with respect to the wishes of others, groveling at the beck and call of authority figures. It gets even worse if schizoid character traits evoke psychotic symptoms in hysterics that lead to egocentric harshness and intolerance. In this type of schizoid illness, hysterics turn into extreme know-it-alls, wrapping themselves in their delusional fantasies and basically letting no one near them. In the worst cases we find querulous and highly aggressive character types who scent potential enemies in every person they encounter. Of course, with such delusional misjudgments of reality, it's always the other guy's fault, with the poor hysteric being the innocent scapegoat.

Obsessive-compulsives develop positively when the compulsive rigidity and the obsession with control are balanced out in favor of a looser attitude and playful lightness, which are part of the essential hysteric character traits. The obsessive-compulsive neurotic will exhibit schizoid characteristics by becoming harsh, unapproachable, and egocentric. Obsessive-compulsives tip over completely into psychosis if depressive traits emerge in them, often showing up as hypochondriac fears or persecution complexes. In case of greater regression, the obsessive-compulsive becomes extremely susceptible to external manipulation, tends to addiction and to total withdrawal into embryonic womb-fantasies. It's no wonder that temperament theory relates the obsessive-compulsive to the phlegmatic type. The most extreme form of stolidity is found in laziness and a total lack of interest in even raising a pinky to attain a goal. The fairy tale about the compliant leprechaun that does all one's work must have been first imagined by an obsessive-compulsive who thus uninhibitedly lived out his fantasies of total womblike care and security. Once you understand psychodynamically that the depressive is the ideal leprechaun, wanting to anticipate the other person's every desire, then you can understand the depressive's deep abhorrence of the immoderateness of the obsessive-compulsive, who would exploit him to the hilt if he could.

At this point, I'd like to break off the description of the character types, so as not to get into overly deep detail and end up detouring into areas that are more of interest to specialists. My intent is to give a brief overview sketch of the positive possibilities that each character type can develop as virtues, which are felt to be sympathetic, likable, and human qualities – just as the opposite can happen, in which bad habits allow the ugly sides of a character type to come to the fore, those which are generally denounced as unfriendly, unsympathetic, and egotistical. Basically, one needs to be clear that our positive characteristics are only worthwhile if they are sincere – since only that which naturally comes from the heart is worth anything over the long run, while feigned and insincere behavior can turn into a dangerous trap for all concerned, leading to entire chain reactions of problems, to psychoenergetic blocks and more "new lies to cover up old lies." **The most important thing of all is to be honest with yourself** – because only then are actions evoked by honest motivations, and only sincere actions lead to long-term positive developments (which, by the way, applies to everyone involved).

Next, I'd like to point out some other therapeutic options that stimulate a person's character type and help positive character traits to mature. A great many different types of therapy and spiritual schools offer to melt away our Central Conflict and increase our positive psychic potential. Which way is right for each character type? Which procedure is the most beneficial? Basically, all current psychotherapies and other widespread forms of self-exploration are invariably tailored to specific character types – i.e., dance therapy and psychodrama for hysterics, group therapy for depressives. Obsessive-compulsives generally prefer therapies with strict rules and structured developmental pathways such as found most clearly in Yoga and similar methods, whereas schizoids feel themselves drawn to ecstatic experiences that they can do all by themselves in their own uniquely individual manner, such as sensory deprivation in *Samadhi Tanks* or solitary meditation using holotropic (very rapid and deep) breathing exercises, which leads to intense feelings of becoming one with the universe, and even to hallucinations.

We see that each character type is attracted to specific types of therapy, correlating with their inmost nature, and

Character Type	Schizoid	Depressive	Obsessive-compulsive	Hysteric
Ideal therapy= *compensatory method & psychotherapy that is optimal for the patient*	*Holotropic breathing, hallucinogens*	*Group therapy*	*Hatha Yoga, Zen Buddhism*	*Gestalt, psychodrama, dance*
Less advisable therapy = *method & psychotherapy that is unfavorable (possibly even harmful) for the patient*	*Gestalt, psychodrama, dance*	*Hatha Yoga, Zen Buddhism*	*Group therapy*	*Holotropic breathing, hallucinogens*

which optimally help them get to know their inner child and enter wholeheartedly into the therapy. My years of experience with many different types of therapy and the most varied character types have enabled me to verify, repeatedly, that the best progress is made when the ideal therapy is selected based on the respective character type. Otherwise the patient is (in the worst case) being "rubbed the wrong way" and won't get much out of it.

But this can be taken a step further, because I have come to the conclusion that the rules for ideal therapy just discussed only apply to the initial phase, when self-exploration has just begun. If one wants to develop further, one shouldn't stay in one place and merely reinforce existing character traits, but rather develop compensating and complementary qualities. However, one shouldn't overdo this by immediately mounting a frontal assault on one's extreme dark side, since this can have very negative repercussions. Thus I noticed among many hysteric patients that methods such as the use of hallucinogens or holotropic breathing, which significantly dissolve ego boundaries, triggered psychotic episodes that led to prolonged negative situations.

In my experience there are only two sensible solutions: at the beginning of self-exploration, one should opt for the type of therapy that ideally matches one's character type, that poses a minimal essential challenge and is innately most sympathetic. This is, however, not a good long-term solution, since it leads to character stagnation – which I'd like to elucidate with the example of the **hysteric**. Hysterics go for expressive, theatrical types of therapy such as Gestalt therapy or expressive dancing. Over the long term, this reinforces their characteristic traits, rather than moderating them –

and the character traits they lack are not trained for at all. To balance out their chaotic nature, hysterics need order, which is why they should do therapy that imparts external structure and discipline, such as Hatha Yoga or Zen meditation.

Conversely, those that belong to the hysteric's complementary type (**obsessive-compulsive**) need a therapy that loosens them up, making them freer and more spontaneous, such as psychodrama or expressive dancing. For them, the strictness of a Zen monastery could be pure poison, since their rigid character traits, over the longer term, would be calamitously reinforced. Of the western Zen adepts I have known, a disproportionate number of them have been obsessive-compulsive persons for whom, from a characterological standpoint, the method has been no help at all. After all, compulsives are by nature way too rigid and strict, so to harmonize their nature they need spontaneity, to "lighten up" and be happy – i.e., loosening-up and liberating therapies such as expressive dancing.

With **schizoids**, the tendency to isolation is reinforced if reclusive therapies are favored in which they concern themselves only with themselves and the empty, impersonal cosmos. Schizoids tend to become eccentric loners, always searching for the answer to the riddle of the universe. Yet schizoids will find their answer precisely where they least suspect it, namely in the social group and its emotional bonds, because emotional warmth and nearness to others will help them rediscover their emotional center. For example, the famous "primeval forest doctor," Dr. Albert SCHWEITZER, went (in my opinion) to Lambarene in "darkest Africa" to help sick natives because he intuited that he needed to experience empathic emotional group processes in order to become personally rounded and whole. SCHWEITZER was, without a doubt, a schizoid who sought the emotional warmth of others, which he received in the form of his patients' gratefulness and love.

Depressives, the complementary type, by nature opt for therapies that speak to their strong points – i.e., dissolving into the group and resonating with the feelings of the others. Yet what depressives need to learn is to be alone, with and for themselves, to set personal boundaries and find their inner center. I recently read about a nurse who had set out, alone, on a world tour by bicycle, and I had no trouble determining, based on certain characteristic traits of this globetrotter, that she had to be a depressive. For example, she intended to mail postcards regularly to those back home, so that they wouldn't worry too much about her – and here we sense the depressive's efforts to see to the well-being of others. At first, I was puzzled that a depressive would want to travel solo around the world, since this goes completely "against the grain," until I realized that this was her chosen form of self-therapy. This woman had also learned Karate which, as it represents a physical (and thus externalized) form of the ability to demarcate oneself from other people, can be a form of self-therapy.

In short, not every therapy is right for every person; usually, people instinctively choose those kinds with which they feel most comfortable. But of course mistakes are made, with consequent undesirable developments, which can be recognized by the fact that someone is trapped in never-ending therapy, or that the therapy is actually favoring the development of negative character traits – or ailments persist (or actually get worse) because the therapy has absolutely no healing effect, but rather leaves everything as it is or, in the worst case, aggravates symptoms. The right therapy, on the other hand, makes us emotionally more rounded, freer, and more relaxed. To those around us, we seem fresher, more grounded and centered. The Bible passage "by their works shall ye know them" thus applies to all forms of therapy as well. Since it's much wiser to choose the right therapy in advance, one first needs to know one's character type and then select the right one, instead of taking unnecessary detours.

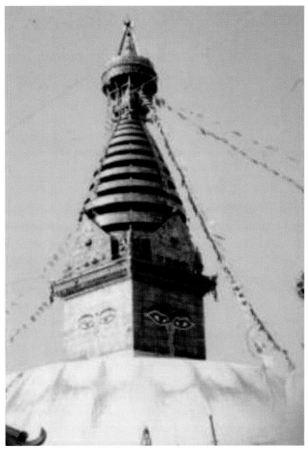

The Swayambunath Stupa in Nepal (5th century AD) shows the eyes of Buddha – symbols of wisdom and enlightenment – gazing out along the four points of the compass. In like manner, we need to develop the facets of all four character types in order to become spiritually well-rounded and whole.

Self-Analysis and Aura Healing

He who truly knows himself can very quickly get to know other people.

(Georg Christoph Lichtenberg)

From the point of view of the healing process, I concentrated on the psychic realm in the preceding chapter, namely on the True Self and the character. Many people who have undergone all manner of therapy believe (wrongly) that they need not concern themselves with the energetic dissolution of their conflicts. One fine day, they'll have to face the fact that, despite their best efforts, the reincarnated subconscious psychological problems haven't changed one bit! The reason that psychological problems are so stubborn is due not so much to a lack of will (as is often erroneously alleged) as the energetic structure of the person's subconscious conflicts. **Because conflicts in the Aura behave like burned-in blockages, they'll obviously not disappear until they're energetically dissolved!**

Because so few therapists dissolve conflicts energetically, their healing results are very unsatisfactory. I can say that because I have run energy tests on hundreds of people who had undergone years of psychoanalysis, or meditated, done pottery, been Rolfed or subjected to countless other types of therapy – always with the same results: in the energy tests, their psychoenergetic conflicts remained clearly detectable and had not been dissolved. To my mind, the only possible conclusion is that most of the current therapies do not act strongly enough to melt and dissolve conflicts energetically.

Critics will accuse me of biased perception, but I can respond that hundreds of other energy testers have come to 100% identical results. Actually, things get even worse for the critics, because psychoenergetic conflicts have been detected even in acknowledged experts such as psychoanalysts and meditation instructors, even though one would normally assume that – because of their role-model function – such people would naturally be healthier than average. Evidently, all of their self-analysis and meditation hasn't been enough to rid them of their own conflicts.

Only energetic dissolution can permanently eliminate conflicts, as numerous examinations of thousands of people have demonstrated. In the present chapter I will deal with how conflicts are extinguished energetically, including discussion of the methods known as Aura Healing and faith healing. In addition, I provide information on unaided self-help (no specialist needed). Then, in the following chapter I introduce Psychosomatic Energetics, the procedure with which I have been able to achieve my best and most lasting therapeutic results.

First I'd like to impart some practical advice on how to recognize – and (in part) heal – one's own conflicts. In order to make contact with one's subconscious conflicts, one needs to understand that this is a sophisticated game of hide-and-seek in which subconscious resistance plays a major role. Subconsciously governed processes such as posture and gestures (body language) are the hardest to manipulate or "fake," so that meticulous self-observation of facial expressions, body positions, and movements provide a relatively easy avenue for establishing contact with one's deep subconscious.

The healing process is based on the profound alteration of negative emotional programs that find expression in gestures and posture, even though in reality one is having completely different feelings. For instance, if you notice that your facial expressions are hard and bitter, you can work on making them softer, more open and friendlier. Of course, you also have to work through the feeling of hardening and defensive bitterness which represents the Persona's first line of defense, behind which lie hidden feelings of having been injured – and the fear that one conceals from oneself and others with the harsh protective expression. Changing one's expression brings one automatically into contact with the softer and more vulnerable parts of the psyche, as one once again experiences the pain and vitality hidden behind the defensive bastion.

Of course, a merely superficial attitude change or an external gestural affectation does effect a certain degree of change, but it doesn't last. The psychic program in the Central Conflict needs to be changed – which I like to paraphrase as *self-analysis*, and which can best be compared to Buddhist attentiveness exercises. **Self-analysis** is by no means a difficult undertaking, it's simply another way of putting to use something that goes on in us all the time anyway. We thus need nothing more than heightened awareness in order to observe ourselves accurately and register our moods and behavioral patterns. Those who want a friendlier and softer demeanor (as in the above example) first have to get a feel for their current harsh facial expressions, since only this awareness enables them to exert a direct influence on their expressions and to learn, in time, to be more open and friendlier once more.

The fact that **unawareness and emotional conflicts are closely related** is one of the best-known and most important basic principles of psychoanalysis. I'd like to go into some detail on what this involves. Up to a point, we're normally aware of what's going on inside us. However, the more we are influenced by a mentally unhealthy, neurosis-inducing environment, the more restricted our self-awareness becomes. In the extreme case, this can go so far that one refers to oneself in the third person, as a stranger. One can see this quite well in some mentally handicapped persons who, when hungry, will say, e.g., "Willie want food." Yet this lack of feeling, dullness, and alienation from oneself is not encountered just among the mentally handicapped, but also in apparently normal people who suffer to some degree from an (often unnoticed) inability to experience themselves as sentient beings with their own mental life. The technical term for the most extreme form of this lack of feeling is *alexithymia* – which has lately become what one could consider to be a collective disease since, in our high civilization, we all live in a relatively feeling-impoverished society.

The real reason for the dullness and feeling-impoverishment of consciousness is our subconscious effort to avoid feeling psychic pain in the form of subconscious conflicts. One acts dead inside, and the conflict is the main reason, in that it distracts us from ourselves and clouds our perceptions – in the worst case making perception completely impossible. A good example of this is psychotics, who often have a sharply restricted proprioceptive sense and thus go out in the middle of winter without adequate cold-weather clothing. The psychotic's enormous Central Conflict leads to a failure to perceive the body's coldness, since the internal feelings distract away from these physical sensations.

There are, of course, numberless kinds of resistance and denial mechanisms that inhibit self-awareness, such as "playing dumb," "going along with the crowd," "not getting it," and so forth. **Therefore, dumbness and clouded perceptions are all repression – i.e., denial – mechanisms!** Now, the last thing I want to do is give the impression that this means that smart people are thus automatically mentally sound. In this context, dumbness is not the opposite of intelligence, since intelligent people can also be "dumb" in a wider sense of the word – i.e., in the sense of any kind of refusal to acknowledge the actual situation and deal with it rationally. *Dumbness* is just another way of saying "not wanting to take notice of facts" or "misclassifying or even shutting out reality." Ultimately, all this is nothing but lack of feeling – which brings us back to self-analysis, the best antidote for lack of feeling.

Through self-analysis, one can learn to deal with oneself and one's environment in an increasingly more conscious and realistic manner. Experience tells us that becoming psychoenergetically more open, aware and clear in one's perceptions – while at the same time becoming more aware of one's subconscious resistance – is a lifelong process. There are many good therapies that aid self-analysis, such as Buddhist attentiveness exercises, various different types of meditation, Fritz PERLS' Gestalt Therapy, motion exercises such as Feldenkrais, *Tai Chi,* and many others.

Considering the broad range of therapeutic options, one basically needs to understand that self-analysis can also function independently of any particular therapy. Life is the best teacher, and one can learn quite a lot about oneself simply through one's own efforts, and by living simply while observing closely. A few simple questions can intensify and accelerate the process of self-discovery; I like to call them the fundamental questions of self-discovery. The questions are always the same and, as simple as they might sound, it's hard for most people to answer them sensibly right off the bat. It calls for a great deal of patience, this working on oneself and dissolving inner resistances (conflicts) so that, after a while, one is able to answer satisfactorily the fundamental questions of self-discovery:

- How do I become more aware of my thoughts and feelings?
- What is it that is blocking my awareness?
- What is real and what is just my imagination?
- What are my true feelings?
- What is it that I really want, way down deep?
- Where is my deepest longing taking me?
- Who am I really … behind the facade, the pain, the illness, the preconceived notions?

Being self-aware and honest with yourself, you can make great strides, and the above questions can be a big help in the process. I boiled them down from the teachings of mankind's great religious/metaphysical traditions, in particular Christianity, Buddhism, and Aldous HUXLEY's *Perennial Philosophy.* You can pose your own questions and let yourself be led by your inner voice.

At some point, however, the personal maturation process comes to an end. Thus, the majority of attentiveness exercises and most therapies eventually hit their limits, which have to do with the subconscious nature of the conflicts and their energetic obstinacy – no matter how hard we may try. At some point we wind up saying to ourselves: "I'm just going around in circles!" The reason for the stagnation is the conflict itself, whose resistance holds us back – like an invisible yet insuperable barrier that shields the conflict from discovery and dissolution. At this point, the usual therapies are simply not enough; it takes powerful energy and outside help to make further progress.

In my experience, there are four possible avenues to helping others heal their conflicts:
- **Supplying high-frequency energy** (causal body energy, e.g., in the form of prayer, intercession, religious ceremonies, faith healing)
- **Working in the Aura** of the patient with one's own healing energy (supplying vital and emotional energy and applying psychoenergetic techniques, e.g., Gerda BOYESEN's Spiral Rotation, Mudras, sketching symbols, shamanistic techniques such as siphoning off the conflict "demon," sweeping away with fans, etc.)

323

- **Confrontational techniques** for the short-term activation of deep subconscious mental problems so as to make the conflict emotionally conscious and guide it in a beneficial direction, i.e. set it on a new positive course (e.g., with cathartic therapies such as primary therapy, LSD therapy, hyperventilation, provocation in group sessions, and so on.)
- **Psychosomatic Energetics** (precise testing of the conflict and dissolution with specific homeopathic compound remedies [emotional remedies])

I'd like to discuss these four possibilities in order, starting with supplying high-frequency "heavenly" healing energy. Prayer as a petition to higher powers – healing diseases and the underlying "conflict demons" (as a kind of act of mercy) by means of high-frequency energy – surely represents the oldest therapy of all, practiced since time immemorial by all the major religions. Many icons of gratitude (votive candles) in pilgrimage shrines confirm that, time and again, unexpected cures take place through the intercession of higher powers. We generally speak of *miracles* when confronted with unexpected cures or rescues from desperate situations which, by any reasonable standards, would not normally have taken place.

Miracles heal not only diseases, of course, but also resolve the underlying conflicts, as can be seen in people who have been cured miraculously: they seem utterly transformed by the experience. Faith, as commitment to causal-body energy, indeed helps the person, as Jesus promised. Through faith, the ailing persons open themselves up to the higher vibrations of the divine, which automatically leads to health because, in my opinion, the causal-body energy incorporates full health within itself, like an ideal form that just needs to be reactivated[77]. However, it requires openness from the people it is to enter into. All limiting ideas and doubts block causal-body energy. Faith – which is a precondition for miracles – is a voluntary act of total commitment and trust, through which the causal-body energy can flow full strength so that miracles become possible.

I myself have as yet examined no patients psychoenergetically before and after miracle cures, because such patients are quite rare and tend naturally not to seek out physicians such as myself, for the simple reason that they have no more need of my services after having been cured miraculously. Yet I am positive that, after instant or miracle cures, the conflicts have been completely and lastingly dissolved. Basically, it seems to be due to the strong healing power of high-vibration healing energy, which melts away conflicts, much like the sun makes short work of ice and snow on a sunny day.

The rational mind considers (belief in) miracle cures to be rank superstition, yet the annals of the renowned pilgrimage sites, such as Lourdes in southern France, document countless cures that medical specialists have checked out scrupulously and pronounced to be genuine. Prayer and miracle cures are thus established fact – that, to be sure, don't tend to occur as a matter of course, but that also aren't all that terribly rare. The American physicians Daniel J. BENOR and Larry DOSSEY have researched prayer intensively, and have statistically confirmed its effectiveness, which seems to be around 30% (i.e., approximately every third patient improves after intercessory prayer). Everyday experience also teaches us that prayer is never amiss, but that – because of its uncertainty factor – it should never be the only means resorted to. The uncertainty means that it makes sense to look to other kinds of help – which immediately brings us to the next point: supplying healing energy from other persons.

One conflict healing option is based on working in the Aura, where therapists make use of their own healing energies. In the foreword to this book, I gave the example of the mother who instinctively sought to heal her child by blowing on the injured knee while talking lovingly and soothingly. The blowing and the loving care are nothing other than Aura work, in which the mother attempts to get her child's blocked energy flowing again. Spiritual healers and others who, with their hands, work in the patient's Aura (laying on of hands, faith healing, Reiki, shamanism, and so on) consistently confirm that their work is a kind of loving care very much like a mother with her child. Thus, despite complicated-sounding theories of healing, faith healers are actually not doing anything substantially different than what the mother did with her injured child.

In contrast to mothers, who in consoling their children must of course be regarded as "amateurs," faith healers have a certain potentiation of their powers and numerous professional-caliber capabilities. In their books and courses, Prana

---

[77] I'd like to add that conventional religious belief by no means leads to improved health. Even religious ecstasy and flagellating exercises don't always promote good health – as I have observed in numerous patients whom one would consider deeply religious. For example, one female patient had a religious delusion coupled with compulsive cleanliness and anorexia, which my examination revealed to be based on an enormous Wrong thinking Central Conflict that in all likelihood correlated with ancient religious dogma, with its roots in prior incarnations, in which the young patient must likewise have been religious in precisely the same delusional way, possibly as a Christian nun.

A very devout man with sexual problems considered sensuality to be pure sin, yet he very much wanted to raise a family, which spoiled his ideas of sinfulness. It was hard to get him to understand that God had created sexuality and intended for us to enjoy it. Ultra-religious delusional ideas were mixed up in this patient into a total blockage of life that ruined his entire existence. These kinds of examples can be multiplied endlessly – and one gets the impression that such deeply religious people need to lose their religiosity to come to their senses and allow themselves to have normal thoughts and feelings again. To some extent, religious faith is a two-edged sword, and religion in the conventional sense can often turn into a barrier that separates the person from true religiosity.

healers such as Mantak CHIA (Thailand) give valuable information on applying faith healing. Also well-known is the Reiki method of the Japanese doctor Mikao USUI, which has various initiation levels and is based on a blend of Christian and far-eastern teachings. British spiritual healers are world leaders, working in state-run hospitals in collaboration with orthodox physicians.

Spiritual healing is one of the oldest medical therapeutic methods, if you include the activities of shamans who, in their healing trances, visualize psychic conflicts as energy-sucking destructive demons, or perceive them as holes in the Aura through which the patient is drained of life force. In my experience, shamanistic visions depict realistically subtle-body events in disease cases, once you subtract the (imaginative) decorative exaggeration. Historically, shamans are the oldest healers there are and, despite their thousands of years of tradition, their healing methods have remained largely unchanged, which speaks well for the effectiveness of their system.

Although I have little personal experience with the dissolution of conflicts in the Aura, I have examined people who had previously submitted to various kinds of spiritual healing practices. Since they continued to have medium to large conflicts, I'd like to assert that, in general, faith healers are only able to heal smaller conflicts of relatively recent origin. Of course, before making more precise statements, I'd have to do further research with certain kinds of healers and their various techniques, but I predict that this would bring no substantially new results to light – apart from the indisputable fact that a few highly talented "superhealers" will get better results. These few very talented healers can also dissolve larger conflicts through the application of strong and especially high-vibration healing energy.

As valuable and useful as I consider Aura work to be in general, it has a number of crucial drawbacks of which one needs to be aware. One big danger for therapists is the depletion of their own energy reserves. I have treated a number of healers who have had to struggle with such problems, and who had themselves fallen ill due to spiritual healing. In fact, healers often become physically ill, looking exhausted and having a gray pallor, with deep rings around their eyes – or they go to the opposite extreme of manic activity, in which process (if they keep it up) they all too often wear themselves out completely. Healers and therapists who work with energy thus need a lot of regeneration, green nature and leisure time to recharge their batteries.

Another (much more hidden) problem lies in the inadvertent transmission of the patient's conflicts to the therapist. I often find unusually large conflicts in healers that, in my estimation – even though they don't come from their patients (as one might think) because conflicts seldom migrate from one person to another – are amplified by the patient's conflicts. It's a very simple matter, and the basis of many a psychiatrist joke. Anyone who deals on a daily basis

with sick people – as healers and therapists do – can easily become infected psychoenergetically. In order to ground and psychically re-center themselves, healers should regularly cleanse themselves of their conflicts and do simple tasks such as weeding the garden and suchlike.

Another downside is the lack of control and certainty with faith healing. Because you don't know exactly what you're doing, therapy is either not effective enough, or there is no healing at all, or (with hypersensitive patients) the situation gets worse, not better. Time and again, I get patients who have fallen seriously ill from healing applications such as pyramid energy, tachyons, or just the laying on of hands. In my experience, it would therefore be a good idea to start monitoring faith healers with energetic test procedures such as Psychosomatic Energetics, and training them better so that they can make optimal use of their healing powers. With the REBA® Test Device, for instance, you can dissolve healers' conflicts and in addition measure their energy strength and see what goes on during and after the curative procedure. You can then check to see if healers are too severely exhausted and how long they take to recuperate – and whether they might not have better luck with other techniques.

In short, faith healing is a very subjective procedure that should only be practiced by trained and psychoenergetically harmonized healers. The best and fullest healing seems to come about because high-vibration healing energy dissolves conflicts, which seems relatively seldom to be the case (for instance with outstanding healing personalities). When the healing energy is not so high-vibration – which is likely the case with most healers – it takes several sessions, because the patient's Aura discharges over time (because the conflicts haven't been dissolved). In most cases, faith healing is a useful aid for convalescence, as documented by the fact that more and more Anglo-American clinics work with faith healers after surgical operations. I'm a big fan of faith healing, yet I'd like to repeat that it should usually play only a supporting role. With rare exception (so-called "super-healers"), faith healing doesn't heal causally, nor does it eliminate the associated conflicts!

Finally, I'd like to talk a little about **confrontational techniques** before (in the next chapter) delving into Psychosomatic Energetics in detail. These are procedures that drastically and unrelentingly confront patients with deep psychic levels. The best-known example of this is Arthur JANOV's *Primal Scream* therapy, in which patients scream something like "Mommy! Daddy!" for a few minutes, until they break out, as they often do, in intense weeping. Confrontational techniques provoke patients until they come into contact with their deepest psychic levels, where the biggest conflicts and the strong emotional pain they contain are found.

Confrontational techniques activate conflicts very strongly, as I was able to demonstrate in sessions of systemic family therapy. The emotionally churning experiences at the sessions made the conflicts substantially bigger. I'd like to mention peripherally that patients' large Central Conflicts are usually perfectly mirrored in the family dynamics. Thus, when we deal with problems within the family, we tend to get our own conflicts reflected back at us (especially the Central Conflict). This is very useful for self-knowledge and can set in motion changes that ameliorate inner emotional conflicts. Still, I have noticed that confrontational techniques usually can't lastingly dissolve conflicts, so that their usefulness seems to be limited to making conflicts visible and bringing them into the light of day; you then have to dissolve them psychoenergetically using other techniques.

For this there are a number of ways that I've already touched upon and whose modes of actions I've explained. I have the most personal experience with Psychosomatic Energetics, a method I discovered and developed, with which conflicts can be easily recognized and extinguished. In this way, the patients' energies then flow full-strength once more, and numerous complaints, diseases, behavioral disorders, and psychological problems dissolve completely. If the disorders are irreversible, because cells are too severely damaged and/or behavioral patterns too deeply engraved, then there is at least some improvement, but no complete cure. So, like every method, Psychosomatic Energetics has its limits as well.

Psychosomatic Energetics

Every disease is a musical problem – and healing its musical resolution. The shorter (yet fuller) the resolution, the greater are the doctor's musical talents.

(Novalis)

Psychosomatic Energetics is a new holistic medical course of treatment which proceeds from the assumption that only the harmonious interaction of the three most important components of our organism, namely

- Body (Soma),
- Mind (Psyche), and
- Life energy (energetics)

can be the basis of genuine health.

Psyche and energy cooperate closely as subtle-body director and dispenser of life, respectively, that supply the coarse-body physical organism with life force and harmonious vibrations. The harmonization of psyche and energy can therefore improve or heal many somatic diseases, as it makes healthy the body's superordinate pacemaker (internal metronome) – i.e., the mind and life energy. One can figuratively compare life energy with the sun, water, and nutrients that maintain the life of a wildflower meadow. Just as flowers wilt and fade if deprived of water, sun, and nutrients (the actual givers of life and "metronomes" of the flowered meadow), so too does the human body need an adequate supply of life energy and psychic harmony to stay healthy.

All three parts of the organism – body, mind, and life energy – are inseparably bound together and cannot be considered independently of each other. It is only their harmonious cooperation that enables physical health and leads to a meaningful, enjoyable life full of zest. The name *Psychosomatic Energetics* is intended to convey the simple truth that, in order to be truly healthy, we need not only physical health but also psychic harmony and life force. The old saying about "a healthy mind in a healthy body" (*Mens sana in corpore sano*) is thus only partly right, since you have to include subtle-body life energy in the mix, so that it should read (correctly now): "Healthy body, healthy mind, healthy life energy." **True health means that we need not only a healthy body and mind, but above all freely flowing unblocked life energy if we are to be really healthy.**

I have been developing and improving Psychosomatic Energetics over the course of the last thirty years, because I wasn't happy with conventional diagnostic methods and therapies. The actual development of the method itself began in 1995 – preceded by years and years of preliminary work in the area of energy medicine and intensive prepara-tory study of entire libraries of the literature in various different fields, ranging from Buddhism to the journals of various medical specialties. My former partner and friend, Dr. Ulrike Banis, also active in general medicine, was a great help in developing the method in the common practice we had shared. I am grateful to her for many important intellectual stimuli, not to mention the emotional support that is so indispensable when daring to tackle such a mammoth undertaking.

I'm also very much indebted to the biophysicist Dieter Jossner, who built the REBA® Test Device and who was the first one to come up with the brilliant idea of bringing together brainwaves and the Aura. In addition, countless colleagues and healers have kept me supplied with valuable inspirations, starting with the Cypriot healer DASKALOS, the British sensitive David TANSLEY, and the doctor and dentist Helmut SCHIMMEL – so that, to be honest, it isn't I who founded this method, but rather the method that found me, with the support of numerous others who showed me the right way and to whom I am eternally grateful. At bottom, Psychosomatic Energetics represents the continuation of ancient spiritual insights and ancient shamanistic and medical experience paired with modern medical and psychological knowledge. What's new about the method is the combination of all this into a practical, logically easy to grasp holistic method that unites psychoanalysis, spirituality, medicine, and energy medicine in a new synthesis.

In the next few pages, I'd like to describe the concrete procedure for the application of Psychosomatic Energetics. As a practicing physician, I need a method that's not only fast, simple, and able to be performed with a minimum of extra equipment, but also effective in providing crucial background information on most diseases and disorders and in offering the simplest and best solution for achieving lasting optimum health for my patients. In particular, I need a method that measures life force, since this has been considered (quite correctly) since time immemorial to be the actual source of health (just think about the teachings of Indian Yoga and Chinese acupuncture).

Because, empirically, spirit and energy are disturbed much earlier than the coarse-body Soma – at least in the case of many chronic and most infectious diseases – it is deeply important to concern oneself with psychoenergy. We know from experience that we're more likely to catch cold when in a weakened state or under nervous stress. The change for the worse of our mental attitude toward a dispirited and blocked condition, and the simultaneous weakening of life force, are essential preconditions for catching a cold or becoming otherwise physically ill. Surprisingly, this applies to seemingly accidental ailments as well. I often see large energy blocks in segments in whose region accident consequences seem particularly to concentrate. Thus, people with a disturbed Neck Chakra often get whiplash, or those with a disturbed Heart Chakra get a contusion trauma in the chest. The energetic weakening of certain body regions seems magically to attract specific types of injuries (Indians speak of *Karma*). Here, the primary factors are psychic and life-force disorders, whereupon somatic diseases soon follow, which very often reflect the psychoenergetic disturbance.

Disturbances of life force and the psyche are important preconditions for becoming susceptible to disease. If we liken man to a computer, life force and psyche correspond to the software that controls the material body (hardware) along with its metabolism and immune system. Psychoenergetic disorders lead to dysregulation, giving rise to longer-term diseases. Disturbances of life force and psyche are thus significant precursors of disease. Our life energy and psyche are disturbed long before we fall physically ill. This is why clairvoyants can detect disturbances in a person's Aura long before the outbreak of disease. **Therefore, if we wish to practice effective prophylaxis, we should make sure that the unseen parts of the organism – energy and psyche – are healthy and undisturbed.**

The determination of disturbances in hidden regions is a difficult matter, because (for one thing) clairvoyants can come up with very subjective – and to some extent contradictory – statements. At this point, many critics "throw out the baby with the bathwater" by coming to the hasty conclusion that every subtle-energy diagnosis is purely subjective. However, this is not so, because my own experience, as well as that of dozens of medical colleagues, has shown that diagnosis of the Aura can be a reliable and solid method – as long as one observes certain conditions.

The important basic rules are taught in our specialist seminars, but the most important point to emphasize is that energy testers cannot have any significant energy blocks of their own, otherwise they can wind up testing their own disturbances in their patients. In addition, therapists should not enter into the testing situation with a critical attitude or any other preconceptions, but rather should empty their minds of such thoughts. If this is done, then one gets very reliable and reproducible readings, such that different examiners will come up with virtually identical results. Moreover, the splendid therapeutic results confirm the correctness of the testing, because when "baloney" is tested, healing goes out the window. Only when certain testing disturbance

sources are deactivated can one again obtain good and reliable healing results.

As a general practitioner, I'm the kind of therapist that is referred to sneeringly as a mere "practitioner" by my more academic colleagues – since healers running a practice are not interested in whether a theory is elegant, but rather whether it works, whether it actually makes people healthy. This is precisely the case with Psychosomatic Energetics! After more than a quarter of a century of therapeutic practice and the accumulated experiences from thousands of patients – also, of course, experiencing what general medicine accomplishes daily – I have come to the firm conclusion that Psychosomatic Energetics, because of its great explanatory power, its uncomplicated operation, and its gentle, inexpensive, and extraordinarily great effectiveness, will be one of the standard procedures in any future energy medicine.

I'd like to demonstrate this with the simple example of a little boy:

A boy is brought in to be treated for bedwetting. Psychologically speaking, his bedwetting represents "weeping via the bladder" because, a while ago, his father divorced his mother. The conflict theme I found has to do with feelings of inferiority and is associated with the 1st Chakra, located in the pelvis, where the bladder sphincter is also situated, which also explains the bedwetting. Just about everything had been tried that tends to cure bedwetting – to no avail. On the very first night after starting the Emvita® 1 drops, the bedwetting stopped! Since then, we've had the same results with dozens of bedwetters. The bedwetting often stops in the first night after the beginning of treatment! But the best part was that the young patient made a great developmental leap forward and acted markedly more self-confident and contented. His grades at school also improved a lot.

We have similar experiences in clinical practice, day after day – in fact, we're starting to get used to it. Still, even we experienced therapists rub our eyes in wonder at how marvelous and extraordinary this healing process is. Summing up, I'd like to point out once more that Psychosomatic Energetics is not an exclusively psychotherapeutic treatment, but rather a holistic procedure that takes in the entire person, encompassing the psychoenergetic aspect along with the body. It is therefore suitable for one and all and, in my opinion, an extremely valuable instrument for permanently eliminating many ailments and complaints, keeping people healthy, and performing genuine psychoenergetic prophylaxis.

Next, I'd like to describe the actual testing procedure of Psychosomatic Energetics. This methods offers, for the first time, the possibility of measuring the otherwise undetectable subtle-body energy field (Aura) with great precision and determining the Aura's percentage energy level (with

100% being ideal health, 50% moderate and 20% severe reduction of the life force). Using a REBA® Test Device, the four Aura levels are exposed to predefined vibrations in the frequency range of the most important brain waves (EEG). The vibrations generated by the REBA® Test Device are extremely fine and do not harm the body in any way, so that even small children and pacemaker wearers can be examined.

Therapists can use whatever energetic examination technique they're familiar with (Kinesiology, Electroacupuncture, and so on). As soon as the vibrations of the REBA® test device resonate with the vibrations of the Aura (like a guitar string that begins to vibrate as one approaches its resonant frequency), then the patient exhibits a test reaction. Thus, with the REBA® Test Device, one can ascertain the "mood" of the four Aura levels and thereby get an accurate value of the "charge state" of each energy level. The more weakly a person vibrates on an Aura level, the less signal the REBA® Test Device needs to emit in order to get a test reaction. Conversely, the healthier the test subject, the more signal the body can withstand without reacting.

This measurement with the REBA® Test Device can be thought of as the "energetic blood pressure." Like a thermometer or sphygmomanometer, with the REBA® Test Device we can measure how much charge a person has on a given energy level. The entire testing process takes about ten minutes and stresses neither the examiner nor the examinee. Testing can be performed with the subject seated or lying down, and I have been able to get reliable test results even with small children (above the age of three). The basic precondition of energy testing is that the patient not give off nervous or restless vibes, but just sit calmly and relaxed, and that the testing room be quiet and peaceful, with a minimum of unnecessary disturbances such as background noise, anxious family members, telephones ringing, and the like.

For the sake of simplicity, readings are expressed in percent. A person just back from a vacation should have a 100% Vitality reading, assuming he was able to rest and relax and recover. Every once in a while, though, I notice (to my consternation) that a patient, just back from vacation, will for some reason have relatively poor energy readings. Psychologists speak of "leisure-time stress" in people trying too hard to extract maximum enjoyment from their vacations – but I've come to the conclusion that the actual cause of vacation frustration is large conflicts, whose energy theft and frustration generation often just get worse during a vacation. Instead of recuperating, the overall condition gets worse during a vacation, because they are profoundly unhappy deep inside, so that not even the joy of a vacation can give them the longed-for satisfaction – for the cause of the inner frustration is psychic in origin and must first be resolved there.

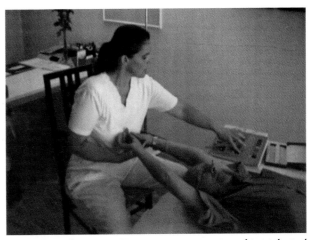

Typical Psychosomatic Energetics test situation: kinesiological arm-length measurement and registering the energy readings with the REBA® Test Device.

With the REBA® Test Device, you can measure how the patient is doing psychoenergetically. Health in the psychoenergetic sense can be quantified with the REBA® test device, because readings of around 100% are obtained with great regularity from healthy persons, while lower measurement values indicate (eventual) disease. Spry seniors who remain healthy well into old age always have high Vitality readings over 90% and even 100%! We can only become and remain long-term healthy with full energy readings. Amazingly, many seemingly healthy persons are sick from an energetic standpoint, without having the slightest inkling of their situation. Energetically, these people only look healthy; upon closer inspection, they have to be considered to be sick.

Thus, in our latitudes, most people's vital readings measure out to 50–80%, which corresponds to a light to moderate weakening of their life force – so it's hardly a surprise (based on these low vital readings) that people age more quickly and eventually become seriously ill. All the diseases of civilization can be found in the majority of our senior citizens, and in fact these days they're considered normal: cataracts, hardening of the arteries, joint attrition, and so on. People think these are a normal part of the aging process, not suspecting that the real reason for the diseases of civilization in older people is to be found in the lowered vital readings that they have had to bear, unknowingly, all their lives.

There's a fundamental distinction between exogenous and endogenous energy disturbances, both of which diminish Aural charge and, over the longer term, make us seriously ill. Exogenous disturbances include primarily georadiation (geopathic stress zones) and its associated problems, such as electrosmog. For these stresses, in our practice we use a small test ampoule of homeopathic mixtures (Geovita®) that correlate with the vibrations of geo-radiation. If, in kinesiological testing, the patient exhibits a reaction to this ampoule, then there is often geopathic or electrosmog stress present. Approximately a quarter of all people who are chronically ill and feel unwell are suffering from severe geopathic stress. Geo-radiation is thus a number-one health problem that, unfortunately, continues to be largely ignored (see the earlier chapter on geopathic stress zones).

The most common cause of disturbed energy readings is located within the organism, in the form of deep-rooted subconscious psychic conflicts. These conflicts can be regarded as energy disturbances that block the energy system to a greater or lesser degree and siphon off a portion of the energy. As energy thieves, conflicts are constantly stealing part of the life force. The majority of people with low vital readings have subconscious psychic conflicts that block the flow of their life force, and in addition use up life force since, like vampires, they suck energy from their victims – who then say things like "I feel like I've been sucked dry" or "something's eating at me" or "I feel blocked up inside." Amazingly, the great majority of people only notice their lack of energy and not the underlying conflicts, which remain largely subconscious.

Using Psychosomatic Energetics, these conflicts can be quickly detected – keeping in mind that only mature conflicts are detected, i.e., those needing treatment. Conflict maturity is signaled by the fact that, besides the activated conflict, the associated Chakra has been thrown out of harmony as well. To test the Chakras, therapists make use of certain homeopathic mixtures (the *Chakra remedies* – Chavita®). The test is performed by checking the patient's kinesiological reaction to specific homeopathic test ampoules (small test-tubes) as they are placed in the REBA® Test Device, to which the patient is connected via a spiral cable that connects his energy system with each test-tube placed in the device. A positive test reaction means that the test ampoule has triggered (resonated with) something in the patient. When a Chakra is disturbed – i.e., when a Chakra ampoule responds – one then looks for the conflict associated with that Chakra. To test conflicts, ones uses certain homeopathic compound remedies (the *emotional remedies* – Emvita®) to identify the conflict. Each of the 28 test-tubes contains a particular homeopathic compound remedy that corresponds to a particular conflict. Now, when a patient reacts to a particular test-tube, that indicates the presence of the corresponding subconscious conflict.

Now, the significance of a conflict for a particular person is determined primarily by the size of the conflict and its "subconsciousness." To get more detailed information, the conflict size is surveyed on four levels. Special test ampoules are used for this purpose, which contain mostly social drugs such as tobacco, Coca-Cola, and so on, that, for a short time, energetically enlarge the conflict enormously, as if with a magnifying glass, so that, at that moment, one is no longer measuring the patient, but rather the Aura of the enlarged conflict. In just a few minutes, the therapist can tell how much life force and emotional energy the conflict has robbed its victim of (**vital and emotional reading of the conflict**). Thus, in the case of severely exhausted patients with low vital and emotional readings, the conflict usually has correspondingly high vital and emotional readings – just as a thief's "net worth" increases in direct proportion to how much he's stolen from his victim.

Next, the **conflict's mental charge** is measured. Its magnitude indicates how conscious the patient has become of the conflict. Experience has shown that the greater the conflict's mental reading (above 20%), the greater the tendency of the conflict to dissolve and heal itself. Conversely, strong subconscious conflicts with little spontaneous healing tendency have mental readings below 10%. The low mental reading means that a conflict's secret (subconscious) influence on the patient's psyche is much greater than for high mental readings. The mental reading thus reveals both the influence that a conflict has on the subconscious and its healing tendency.

Lastly, the **conflict's causal charge** is measured, which corresponds to the conflict's repetitive tendency or stubbornness (like a simple-minded robot that reiterates the same motion sequence over and over again). This applies especially to the Central Conflict, which usually has causal readings in excess of 70–80%. A high causal reading means a large and particularly stubborn conflict. Moreover, high causal readings reveal when a conflict arose. The Central

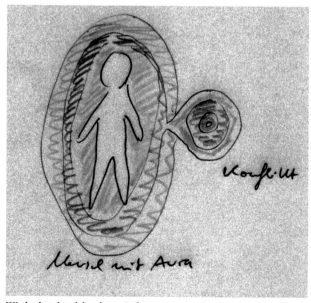

With sketches like these, I show my patients how the conflict is located in the Aura.

Conflict is usually karmically conditioned and originates in a previous life, while young conflicts with causal readings below 70% originate in early childhood. Conflicts with causal readings in the 50% range and below are mainly of recent provenance, having arisen during adolescence or adulthood.

I'd next like to talk about **conflict healing**. Basically, it's a simple matter of extinguishing the conflict with energy vibrations, as the conflict is melted away by means of a family of kindred homeopathic compound remedies (the *emotional remedies* – Emvita®). Usually, this occurs in a completely soundless and side-effect-free manner. Sometimes, the subconscious reacts with vivid dreams, and (rarely) there is short-term aggravation or somatic reactions. As a rule, the patient takes 12 drops of the prescribed homeopathic on the tongue every morning and evening. Then, over the course of a few weeks or months (usually 2–4 months) the conflict completely melts away. Once the conflict has been dissolved, our experience to date has been that it does not return – so we are speaking here in terms of a lasting healing of the conflict.

I'm often asked, with amazement, whether it can really be that simple, that – with a couple of homeopathic droplets – conflicts can be made to disappear permanently. Actually, the healing procedure only looks that simple on the surface, since the profound changes due to conflict dissolution are taking place deep within the psyche – but since these things occur largely in the subconscious, the patient is very rarely aware of any of it. Often the only perceptible reaction consists of vivid emotionally-charged dreams full of deep significance, in which the psyche gradually realizes which conflict contents it had been repressing and failed to recognize. Energetic conflict healing using Psychosomatic Energetics is an extraordinarily gentle procedure that, in the great majority of cases, does not have to be purchased at the price of additional suffering or strenuous effort, but rather plays out, effortlessly and unnoticed, in the background.

Yet another big advantage to energy testing with the REBA® Test Device is that the therapist can check, during the course of treatment, that the conflict is diminishing – and in fact measure precisely how much. This therapeutic monitoring gives the therapist the greatest possible assurance, since he can know exactly to what extent the conflict is getting smaller – and that the patient's energy readings are getting larger. This isn't hard to understand, since the energy thief keeps shrinking, which means that the patient will have more energy available. At the end of treatment, which usually lasts a few months, the patient once again has normal energy readings and the conflict has permanently disappeared.

In about 50–60% of the cases, additional conflicts subsequently emerge, which must also be identified and healed, so that the patient may continue to improve. Experience has shown that healing progress, once achieved, hardly ever is lost; rather, attained higher vibration levels are retained even if new conflicts turn up. Most people's causal readings rise steadily during the course of treatment, which is manifested in greater emotional openness and a more buoyant mood. Conflict healing thus leads to psychic growth (recognizable in the higher causal readings), which I'd like to describe in greater detail in the next chapter, by way of some practical examples and experiences.

Psychosomatic Energetics offers yet more possibilities of great medicinal worth, most of which are of interest primarily to therapists and are part of the special training we provide in our seminars. However, I'd like to point out some testing options that might also interest the lay reader of this book. First of all, the REBA® Test Device can measure what things are beneficial to us, which of them are neutral and which do us harm. This includes medications, foods, certain interference sources such as cell phones, and even various therapeutic procedures. I'd like to report briefly on an experimental measurement of twenty Yoga students before and after Yoga class:

For instance, if students had vital readings of ca. 60% before Yoga practice, we would measure higher values of around 80% in about a third of the participants, while two-thirds of them showed little or no improvement. We concluded from this that, although Yoga harmed no one in the group, it only benefited about a third of them. It might be interesting to find out what would have to be done so that the other two-thirds (those that it didn't affect) would profit from the exercises (i.e., variant forms of Yoga or some completely different kind of therapy).

Another investigative possibility with Psychosomatic Energetics is based on the measurement of higher psychic components. With two more test steps, one can ascertain how highly developed a person is spiritually: the causal reading and the Brunler-Bovis reading (the latter is a special measurement of the total energy of all four Aura levels). The simplest way of ascertaining a person's vibrational level is on the basis of the causal reading, which most clearly reflects the state of spiritual development. People with a causal reading above 60% (30–40% the norm) belong to the class of spiritually more advanced persons who tend to be more creative, intuitive, and sensitive than average. At causal readings above 80%, more parapsychological abilities develop, such as clairvoyance, training in healing powers in the context of faith healing, increased intuition, and even more refined sensitivity. In the next chapter, I'll report on my experiences with such spiritually advanced persons.

In closing, I'd like to touch on two important points with which I am often confronted in daily practice. Because of their importance, I'd like to call particular attention to them:

1. **Resistance to the dissolution of conflicts** (sometimes observed)
2. **The Central Conflict and its healing**

Sigmund FREUD knew about and reported the remarkable circumstance that patients would subconsciously resist their own healing. FREUD ascribed this absurd self-destructive tendency to want to stay sick to a subconscious "death instinct." You would think that all dissatisfied or sick people (or anyone trapped in any kind of problematic situation) would be greatly interested in recognizing their conflicts and being freed of them – and this is indeed the case for the majority of people, if offered the opportunity. Yet (astonishingly) there are a few "rebels" who have evidently built up such an intense love-relationship with their conflicts that they reject all efforts to heal them.

Interestingly, such people open up to therapy once the conflict gets smaller (e.g., by melting the energetic conflict component with homeopathic complex remedies – the Emvita® *emotional remedies*), so that it becomes clear that the real reason for therapy resistance is the conflict itself. There is no need, therefore, to conjure up an ominous "death instinct" since the explanation for the resistance lies in the conflict itself – because, as a semi-autonomous living being, the conflict has little motivation to be dissolved and "healed." It therefore subconsciously suggests to its host, like the prompter in a stage play, that it break off the therapy. Only after the conflict has gotten smaller does its baneful influence diminish, and most patients then make serious efforts to help bring about their own healing, since the inner resistance is diminishing.

I'd next like to talk about **healing the Central Conflict**. More and more people suffer from an active Central Conflict without realizing the true cause of their symptoms. I find an active Central Conflict in about 50–60% of my patients, which makes me strongly suspect that this is an extraordinarily frequent and important health problem. I'd like to call particular attention to the agonizing circumstance in which the Central Conflict has been activated and will no longer disappear on its own, for instance in children with behavioral disorders, or persons with severe chronic ailments. Empirically, the real cause of the disease almost always remains obscured (and thus untreated), so that most children with learning disorders (legasthenia, ADS, and such) face a difficult future. If the Central Conflict can be eliminated before a chain-reaction of low marks, repeating a grade, and general defiance ensue, one can forestall a lot of misery in the lives of such children, and enable them to live a normal life with good scholastic performance.

In children with behavioral disorders and immature personalities, psychoenergetic testing almost always reveals an enormous Central Conflict that is keeping part of the personality under wraps. I call this concealment of the true personality "pupation." In a (psychic) sense, such children are not fully born yet, so a part of their being is missing, off in a dream-world far removed from reality. These dreamers and insecure children often exhibit disturbed concentration, restlessness, fidgetiness, asocial behavior, and the like. In cases of severe handicap, the psyche has chosen a handicapped body at the moment of reincarnation in order to avoid having to be fully present in the world right from the outset (along the lines of "I'll be more careful this time!"). Even these children can be persuaded, through gradual melting away of their Central Conflict, that the world can be a place worth living in, that life is indeed worth living, leading to improvement one step at a time.

In healthy persons, the Central Conflict is usually inactive, and thus provokes minimal or no health problems. When it comes **to activation of the Central Conflict**, there are various types of activation to distinguish between, after which I'll deal with why conflicts become active. In the first type, the process slinks in, virtually unnoticed. At first, the victim no longer recovers from certain kinds of painful emotional distress because the awakened conflict doesn't allow him any peace. Then the conflict becomes so dominant that it disrupts overall equilibrium and the victim feels worse and worse. Disturbed well-being and diminished stress resistance make it clear that the person has gotten substantially out of kilter.

The most conspicuous type of Central Conflict origin, involving post-traumatic conditions in which the Central Conflict is abruptly activated, illustrates particularly well the awakening of conflicts and the incapacity for self-healing. A shocking traumatic experience will appear literally to destroy a person's life: being in a serious car accident, living through an atrocity, being raped, and so on. For younger minds, even watching violent scenes in movies or on TV might activate Central Conflicts (I consider this to be very likely, and it's something that should be looked into more closely). In principle, a severe psychic trauma triggers an emotional existential crisis that activates the Central Conflict in the depths of the psyche, like a bomb being primed. Next, the active Central Conflict sucks a great deal of the life force and personal integrity into itself, much like a black hole out in space attracts all nearby matter (and even light quanta). Using vivid imagery, people with *Post-Traumatic Stress Disorder* (PTSD) report that they feel like they have a heavy stone on their chest, or that evil thoughts are sucking away all their strength. Thus do they describe, graphically and accurately, the conflicts that burden them and vampirically sap their vitality.

There are many possible gradations between the two poles of abrupt conflict arousal by traumatic incidents and a slowly creeping activation – which, however, matters little in the end since, once the Central Conflict has made its appearance, the resulting symptoms and diseases are quite similar. For certain diseases and problems, an active Central Conflict can be identified with great regularity; for these poor unfortunates, the Central Conflict is a menacing entity whose fateful basic tendency has destructive consequences: psychosis (destruction of the Self), addiction (systemic destruction), cancer (destruction of the body), or severe rheumatoid arthritis (destruction of the joints). The monstrous conflict is the victim's worst enemy – and yet, remarkably often, these people put up a baffling resistance to being healed (which led Sigmund FREUD to postulate an independent biological will – a death instinct). Actually, it's simply the destructive nature of the Central Conflict, which ruins and destroys its victims.

In my experience, the Central Conflict is above all activated when people get into certain existential crises. It might be a psychosocial crisis such as the loss of a loved one, workplace harassment, rape, or neglect, which leads to severe psychic concussions. Or it might be a severe disease such as cancer, agonizing skin disease, or long-term chronic pain, all extreme psychic challenges that drive the victims "out of their minds." In these cases, the Central Conflict then confronts them in its incorporated aspect. The personality can be altered in the process, although it needn't be (it depends mostly on the personality's existing strengths and their degree of maturity). You almost always find the Central Conflict in psychoses and other grave psychiatric illnesses that severely alter personality. In cases I've personally known, the personality (of those patients I knew before they fell ill) seems weirdly deformed.

Significantly, the cancer rate among schizophrenics is markedly below the norm, which points to the different modes of elimination of Central Conflict tension – i.e., conflict tension relief either takes place via the psyche (mind) or the soma (body). It has been my experience that the Central Conflict does not all that often manifest itself both somatically and psychically. Psychosomatic disorders in the sense of a common tension reduction of body and mind are more the domain of medium-sized conflicts, being found in neurotic disorders – or, more tritely, when the mentally ill make life unnecessarily hard for themselves, in which process inner emotional blocks inhibit them (known medically as neurosis).

Unlike the neurotic hodgepodge of psychosomatic symptoms such as cardiac arrhythmia, tension headaches, and nervous tension, the activated Central Conflict seems to have such a powerful dynamism that only a single "discharge path" or projection surface is sought out – which means (monomaniacally) eliminating psychic energetic tensions via the body or the mind exclusively, but not both. To a certain degree, the subtle games of the neurotic psyche are not applicable to the Central Conflict since – because of the enormous fears involved – it's an all-out matter of "to be or not to be." Like a tornado, the activated Central Conflict sucks all available energy in a single direction.

When purging via the mind or the body, the ability of the invalid's psyche to cope with the eliminatory output will vary. With somatically expressed diseases such as cancer, repression of the Central Conflict's psychic contents can become so extensive that the victim is totally unaware of the conflict and its theme complex. In many cases, the entire problem becomes so somatized that it results in total forgetting and repression of conflict contents. At the opposite end of the repression spectrum we find the psychotics, who are almost always aware of their conflicts. We may conclude from this that the popular equation – namely that *conflict awareness = conflict healing* (at least when it comes to the Central Conflict) – is wrong, and doesn't go nearly far enough, especially as regards purely somatic diseases since, in many of these cases, patients know nothing whatsoever about their Central Conflict and its devastating significance as a major (but hidden) disease cause.

One normally treats the Central Conflict when it is mature and can be identified naturally in energy testing – but there are some cases in which a passive background Central Conflict can be treated, e.g., when a secure and stable personality desires to grow spiritually. Here, the dissolution of the Central Conflict leads to more vigorous confrontation of deep fears and repressed personality components. There's virtually no spiritual method that I know of that results in such clear-cut and rapid personality progress as treating the Central Conflict. The precondition, of course – and I'd like to underscore this point once more – is a stable personality structure. Because this kind of structure usually only develops in adults, I would exclude adolescents from this treatment, just as I would emotionally unstable adults.

Whereas the preceding applies to healthy people, therapizing the Central Conflict of patients with chronic and extremely hard-to-treat diseases often takes on a life-saving aspect, even when the Central Conflict does not at first show up in energy testing. Particularly the self-destructive psychological tendencies of the severely ill often derive from the Central Conflict, e.g., cancer and auto-aggressive diseases such as *Lupus erythematosus*. Sigmund FREUD sensed the death-wish of many patients so overpoweringly that he was moved to postulate a "death instinct." To the extent that the conscious personality components are overpowered and utterly possessed by this death instinct, the patient has to make a conscious decision to say Yes to life if treatment is to have any chance of success. Experience has shown that as soon as the Central Conflict begins to diminish under the influence of the appropriate *emotional remedy*, the critically ill patient's (often unconscious) death-wish also subsides and eventually disappears completely – only then can the organism's self-healing powers become fully active again.

In cases of chronic disease and of severe behavioral disorder, one often finds inner feelings of guilt and self-castigation which – like the death-wish – contain a negative program with which the person is trying to atone for something. The conscious part of this negative program makes these patients unable to "give up" their disease and "let it go." Even among religious persons, this ancient dogma of the punitive god cannot be rooted out. The solution is – always, only, and forever: Love, with its attendant forgiveness and humility. **Only when we are convinced, in the deepest depths of our soul, that we are deserving of God's love and are indeed a creature beloved of the Creator, can we become really and truly whole and healthy**. The Central Conflict often (demonically) displaces the feeling of truly being loved by the Creator and by Life. If the Central Conflict can be reduced, then new courage can develop and hope for improvement can germinate, which the invalid must accept in a conscious act of will ("Thy faith hath made thee whole!" said Jesus in this context.).

In conclusion, I'd like to report on some other experiences related to healing the Central Conflict. With Psychosomatic Energetics, we attempt to heal the Central Conflict in an especially deep, gentle, and lasting manner. The primary principle consists of several months of melting away the Central Conflict with specific homeopathic compound remedies (emotional remedies). These are homeopathic compound remedies that I developed to dissolve conflicts, and whose individual homeopathic ingredients correlate with psychic contents which are the basis of the 28 conflicts described earlier in the book. Treatment is quite simple and consists of simply taking the appropriate drops for several months.

The energetic dissolution of conflicts brings one – playfully and by-the-way as it were – into contact with conflict contents, which primarily surface in vivid dreams. In addition, in many cases negative character elements erupt now and again, like a monstrous beast, mortally wounded, trying to raise its head one last time. In a most unlovely manner, people exhibit their negative character traits, in the process exaggerating both the ugly parts and the underlying feelings and longings that are trying to surface. Such phases can be hard to endure, both for patients and their friends and family. Therefore, during the Central Conflict treatment phase, one should take to heart the basic rule of thumb of many psychoanalytic methods: don't make any far-reaching decisions, but wait until you have regained a measure of psychological stability.

The diminution of the Central Conflict leads to a gradual enlargement of one's True Self, such that one can better answer the core questions: "What do I truly want? What am I actually feeling? What are my real thoughts?" One begins once again to feel centered and truly well. Besides the feeling of again becoming emotionally genuine and living a whole and fulfilled life, body perception also improves and overall energy increases, so that one feels fresher, more energetic and more at home in one's body. Healing processes start up that had previously been psychoenergetically blocked.

Of course, the primary healing process pertains to the psyche, but these deeper psychic processes are hard to articulate, since the main action takes place in a nonverbal environment which relates to a fundamental standpoint. To use a graphic analogy, you might say that our emotional center gets shifted, which in turn re-orients the axes of our real-world experience – like the Earth's axis of rotation undergoes gradual (and thus unnoticed) precession, thereby giving rise to an altered world. Our center thus gradually wanders from the Ego over to the Self, which houses our genuine drives and desires. The great majority of people – often for the first time in their adult lives – get the feeling of having returned to an old familiar landscape, a homeland they last inhabited in their childhood.

Once the Central Conflict is eliminated, we make a tremendous developmental leap forward, visible to others in altered posture, gestures, and facial expressions. People will compliment us by saying things like "You look years younger and seem much healthier." We feel much more authentic and "with it," and have a deeper body feeling and sense more energy and vigor than ever before. Of course, these are all potentials that we need to relearn how to use. Since most of us have forgotten how to develop their potentials – much less enjoy them to their utmost – we often need developmental assistance to get the process in gear.

Even though melting away the Central Conflict makes us more open, if we don't make use of the energies that this releases and makes available, then not much will change. The nice initial success that manifested itself in our (fleeting) glowing appearance and demeanor, will rapidly fade out. We need a "User's Manual" to learn how to exploit our new potentials. It's here that I see a great challenge for therapists to help the Self being liberated to its feet, so to speak, to develop on its own initiative – especially for the mentally ill who exhibit neurotic personality disorders. Of course, most people are able to take the necessary developmental steps on their own. In 90–95% of the cases, melting away the Central Conflict is enough to initiate psychological healing without outside aid. I'm always surprised at how enormously strong the self-healing powers are that kick in spontaneously and bring everything to a favorable conclusion once the disruptive Central Conflict has been dissolved.

Spiritual Growth and New Liveliness

There is only one sign of wisdom: persistent good humor.
(Michel de Montaigne)

It has lately dawned on many people that, from the viewpoint of a higher spiritual realm, our most important task is to develop as spiritual beings. As the Bible says in this context: "*What is a man profited, if he shall gain the whole world, and lose his own soul?*" The soul has a sublime significance for each and every person – which those with a religious orientation, or who believe in life after death, have always known. All religions point out the need to take frequent breaks in the headlong rush of our hectic daily lives, to lament our tarnished souls and the evil deeds that proceed therefrom. We want to change for the better because, after death, only the spiritual will endure, will be what remains of us. Why bother to accumulate knowledge in this earthly life, and wealth and power, if we can't do anything with them in our life after death?

Because of the millennia of sins that religions have been blamed for, spirituality has for many – especially critical – contemporaries acquired an unpleasant aftertaste. In my psychoenergetic examinations, I've observed, in our secularized world, that spiritual growth takes place in different places entirely, where one would have least expected it. And when we seek out spiritually highly developed people and places using the methods of Psychosomatic Energetics, there's no need to restrict the search to areas of power, Tibetan lamas, and pious hermits. I'd thus like to try to prove in what follows that the churches and sects have no monopoly on spiritual growth – indeed, it can be an ordinary everyday process.

With Psychosomatic Energetics, we can determine in a few minutes where a person stands psychoenergetically and how spiritually advanced that person is. One option consists in measuring the Brunler-Bovis value, which represents a cross-section of all vibrational readings and accurately characterizes a person's spiritual progress. Also, the size of the Central Conflict lets us know how long and intensively a person has been working on self-improvement. The vitality of the energy levels likewise reveals how spiritually advanced someone is, with the causal readings providing the most accurate results. We can thus quickly determine where a person stands spiritually and psychoenergetically. Obviously, I as a doctor have looked more closely at people who have particularly high vibrational readings. I'd like to talk about these people a little more, with an emphasis on what they have in common.

In some people with high vibrational readings, I have found behavioral disorders that are misinterpreted by others. For instance, many people with high energy readings and advanced spiritual maturity (recognizable by the high causal readings) are downright difficult, and hard to integrate socially. When it comes to children, people often falsely assume they're "less gifted" or neurotically fidgety (the so-called "hyperkinetic disorder" with attention deficit). However, these kids are often so mentally agile that everything bores them and, conversely, anything new (and any external stimulus) quickly captures their interest, which is why they seem unconcentrated and easily distracted.

With adolescents and adults, this often leads to behavioral disorders. Because of their high vibrational readings, they feel out of place and misunderstood. The following example of a young man illustrates this quite clearly:

With a puffy face and in a flat monotone voice, the 19-year-old tells me that his parents sent him to see me. When asked what's wrong he says that everything's just fine by him. There's just one problem: for about a year and a half – ever since he finished school – he's been totally lacking in orientation and interest. He sleeps until noon and sits in front of the computer a lot. I measure very low emotional readings of 30% coupled with a very large Central Conflict with the theme Disinterestedness, isolation, laziness *in the 3rd Chakra. Later, the mother tells me that the boy hasn't spoken to anybody in the family for months, and just broods all day long in his room. I find no indication of any psychiatric or other disturbance, so the neurotic development due to the enormous Central Conflict fully explains his behavior. There is also an extremely high causal reading of 90%. As I explain to him what is so unusual about him and point out his high spiritual development, he slowly emerges from his shell as he begins to understand that I mean him well.*

Now, the majority of people with higher vibrational readings are well integrated socially. Their psychoenergetically high vibration, however, expresses itself in unexpected ways. Amazingly enough, cultural qualities, luxury characteristics of civilization, and social refinements (such as gourmet restaurants with excellent food, soft piano music, cleanliness, and good manners) are, in my experience, an expression of psychoenergetically higher vibrations. It took a long time – and it thoroughly turned my basic personal convictions topsy-turvy – before I arrived at this uncommon worldview.

Based on common sense alone, I would normally count highly ascetic people and those averse to sensory stimulus as belonging to the spiritually highly advanced class. I'd like to point out in advance that I am by no means one of those people with a "sweet tooth" who talk about "gourmet temples" and celebrate fine dining as if it were a religious experience, so I might be susceptible to a bit of self-deception here. But I have indeed noticed a **refined sensuality** in many people who, according to my examinations, have relatively high vibrations. The resulting lifestyle would then be a consequence, not a cause – and most certainly not an end in itself – of more advanced spirituality. Such people are drawn to a refined lifestyle, which they consider quite natural and normal.

The same goes for many occupations; among factory owners and those generally derided as "capitalists," I have found many spiritually unusually advanced persons, which I would not have expected to be the case. Such people often work so hard that it amounts to **self-sacrifice**, which is superficially passed off as workaholism. Evidently underlying this is a passion to devote themselves wholeheartedly to a task and place their Self completely in the service of a cause. Critics will object that the capitalist, by nature egotistical, is only concerned with his own interests and benefit – but this seems not at all to be the case with spiritually more advanced individuals. And I'd like further to add that, empirically, a well-hidden covert egotism is totally incompatible with spiritual advancement and, over the long run, leads to illness. Therefore, spiritually more highly advanced persons can't possibly be egotists (and, vice-versa, egotists can't possibly be spiritually advanced!).

Even ordinary people can be angels from a vibrational standpoint, although one wouldn't think it of them at first glance. All these people have in common that, within their social group, they act as a calming and conciliatory center around whom daily life rages and roils on. At a superficial glance, they seem like people such as you and me, and can have all the usual contradictions and shortcomings. They often gripe and grumble, occasionally behave badly and in general act like the rest of our contemporaries. But when you consider carefully what it is that makes them different from the run-of-the-mill person, it is their basic **altruistic** attitude and sociability that becomes so strikingly evident, which comes from the heart and is totally genuine. Other characteristics that people with high psychoenergetic vibrational values have in common include a disarming **modesty** and decency, a profound **humaneness** – and something that's at bottom quite normal and unspectacular: a **positive mental attitude**.

Many serious diseases lead directly to phases in which **death** comes ever closer, to a psychological detachment and supernatural-seeming sublimity that is quite incomprehensible and appears enormously admirable from the outside. My remark to patients that they've made enormous spiritual progress in the course of their illness is usually met with a peculiar indifference. To the family members, however – steeling themselves for the imminent end and, wringing their hands, trying to discover some meaning in the tragedy they're being forced to witness without being able to do anything about it – such a statement is often a big relief: all of a sudden there's a glimmer of hope after all amidst the suffering and grief, which points to a deeper meaning behind it all.

Having made these observations, the meaningfulness of a deeply religious life shaped by religious ritual seemed more and more questionable. All the traditional models of spiritual growth such as meditation, pious moral conduct, and asceticism seem to have far too little effect. Priests, Yogis, and a few famous authors who have come to my practice, and who are respected and admired as spiritual leaders, often did not have the high vibrational values I expected. Since it's not my job as a doctor to draw up a psychoenergetic "Hit Parade" of my fellow humans – and hurt the feelings of those whose readings aren't all that great – I've always conducted these Psychosomatic Energetics measurements discreetly and unobtrusively. I seldom told the person in question straight out, mincing no words, what had turned up in the way of secondary findings. But it made me think that spiritual progress really is different from what the average person tends to think it is.

I got my next surprise when I began to dissolve Side and Central Conflicts with appropriate homeopathics. To this end, I developed the aforementioned *emotional remedies* that cause the subconscious conflicts to disappear completely within weeks or months. Some patients' vibrational levels shot up dramatically in a way that I had never seen with any other method. When you take a closer look at these people, it turns out that they're the kind that are more developed in many parts of their personality than they let on to the outside world. One is thus simply uncovering a psychic treasure trove that was already there, but covered up by conflicts and other adverse environmental influences. I get the impression that, in their reincarnation, they exhibit a kind of *pupation* – like a caterpillar turning, through therapy, into a butterfly. These "pupated people" give the appearance of being silly, legasthenic, handicapped, awkward, shy, and so on. In all likelihood, they use these strategies – after particularly painful experiences in earlier incarnations – in order to live in a protected niche.

As I gained experience, I was able to classify people based on what conflicts they carry around with them. Like Santa Claus with his huge, heavy gift bag, at the beginning of the spiritual journey we find a subconscious filled to the brim with conflicts that are perfectly concealed by the *persona* mask ("… so that nobody shall know that my name is Rumpelstiltskin!"). Like a thief living a double life, the sub-

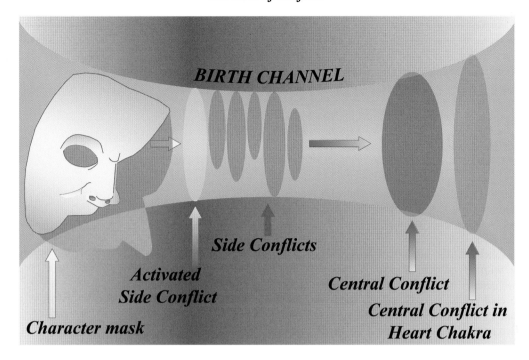

conscious tries to conceal its baseness, "swinishness," and taboo feelings from the outside world. If the *persona* mask is particularly strong and inflexible, these people seem at first glance to be robust, full of life, and normal, since they meet the expected criteria of the *persona* mask exceptionally well – i.e., acting socially adjusted and, to those around them, acting very friendly and like "just plain folks."

As the mask begins to loosen and slip due to conversations, relaxation exercises, Bach Flowers and homeopathics, the first Side Conflicts begin to emerge; repressed and unpleasant feelings crowd to the surface. Gradually, one **Side Conflict** after another appears. One is reminded of a birthing process in which the subconscious brings forth one conflict after another, or peeling the layers of an onion. Normally, this takes place such that only a single conflict is active at a time, but the problem with many chronic illnesses and long-term complaints is that some of these sufferers "give birth to" two or three conflicts at once. Clearly, this is not a good development, and the psyche gets completely confused and overtaxed by this. A person tormented by too many conflicts does not get relief until these multiple conflicts are dissolved – i.e., by administering *emotional remedies* (see Supplement).

With sufficient psychic maturity, the Central Conflict will eventually surface. Often, a person will, for a longish time, inexplicably feel listless and somehow unwell. As during the birth of an unusually large baby, the affected person gets regular "bearing-down pains" in the form of episodical-ly feeling particularly bad. Many people have either night-mares, restlessness, or various kinds of dysesthesia, including all facets from headaches to lumbago – or develop, in these phases, severe chronic diseases all the way up to psychoses. The cancer rate is known (inexplicably) to be dramatically lower among schizophrenics – which has to do, in my opinion, with the fact that the Central Conflict only needs a single stage on which to have its fling, i.e., *either* cancer *or* psychosis. Both diseases together are seldom necessary to "flare off" the Central Conflict.

As personal growth proceeds, the Central Conflict heals up and a new, final large conflict makes its appearance: that of the Heart Chakra. People who are especially spiritually advanced often have a Central Conflict in the Heart Chakra, which is either exactly the same as their character type (i.e., recapitulates the theme of the Central Conflict) or else belongs to the essentially identical type. In the latter case, in working out the last big fears, the psyche evidently tries to come up with a particularly good harmony and character balance. I'd like to present a typical example of this:

Ms. S., a 67-year-old meditation guide, has led a Christian-esoteric life for decades. Psychoenergetic testing shows optimal readings at all four Aura levels, and the overall vibrational values are amazingly high, which indicate that Ms. S. is a spiritually highly developed personality. Nevertheless, she has for a while felt inexplicably weak, has an excessive need for sleep, complains of neck pains and a bloated feeling in the abdomen. Character-wise, she belongs to the hysteric type who enjoys self-expression and display; she dresses and makes herself up elegantly and always wants to be the center of attention. In the disturbed Heart Chakra, the Central Conflict found is Theme 16 (Panic, mortal fear). It is an enormous conflict that sucks a lot of life energy out of Ms. S. After taking emotional remedy #16, she begins to remember early childhood experiences dealing with being separated from her mother. After taking the remedy for several months, Ms. S. feels as if she has been reborn, and reports that the paralyzing weakness and other complaints have vanished without a trace.

We can see that Heart Chakra conflicts deal with themes that remain hidden for a long time and that we especially "take to heart." However, once a conflict is "ripe" and ready to be born, there's no turning back – the painful birth can no longer be cancelled. Yet instead of getting the whole business over with as quickly as possible, subconscious repression mechanisms keep it in an agonizing state of limbo. The overall psychoenergetic system wants to avoid the pain of conflict at all costs. This includes *somatization* of the conflict, as a result of which appear diverse disorders and diseases. In the above example, it is easy to see that Ms. S. suffered from the agonizing fear of being abandoned, which fear then needed to be repressed. Once the fears have been allayed and the conflict melts away, the somatized symptoms and the weakness go away, since the conflict is no longer draining off energy and no longer needs to be abreacted with somatic illnesses.

The psychic wounds that we all have in some form or other generally act as troublemakers, blocking genuine drives and desires and inhibiting personal development. More and more people are recognizing that their subconscious blocks are the main obstacle to psychic progress. Psychosomatic Energetics is thus also an outstanding supplementary aid for healthy people who want to make further progress, by helping them shed dead weight more quickly and thereby vibrate psychoenergetically at a higher level. We're talking here about the desire to make spiritual progress, which springs from people's deep longing for their true spiritual homeland. Like salmon impelled by an enormously powerful drive and making their arduous way upstream to their ancestral spawning grounds, more and more people are driven to seek out their True Self.

Many experiences in life are utterly paradoxical – including the fact that our life becomes ever richer the more we live it in service of a higher purpose. Psychosomatic Energetics is an ideal instrument, through which the patient's mind and body (energetic system) reveals what the patient at bottom really wants and needs – and we become mere servants, allowed to help the patient's psyche along the path of spiritual progress. In this process, we therapists never impose our opinions and verities on patients; instead, patients and their reactions reveal to us what is best. To that extent, it's a gentle unobtrusive healing method that teaches modesty and casts the therapist in the role of a servant who must learn anew what the next problem is to be solved.

Spiritual Medicine

It has recently become fashionable for authors of esoterica to invoke higher spiritual sources, for which the author serves as a kind of cosmic speaking tube. If one does this in a medical-psychological context, the author is considered to have "flipped out." Well, I'm willing to take that risk, because I'm convinced that, for parts of this book and its insights, I have not myself to thank, but rather a being that has made me its instrument. As rational 20th-century people, we tend to call this *intuition* or *inspiration* because we presume that we're the originators of our brilliant ideas. If we take a closer look, we'll notice that we're just the useful tool of an unknown power that channels the course of events. In that sense, I consider Psychosomatic Energetics also to be the gift of well-disposed spiritual beings who have evidently seen in me a faithful conduit for getting the whole thing down on paper.

My personal experience with a number spiritually advanced persons is that more and more of them sense that they're being "led by benevolent spirits" and "guided from above." I'd like to use the renowned Swiss nuclear physicist Wolfgang PAULI as an example of the fact that even scientifically-recognized authorities have noticed this guidance. PAULI was once placed in a hospital room whose room number was identical to a certain three-digit physical constant; when he noticed this, it immediately became intuitively clear to him that he would die in this room. So, was PAULI at that moment no more than a superstitious simpleton, or perhaps no longer in his right mind? I think that this scientist, normally so devoted to rationality, had become aware of the phenomenon of the unlikely coincidence – very likely due to the influence of C.G. JUNG, with whom he had undergone depth-psychological therapy. JUNG, along with PAULI, termed this incredible-seeming co-incidence of things and events *Synchronicity*. It was only because PAULI had trained his attention that he was able to perceive the phenomenon at all.

Empirically, we can only "see" what we're expecting to see, based on our experience. In my estimation, this is why we in modern science are more and more spinning our wheels, as our rationalistic orientation and rigid fixation on traditional concepts causes us to get distracted by trivial details – and miss the larger context. Especially when it comes to such an extraordinarily complex and multi-layered matter as our soul, I think it's a good idea to expand our rational understanding through intuitive and psychoener-

getic perceptions. This does not mean disconnecting our rational mind: critics suspiciously take such statements as an attempt to disguise intellectual sloppiness or (even worse!) to pull an ideological fast one. I'd like to counter that by saying that I'm not affiliated with any ideology or sect, but rather am beholden to the eternal truths. In its simplest form, I call this eternal verity Love.

The strict logical consistency and simplicity of the psychoenergetic model presented here speaks for its veracity, because all great ideas exhibit these attributes. Psychosomatic Energetics can effortlessly integrate such varied perspectives as modern science, ancient energetic models, and religious concepts into a consolidated point of view. Everything points to its being an important model with a promising future that basically does no more than bring together old and new well-known truths and insights into a common vision. There's thus no need to give up our medical know-how, our acquired knowledge, and our rational criticality; we just need to learn the right times to deploy rationality or intuition. Common sense will reveal to us how to do that as we, heeding the Kantian categorical imperative, apply to the patient that which we would want were we in the patient's place.

Scientific models leave out of consideration the question as to the meaning of life. I wonder why we feel we have to impose such a taboo on these most personal and subjective questions about God and our destiny. Anyone who raises these questions outside the context of a theological seminar is considered by scientists and rationalists to be a woolly-headed dreamer, not to be taken seriously. But in the healing arts there's no getting around these questions. Even an atheistic doctor, caring for a dying patient, has to come up with some kind of meaningful answer to what happens in the dying process. Ultimately, the dying person's basic question is: "Does the universe still love me, even though it's letting me die?"

As therapist and healer, I am the torchbearer of hope and life. This manifests, at bottom, a religious attitude that assumes that Life is fundamentally benevolent. How can I give consolation and hopefulness if, in my heart of hearts, I simply don't believe in the goodness of this world? The ancient rift between priests and healers only opened up because the joint exercise of both professions had become more and more difficult for logistical reasons. Nevertheless, healers are still priests way down deep – or at least that's been my lifelong experience as a doctor, in which I have had to learn what patients' true spiritual needs are.

There are still more reasons for believing in a spiritual dimension to our earthly existence. For one, we see in our psychoenergetic structure – as revealed in the Aura levels and the Chakras – that we are a cleverly and wisely put together mechanism. Plus, we – this is psychoenergetically interesting – continue to grow, advance to higher vibrational levels, and develop spiritually. Why should Creation take so much trouble with us if our soul didn't have a mission, one that extends beyond our current life and transcends death itself? My experience with biological-psychological structures of this kind has shown that nature doesn't create meaningless objects that are so complex and well-adapted. Therefore, even from a scientific viewpoint, there is more and more reason to believe in the existence of a higher intelligence in the cosmos.

At its core, spiritual medicine is a truly humane medicine. Because many fields of modern medicine have an atheistic, unspiritual, and mundane worldview, one can't help wondering if the colleagues representing these fields aren't in some way "in-human beings." In the intensive care units (ICUs) we find brain-dead patients connected to respirators for months, whimpering to themselves, in all likelihood dying sooner or later, or continuing to live extraordinarily handicapped lives.

A similar fate awaits the many babies born with severe birth defects, whose parents often don't want the newborn at all once they're aware of the extent of the tragedy. After a couple of years, the abandoned orphan will die in an orphanage. As a young med student, I would ask the attending physicians and professors what they thought of the needless suffering of these poor creatures, but I never got a satisfactory answer. They'd always trot out that one-in-a-million case of totally unexpected recovery. I have virtually never come across these "mythological creatures," and, if we're honest, we have to admit that far too many people have to suffer for the sake of these miracle cases. Looking back, for me the worst thing about it was that the attending physicians were completely incapable of recognizing the inhumanity of their actions. Where has humanity gone, if we doctors commit such acts? To knock down in advance all discussions on this topic with the "euthanasia" club seems to me especially perfidious and inhumane!

As modern humans with the undreamt-of possibilities of our advanced civilization, we're still constantly being forced to deal with limits that were inconceivable in earlier times. Many of these "border crossings" lead to inhuman acts – as I have described above in the (at times appalling) repercussions of modern medicine. Is it possible that a spiritually-oriented medicine can help us out here, to come to a deeper understanding of the connections, to wiser decisions and more humane behavior? I think it can – if we start with ourselves and self-exploration. For this, we don't need any great

big ethics commission and hard-to-implement external preconditions – just the courage, as caregivers, to grapple with our dark side. Why do we doctors allow some people to suffer needlessly when there is so little hope for them? Is it because of our reputation as, say, a miracle-working university professor that we so lust after these wonders – that, for instance, a brain-dead patient might return to the land of the living – and are willing to pay a high price for (a chance at) this? Is it maybe emotional sclerosis – or the desire to be punished, projected outward?

The expansion of material possibilities that modern medical progress makes possible ought to be accompanied by a corresponding increase in wisdom and tender loving understanding. But how does that work on the practical level? I think that doctors should have to take encounter-group and sensitivity training before being let loose on mankind. But even without any additional rules and regulations, more and more therapists are trying to follow the path of a more spiritualized medicine – partly on their own and partly at the urging of patients. Often – due of course to the psychological distress associated with the medical profession itself – they try to practice medicine in a way that encompasses the search for meaning and self-discovery.

I consider any medical discipline that includes religion to be *spiritual medicine*. I understand *religion* as the effort to see, behind the façade of everyday reality, a benevolent higher spiritual power that endows our individual lives with a deeper meaning and purpose. A deeper meaning *without* life after death seems inconceivable, regardless of whether we imagine it as a one-time event or a cyclic process with numerous future earthly lives. If we acknowledge a deeper meaning to life, then we'll ask ourselves: what is this deeper meaning supposed to consist of? Probably **not** just getting up in the morning, going to work, dozing off in front of the TV after supper. And few people, anymore, are content to believe in a distant God who will, someday, magnanimously admit them into Heaven. We have become ever more clearly aware that the deeper meaning of life must have something to do with our inmost essential core – if it is to be truly significant.

The deeper meaning of life includes reuniting our individual personality with our True Self and making them congruent, as I have attempted to show in this book in great detail. All great esoteric spiritual disciplines come to the same point regarding what purpose our life really serves: to mature, on our spiritual journey, into better human beings and, ultimately, to discover our True Self. From this viewpoint, we healers acquire a new and extended significance, since disease, life crises, and mental anguish are important way-stations on the spiritual journey, whose meaning we need to puzzle out. What does our soul want when disease and difficulty come our way? What meaning do subconscious emotional conflicts have? What is our True Self behind all the façades, repressions, and shadow-boxing?

Besides the methods presented in this book, which can be a great help in answering such difficult questions, there exists yet another important possibility for us healers to function as a channel for higher beings and wisdoms: we open ourselves up humbly to a higher spiritual power whose wishes, intentions, and healing powers are mediated through us, as healers. Usually, such powers are constantly active in us without our being consciously aware of it. The difference – between this and orthodox physicians – is that, in an act of humble devotion, we turn ourselves into an instrument that makes the work of the higher powers easier. This can be: a special sensitivity and psychoenergetic openness; the reception of intuitive messages; or a prayer in the name of the ailing person.

A Closing Personal Note

*I believe that the most important thing in life for all people
is to summon up the courage to have great dreams!*

(Golda Meir)

Wise men say that you must be extremely careful with your dreams, because they might someday be fulfilled – but maybe not the way you thought they would be. When I was growing up, I dreamed of being a famous author, able to live a peaceful life through the simple activity of transcribing my thoughts, feelings, inner images, and outer experiences into words. Since then, this dream has come true in a quite unexpected way, but a different one than I had expected. I was forced, namely, to learn the painful lesson that writing books is an extraordinarily difficult undertaking. Plus, there were other lessons, which I'd like to describe briefly.

First off, I got a lesson in *diligence*, evidently because a higher power thought I needed such a lesson. As I was growing up, I was a lazybones, and didn't have the slightest idea how much hard work was involved in writing a book. This book took three long years to write, at various places around the planet. For instance, while outside a sunny Caribbean day was dawning, and normal folk took a beach towel and relaxed under a palm tree, I would sit for hours in front of my laptop, sweating over how to formulate a tricky concept. Or weeks would pass with the finest powder snow outside, without my going skiing even once, even though the ski slopes of central Switzerland were right outside my front door (the greater part of this book was written in the Canton of Nidwalden on Lake Lucerne). In my head and heart, the *idée fixe* had taken root that I'd write the book as perfectly and quickly as possible. And so mountains of work piled up, with no end in sight.

The next lesson had to do with my *Ego* – which is of course the secret motive behind many an ambitious project. At first, I was flattered to have people asking me when the book would be finished. They had heard about the project and wanted to learn more about energy medicine, spiritual topics, and associated diseases. As time passed, it became clearer that my fame as an author in the eyes of my fellow man was far less than I had led myself to believe. In point of fact, I was a torchbearer, carrying various ancient wisdoms into the present day, just mixed together in something other than the usual way. It became increasingly clear to me that the inquisitive readers of my book were not interested in me at all, but rather in themselves and in insights into their own problems. Like all people, readers are for the most part egotists concerned, first and foremost, with their own welfare.

Another lesson had to do with the *professional pride* that twines around the professions of physician and scientist. I had originally intended to write a tremendous philosophical *magnum opus* that would astound specialists – but the more world-famous specialists I got to know, the clearer it became that they had little or no interest in my theories: they're interested primarily in their own theories and – at the most – how other theories might relate to theirs. Specialists are the most uninterested readers you can possibly imagine. What's more, difficult philosophical treatises are understood by very few readers. Even top-ranked specialists seemed not to grasp what extremely important knowledge I had found.

Therefore, I was forced to re-evaluate – and realize (with the generous assistance of my former partner, Dr. Ulrike Banis, who is a thoroughly practical person) that the world has more than enough philosophical tomes, but way too few clearly understandable books that can change people for the better and enrich their lives. Much more important than conveying grandiose philosophies is that as many readers as possible understand what this book is about. And the more sad children's eyes I look into, whose lives threaten to be ruined because of behavioral disorders and ailments – and this only because an enormous psychoenergetic conflict is behind it all, which can be detected and dissolved with simple methods – the clearer my mission became to me: to help people attain better psychoenergetic health and more joy in life.

A typical example of this involves a ten-year-old boy:

Paul is the oldest of three children and he's supposed to attend high school, because the plan is for him eventually to take over his father's business, for which he needs a good education. Paul longs to attain this goal, and his scholastic aptitude tests show that he has the necessary intelligence. His biggest problems are, however, concentration disorders and a poor memory. In exams he's a "blockhead." The parents are also worried about Paul's inferiority complex and his shyness, which makes it very hard for him to assert himself with his peers. Lately, he's begun to stutter and, on some mornings, has refused to go to school out of shame.

Energy testing reveals strikingly low Vital and Emotional Levels of less than 20%. In children, this almost always leads to severe disturbance of scholastic performance, since the lack of energy makes it hard to concentrate, while the low Emotional Level is responsible for poor memory. Paul has unusually high causal readings of 80%, indicating high creative and intuitive abilities. A geopathy is found (the corresponding Geovita® test ampoule responds) and shortly thereafter confirmed by an experienced dowser. The conflict theme Wrong thinking *tests out as an enormous Central Conflict in the 7th Chakra, which in my experience often leads to shyness and mental blocks.*

After three months of treating the Central Conflict with homeopathic compound remedies (emotional remedy Emvita® 28) and relocating the bed away from the geopathic stress zone, a completely transformed youth enters the consulting room. Paul has an open and self-confident facial expression, seems happy and his face has a healthy rosy glow, where he had been quite pale before. He has passed a number of exams with flying colors, so he'll be able to attend high school. He gave the strongest boy in class a good drubbing, he confesses to me, for constantly teasing him, which he was no longer prepared to put up with.

To show that not only humans but also animals can benefit from the dissolution of their psychoenergetic conflicts, I'd like to describe the revealing case of a Spanish dog:

This dog was a walking disaster! It would jump onto the dinner table and, in wild abandon, gobble down everything edible. At some point, this ill-mannered dog lay next to me, I had the Test Kit to hand and was testing it in sequence by placing the ampoules in the dog's vicinity and watching to see for which ampoule I noticed an altered kinesiological reaction in myself. At last, I found the conflict Emotional emptiness, shock *in the dog's Neck Chakra.*

The dog's mistress told me an interesting story that explained the cause of its emotional trauma. The dog used to belonged to a woman with incurable cancer, who had asked her friend – its current mistress – to adopt it after she died. Evidently, the sudden death of its former owner had severely traumatized the dog, being a tragedy that it "couldn't swallow," as it were. The energy vacuum in the Heart Chakra turned it into a ravenous monster that tried to fill the emotional void with food orgies – a safety-valve function of eating that can be observed in people as well. The next part of the story gets even more exciting: after taking the homeopathic drops (to dissolve the shock) for only a few days, the dog was once again completely well-behaved, ate normal portions, and no longer acted hectic and driven, but rather normal and peaceable once more.

The two examples of the boy and the dog show us what tremendous healing opportunities open up when you do something as ordinary as unblock a patient's energy field. Shamans have known this forever, and their success in healing psychosomatic problems is undisputed, even by experts. "Can it really be that simple?" I'm often asked by patients who are amazed at being cured by a few homeopathic drops, after a lifetime of being "poked and prodded and experimented on" by others. I have to admit that, even after thousands of cures, I'm still amazed that healing can be achieved so simply.

In closing, I'd like to point out that the elimination of inner emotional conflicts does not resolve all problems and responsibilities, so you don't by any means wind up automatically in Paradise. Once the conflicts are dissolved, real life begins, i.e., only then does the real work start! After their psychic energy blocks are dissolved, many people get a new and completely unexpected challenge, one that can be discerned in my own personal example. The challenge is to recognize one's true mission in life and to heed its stipulations. Everyone seems to have such a mission, which can seem completely insignificant from the outside – e.g., being a good letter-carrier, performing one's duties with devotion and zeal, or being a warm-hearted mother and giving one's children a lot of love. Of course there are also people with spectacular missions who attract a great deal more attention, such as artists or inventors with special missions. However, the important thing is to follow one's heart and listen to one's inner voice.

Realizing your true mission in life is by no means a normal everyday matter, but rather is an urgent, driving need that you should obey unconditionally – because if you don't, you'll become energetically blocked, most likely because you're no longer attuned to the rhythm of the cosmic unity. So if you want to stay physically and mentally healthy, you have to follow the melody of your own life-meaning, whatever that might be. Over the years, many people have confirmed this observation and found their life's happiness and fortune by recognizing their true mission in life and being wise enough to pursue it.

Finally, I'd like to point out something quite ordinary having to do with the realization of one's life-meaning, which is completely contrary to the egotistical concept of a materialistic world. The more open we become psychoenergetically, the more we experience the world as a unified whole, and our true meaning manifests itself to us as part of the whole. Therefore, we cannot ever be enduringly happy as long as we act counter to the world's unity – but it's just as true that we can never be happy if we don't also see to our own happiness and well-being. It seems to me that the happiest people of all are egotists who act in a social and altruistic manner simply because it comes from the heart. This is why the realization of one's life-meaning is something that at first benefits oneself but, looked at more closely, also benefits everyone else.

Appendix
(With Some Practical Advice)

1. Practical Tips for Psychoenergetic Harmony in Everyday Life

It's worth the effort to take some basic rules to heart in order to stay in tiptop energetic shape:

Regarding diet, you should favor Mediterranean and Asian cuisine (e.g., Japanese or Thai). Have ocean fish at least once or twice a week. Low protein is best, with little meat and a lot of seasoning – and above all: stop eating when satiated (you have to train your "gut feeling" for this). Good white bread and fine-ground flours are more healthful than whole grains (check out the readable book by master baker Wilhelm Kanne). A lot of garlic and anti-bacterial spices such as Curcuma are good for you. Sea salt ensures a balanced mineral intake (better to over- than under-salt!). I personally think vitamin and mineral supplements don't do all that much good. More but smaller meals throughout the day are better than one big meal; eat as little as possible in the evening. Indulge yourself with a feast every now and then, and – for those who are instinctively drawn to this – once a year, do a moderate fast (e.g., a half to a third of your normal caloric intake) for a few weeks. Body weight (in kg) should not exceed body height (in cm) minus 100 – and it's better to be 5–10% below this figure.

The best thing to drink is good spring water, at least 1–1.5 liters per day. Water treatment systems don't seem so beneficial to me. Green and black teas, as well as coffee in small doses (after meals) are known to be good. Sour-milk drinks are very healthful, as is Kefir and Yoghurt. Fruit juices should be greatly diluted.

"Early to bed" is best, and you should get enough sleep so that you feel refreshed and rested. Children especially need a lot of sleep, but adults also get way too little sleep: 6–7 hours is the minimum, in my opinion. As to bed location, see the chapter dealing with geopathic stress zones. Children should watch as little TV as possible (at the most 30–60 minutes daily), and adults no more than 2 hours. I think banning TV makes no sense, since it's our society's most important source of information – but the "dosage" is crucial. In general, try to maintain a low-noise environment (especially at night). Substances such as nicotine and drugs should be avoided entirely or at least kept to an absolute minimum. In biologically tolerable amounts, wine helps prolong life (1 glass daily for women, 2 for men).

As to clothing, sports and other behavioral aspects, see the chapter Body Energy – its Everyday Significance ... Physical activity/exercise is one of the most important suppliers of subtle energy, likewise fresh air, sun, and nature itself. Sports should be done in a playful spirit and not over-done (this applies equally to all the other factors). Once a week, you should spend a few hours lazing about and doing nothing, for R&R (rest and recuperation). You should have some activity you enjoy doing a lot, i.e., a hobby, for regeneration.

Above and beyond all the advice that I might yet dispense, it seems to me that there are two mental attitudes that are of fundamental significance – which seem, at first glance, to contradict each other: you should live your life with as much modesty as possible *and* also with much egotism. How does that work? – I hear you ask. I can't give you a satisfactory answer, and can only encourage you, the reader, to try out, in your own life, these seemingly opposed positions, which I have encountered in the great majority of people that I consider to be wise, full of energy, healthy, and happy. What is these people's secret? Well, that one should exercise humility in thanking the divine force every day that you're alive and can work. But you should also see to it that you live like a king (or queen). To be humble and also to live with 100% enthusiasm thus seems to me the most important key to psychoenergetic harmony. Whether this in fact is so is of course something that you, dear reader, will have to try out and find out for yourself.

2. Information about therapists and *Psychosomatic Energetics* (please include stamped self-addressed envelope):

Central office:

Rubimed AG, Grossmatt 3, 6052 Hergiswil
SWITZERLAND
Tel. 0 41 – 630 08 88 (Country code for Switzerland: 0041 from the USA ++141)
www.rubimed.com (with list of therapists)

USA:

Terra Medica
3873 Airport Way
Bellingham, WA 98227-9754
toll free: (888) 415- 0535
toll free fax: (866) 881-2888
email: order@terra-medica.com

Canada:

Biomed
Unit 102 - 3738 N. Fraser Way
Burnaby, B.C. V5J 5G7
Canada
ph: (604) 415-0535
toll free: (800) 665-8308
toll free fax: (866) 881-2888
order desk: order@biomedicine.com

3. Books about *Psychosomatic Energetics*:

Banis, Reimar: *Psychosomatic Energetics Reader*, Amazon.com, 1st Ed. 2008

Banis, Reimar: *Manual of Psychosomatic Energetics*, Chrystyne Jackson Enterprises, Prescott, AZ, 2005

Banis, U.: *Handbook of Psychosomatic Energetics*, Comed Publications, Hochheim/Germany, 2004

Banis, U.: *Geopathic Stress – and What You Can Do About It*, Hochheim/Germany, 2003

For current information on the availability of these titles, contact any of the offices listed under 2. above, or the publisher:

Artemis Books
P. O. Box 482
Penn Valley, CA 95946
(530) 477-8101
www.artemis-books.com

Selected Bibliography

(important and supplementary books in boldface)

Ackerknecht, Erwin, *A Short History of Medicine.* (Baltimore: Johns Hopkins, 1982)

Adler, Ernesto, *Neural focal dentistry: Illness Caused by Interference Fields in the Trigeminal.* (Multi-Discipline Research Foundation, 1984)

Asbeck, Friedrich, *Naturmedizin in Lebensbildern.* (Leer: Verlag Grundlagen und Praxis, 1977)

Atthesli, Stylianos (Daskalos), *The Symbol of Life* (The Stoa Series). (P.O. Box 8347, 2020 Nikosia, Cyprus: 1998)

Atthesli, Stylianos (Daskalos), *Joshua Immanuel the Christ* (The Stoa Series). (P.O. Box 8347, 2020 Nikosia, Cyprus: 2001)

Banis, Reimar, *Psychosomatic Energetics.* (Hochheim: Co`med Verlag, 1998)

Banis, Ulrike, *The Practice of Psychosomatic Energetics.* (Hochheim: Co`med Verlag, 1999)

Banis, Ulrike, *Geopathic Stress & Co.* (Heidelberg: Haug, 2001)

Barbados – *APA Guide.* (Munich: Travel Media, 1995)

Berendt, Joachim-Ernst, *Nada Brahma: Music and the Landscape of Consciousness.* (Rochester/Vermont: Destiny Books, 1991)

Bender, Hans, *Unser sechster Sinn.* (Stuttgart: DVA, 1967)

Bergsmann, Otto, *Risikofaktor Standort – Rutengängerzone und Mensch.* (Vienna: Facultas Universitätsverlag, 1990)

Beuchelt, Hellmuth, *Konstitutions- und Reaktionstypen in der Medizin mit Berücksichtigung ihrer therapeutischen Auswertbarkeit in Wort und Bild.* (Heidelberg: Haug, 1971)

Blofeld, John, *Wheel of Life: The Autobiography of a Western Buddhist.* (Boston: Shambhala, 1988)

Boerner, Moritz, *Byron Katie's The Work.* (Munich: Goldmann Taschenbuchverlag, 1999)

Bösch, Jakob, *Spirituelles Heilen und Schulmedizin.* (Bern: Lokwort Verlag, 2002)

Bohm, Werner, *Chakras: Roots of Power.* (Newburyport, Massachusetts: Red Wheel Weiser, 1991)

Boorstein, Seymour, *Transpersonal Psychotherapy.* (Albany: SUNY Press, 1996)

Borck, Cornelius, *Anatomien medizinischen Wissens.* (Frankfurt: Fischer Verlag, 1996)

Boyesen, Gerda und Mona-Lisa, *Biodynamik des Lebens – Grundlagen der biodynamischen Psychologie.* (Essen: Synthesis-Verlag, 1987)

Boyesen, Gerda, *Über den Körper die Seele heilen.* (Munich: Kösel, 1988)

Boyesen, Gerda, *Von der Lust am Heilen.* (Munich: Kösel, 1995)

Bozzano, Ernesto, *Übersinnliche Erscheinungen bei Naturvölkern.* (Bern: A. Francke Verlag, 1948)

Brugh Joy, W., *Joy's Way.* (New York: Tarcher, 1979)

Campbell, Joseph, *Transformations of Myth Through Time.* (New York: Harper Perennial, 1990)

Candi, *Radiästhetische Studien.* (St. Gallen: Verlag RGS, 1982)

Choa Kok Sui, *Pranic Healing.* (Newburyport, Massachusetts: Red Wheel Weiser, 1990)

Dalai Lama, *How to Expand Love: Widening the Circle of Loving Relationships.* (New York, Atria, 2005)

Daskalos (Stylianos Atteshlis), *Die esoterische Praxis.* (Duisburg: Edel-Verlag, 1994)

Dethlefsen, Thorwald, *The Healing Power of Illness.* (Vega, 2002)

Diamond, John, *Your Body Doesn't Lie.* (New York: Warner Books, 1989)

Diamond, John, *Life Energy: Using the Meridians to Unlock the Hidden Power of Your Emotions.* (New York: Continuum International Publishing Group, 1990)

Duerr, Hans Peter, *Der Mythos vom Zivilisationsprozess 2: Intimität.* (Frankfurt: Suhrkamp, 1994)

Dürckheim, Karlfried, *Hara – The Vital Centre of Man.* (Ludlow/England: Unwin Books, 1977)

Emoto, Masaru, *Messages from Water.* (Tokyo: Hado Publishing, 1999)

Evans-Wentz, W.Y., *The Tibetan Book of the Dead – Or the After-Death Experiences on the Bardo Plane.* (New York: Oxford, 2000)

Fisch, Guido, *Akupunktur – Chinesische Heilkunde als Medizin der Zukunft.* (Stuttgart: DVA, 1973)

von Franz, Marie-Luise et al, *Das Böse.* (Zurich & Stuttgart: Rascher Verlag, 1961)

von Franz, Marie-Luise, *Shadow and Evil in Fairy Tales.* (Putnam/Connecticut: Spring Publications, 1980)

von Franz, Marie-Luise, *Spiegelungen der Seele.* (Munich: Kösel, 1988)

Fromm, Erich, *The Anatomy of Human Destructiveness.* (Owl Books, 1992)

Fromm, Erich, Suzuki, D.T. & DeMartino, Richard, *Zen Buddhism and Psychoanalysis.* (New York: HarperCollins, 1970)

Fuchs, Christian, *Yoga in Deutschland.* (Stuttgart: Kohlhammer, 1990)

Gedeon, Wolfgang, *Von der biologischen Medizin zur Ganzheitsmedizin – eine Gesamtschau der Heilkunde.* (Heidelberg: Haug, 1991)

Gelpke, Rudolf, *Drogen und Seelenerweiterung*. (Munich: Kindler, 1966)

Gerber, Richard, *Vibrational Medicine for the 21st Century*. (New York: Harper & Collins, 2000)

Gleditsch, Anneliese, *Vom Bewusstsein zum Gewisssein*. (Augsburg: Opal Friedberg, 1991)

Gopi Krishna, *Kundalini – the Evolutionary Energy in Man*. (Boston: Shambhala, 1997)

Govinda, Lama Anagarika, *Psychological Attitude of Early Buddhist Philosophy*. (Delhi: Motilal Banarsidass Pub, 1998)

Grof, Stanislav, *The Adventure of Self-Discovery – I : Dimensions of Consciousness – II : New Perspectives in Psychotherapy*. (Albany: SUNY Press, 1988)

Grof, Stanislav, *Beyond the Brain: Birth, Death, and Transcendence in Psychotherapy*. (Albany: SUNY Press, 1986)

Grossarth-Maticek, Ronald, *Systemische Epidemiologie und präventive Verhaltensmedizin chronischer Erkrankungen: Strategien zur Aufrechterhaltung der Gesundheit*. (Berlin & New York: de Gruyter, 1999)

Grossmann, David, *On Killing – The Psychological Cost of Learning to Kill in War and Society*. (Boston: Back Bay Books, 1996)

Hammer, Leon, *Dragon Rises, Red Bird Flies – Psychology, Energy and Chinese Medicine*. (Barrytown, New York: Station Hill Press, 1991)

Harner, Michael, *The Way of the Shaman*. (San Francisco: HarperSanFrancisco, 1990)

Hartmann, Ernst, *Krankheit als Standortproblem*. (Heidelberg: Haug, 1986)

Hartmann, Ernst, *Yin Yang: Über Konstitutionen und Reaktionstypen*. (Waldbrunn: Forschungskreis für Geobiologie, 1986)

Hellinger, Bert, *Love's Hidden Symmetry: What Makes Love Work in Relationships*. (Zeig, Tucker & Theisen, 1998)

Hoffmann, Sven, *Neurosenlehre, psychotherapeutische und psychosomatische Medizin*. (Stuttgart: Schattauer, 1999)

Hofmann, Albert, *LSD – My Problem Child*. (MAPS, 2005)

Huxley, Aldous, *The Doors of Perception*. (New York: Harper Perennial, 2004)

Huxley, Aldous, *The Perennial Philosophy*. (New York: Harper Perennial, 2004)

Jaeger, Willigis, *Search for the Meaning of Life: Essays and Reflections on the Mystical Experience*. (Liguori, Missouri: Liguori/Triumph, 2003)

Johari, Harish, *Chakras: Energy Centers of Transformation*. (Destiny Books; Rev&Expand edition, 2000)

Jones, Constance, *R.I.P.: The Complete Book of Death and Dying*. (New York: HarperCollins, 1997)

Jordan, Michael, Cults: *Prophecies, Practices and Personalities*. (Carlton Books Ltd, 1996)

Jung, C.G., *Man and His Symbols*. (Dell Publishing, 1968)

Jung, C.G., *The Psychology of Kundalini Yoga*. (Princeton, 1999)

Jung, C.G., *Über psychische Energetik und das Wesen der Träume*. (Zurich: Rascher Verlag, 1948)

Jung, Hans, *Persönlichkeitstypologie – Instrument der Mitarbeiterführung*. (Munich & Vienna: R. Oldenbourg-Verlag, 2000)

Kafkalides, Athanassios, *The Knowledge of the Womb*. (Heidelberg: Mattes, 1995)

Kanne, Wilhelm, *Krebs ist vermeidbar! Krebs ist heilbar! Aktiver Gesundheitsschutz durch richtige Ernährung*. (Thannhausen: Deni Druck, 2002)

Keleman, Stanley, *Your Body Speaks its Mind*. (Berkeley: Center Press, 1981)

Klussmann, Rudolf, *Psychosomatische Medizin*. (Heidelberg: Springer, 1998)

König, Karl, *Mit dem eigenen Charakter umgehen*. (Dusseldorf & Zurich: Walter Verlag, 2001)

Krapp, Holger & Wägenbaur, Thomas, *Komplexität und Selbstorganisation- "Chaos" in den Natur- und Kulturwissenschaften*. (Munich: Wilhelm Fink Verlag, 1997)

Krishnamurti, J., Living: *Down to Earth Observations on the Meaning of Life*. (What-Is Press, 1987)

Kübler-Ross, Elisabeth, *On Death and Dying*. (Basingstoke, England: MacMillan, 1969)

Kurtz, Ron, *The Body Reveals: An Illustrated Guide to the Psychology of the Body*. (New York: Harper & Row/Quicksilver, 1976)

Leadbeater, C.W., *Chakras: A Monograph*. (Whitefish, Montana: Kessinger Publishing, 2003)

Leadbeater, C.W., *Man Visible and Invisible: Examples of Different Types of Men as Seen by Means of Trained Clairvoyance*. (Whitefish, Montana: Kessinger Publishing, 1942)

Leary, Timothy, *Psychedelic Experience – A Manual Based on the Tibetan Book of the Dead*. (Sacramento, California: Citadel Press, 1995)

Leuner, Hanscarl, *Lehrbuch der Katathym-imaginativen Psychotherapie*. (Bern: Hans Huber Verlag, 1994)

Levin, Michal, introduction by Ken Wilber, *Meditation: Path to the Deepest Self*. (London: Dorling Kindersley, 2002)

Lévy-Bruhl, Lucien & Hamburger Margarethe, *Primitive Mentality*. (Brooklyn: AMS Press, 1975)

Lowen, Alexander, *The Betrayal of the Body*. (Alachua/Florida: Bioenergetics Press, 2005)

Malin, Lisa, *Die schönen Kräfte – eine Arbeit über Heilen in verschiedenen Dimensionen*. (Frankfurt: Zweitausendeins, 1986)

Mann, A.T., *The Elements of Reincarnation*. (Element Books Ltd, 1995)

Markides, Kyriakos, *The Magus of Strovolos – The Extraordinary World of a Spiritual Healer*. (London: Penguin, 1989)

McDougall, Joyce, *Theaters of the Body – A Psychoanalytic Approach to Psychosomatic Illness*. (New York: Norton, 1989)

Meier, Pirmin, *Paracelsus – Arzt und Prophet*. (Zurich: Pendo Verlag, 1998)

Meinhold, Werner J., *Krebs – eine mystifizierte Krankheit.* (Dusseldorf: Walter Verlag, 1996)

Meinhold, Werner J., *Der Wieder-Verkörperungsweg eines Menschen durch die Jahrtausende – Reinkarnationserfahrung in Hypnose.* (Freiburg: Aurum Verlag, 1989)

Meinhold, Werner J., *Das grosse Handbuch der Hypnose.* (Kreuzlingen & Munich: Ariston, 1997)

Meinhold, Werner J., *Das menschliche Bewusstsein.* (Zurich & Dusseldorf: Walter Verlag, 1998)

Mertens, Wolfgang, *Einführung in die psychoanalytische Therapie,* 3 Vols. (Stuttgart: Kohlhammer, 1990)

Milgram, Stanley, *Obedience to Authority: An Experimental View.* (Hamburg: Rowohlt, 1982)

Mlaker, Rudolf, *Geistiges Pendeln.* (Berlin: Verlag Richard Schikoswki, 1974)

Motoyama, Hiroshi, Chakra, *Nadi of Yoga and Meridians, Points of Acupuncture.* (Tokyo: Institute of Religious Psychology, 1972)

Motoyama, Hiroshi, *Chakras – Bridge to Higher Consciousness.* (Wheaton, Illinois: Quest Books, 1995)

Motoyama, Hiroshi, *Diagnostic Methods in Western & Eastern Medicine – a Correlation Between Ki Energy and Environmental Conditions.* (Tokyo: Human Science Press, 1999)

Motoyama, Hiroshi, *Measurements of Ki Energy Diagnoses & Treatment – Treatment Principles of Oriental Medicine from an Electrophysiological Point of View.* (Tokyo: Human Science Press, 1997)

Murphy, Michael, *The Future of the Body* (Tarcher: Reprint edition, 1993)

Panikkar, Raimon, *Gott, Mensch und Welt – Die Drei-Einheit der Wirklichkeit.* (Petersberg: Verlag Via Nova, 1999)

Perspektiva (Ed.), *Sinnlichkeit und Sexualität – Beiträge zu den Luzerner Psychotherapietagen 1996.* (Rheinfelden, Switzerland: Mandala Media, 1996)

Pierrakos, John, *Core Energetics: Developing the Capacity to Love And Heal.* (Mendocino, California: Core Evolution Publishing, 2005)

Popp, Fritz-Albert, *Neue Horizonte in der Medizin.* (Heidelberg: Haug, 1983)

Popper, Karl & Eccles, John, *The Self and Its Brain.* (London: Routledge, 1984)

Powers, Rhea, *Reinkarnation oder die Illusion der persönlichen Identität.* (Schliersee: Falk-Verlag, 1989)

Preusser, Wilhelm, *Regulationstherapie über palpable Kolloidveränderungen im Bindegewebe (Gelosenbehandlung).* (Heidelberg: Haug, 1987)

Rademacher, P.G., *Handbuch der Vegatest-Methode.* (Schiltach, Germany: Vega Grieshaber, 1982)

Rätsch, Christian, *Ethnotherapien.* (Berlin: VWB, 1998)

Raknes, Ola, *Wilhelm Reich and Orgonomy.* (Oslo: Universitetsforlaget, 1970)

Reich, Wilhelm, *Character Analysis,* 3rd Ed. (New York: Farrar, Strauss Giroux, 1980)

Reich, Wilhelm, *The Cancer Biopathy.* (Doubleday, 1973)

Resch, Andreas, *Kosmopathie – Imago Mundi,* Vol. 8. (Innsbruck: Resch Verlag, 1981)

Resch, Andreas, *Psyche und Geist.* (Innsbruck: Resch Verlag, 1986)

Riemann, Fritz, *Grundformen der Angst.* (Munich: Ernst Reinhard Verlag, 1968)

Rodewyk, Adolf, *Dämonische Besessenheit heute.* (Aschaffenburg: Pattloch-Verlag, 1966)

Rosenberg, Alfons, *Die Seelenreise.* (Olten/Switzerland & Freiburg: Walter-Verlag, 1952)

Sanders, Lea, *Rainbows of Your Aura.* (Piermont, New York: Riverrun Press, 1987)

Schäfer, Hans, *Gott im Kosmos und im Menschen.* (Graz & Vienna: Topos Styria Verlag, 2000)

Schedlowski, Manfred, *Pyschoneuroimmunology – An Interdisciplinary Introduction.* (New York: Springer, 2001)

Scheffer, Mechthild, *Keys to the Soul: A Workbook for Self-Diagnosis Using the Bach Flowers.* (London: C.W. Daniel Co. Ltd, 2004)

Schleich, Carl Ludwig, *Das Ich und die Dämonien.* (Berlin: S. Fischer, 1922)

Schönenberger, M., *Weltformel I-Ching im genetischen Code.* (Weilheim: Otto-Wilhelm Barth Verlag, 1973)

Schroeder, Burkhard, Atem, *Ekstase – Rebirthing.* (Essen: Synthesis-Verlag)

Schuhmacher, Guido, *Diagnose und Therapie für eine neue Zeit.* (Babenhausen: Eigenverlag Schuhma-Verlag, 1997)

Schweitzer, Albert, *Selbstzeugnisse.* (Stuttgart & Hamburg: Deutscher Bücherbund, 1959)

Seeger, P.G., *Krebs – Problem ohne Ausweg.* (Heidelberg: Verlag für Medizin Ewald Fischer, 1974)

Sheldrake, Rupert, *A New Science of Life – The Hypothesis of Morphic Resonance* (Par Street Press; Reprint edition, 1995)

Spierling, Volker, *Kleine Geschichte der Philosophie.* (Munich: Piper, 1992)

Stein, Murray, *Jung's Map of the Soul – An Introduction.* (Chicago: Open Court Publishing, 1998)

Stevenson, Ian, *Children Who Remember Previous Lives – A Question of Reincarnation.* (Jefferson, North Carolina: McFarland & Company, 2000)

Stierlin, Helm, *Das Tun des Einen ist das Tun des Anderen.* (Frankfurt: Suhrkamp, 1978)

Suzuki, D.T., Fromm, Erich, & de Martino, Richard, *Zen Buddhism and Psychoanalysis.* (New York: Harper Colophon, 1970)

Swedenborg, Emanuel, *Homo maximus.* (Weilheim: Otto-Wilhelm Barth Verlag, 1962)

Tansley, David, *Dimensions of Radionics.* (Health Sci P, 1977)

Tansley, David, *Subtle Body – Essence and Shadow* (London: Thames & Hudson Ltd, 1977)

Tansley, David, Aura, *Chakras – Rays and Radionics.* (London: C.W. Daniel Co. Ltd, 2004)

Tarthang Tulku, *Gesture of Balance – A Guide to Awareness, Self-Healing and Meditation.* (Berkeley: Dharma Publishing, 1977)

Thakkur, Chandrashekhar Gopalji, *Introduction to Ayurveda.* (New Delhi: Times of India Press, 1965)

Thie, John, *Touch for Health.* (Camarillo, California: DeVorss & Company, 1973)

Tolle, Eckhart, *The Power of Now – A Guide to Spiritual Enlightenment.* (Novato, California: New World Library, 1999)

Tomatis, Alfred, *The Conscious Ear: My Life of Transformation Through Listening.* (Barrytown: Station Hill, 1992)

Tompkins, Peter, *The Secret Life of Plants.* (New York: Harper, 1989)

Ulmer, Eberhard, *Herddiagnostik und Therapie mit BFD.* (Schorndorf: WBV, 1988)

Voll, Reinhold, *Electro-acupuncture Primer.* (Uelzen, Germany: ML-Verlag, 1979)

Watts, Alan, *The Way of Zen.* (New York: Vintage Books, 1989)

Weiss, Jordan P., *Selbsterkenntnis und Heilung – Die Auflösung emotionaler Energieblockaden.* (Petersberg: Verlag Via Nova, 1997)

Westlake, Aubrey T., *The Pattern of Health.* (Boulder: Shambala 1974)

Whitrow, G.J., Soulsby, Marlene & Fraser, J.T., *What Is Time? – The Classic Account of the Nature of Time.* (New York: Oxford USA, 2004)

Wilber, Ken: *Sex, Ecology, Spirituality.* (Boulder: Shambala; 2nd Rev edition, 2001)

Wilber, Ken: *Holographic Paradigm.* (Boulder: Shambala, 1982)

Woolger, Roger: *Healing Your Past Lives: Exploring the Many Lives of the Soul.* (Sounds True; Book & CD edition, 2005)

Relevant reference works and basic literature (a small selection):

Lexikon der östlichen Weisheitslehren. (Bern: Scherz-Verlag, 1986)

Bowker, John, *The Oxford Dictionary of World Religions.* (New York: Oxford, 1997)

DTV-Lexikon, Vols. 1–20. (Leipzig: Brockhaus, 1992)

Knaurs Lexikon der Symbole. (Munich: Knaur, 1998)

Harrison, *Internal Medicine*, 2 Vols. (New York: McGraw-Hill, 13th Ed. 1995)

Pschyrembel, Willibald, *Clinical Dictionary – Klinisches Wörterbuch.* (French & European Publications, 1993)

Birbaumer, Niels & Schmidt, Robert, *Biologische Psychologie.* (Heidelberg: Springer, 4th Ed. 1999)

Zentrum zur Dokumentation für Naturheilverfahren (Ed.), *Dokumentation der besonderen Therapierichtungen und natürlichem Heilweisen in Europa.* (Lüneburg: Verlag für Ganzheitsmedizin, 1993)

Contact Information

For information about therapists and about *Psychosomatic Energetics*, contact any of the offices listed below (please include self-addressed, stamped envelope):

Central office:

Rubimed AG
Grossmatt 3
6052 Hergiswil
Switzerland
ph: +41 (630) 08 88
www.rubimed.com

USA:

Terra Medica
3873 Airport Way
Bellingham, WA 98227-9754
ph: (888) 415- 0535
toll free fax: (866) 881-2888
email: order@terra-medica.com

Canada:

Biomed
Unit 102 - 3738 N. Fraser Way
Burnaby, B.C. V5J 5G7
Canada
ph: (604) 415-0535
toll free: (800) 665-8308
toll free fax: (866) 881-2888
order desk: order@biomedicine.com

For current information on the availability of this book in the United States or Canada, and for other titles related to Psychosomatic Energetics, contact any of the offices listed above, or contact the publisher directly:

Artemis Books
P. O. Box 482
Penn Valley, CA 95946 USA
(530) 477-8101
www.artemis-books.com